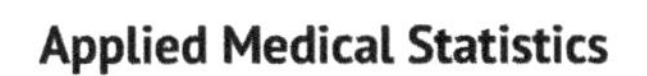
Applied Medical Statistics

Applied Medical Statistics

Jingmei Jiang

Department of Epidemiology and Biostatistics,
Institute of Basic Medical Sciences,
Chinese Academy of Medical Sciences
School of Basic Medicine,
Peking Union Medical College,
Beijing, China

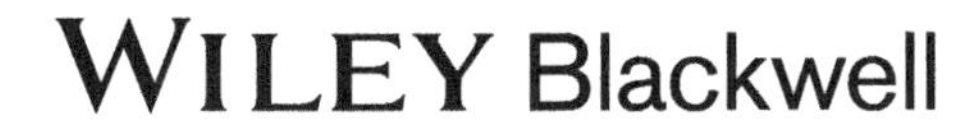

This edition first published 2022

Registered Office
John Wiley & Sons, Inc., 111 River Street, Hoboken, NJ 07030, USA

Editorial Office
9600 Garsington Road, Oxford, OX4 2DQ, UK

For details of our global editorial offices, customer services, and more information about Wiley products visit us at www.wiley.com.

Wiley also publishes its books in a variety of electronic formats and by print-on-demand. Some content that appears in standard print versions of this book may not be available in other formats.

Library of Congress Cataloging-in-Publication Data
Names: Jiang, Jingmei, 1958- author.
Title: Applied medical statistics / Jingmei Jiang.
Description: Hoboken, NJ : John Wiley & Sons, Inc., 2022. | Includes bibliographical references and index.
Identifiers: LCCN 2021021097 (print) | LCCN 2021021098 (ebook) | ISBN 9781119716709 (hardback) | ISBN 9781119716778 (pdf) | ISBN 9781119716792 (epub) | ISBN 9781119716822 (ebook)
Subjects: LCSH: Medicine--Research--Statistical methods--Textbooks. | Medical statistics--Textbooks. | Biometry--Textbooks.
Classification: LCC R853.S7 J53 2022 (print) | LCC R853.S7 (ebook) | DDC 610.72/7--dc23
LC record available at https://lccn.loc.gov/2021021097
LC ebook record available at https://lccn.loc.gov/2021021098

Cover image: © Andriy Onufriyenko/Getty Images
Cover design by Wiley

Set in 9.5/12pt STIXTwoText by Integra Software Services Pvt. Ltd, Pondicherry, India

10 9 8 7 6 5 4 3 2 1

Contents

Preface

Over the past few decades, biomedical data have proliferated rapidly, and opportunities have arisen to use this data to improve human health. Burgeoning methods, such as machine learning techniques, have emerged to respond to the rapid growth of the volume of data, and to exploit data in an effective and efficient manner. These methods were founded on statistical learning theory, which is an expansion of traditional statistics. Therefore, cultivating basic statistical thinking capability plays an important and fundamental role in mastering these state-of-the-art methods and embracing the upcoming big data era, which makes a course of introductory biostatistics an indispensable part of the curriculum for medical students. However, as a branch of mathematics, statistics is characterized by hierarchically organized concepts, but a conceptual understanding of statistics is not always intuitive, which makes biostatistics an obstacle that is regarded as a burden for most medical students. During almost 30 years of teaching statistics at the Chinese Academy of Medical Sciences & Peking Union Medical College, China, I have experienced too many occasions on which generations of students, both undergraduate and postgraduate, have felt that they are struggling to grasp the essence of statistical concepts and the implications of mathematical formulas, and to master complex analytical methods. Moreover, their motivation to learn biostatistics has also been dampened by abstruse formulas and derivation processes. Therefore, a reader-friendly text that can provide sufficient help for developing statistical thinking and building propositional knowledge, as well as understanding and mastering analytical skills, is of great necessity, which was my motivation for writing this book.

Applied Medical Statistics is an introductory-level textbook written for postgraduate students in the human life-science field, with most topics also being suitable for undergraduate medical students. The ultimate objective of this book is to provide help in developing "habits of mind" for statistical thinking, and to establish a trade-off between mathematical derivation and know-how application among medical students. The most distinctive features of this book are summarized as follows: First, emphasis is placed on the most basic probability theory at the start of the book because, as the theoretical pillar for almost all statistical methods, strengthening these fundamental concepts is of great importance for laying a solid theoretical foundation for understanding subsequent chapters. However, for students to benefit from a practical and intuitive understanding of principles, rather than presenting abstract concepts, I have minimized the mathematical sophistication, and introduced content in a user-friendly style to nurture interest and motivate learning. Second, I have based most of the

Applied Medical Statistics, First Edition. Jingmei Jiang.

Companion website: www.wiley.com\go\jiang\appliedmedicalstatistics

working examples on research projects that I have conducted or participated in, and such real-world settings, in my view, are more helpful for stimulating students' interest, as well as helping them to learn how to use statistical procedures in practice. Finally, although this is an elementary applied statistics textbook, it covers some commonly used advanced statistical techniques, such as survival analysis and logistic regression. I also discuss fundamental issues in research design, and the inclusion of this content will greatly enhance the applicability and benefit to students who need to reference this book while performing day-to-day medical research.

I have organized the content of this book in a cohesive manner that links all the relevant foundation concepts as building blocks. Chapter 1 starts with an introduction to the basic concepts of biostatistics, and a section called "statistical thinking" strengthens the importance of statistical thinking in solving real-world problems. Chapter 2 contains an introduction to the basic concepts and application of some fundamental summary statistics. Moreover, it also covers how to organize data and display data using graphical methods. Chapters 3 to 5 are compact, and provide background supporting information to enable students to understand the basic rationale of biostatistics, in addition to laying a theoretical foundation for subsequent chapters. Chapter 3 contains the development of the basic principles of probability, with suitable examples. Chapter 4 covers the fundamental concepts of random variables and discrete probability distribution, including binomial distribution, multinomial probability distribution, and Poisson distribution. Chapter 5 briefly introduces the most commonly used continuous probability distributions: mainly normal and standard normal distributions. Chapter 6 mainly focuses on an introduction to the sampling distribution, as well as parameter estimation, and plays a unique role in linking descriptive statistics to inferential statistics. This chapter starts the formal discussion of the theoretical background, as well as the application of inferential statistics. Chapters 7 to 10 contain the basic principles of hypothesis testing and the elementary parametric hypothesis testing methods for normally distributed data in two-sample and multiple-sample scenarios, such as the t-test and analysis of variance methods. The common requirement for implementing these methods is the assumption that the underlying population should be normally distributed. Chapter 11 contains an introduction to the fundamental concepts of hypothesis testing methods for categorical data, the chi-square test, and Fisher's exact test, which are widely used in statistical analysis. Chapter 12 contains an overview of some of the most well-known non-parametric tests suitable for scenarios in which assumptions of normality can be relaxed. Chapters 13 and 15 contain introductions to extensively used models and techniques for exploring the association between risk or predictor factors and continuous response variables. Chapter 13 mainly focuses on the basic concepts and application of simple linear regression, and Chapter 15 covers its extension: multiple linear regression. Additionally, Chapter 14 contains an introduction to simple correlation and rank correlation, which measure the strength of the relationship between two variables. Chapters 16 and 17 contain an introduction to some essential analysis techniques for modeling the binary and time-to-event response variables, such as unconditional and conditional logistic regression, and the Cox proportional hazards model used in processing time-to-event data. Chapter 18 then covers the most commonly used statistical evaluation indices and methods in diagnostic tests. Chapters 19 and 20, as the concluding chapters of this textbook, contain a discussion of methods for design and sample size estimation issues for observational and experimental studies.

Acknowledgments

I am grateful for the support I received from many people and institutions during the writing of this book. First and foremost, I express my deepest gratitude to an expert and consultant team, which included professors Youshang Zhou, Songlin Yu, Konglai Zhang, and Hui Li, all of whom are well-known Chinese statisticians and epidemiologists. Their unconditional support and encouragement at every stage of the writing of this book made it possible for me to complete this work.

I am also grateful for the immense help that I received from my colleagues at the School of Basic Medicine of Peking Union Medical College. Professor Tao Xu and Dr. Fang Xue deserve special acknowledgement for providing assistance through conducting a professional review of my work, and their constructive comments greatly improved the manuscript. I also want to acknowledge help from Doctors Wei Han, Zixing Wang, Yaoda Hu, and Haiyu Pang, who provided assistance in the production of this book through copyediting, reviewing, and correcting many subtle errors. Fruitful discussions with them also improved how the manuscript treated certain topics.

In particular, I appreciate the help of my post-graduate students in putting together this book. Peng Wu help me in organizing much of the material and analyzing the data in the examples; Ning Li and Cuihong Yang produced accurate figures and diagrams; Yubing Shen and Luwen Zhang checked the accuracy of all the formulae; Yali Chen and Lei Wang constructed the index and checked the accuracy of terminology and reference sources; Jin Du and Yujie Zhao checked the answers to exercises; and Wentao Gu improved the quality of the mathematical formulas. Without their help, this work would have been far more difficult to complete.

Much of the motivation of writing comes from teaching and supervising post-graduate students at Peking Union Medical College. I am grateful for their inquisitive questions and useful feedback on a draft version of this manuscript, which allowed me to improve the final version.

I express my gratitude to the research projects from which I obtained the data and background for the examples and exercises; these projects were funded by the National Natural Science Foundation of China, Ministry of Science and Technology Fund, Chinese Academy of Medical Sciences Innovation Fund for Medical Sciences, Cancer Research UK, UK Medical Research Council, and US National Institutes of Health.

Applied Medical Statistics, First Edition. Jingmei Jiang.

Companion website: www.wiley.com\go\jiang\appliedmedicalstatistics

I would like express my deep and sincere gratitude to managing editor Kimberly Monroe-Hill for the professional guidance, coordinating effort and continued support during the entire drafting and publication process. I also wish to thank commissioning editor James Watson for assisting us in many ways with this book. I would also like to thank Arthi Kangeyan and Dilip Varma, the content refinement specialists, for the professional help in getting the manuscript ready for production.

I thank the School of Basic Medicine of Peking Union Medical College for making available all the support that I needed in the writing process.

Thanks are owed to Dr. Maxine Garcia, Dr. Jennifer Barrett, and the team at Edanz Group China for their dedicated and professional language editing support.

Finally, I thank my family for their understanding and encouragement while I was writing this book.

About the Companion Website

This book is accompanied by a companion website:

www.wiley.com\go\jiang\appliedmedicalstatistics

The website includes the solutions manual and data sets.

Applied Medical Statistics, First Edition. Jingmei Jiang.

Companion website: www.wiley.com\go\jiang\appliedmedicalstatistics

1

What is Biostatistics?

CONTENTS

1.1 Overview

Data are present everywhere in our lives, and almost all types of scientific research have to deal with the collection, description, or analysis of data. This makes statistics one of the most powerful methodologies across all disciplines for exploring the unknown world. Statistics is a discipline on its own and has a wide spectrum of theories, methods, and applications. A prerequisite for discussing the theory and application of statistics is the definition and statement of its objectives. According to *Merriam–Webster's Collegiate Dictionary*, statistics is "a branch of mathematics dealing with the collection, analysis, interpretation, and presentation of masses of numerical data." According to the *Random House College Dictionary*, it is "the science that deals with the collection, classification, analysis, and interpretation of information or data." According to *The New Oxford English–Chinese Dictionary*, it is "the practice or science of collecting and analyzing numerical data in large quantities, especially for the purpose of inferring proportions in a whole from those in a representative sample." Although there are some differences among these definitions, each definition implies that statistics is a science of data and uses the theory of mathematical statistics to make inferences.

Applied Medical Statistics, First Edition. Jingmei Jiang.

Companion website: www.wiley.com\go\jiang\appliedmedicalstatistics

The application of statistical theories and methods to medical research fields is termed "medical statistics," or more broadly, biostatistics when applied to life sciences.

There are two branches of biostatistics based on its functions: (i) *statistical description* is concerned with the organization, summarization, and description of data; and (ii) *statistical inference* is concerned with the use of sample data to make inferences about the characteristics of a larger set of data. This division of descriptive and inferential statistics helps us to establish a progressive learning framework for statistics. However, this division is not always necessary in scientific activities where the two branches complement each other in deepening our knowledge of the real world.

We briefly review the development of biostatistics. In London in 1603, the Bills of Mortality began to be published weekly, which is generally considered to mark the beginning of biostatistics. Since then, related theories have continued to emerge, and the early twentieth century ushered in the peak of development of biostatistics. Several pioneers played a crucial role in the development of the theoretical framework and applications of biostatistics. G.J. Mendel (1822–1884), the father of modern genetics, used probability rules to discover the basic laws of biogenetics in the 1860s. He is considered to be one of the first to apply mathematical methods to biology. K. Pearson (1857–1936), the founding father of modern statistics, established the world's first department of statistics at University College London in 1911, and developed several key statistical theories (e.g., measure of correlation and χ^2 distribution). W.S. Gosset (1876–1937) proposed the t distribution and t-test in 1908, which laid the foundation for the sampling distribution of the sample mean, and signified the establishment of small sample theory and methodology. R.A. Fisher (1890–1962) developed statistical significance tests, and various sampling distributions, and established the experimental design method and related statistical analysis technique. These were collected in Design of Experiments, which was first published in 1935. With the efforts of these pioneers and other statisticians, after hundreds of years, a complete theoretical system of biostatistics had formed.

At the present time, the development of biostatistics is being driven by the unprecedented and still growing range of life science applications using advances in computing power and computer technology, and new formats of data that continue to emerge. Despite this, the ideas of basic statistics have not changed: to make an inference about a population based on information contained in a sample from that population and to provide an associated measure of goodness for the inference.

1.2 Some Statistical Terminology

In this text, we aim to explain basic statistical methods commonly applied in biomedical research. Before this, we provide an overview of several statistical terms, which are the premise for further learning.

1.2.1 Population and Sample

A *population* (*statistical population* or *target population*) is a certain or some characteristics of study subjects that are our target of interest. Population is usually denoted by X (also called random variable), and can be viewed as a dataset. The basic unit that constitutes the population is called the *individual*.

The dataset that defines a population is typically large or conceptual. The former suggests a *finite population* because it has a finite number of individuals regardless of how large it is. For example, the dataset of the heights of all the college freshman boys in Beijing in 2020 is a finite population (though very large). When the dataset only exists conceptually, we call it an *infinite population*, for example, the weights of infants and the antihypertensive treatment effects of a certain drug. The sampling theory and statistical inference principle introduced in this text are based on an infinite population.

A *sample*, denoted by $X_1, X_2, \ldots, X_n$ (n is the sample size), is a subset of data selected from a population. The purpose of obtaining a sample is to infer about the characteristics of its underlying unknown population.

The process of drawing a sample from a population is termed sampling. In practice, depending on the research objectives and feasibility, samples can be obtained using random or non-random sampling. A random sample is obtained through probability sampling. In this text, we generally assume the use of a *simple random sample* in which each individual in the population has an equal chance of being sampled. Non-random sampling relies on the subjective judgment of the researcher and is beyond the scope of this text.

Note the following: (i) The concept of population is different in biomedical research and statistical terminology. In biomedical research, the term "study population" (or study subject) typically refers to a group of humans or other species of organism, whereas the characteristics of the study subjects are the population we are interested in statistics. For example, in a study of blood glucose concentrations among 3-year-old children, all children of that age are regarded as the study population. However, from a statistical point of view, all blood glucose concentrations in children of that age constitute the population of interest. (ii) Although the dataset of a population is typically large, the essential difference between the population and the sample is not the amount of data we have, but the objective of the research. If the objective is to provide a description only, then the data we have can be regarded as a population, regardless of how small it is, whereas if the objective is to draw an inference, then we need to clarify what population we are interested in, and consider how to obtain a representative sample, or how good the sample at hand is. The representativeness of the sample of the population is a very important basis for a reasonable inference.

1.2.2 Homogeneity and Variation

In statistics, *homogeneity* means the similarity among individuals within a population. In fact, without homogeneity, we can rarely define a population. The individual differences in a homogenous population are termed *variation*.

Example 1.1 Survey of the height of college freshman boys in Beijing in 2020.
Homogeneity: College freshman boys in Beijing in 2020.
Variation: Individual differences in height.

Example 1.2 Study of the antihypertensive treatment effects of a drug.
Homogeneity: Hypertensive patients taking this drug.
Variation: Individual differences in the treatment effects.

From Examples 1.1 and 1.2, we can see that homogeneity refers to similarities in the nature, condition, or background of individuals in a population. The mission of statistics can be interpreted as describing the features of a homogenous population and identifying the heterogeneity of different populations. Variation is an inherent attribute of life sciences, and biomedical researchers should learn to use statistical methods to reveal the laws of biological phenomena in the context of variation.

1.2.3 Parameter and Statistic

A descriptive measure of the characteristics calculated on a population is called a *population parameter*, or simply, a *parameter*, generally denoted by the Greek letter θ. For example, in the survey of the height of freshman boys, the population mean (average height, typically denoted by μ) is a parameter. However, it is difficult to have data for the entire population most of the time, so a sample is used instead. Correspondingly, a descriptive measure based on a sample is called a *sample statistic*, or simply, a *statistic*. For example, if we draw a sample (typically a random sample) from the population and calculate the average height, the sample mean is a statistic and is typically denoted by $\bar{x}$. The mathematical definition and roles of statistics are elaborated on in Chapter 6. Because most populations are theoretical, the parameters are constants that are usually unknown, whereas the statistics are calculated from samples, which are indeterminate, and the values of statistics could be different for different samples.

1.2.4 Types of Data

Data are the representation or observation of the characteristic population. Data can be classified as numerical and categorical, depending on their properties:

(1) *Numerical data*, also known as quantitative data, are the data expressed in numbers and are obtained by measuring each research subject's indices, that is, the quantity or number of things. Numerical data differentiate themselves from other number-form data types as a result of the ability to perform arithmetic operations using these numbers. We can subdivide numerical data into two types:

Continuous data occur when data can be measured on a continuum or scale, i.e., there is a possible value between any other two values.

Most numerical data in biomedical research are continuous or can be viewed as continuous. For instance, if we conduct a survey on the health and nutritional status of 7-year-old boys in a less developed region in 2020, the measurement results of their heights (cm), weights (kg), and hemoglobin (g/L) can be viewed as continuous data because their values can assume, in theory, any value in a certain range.

Discrete data occur when the data can only take certain values. The possible values of discrete data are generally integers. For instance, if we also collect data on the number of cases of cold $(0,1,2,\ldots)$ in 2020 for the 7-year-old boys, then they are discrete data.

(2) *Categorical data*, also known as qualitative data, include two subtypes:

Unordered categorical data are obtained by dividing research subjects into two or more unordered groups. For instance, we can denote a man and woman as 1 and 2 for sex and denote A, B, O, and AB as 1, 2, 3, and 4 for blood type. Unlike numerical data, the numbers representing different categories do not have mathematical meanings.

Individual values do not have a quantitative difference if they belong to the same category and have qualitative differences if they belong to different categories.

Ordinal categorical data are obtained by dividing research subjects into orderings of an attribute. They are not measured; nonetheless, they have a potential ordering. For instance, the treatment effect of a disease can be ordered as cured, effective, improved, ineffective, and deteriorated. The laboratory test results of urine protein determination can be ordered as $-$, $\pm$, $+$, $++$, and $+++$. We can also use numerical values such as 1,2,3,... to represent the potential grades, although the numbers do not have numerical meanings.

Numerical data and categorical data are not set in stone; under certain conditions, they can be exchanged according to the research objectives and statistical methods used. For example, in a large survey on hypertension, the blood pressure values collected are numerical data. If we want to estimate the prevalence of hypertension, we could group survey participants according to whether they are hypertensive (1 for hypertensive and 0 for not hypertensive), and the data become unordered categorical data (*binary data*). If we want to know the degrees of hypertension, the blood pressure measurements can be reclassified into ordinal categorical data. Conversely, categorical data can also be changed to numerical data. For example, if we want to compare the epidemic of hypertension in different regions, we could use binary data to calculate the hypertension prevalence p, which ranges from 0 to 1 and belongs to the scope of numerical data. In the study design, we should collect as much raw data (original data) as possible in numerical form to minimize the loss of information and allow for flexible transformation.

1.2.5 Error

Error refers to the difference between the observed value and real value (parameter). The following formula defines the relation between them:

$$x = \theta + \varepsilon, \tag{1.1}$$

where x denotes the observed value; θ denotes the real value, theoretically; and ε denotes the error, which can represent a random error or systematic error.

(1) A *random error*, as the name suggests, is completely random, that is, the magnitude and sign of ε cannot be predetermined, and the scope $\varepsilon \in (-\infty, +\infty)$. A random error is caused by the influence of many uncertain factors in the actual observation or measurement process.

As shown in Formula 1.1, a random error can be interpreted in many ways. For example, if x is the measured value in an experiment, then $\varepsilon = x - \theta$ reflects the measurement error in the results of each measurement. Additionally, the sampling error is the most typical type of random error. If x is a sample statistic, then $\varepsilon = x - \theta$ reflects the difference between statistic x and the parameter θ resulting from the sampling process, which is fundamental to the study of statistical inference introduced in Chapter 6.

(2) A *systematic error*, also known as bias in epidemiology, is another type of error that has a fixed magnitude and directional systematic deviation from a real number, that is, $\varepsilon = a(a \neq 0)$, where a is a constant. A systematic error is caused by the influence

of certain factors, for example, an uncorrected instrument, the sensory disturbance of the measurer, or high or low standards in evaluating a treatment effect.

Random errors are unavoidable but could manifest some laws of regularity in some conditions. The study and application of the law of random errors is one of the most important elements of statistics. In practice, random and systematic errors often coexist, both requiring considerations in the study design and data analysis.

1.3 Workflow of Applied Statistics

The following four steps in applied statistical workflow are indispensable in practice:

Statistical design: This marks the beginning of scientific research, and is directly responsible for the accuracy and reliability of the research results. Statistical design should be conducted with specific research objectives and domain knowledge. This means that good research design is inevitably based on interactions between domain experts and statisticians. Two categories of research design exist in general, observational design and experimental design, which we discuss in Chapters 19 and 20, respectively.

Data collection: Data collection is used to obtain the raw data required by research through a reasonable and reliable approach. The collection of representative data is important for obtaining reliable conclusions. Regardless of which method is used, the accuracy and integrity of the data should be given high priority.

Statistical analysis: The next step is the management and analysis of the raw data according to the research objectives and types of data. This step typically includes the statistical description, statistical inference, and (or) statistical modeling for mining the information hidden in the data.

Statistical reporting: After all the steps are executed, the analysis results are displayed. Appropriate statistical tables and graphs can be used to enhance the presentation of results. Final conclusions and suggestions are drawn, guided by domain knowledge. A key feature of statistical reporting is that all conclusions are probabilistic.

1.4 Statistics and Its Related Disciplines

The discipline of statistics does not stand alone. Instead, it is closely related to the development of other disciplines.

Statistics and medicine: Statistics not only helps to solve practical problems, but also promotes its own development during the process. Its application to the biomedical sciences is a typical demonstration of this. With the further understanding of data in the twenty-first century, evidence-based medicine, precision medicine, and other quantitative methods will provide a broader space for applying statistics.

Statistics and mathematics: Statistics is a branch of mathematics. The mathematical basis of statistics is the theory of probability and calculus. However, this does not mean that learning statistics must be based on knowledge of advanced mathematics. In fact, the objective of learning statistics is not to master complicated mathematical proofs but the application of statistical thinking and methods to solve problems that arise in scientific research.

Statistics and computer science: Modern statistics cannot be separated from developments in computer science. The field of statistics has benefited greatly from advances in computing power. In the digital era, computer science and information technology are as important to statistics as the theory of probability. Computer software has become an important auxiliary tool for statistical analysis. The conclusions are largely the same using different statistical software, even if the numerical results have minor differences. To avoid any distraction caused by these technical issues in learning statistical ideas and methods, in this text, we present results mainly using SPSS, among other alternatives.

1.5 Statistical Thinking

Statistical thinking includes applying rational thinking and statistical science to critically evaluate data and the resultant correct and false inferences. How does statistical thinking play its role in scientific research practice? To answer this question, we must note that inferences based on sample data are almost always subject to error because a sample does not provide an exact image of the population.

The population is typically a theoretical and conceptual truth of interest. The science of statistics helps us to establish a methodological framework or workflow to draw inferences about the unknown characteristics of the population using the sample of limited data at hand, based on one or a few assumptions. The statistical inference process is an important part of the scientific method. Inference based on experimental or observational data is first used to develop a theory about some phenomenon. Then the theory is tested against additional sample data.

Errors may occur in the inference process based on a sample. What matters is how we quantify and evaluate the error. Statistics connects the quantification of errors with the measurement of the reliability of inference using probability. This connection provides a solid theoretical basis for reasonable statistical inference.

Statistics builds a bridge between abstract theoretical concepts and the solution of specific problems. It enables researchers to make inferences (estimates and decisions about the target population) with a known measurement of reliability. With this ability, a researcher can make intelligent decisions and inferences from data; that is, statistics helps researchers to think critically about their results.

We end this chapter with remarks from the famous statistician, C.R. Rao.

All knowledge is, in the final analysis, history.
All sciences are, in the abstract, mathematics.
All judgments are, in their rationale, statistics.

1.6 Summary

The learning objective of this chapter is to understand some basic concepts in statistics and the role of statistics in biomedical research, which are the basis for future learning.

Statistics is a science about data, and its basic characteristic is that it is a quantitative science.

Two branches, statistical description and statistical inference, constitute the main content of statistics.

The application of statistics to biomedical research generally includes the following four steps: statistical design, data collection, statistical analysis, and statistical reporting.

Statistical thinking includes the application of rational thinking and statistical science to critically evaluate data and make inferences from them.

1.7 Exercises

1. Suppose you were so interested in the waist circumference of your schoolmates that you prepared a tape measure in a statistics class and measured the waist circumference of all your classmates who were present. Answer the following questions:
   (a) Decide whether the data you obtained is a sample or population? For what research objectives should it be considered a sample or population?
   (b) If it is considered a sample, what is the population you are drawing an inference about? How representative of the population is it?
   (c) How do you determine the homogeneity of your population? Is there heterogeneity? If yes, how can you improve the homogeneity? Is there variation? What may lead to this variation?
   (d) Are there errors in the obtained data? What are the random errors and systematic errors? Can you tell the difference between them? Can you, and how do you, minimize the errors?
   (e) What steps do you need to follow to complete a report on your survey?

2. Choose a quantitative research article in clinical medicine, basic medicine, public health, or any biomedical research topic you are interested in and answer the following questions:
   (a) What is the population and how is it defined from the perspectives of the research and statistics, respectively? What are the differences between the concepts of population using different perspectives?
   (b) Is the sample presented in the research a random sample? What are the advantages of a random sample and non-random sample?
   (c) Illustrate the relationship between the population and sample, and between homogeneity and variation using your selected paper.
   (d) Is there any factor that may lead to random or systematic errors in the research? How do you distinguish them? How have they been minimized? Can you think of ways to further minimize the errors?
   (e) What data are collected? What are the types of data? How do you determine the type of data? Which type of data contains more information? Do these types of data allow for further transformation?
   (f) How many steps are involved in the statistical plan? What are the specific roles of these steps and what is the relation between these steps?

(g) Are the conclusions obtained from the research correct? How does the knowledge of statistics learned from this chapter help you with critical thinking?

(h) Can you follow the conceptual path as laid out by the research and use statistical critical thinking to solve a problem that interests you in your daily life? Try to create a statistical design as you deepen your knowledge and skills through further learning.

2

Descriptive Statistics

CONTENTS

In the previous chapter, we learned that there are two branches in statistics – description and inference. Statistical description, as the basis of statistical inference, provides a way to organize and summarize data in a meaningful and intuitive manner. In this chapter, we introduce several basic statistical tools for describing data. These tools include tables and graphs that rapidly convey a concise presentation or visual picture of the data, as well as numerical measures that describe certain characteristics of the data. The appropriate tool depends on the type of data (numerical or categorical) that we want to describe.

Example 2.1 In a survey on the physiological characteristics of school-age children in a certain region in 2010, 153 10-year-old girls were randomly selected, and several physiological indicators were measured and recorded. The raw data of girls' height are shown in Table 2.1.

The data shown in Table 2.1 are raw data presented in an unorganized manner. Although it would be easy to find the highest and lowest values in this sample, it would be very difficult to extract more useful information from this set of data without organizing them using descriptive statistical techniques.

Applied Medical Statistics, First Edition. Jingmei Jiang.

Companion website: www.wiley.com\go\jiang\appliedmedicalstatistics

Table 2.1 Raw data on the height (cm) of 153 10-year-old girls.

139.9	141.6	150.5	146.0	143.0	148.0	142.5	152.0
131.3	147.9	147.6	145.0	150.0	149.0	138.0	137.8
128.8	143.8	138.7	142.0	138.0	142.0	151.0	134.9
128.6	141.8	143.3	131.8	139.0	140.0	149.0	135.1
130.5	140.1	139.8	132.0	142.6	144.0	147.0	147.0
142.2	135.9	149.1	136.7	140.0	137.0	138.2	137.0
144.0	141.3	148.5	132.0	146.0	148.0	148.0	149.6
129.4	143.8	153.5	143.0	145.2	134.6	146.7	146.8
138.5	146.6	143.3	137.4	145.0	143.0	149.0	142.0
140.8	138.0	144.2	126.7	130.0	154.0	138.0	**158.0**
136.5	141.3	154.0	146.0	154.0	140.0	156.0	129.0
135.1	135.0	146.0	148.5	141.2	145.0	139.0	151.0
140.2	139.5	140.0	157.0	149.0	137.0	152.0	143.0
138.2	141.2	135.0	131.9	134.0	142.9	140.5	142.0
139.0	138.7	138.0	148.0	134.7	153.0	146.0	137.6
143.3	143.6	**125.3**	132.0	139.5	135.0	154.0	131.0
137.6	142.7	131.0	146.0	132.4	151.0	152.0	147.0
140.5	143.8	138.0	152.0	141.0	157.7	149.0	143.0
134.2	142.0	140.0	134.0	139.0	154.4	134.1	141.3
145.0							

2.1 Frequency Tables and Graphs

The frequency distribution table and the frequency distribution diagram are starting points for summarizing data and provide a basis for observing the characteristics of the distribution. They are made by grouping observations and obtaining the frequency distribution by counting the number of observations in each group.

2.1.1 Frequency Distribution of Numerical Data

Most of numerical data can be regarded as continuous, theoretically taking on an infinite number of values. Thus, one is essentially always dealing with a frequency distribution tabulated by group (i.e., the data are grouped into several non-overlapping intervals). Therefore, the number of observations falling into each interval, which we call the frequency, can be determined. We use these numbers to construct the frequency distribution table and the frequency distribution diagram.

In the following steps, we use the data shown in Table 2.1 to illustrate the procedures for organizing a frequency table.

Steps to follow in constructing a frequency distribution table:

(1) Calculate the range of the data. *Range* (R) is defined as the difference between the largest and smallest observation values in the sample

$$R = x_{max} - x_{min}. \tag{2.1}$$

For example, using the data shown in Table 2.1, $x_{max} = 158.0$ and $x_{min} = 125.3$. The range is then calculated as

$$R = 158.0 - 125.3 = 32.7$$

Thus, the range of height for the girls is about 33 cm.

(2) Determine the specific group interval. The range is usually divided into 5 to 15 intervals of equal width, and the number of intervals can be determined according to the sample size. A small number of groups is suitable for a small dataset, and vice versa. The lowest (or first) interval boundary should be located below the smallest value, and the interval width should be chosen so that no observation can fall on the lowest boundary. In practice, the width of the interval is usually set to be 1/10 of the range. Using the data presented in Table 2.1, the width of each interval is $32.7/10 = 3.27$, which is approximately equal to 3 cm. Except the last interval, the intervals are generally denoted by the lower boundary followed by "–", which indicates that the values within the interval are no smaller than the lower boundary of that interval but that they are smaller than the lower boundary of the next interval. For instance, "125.0–" means that the range is $[125.0, 128.0)$. The last interval is closed (i.e., "155.0–158.0," corresponding to a range of $[155.0, 158.0]$).

(3) For each group interval, count the number of observations that fall in that group. The construction of the frequency distribution table, which consists of the group interval and the count corresponding to each group (the first two columns of Table 2.2), is then completed.

For convenience of comparison, we also include the relative frequency (proportion) in Table 2.2.

$$\text{relative frequency} = \frac{\text{frequency}}{\text{total number of measurements}}. \tag{2.2}$$

Because the denominators used to calculate the relative frequencies (sample size n) are the same for all groups, the distribution shapes of frequency and relative frequency are similar.

Table 2.2 shows the frequencies and relative frequencies for the heights of the girls in Example 2.1. The total of all the frequencies is n, and the total of all the relative frequencies is 100%.

The highest frequency (28) is in the "140.0–" interval, and the relative frequency for this interval is also the highest (18.3%). Moreover, we could easily find that the relative frequency distribution is symmetric around the "140.0–" group. The advantage of the relative frequency is that it allows us to freely compare frequency distributions across two or more groups of individuals.

Table 2.2 Frequency distribution for height (cm) of 153 10-year-old girls in Example 2.1.

Group (1)	Frequency (2)	Relative frequency (%) (3)
125.0–	2	1.3
128.0–	6	3.9
131.0–	9	5.9
134.0–	15	9.8
137.0–	26	17.0
140.0–	28	18.3
143.0–	20	13.1
146.0–	20	13.1
149.0–	12	7.8
152.0–	11	7.2
155.0–158.0	4	2.6
Total	153	100.0

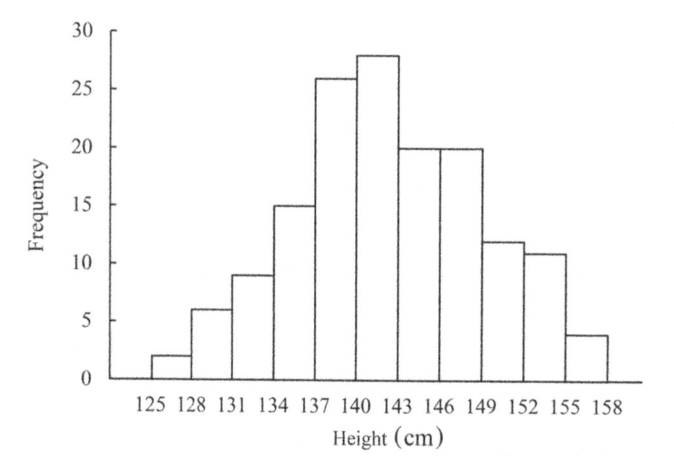

Figure 2.1 Histogram for the height of the 153 10-year-old girls in Example 2.1.

After the frequencies (or relative frequencies) have been obtained, a more intuitive way to depict the frequency (or relative frequency) distribution is to plot a histogram. Figure 2.1 presents a histogram using the data shown in Table 2.2.

The *x*-axis in Figure 2.1, which shows the height of the 10-year-old girls, is divided into group intervals commencing with the interval of 125.0– and proceeding in intervals of equal size (3.0 cm). The *y*-axis (frequency) gives the number of the 153 readings that fall in each interval. The data appear to have a bell-shaped distribution. About 28 of the 153 girls, or 18.3%, had a height of 140.0–142.9 cm. This group interval contains the highest frequency, and the intervals tend to contain smaller numbers of measurements as height gets smaller or larger.

Histograms can be used to display either the frequency or the relative frequency of the measurements falling into the group intervals. The graph is generally constructed by dividing the x-axis into intervals of equal width. A rectangle is then drawn over each interval, such that the height of the rectangle is proportional to the fraction of the total number of measurements falling in each interval. Notice that when constructing a frequency table (or a histogram), using many intervals with a small amount of data results in little summarization and presents a picture very similar to the data in their original form. Now, computer software can be used to produce any desired histograms. These software packages all produce histograms that conform to widely agreed-upon constraints on scaling, the number of intervals used, the widths of intervals, and the like.

Example 2.2 Referring to Example 2.1, the triglyceride levels of the 153 10-year-old girls were also measured. The distribution of the triglyceride data is shown in Table 2.3.

Table 2.3 could be constructed in the same way described for building Table 2.2, except for the newly added *cumulative relative frequency*, which is obtained simply by adding all previous relative frequencies to the relative frequency for the current group. For example, if we wished to know what percentage of the girls had a triglyceride level under 1.2 mmol/L, we would sum all frequencies from the smallest group 0.3– through the third group 0.9–. We would then arrive at the answer of 71.2%.

Cumulative relative frequency is useful in determining medians, percentiles, and other quantiles, which will be used frequently in subsequent analysis.

Likewise, we could convert the frequency distribution table to the corresponding histogram, as shown in Figure 2.2.

Figure 2.2 shows the same pattern observed in the frequency table, characterized by a peak that is off center toward the left side and a long tail on the right side. We call

Table 2.3 Frequency distribution of triglycerides (mmol/L) in 153 10-year-old girls.

Group (1)	Frequency (2)	Relative frequency (%) (3)	Cumulative relative frequency (%) (4)
0.3–	22	14.4	14.4
0.6–	42	27.4	41.8
0.9–	45	29.4	71.2
1.2–	26	17.0	88.2
1.5–	11	7.2	95.4
1.8–	4	2.6	98.0
2.1–	2	1.3	99.3
2.4–2.7	1	0.7	100.0
Total	153	100.0	—

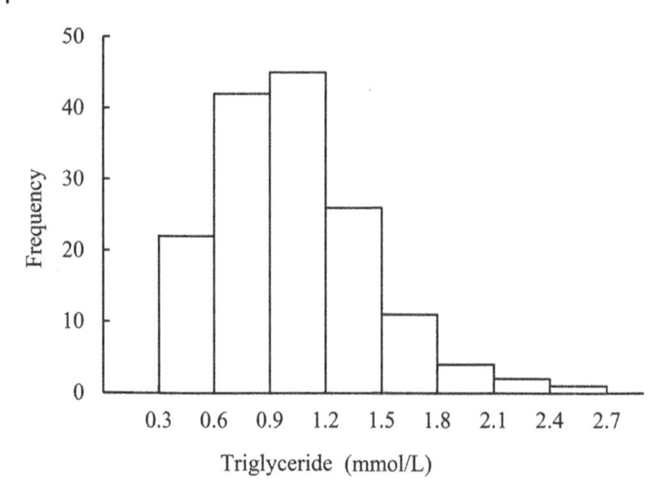

Figure 2.2 Histogram of triglycerides in 153 10-year-old girls.

distributions with such characteristics positively (or right) skewed distributions. Conversely, if the peak of the distribution is pulled to the right and the long tail extends to the left, the distribution is said to be negatively (or left) skewed.

2.1.2 Frequency Distribution of Categorical Data

For categorical data with finite distinct values, we first need to define classes according to the research objective and the characteristics of the data. Each observed value belongs to only one class. The frequency table and frequency diagram can then be constructed by counting the exact number of values within each class.

Example 2.3 A total of 1668 adult (≥30 years old) Kazakh residents in the Altay region of Xinjiang, China, were surveyed on their blood pressure in 2013. According to the "Chinese Guidelines for the Prevention and Treatment of Hypertension," the subjects were classified into five distinct groups: normal, high normal, and grades 1, 2, and 3 hypertension. Using this classification, a frequency table of blood pressure status was constructed, as shown in Table 2.4.

In Table 2.4, we see that more than one-third (34.8%) of the Kazakh residents participating in the survey had high normal blood pressure, and 44.0% of them had grade 1–3 hypertension. The corresponding bar chart is shown in Figure 2.3.

Figure 2.3 is an example of the depiction of the frequency distribution of categorical data. In a bar chart, the frequencies (or relative frequencies) of all groups are represented by the height of bars of equal width. The bar chart can be vertical or horizontal, which does not change the meaning.

The frequency distribution tables and diagrams for both numerical data and categorical data have clear advantages, especially when the sample size is large:

(1) The distribution of the data can be intuitively presented, which is very important because this distribution plays a determinant role in choosing the subsequent statistical analysis methods.

Table 2.4 Frequency distribution of blood pressure group for 1668 adult Kazakh residents.

Blood pressure group (1)	Frequency (2)	Relative frequency (%) (3)	Cumulative frequency (4)	Cumulative relative frequency (%) (5)
Normal	353	21.2	353	21.2
High normal	580	34.8	933	56.0
Grade 1 hypertension	389	23.3	1322	79.3
Grade 2 hypertension	212	12.7	1534	92.0
Grade 3 hypertension	134	8.0	1668	100.0
Total	1668	100.0	—	—

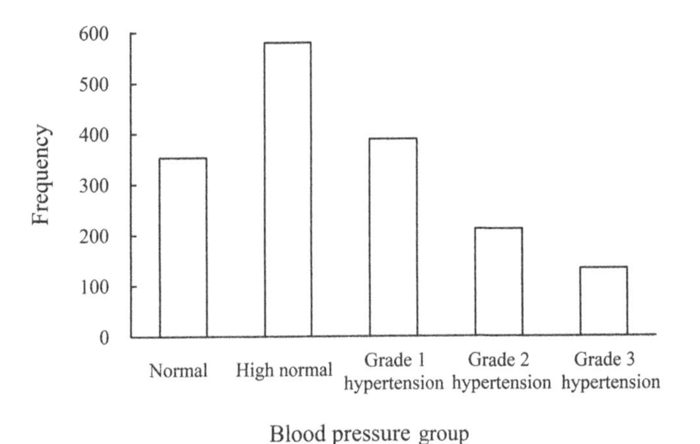

Figure 2.3 Bar chart of blood pressure group for 1668 adult Kazakh residents.

(2) *Central tendency* and *dispersion*, which are two important characteristics of data distribution, can be shown, and outliers can also be observed.

(3) When the sample size is large, the relative frequency of each group can be used to estimate probability (the concept of probability will be introduced in Chapter 3).

2.2 Descriptive Statistics of Numerical Data

2.2.1 Measures of Central Tendency

Although frequency tables and diagrams can be used to visually depict the characteristics of a distribution, they are usually not adequate for the purpose of making inferences. Before making inferences about a population on the basis of information contained in a sample and measuring how good the inferences are, we need to rigorously define the quantities used to summarize information about a sample. In this section, we introduce three commonly used measures to describe the location or center of a sample. They are the arithmetic mean, median, and geometric mean.

1. Arithmetic Mean

The most widely utilized measure of central tendency is the *arithmetic mean* (or simply the mean).

(1) Calculating the mean with an original dataset (the direct method)

Definition 2.1 Let $x_1, x_2, \ldots, x_n$ be a set of n measurements. The sample mean is calculated as follows:

$$\bar{x} = \frac{1}{n}(x_1 + x_2 + \cdots + x_n) = \frac{1}{n}\sum_{i=1}^{n} x_i, \tag{2.3}$$

where $\bar{x}$ refers to the sample mean, Σ means "the sum of," and the subscripts and superscripts to Σ indicate that we sum the values from $i=1$ to $i=n$. This formula can also be written as $\bar{x} = \frac{1}{n}\sum_i x_i$.

Usually, we cannot measure the population mean μ, which is the unknown constant that we want to estimate using the sample mean $\bar{x}$.

Example 2.4 A physician collected an initial measurement of hemoglobin (g/L) after the admission of 10 inpatients to a hospital's department of cardiology. The hemoglobin measurements were

139, 158, 120, 112, 122, 132, 97, 104, 159, and 129.

Calculate the mean hemoglobin level.

Solution

Based on Definition 2.1 and the hemoglobin records shown above, we have:

$$\bar{x} = \frac{1}{n}\sum_i x_i = \frac{1}{10} \times (139 + 158 + \cdots + 129) = \frac{1272}{10} = 127.2$$

Therefore, the mean level of the first hemoglobin measurement after admission for the 10 inpatients was 127.2 g/L.

(2) Calculating the mean with a frequency-table dataset

When large datasets are organized into frequency tables or presented as grouped data, there is a shortcut method to calculate the mean:

$$\bar{x} = \frac{f_1 x_{m1} + f_2 x_{m2} + \cdots + f_k x_{mk} + \cdots + f_g x_{mg}}{f_1 + f_2 + \cdots + f_k + \cdots + f_g} = \frac{\sum_{k=1}^{g} f_k x_{mk}}{\sum_{k=1}^{g} f_k}, \tag{2.4}$$

where g means the number of groups f_k is the frequency, and x_{mk} is the midpoint value of the kth group (i.e., (upper bound of the kth group + lower bound of the kth group)/2), and $\sum_k f_k = n$.

Formula 2.4 is also called the *weighted method*, and the weight is f_k / n.

Obviously, with larger group frequencies, the midpoint value of the group makes a greater contribution in the calculation of the mean. The method in Formula 2.3 can actually be considered a special case of the weighted method, where the weight of the observed values is $1/n$.

Example 2.5 Calculate the mean height of the 153 10-year-old girls using the weighted method with data from frequency table in Example 2.1.

Solution

We first determine the midpoint value for each group (Column 3 of Table 2.5). Then, the mean can be obtained using Formula 2.4:

$$\bar{x} = \frac{\sum_k f_k x_{mk}}{\sum_k f_k} = \frac{2\times126.5+6\times129.5+\cdots+4\times156.5}{2+6+\cdots+4} = \frac{21778.5}{153} = 142.3$$

Thus, the mean height of the girls is 142.3 cm.

If we calculate the mean directly using the raw data (Formula 2.3), the result is 142.0—a difference of 0.3. The reason for this difference is that the weighted method assumes that the midpoint value for each group in the frequency table is exactly the average of that group, which, in most cases, is merely an approximation. In spite of this, such a trivial difference is negligible in practice. Note that statistical analysis

Table 2.5 Calculation of the mean height (cm) of 153 10-year-old girls, using the weighted method.

Group k (1)	Frequency f_k (2)	Midpoint value x_{mk} (3)	$f_k x_{mk}$ (4)
125.0–	2	126.5	253.0
128.0–	6	129.5	777.0
131.0–	9	132.5	1192.5
134.0–	15	135.5	2032.5
137.0–	26	138.5	3601.0
140.0–	28	141.5	3962.0
143.0–	20	144.5	2890.0
146.0–	20	147.5	2950.0
149.0–	12	150.5	1806.0
152.0–	11	153.5	1688.5
155.0–158.0	4	156.5	626.0
Total	153	—	21,778.5

packages employ the direct method to calculate the mean even if the sample size is large, which can greatly improve the calculation accuracy. Nevertheless, knowing the frequency distribution of the data is important because capturing the characteristics of the distribution through the frequency table is crucial for subsequent analyses.

The advantages of the mean are: (i) using all the data values in the calculation; (ii) being algebraically defined and thus mathematically manageable; and (iii) having a known sampling distribution (Chapter 6). The disadvantage of the mean is also obvious: it may be distorted by outliers and by skewed data.

2. Median

The arithmetic mean is very sensitive to very large or very small values. When these values are present, the mean may not be representative of the location of the great majority of the sample points. The *median*, another measure of central tendency, is a value that divides all ordered values equally into two parts, thus more accurately reflects the central position of an ordered list of observations. The formula to calculate the median is presented below.

(1) Calculating the median with an original dataset

Definition 2.2 Let $x_1, x_2, \ldots, x_n$ be a set of n measurements that is arranged in ascending order. The sample median is calculated as follows:

$$\begin{cases} M = x_{(n+1)/2}, & \text{if } n \text{ is odd,} \\ M = \dfrac{1}{2}\left(x_{n/2} + x_{n/2+1}\right), & \text{if } n \text{ is even.} \end{cases} \tag{2.5}$$

Obviously, if the number of observations is odd, the median is the value in the middle. When the number of values is even, strictly, there is no median. However, we usually calculate the median in this case as the arithmetic mean of the two middle observations $\left(x_{n/2} + x_{n/2+1}\right)$ in the ordered set. The rationale for these definitions is to ensure an equal frequency on both sides of the sample median.

Example 2.6 The incubation period (day) for 11 patients with a certain infectious disease was recorded as

4, 2, 3, 6, 17, 8, 4, 15, 2, 10, and 8.

Find the median incubation period for these patients.

Solution

First, arrange the sample values in ascending order:

2, 2, 3, 4, 4, 6, 8, 8, 10, 15, and 17.

Based on Definition 2.2, because n is odd $(n = 11)$, the median is calculated as

$$M = x_{(11+1)/2} = x_6 = 6$$

Thus, the median incubation period of the infectious disease in this group was 6 days, indicating the half of the observations are smaller than 6.

(2) Calculating the median with a frequency-table dataset

$$M = L + \frac{i}{f_M}\left(\frac{n}{2} - \sum f_L\right). \tag{2.6}$$

In Formula 2.6, i denotes the interval width of the group, L represents the lower bound of the group interval that the median falls into, and f_M is the frequency of this group. $\sum f_L$ is the cumulative frequency prior to this group.

Example 2.7 The incubation period (hour) for 84 patients with food poisoning is shown in Table 2.6. Find the median.

Solution

The incubation period values have been sorted in ascending order in Table 2.6. Because the median lies in the first group where the cumulative relative frequency is > 50% (or frequency > n/2), we have

$$L = 10, i = 2, f_M = 7, n = 84, \sum f_L = 36$$

Using Formula 2.6, the median is

$$M = L + \frac{i}{f_M}\left(\frac{n}{2} - \sum f_L\right) = 10 + \frac{2}{7} \times \left(\frac{84}{2} - 36\right) = 11.7$$

Thus, the median incubation period of food poisoning among these patients was 11.7 hours.

We know from Formula 2.6 that the calculation of the median is determined only by the median value and is not susceptible to the influence of extreme values. For data with a heavily skewed distribution, the median might be the only choice for describing the central location of the data. The main weakness of the median is that it is determined mainly by the middle points in a sample and is less sensitive to the actual numerical values of the remaining data points. Thus, it ignores most of the numerical information.

3. Geometric Mean

Many biomedical indicators, such as antibody titers tested in the laboratory, bacterial counts, concentrations of certain drugs, and the incubation period of certain infectious diseases, are distributed asymmetrically. These data often exhibit geometric progression or obvious right skewness. In such cases, the arithmetic mean is not appropriate for measuring central tendency because this statistic would poorly represent the average level of the data. One solution is to convert the original values before calculation, and many options exist for converting the data; the most commonly used of these is the logarithm transformation. Because data with geometric progression and most data with a right-skewed distribution approximate the normal distribution after logarithmic transformation, we call such skewed distributions *log-normal distributions*. The calculation of the *geometric mean* also involves either the direct method or the weighted method.

Table 2.6 Incubation period (hour) for 84 patients with food poisoning.

Group k (1)	Frequency f_k (2)	Cumulative frequency $\sum f_k$ (3)	Cumulative relative frequency (%) (4)
4–	5	5	6.0
6–	12	17	20.2
8–	19	36	42.9
10–	7	43	51.2
12–	7	50	59.5
14–	6	56	66.7
16–	7	63	75.0
18–	5	68	81.0
20–	4	72	85.7
22–	4	76	90.5
24–	3	79	94.0
26–	1	80	95.2
28–	0	80	95.2
30–	1	81	96.4
32–	1	82	97.6
34–	0	82	97.6
36–	0	82	97.6
38–	0	82	97.6
40–	1	83	98.8
42–	0	83	98.8
44–	0	83	98.8
46–48	1	84	100.0
Total	84	—	—

(1) Calculating the geometric mean with an original dataset

Definition 2.3 Let $x_1, x_2, \ldots, x_n$ be a set of n measurements, $x_i > 0 (i = 1, 2, \ldots, n)$. The sample geometric mean is calculated as follows

$$G = \sqrt[n]{x_1 \times x_2 \times \cdots \times x_n}. \tag{2.7}$$

After the logarithmic transformation, the calculation formula is

$$G = \log^{-1}\left(\frac{\log x_1 + \log x_2 + \cdots + \log x_n}{n}\right) = \log^{-1}\left(\frac{\sum_{i=1}^{n} \log x_i}{n}\right). \tag{2.8}$$

The natural constant e or 10 is usually chosen as the base of the logarithm in Formula 2.8, but other options also exist and may be appropriate in practice.

Example 2.8 A physician measured serum hepatitis B surface antibody titer in 8 hepatitis B patients, and the measured values were

1:8, 1:16, 1:16, 1:32, 1:64, 1:128, 1:256, and 1:512.

Find the average titer.

Solution
Because the reciprocal value of the antibody titer increases in geometric series (the common ratio is 2), we calculate the geometric mean based on Definition 2.3. For convenience of calculation, the reciprocal value of the titer is substituted into Formula 2.7

$$G = \sqrt[8]{x_1 \times x_2 \times \cdots \times x_8} = \sqrt[8]{8 \times 16 \times 16 \times 32 \times 64 \times 128 \times 256 \times 512} = 53.8$$

Here, we could also use Formula 2.8

$$G = \lg^{-1}\left(\frac{\sum_i \lg x_i}{n}\right) = \lg^{-1}\left(\frac{\lg 8 + \lg 16 + \cdots + \lg 512}{8}\right)$$
$$= \lg^{-1}\left(\frac{13.8474}{8}\right) = \lg^{-1}(1.7309) = 53.8.$$

The results are the same. The average hepatitis B surface antibody titer in the 8 hepatitis B patients was about 1:54.

(2) Calculating the geometric mean with a frequency-table dataset

Similar to the calculation of the arithmetic mean, the geometric mean can be calculated in the following manner:

$$G = \log^{-1}\left(\frac{\sum_{k=1}^{g} f_k \log x_{mk}}{\sum_{k=1}^{g} f_k}\right). \tag{2.9}$$

Formula 2.9 is self-evident because log-normal distributed data approximate the normal distribution after logarithmic transformation and can then be processed as normally distributed data. That is, first, the logarithmic mean is calculated, and the geometric mean is then obtained by taking the antilog transformation.

Example 2.9 Calculate the average triglyceride levels of the 153 10-year-old girls using the data shown in the frequency table in Example 2.2.

Solution
The distribution of the data is right-skewed, as shown in the frequency distribution table, suggesting that the geometric mean is more appropriate than the arithmetic

Table 2.7 Calculation of the geometric mean of triglyceride levels (mmol/L) for 153 10-year-old girls, using the weighted method.

Group k (1)	Frequency f_k (2)	Midpoint value x_{mk} (3)	$\ln x_{mk}$ (4)	$f_k \ln x_{mk}$ (5)
0.3–	22	0.45	-0.799	-17.567
0.6–	42	0.75	-0.288	-12.083
0.9–	45	1.05	0.049	2.196
1.2–	26	1.35	0.300	7.803
1.5–	11	1.65	0.501	5.509
1.8–	4	1.95	0.668	2.671
2.1–	2	2.25	0.811	1.622
2.4–2.7	1	2.55	0.936	0.936
Total	153	—	—	-8.913

mean for representing the average triglyceride level. The specific solution process is shown in Table 2.7.

Using the data shown in Table 2.7 and Formula 2.9, we have

$$\ln G = \frac{1}{n}\sum_k f_k \ln x_{mk} = \frac{1}{153}\times(-17.567-12.083+\cdots+0.936)$$
$$= -8.913/153 = -0.0583.$$

After taking the antilog,

$$G = \ln^{-1}(-0.0583) = 0.9434$$

Thus, the average triglyceride level for these girls was 0.94 mmol/L.

4. Comparison of Mean, Median, and Geometric Mean

In many cases, the mean, median, and geometric mean can be used to assess the symmetry of a distribution. Figure 2.4 presents an example of this.

In Example 2.1, because the distribution of the girls' heights appeared reasonably symmetrical, the three measures of the "average" all took similar values (Figure 2.4(a)). In particular, the arithmetic mean is approximately the same as the median. If a distribution is positively skewed, as was the case for the triglyceride data in Example 2.2, the arithmetic mean shows a higher "average" than either the median or the geometric mean (Figure 2.4(b)). Given a right skewed distribution, when the median and geometric mean are approximately equal, these two statistics usually give a better description of the central location. Figure 2.4(c) provides another example, which presents the distribution of the Patient Health Questionnaire-9 (PHQ-9) scores of 1072 depressed patients. The distribution is negatively skewed. In this case, only the median can provide a good expression of the central location.

The best measure of central tendency for a dataset depends on the type of descriptive information you want. Most of the inferential statistical methods discussed in

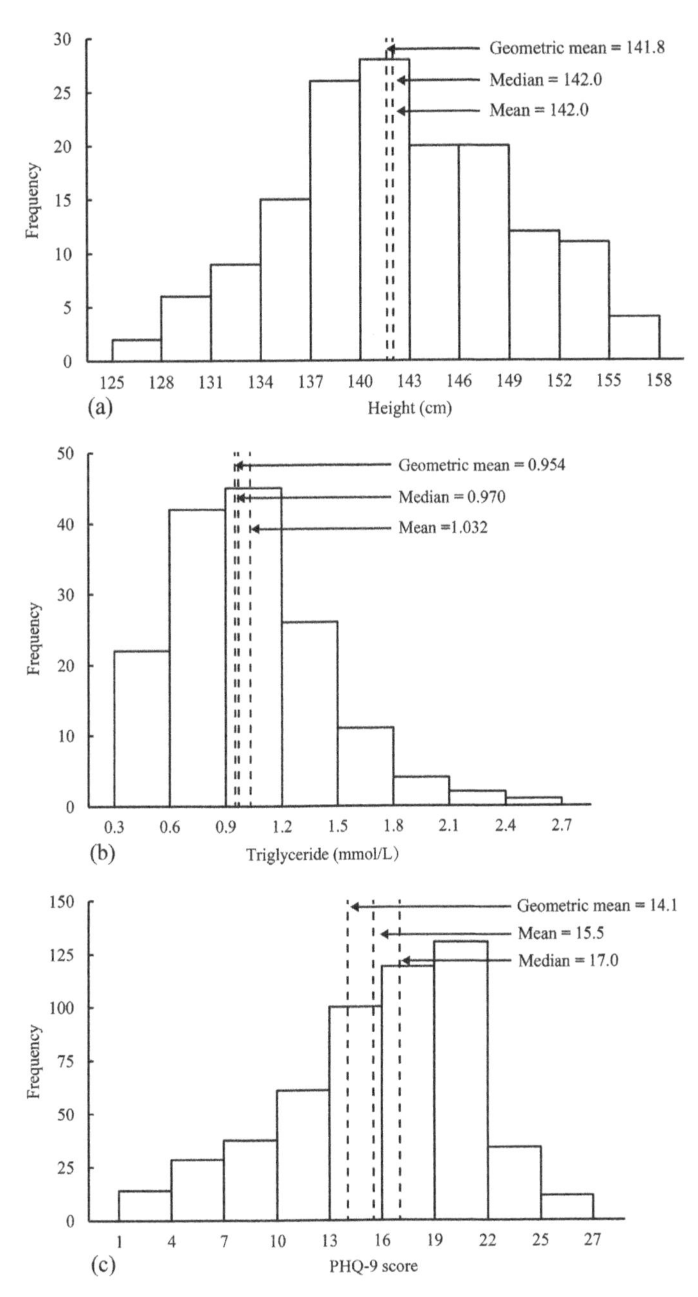

Figure 2.4 Comparison of three "averages" using the height data from Example 2.1 (a), the triglyceride data from Example 2.2 (b), and data on the Patient Health Questionnaire-9 (PHQ-9) scores of 1072 depressed patients (c).

this text are based, theoretically, on bell-shaped distributions of data with little or no skewness. With such data, the mean and the median will be, for all practical purposes, the same. Because the mean has nicer mathematical properties than the median, the mean is the preferred measure of central tendency for these inferential techniques.

2.2.2 Measures of Dispersion

To describe data adequately, we must also define measures of dispersion. We will begin with an illustrative example.

Example 2.10 The platelet counts $\left(\times 10^9 / \mathrm{L}\right)$ of 12 patients in two wards were measured. The resultant values were as follows:

Ward A: 186, 191, 199, 200, 209, and 215 $\bar{x}_A = 200$

Ward B: 160, 185, 190, 204, 217, and 244 $\bar{x}_B = 200$

Both of the groups had a mean platelet count of $200 \times 10^9 / \mathrm{L}$. However, there was a large difference between the two groups in terms of the dispersion of the data. That is, the platelet counts for patients in ward B were more widely spread out compared with those for patients in ward A.

In this section, we introduce several commonly used descriptive statistics that convey information regarding the degree of dispersion present in a set of data: range, percentile and interquartile range, variance and standard deviation, and the coefficient of variation. These statistics, combined with those describing central tendency, have great value in describing the distribution characteristics of a dataset.

1. Range

The definition of range was previously provided in Formula 2.1. Calculating the range from Example 2.10, we have

Range for ward A: $R_A = x_{\max} - x_{\min} = 215 - 186 = 29$

Range for ward B: $R_B = x_{\max} - x_{\min} = 244 - 160 = 84$

The results indicate that the range of platelet count in ward B was larger than that in ward A, although the two wards had the same mean.

A prime advantage of range is that it is easy to calculate. Moreover, range is measured in the same units as the original data; thus, range has a direct interpretation. However, range also has several clear disadvantages: (i) It takes into account only two values (the smallest and the largest), ignoring the variation caused by other observations. (ii) It is very sensitive to variation in sample size; as the sample size increases, the range tends to become larger. (iii) Compared with other dispersion measures, the sampling error (see Chapter 6) of range is relatively large, and therefore the stability of range is poorer.

2. Percentile and Interquartile Range

Formula 2.5 shows that the median divides all ordered values equally into two parts. Similarly, the values can be equally divided into a larger number of parts if desired.

Definition 2.4 If the observations are sorted from smallest to largest and equally divided into 100 parts, the corresponding value of the proportion $p\,\%\ \left(0 \le p \le 100\right)$ is called the *percentile*, which is denoted by the symbol $X_{p\%}$. For frequency-table data, $X_{p\%}$ is calculated as

$$X_{p\%} = L + \frac{i}{f_{p\%}}\left(n \times p\% - \sum f_L\right). \tag{2.10}$$

Percentile is also a location parameter. The pth percentile of a dataset is the value of X located so that the $p\%$ of the area under the relative frequency distribution for the data lies to the left of the pth percentile and $1-p\%$ of this area lies to its right.

Obviously, the median could be shown as $M = X_{50\%}$.

The *interquartile range* may be shown as $Q = X_{75\%} - X_{25\%}$.

Example 2.11 Calculate the interquartile range of the incubation period of food poisoning in Table 2.6.

Solution

Based on **Definition 2.4**:

(1) First, calculate $X_{25\%}$. As shown in Column 4 of Table 2.6, the cumulative relative frequency of the group that the 25th percentile lies in is 42.9%; therefore, $X_{25\%}$ is in the "8–" group. Thus, $L=8$, $i=2$, $f_{25\%}=19$, $n=84$, and $\sum f_L = 17$. Using Formula 2.10, we have

$$X_{25\%} = L + \frac{i}{f_{25\%}}\left(n \times 25\% - \sum f_L\right) = 8 + \frac{2}{19}\left(84 \times 25\% - 17\right) = 8.4$$

(2) Calculate $X_{75\%}$ in the same way. The corresponding cumulative relative frequency is 75%, which is in the "16–" group. Thus, for $i=2$, $f_{75\%}=7$, $n=84$, and $\sum f_L = 56$, we have

$$X_{75\%} = L + \frac{i}{f_{75\%}}\left(n \times 75\% - \sum f_L\right) = 16 + \frac{2}{7}\left(84 \times 75\% - 56\right) = 18.0$$

(3) Thus, the interquartile range is

$$Q = X_{75\%} - X_{25\%} = 18.0 - 8.4 = 9.6$$

indicating that the incubation period was between 8.4 and 18.0 hours for the middle 50% of patients.

Because the calculation of interquartile range is determined only by observations near that location, the ability to utilize the total information remains limited. The interquartile range has the advantage of reflecting the dispersion of the data in a relatively stable manner, especially for data with a skewed distribution.

3. Variance and Standard Deviation

Suppose we have a set of sample data with most of the observations lying close to their mean; it is intuitive to imagine that the dispersion in this case is less than when the observations are spread over a wide range. Therefore, it would be reasonable to measure the dispersion based on the degree of spread of values around their mean. Such a measure is realized in what is known as variance. The calculation of variance also depends on sample size.

(1) Calculating the variance in an original dataset

Definition 2.5 Let $x_1, x_2, \ldots, x_n$ be a set of n measurements. The average squared deviation of each value from the mean of a dataset is defined as the *variance*, which is calculated as follows:

$$s^2 = \frac{\sum_{i=1}^{n}(x_i - \bar{x})^2}{n-1}. \tag{2.11}$$

Variance reflects the average degree of dispersion of the data. Obviously, greater dispersion in the observed data corresponds to greater variance. Here, $n-1$ is called the degrees of freedom. We divide by $n-1$ instead of by n in our definition of variance, s^2. The theoretical reason for this choice of divisor is provided in Chapter 6, where we will show that defining s^2 in this way provides a "better" estimator of the true population variance σ^2.

However, variance is somewhat inconvenient and less interpretable in practice compared with the statistics already discussed, because the squared units are not consistent with the original units. Take height as an example: centimeters (cm) were the unit of the original data, whereas the square of centimeters (cm^2) is the unit of variance. In fact, an appropriate measure of dispersion in the original units can be obtained by merely taking the square root of the variance. The result is called the *standard deviation*, which has more practical implications in application because it has the same units as the mean. Standard deviation, denoted as s, is calculated as follows:

$$s = \sqrt{\frac{\sum_{i=1}^{n}(x_i - \bar{x})^2}{n-1}}. \tag{2.12}$$

For convenience of calculation, we use $\sum_i (x_i - \bar{x})^2 = \sum_i x_i^2 - \left(\sum_i x_i\right)^2 / n$; thus, Formula 2.12 can be written as

$$s = \sqrt{\frac{\sum_{i=1}^{n} x_i^2 - \frac{\left(\sum_{i=1}^{n} x_i\right)^2}{n}}{n-1}}. \tag{2.13}$$

Example 2.12 Calculate the standard deviation of hemoglobin (g/L) after admission for the 10 hospitalized patients in Example 2.4.

Solution

Based on Definition 2.5 and the data shown in Example 2.4, we have

$$\sum_i x_i = 139 + 158 + \cdots + 129 = 1272,$$

$$\sum_i x_i^2 = 139^2 + 158^2 + \cdots + 129^2 = 165684, \text{ and}$$

$$n = 10$$

Using Formula 2.13,

$$s = \sqrt{\frac{\sum_i x_i^2 - \frac{\left(\sum_i x_i\right)^2}{n}}{n-1}} = \sqrt{\frac{165684 - (1272)^2/10}{10-1}} = \sqrt{431.7} = 20.8.$$

Thus, the standard deviation of hemoglobin for these 10 patients was 20.8 g/L.

(2) Calculating the variance in a frequency-table dataset

Similar to the calculation of the mean, the standard deviation can be calculated using the weighted method with data from a frequency table; the formula for this approach is as follows:

$$s = \sqrt{\frac{\sum_{k=1}^{g} f_k x_{mk}^2 - \left(\sum_{k=1}^{g} f_k x_{mk}\right)^2 \Big/ \sum_{k=1}^{g} f_k}{\sum_{k=1}^{g} f_k - 1}} \tag{2.14}$$

where x_{mk} is the midpoint value group k, and f_k is the frequency of the corresponding group.

Example 2.13 Calculate the standard deviation of the height of the 153 10-year-old girls using the data in Table 2.5.

Solution

$$s = \sqrt{\frac{\sum_k f_k x_{mk}^2 - \left(\sum_k f_k x_{mk}\right)^2 \Big/ \sum_k f_k}{\sum_k f_k - 1}}$$

$$= \sqrt{\frac{(32004.50 + \cdots + 97969.00) - (253.0 + \cdots + 626.0)^2/153}{153-1}}$$

$$= \sqrt{\frac{3107084.3 - 21778.5^2/153}{152}} = 6.82.$$

Thus, the standard deviation of the height of the 153 10-year-old girls was 6.82 cm.

Compared with range and interquartile range, variance and standard deviation more sufficiently utilize the information of every observed value in the sample.

4. Coefficient of Variation

Although the standard deviation is useful for measuring the variability within a sample dataset, when a comparison of variability between datasets is needed, it might be inappropriate to use standard deviation to directly compare the degree of dispersion between two groups under the following conditions:

(1) The two means are quite different. For example, if the means of two samples are 100 and 1000, but the standard deviation is 10 in both samples, how can variability be compared between the two samples?
(2) The two indicators are measured in different units. For example, in the measurement of human physiological indicators, the unit of height is usually centimeters, whereas the unit of weight is usually kilograms. How, then, can height and weight be compared?

In both cases, we can use the coefficient of variation. The *coefficient of variation*, referred as *CV*, is a quantity jointly determined by the mean and the standard deviation. The calculation formula for *CV* is as follows:

$$CV = \frac{s}{\bar{x}} \times 100\%, \quad \bar{x} > 0. \tag{2.15}$$

It can be seen in Formula 2.15 that *CV* is a unit-free measure because the standard deviation is standardized by the mean. *CV* is thus more appropriate for comparing the dispersion of data with different units or with a considerable difference in the means.

Example 2.14 Referring to Example 2.1, 140 10-year-old boys were also randomly selected in the same survey. The mean and standard deviation of the height of these boys were 140.8 cm and 7.0 cm, respectively, and the mean and standard deviation for body weight were 35.6 kg and 7.0 kg, respectively. Compare the degree of variation of height and body weight.

Solution

Height: $\bar{x}_1 = 140.8$, $s_1 = 7.0$; weight: $\bar{x}_2 = 35.6$, $s_2 = 7.0$

The *CV* of the height of the boys is

$$CV_{\text{height}} = \frac{s_1}{\bar{x}_1} \times 100\% = \frac{7.0}{140.8} \times 100\% = 5.0\%$$

The *CV* of the weight of the boys is

$$CV_{\text{weight}} = \frac{s_2}{\bar{x}_2} \times 100\% = \frac{7.0}{35.6} \times 100\% = 19.7\%$$

Therefore, the variation of body weight is greater than the variation of height among 10-year-old boys in this sample.

When using the coefficient of variation, it should be noted that it is only meaningful to compare related indicators. Additionally, when the mean is less than the standard deviation, the practical application value of the coefficient of variation should be carefully considered. In this case, the coefficient of variation will be more than 100%, especially when the mean is close to 0, and it should not be used.

2.3 Descriptive Statistics of Categorical Data

2.3.1 Relative Numbers

When dealing with categorical data, relative numbers are often used to describe and compare data characteristics. In this section, we discuss various forms of rates and ratios that are commonly used to describe categorical data.

1. Rates

A *rate* refers to a measure of the relative frequency of occurrence of a phenomenon. In epidemiology, demography, and vital statistics, a rate is an expression of the relative frequency with which an event occurs in a defined population, usually over a specified period of time. The use of rate can be understood in two ways:

(1) Some statisticians restrict use of the term "rate" to measures that are expressed per unit of time. In this case, a rate describes, for instance, how quickly disease occurs in a population (e.g., two new cases of breast cancer per 10,000 women per year). This measure conveys a sense of the speed with which disease occurs in a population and seems to imply that this pattern has occurred and will continue to occur for the foreseeable future.
The formula is

$$\text{rate} = \frac{\text{number of events occuring during the period}}{\text{total person-time units at risk observed during the period}} \times k. \tag{2.16}$$

In Formula 2.16, rate is essentially the relative frequency of an event per unit time. The denominator of rate has a time element, using person-time to sum the periods of time at risk for each of the subjects by combining persons and time. The multiplier k is called the *base* of the proportion; its value could be 100%, 1000‰, 10,000/10,000, and so on; the calculated rate usually retain one to two decimals.

Example 2.15 A total of 3210 person-days of 150 hospitalized patients were observed from 1 to 31 January 2019, to estimate the incidence rate of pneumonia in a general surgery department of a hospital. Six patients developed pneumonia. Calculate the incidence rate of pneumonia for January 2019.

Solution

According to Formula 2.16,

$$\text{incidence rate of pneumonia} = \frac{6}{3210} \times 1000‰ = 1.90‰$$

The incidence rate of pneumonia from 1 to 31 January 2019, was 1.9‰, which means that an average of 1.9‰ of hospitalized patients in the general surgery department developed pneumonia each day in January.

(2) Other statisticians use the term "rate" more loosely to refer to the proportion (see the following section on ratios) calculated with the total number of individuals

who have the condition of interest (e.g., disease, exposure, or attribute) in the numerator and the size of the population in the denominator. Thus, a prevalence is the proportion of the population that has a certain health condition at a particular point in time.

In this case, the formula is

$$\text{rate} = \frac{\text{number of individuals who have the condition}}{\text{total size of the population at risk of having the condition}} \times k. \tag{2.17}$$

In this formula, the denominator of rate has no time element. The base k is the same as that in Formula 2.16.

Example 2.16 A survey conducted in 2015 showed that, among 103,497 adult men aged 30 years or older in a certain area, a total of 31,082 people had hypertension. The prevalence of hypertension in adult men aged 30 years or older in this area is

$$\text{prevalence of hypertension} = \frac{31082}{103497} \times 100\% = 30.0\%$$

It should be noted that, when calculating the rate, the length of the time period must be specified before the calculation is performed because the number of cases varies with the length of the time period. In Example 2.15, the observation period is clearly specified as from 1 January 2019 to 31 January 2019. In Example 2.16, the study was conducted in 2015.

"Rates" are widely used in medical research to indicate, for example, the incidence, prevalence, and infection rate of disease and to describe mortality rates, fatality rates, and survival rates of diseases. When the sample size is sufficiently large, the magnitude of a "rate" is often used to indicate the estimated value of the probability of an event.

2. Ratios

A *ratio* is a value obtained by dividing one quantity by another; these are two similar quantities measured from different groups or under different circumstances. For example, among patients who were vaccinated, the ratio of those who were diagnosed with the flu to those who were not is $154/592 = 0.26$. Later, we will introduce the standardized incidence ratio (SIR) and the standardized mortality ratio (SMR) in Section 2.3.2, and the odds ratio in Chapter 19.

Proportions are another commonly used type of ratio. Proportions, also called relative frequencies, are used to describe the proportion of the distribution structure and the relationship between the whole and the part. Proportion is defined as follows:

$$\text{proportion} = \frac{\text{part of the total number}}{\text{total number}} \times 100\%. \tag{2.18}$$

Formula 2.18 takes 100% as the base, so it is also called a percentage. The proportion has no units of measurement. When calculating a proportion, it is necessary to ensure that the numerator is part of the denominator; thus, the value of a proportion ranges from 0% to 100%. In addition, the proportion is not time-sensitive.

Table 2.8 Proportion of Category B infectious diseases in a certain region in 2015.

Disease	Number of cases	Proportion (%)
Viral hepatitis	124,984	33.6
Tuberculosis	95,151	25.6
Syphilis	36,339	9.8
Gonorrhea	8429	2.3
Scarlet fever	6859	1.8
Bacterial and amoebic dysentery	6703	1.8
Measles	3341	0.9
Other	89,731	24.2
Total	371,537	100.0

Example 2.17 The proportion of Category B infectious diseases in a certain region in 2015 is shown in Table 2.8.

Table 2.8 shows that viral hepatitis and tuberculosis had the largest and second largest proportions. Together, these two diseases accounted for 59.2% of the total cases.

Because the sum of the proportions is 100%, an increase or decrease of a certain component will affect the proportions of other parts.

Notice that: (i) To ensure the stability of relative numbers. It is necessary to confirm that there are enough observations – that is, the denominator should not be too small. This is because having a small number of observations could lead to large sampling errors, making the relative numbers unstable and less reliable. (ii) Proportions and rates should not be misused. The term "rate" is sometimes confused with "proportion"; although they are often used interchangeably, the two terms are not synonymous. If there is a time element involved, this should be expressed as a rate, such as the incidence rate over a certain period of time in a population of 100,000. If there is no time element, the meaning represented by the denominator is important to note when interpreting the result. For instance, in Example 2.17, viral hepatitis accounted for the largest proportion of infectious diseases (33.6%); however, this does not mean that hepatitis was the most serious disease in this region because this proportion does not reflect the severity of the disease. Thus, 33.6% is a proportion because the numerator is the number of hepatitis cases in the population (infectious cases) and the denominator is the number of all infectious cases. For a rate, the numerator would be the number of people experiencing hepatitis and the denominator would be the total population at risk, which can reflect the severity of hepatitis. (iii) Attention should be paid to the background of the data, which is especially important in longitudinal research. If you want to compare the annual incidence of lung cancer among residents of the same area in 1985 and 2015, for example, you should pay attention to changes in objective conditions. In addition to unhealthy habits, environmental pollution, and occupational exposure, the improvement of diagnostic capabilities may be another important factor influencing the incidence rate of lung cancer.

2.3.2 Standardization of Rates

The rate calculated in Example 2.16 can be used to describe the relative frequency of a certain disease in the population. These rates are also called *crude rates*. However, when comparing the rates, it is often inappropriate to use crude rates because some important characteristics of different groups, such as age, gender, occupation, and ethnicity, may vary. Therefore, when comparing rates, standardized methods are usually needed. The basic idea is to use a unified standard to eliminate the influence of differences in internal composition between the groups being compared. The rate after standardization is called the *standardized rate* or the *adjusted rate*. There are two main types of rate standardization methods: direct and indirect standardization. We use the age-standardized rate as an example to introduce the standardized method.

1. Direct Standardization

If the rate of each subgroup in the population to be compared is known, a set of standard population structure data for the reference population can be used to obtain the standardized rate.

Example 2.18 Table 2.9 shows the prevalence of hypertension among adult men in areas A and B. In which area is hypertension more prevalent?

Analysis

In each area, the prevalence of hypertension increases with age. We observe that the age-specific prevalence of hypertension in area B is slightly higher than that in area A; however, the overall prevalence is slightly higher in area A than in area B (26.8% vs. 25.8%). Why are these results so contradictory? With a closer look at the data, we find that the proportion of the population that is middle-aged or older (age ≥ 55 years) is higher in area A than in area B. Because the prevalence of hypertension is usually higher within this age group, the difference in age structure leads to a potentially misleading result. To eliminate the influence of age structure, the standardized rates should be used for comparison.

Table 2.9 The prevalence of hypertension among adult men in areas A and B.

Age group (years)	Area A			Area B		
	Participants	Cases	Prevalence (%)	Participants	Cases	Prevalence (%)
18–	4105	394	9.6	4818	477	9.9
25–	3056	452	14.8	2507	444	17.7
35–	1730	446	25.8	2519	678	26.9
45–	1501	627	41.8	2584	1085	42.0
55–	1222	675	55.2	1100	623	56.6
65–	880	567	64.4	346	236	68.2
75–	411	292	71.0	74	55	74.3
Total	12,905	3453	26.8	13,948	3598	25.8

The direct standardized rate calculation formula is

$$p' = \frac{\sum_{k=1}^{g} N_k p_k}{N}, \tag{2.19}$$

where p' denotes the standardized rate, $N_k\ (k = 1, 2, \ldots, g)$ denotes the size of the standard population of the kth age group, N represents the size of the total standard population, and p_k represents the actual prevalence of the kth age group.
The direct method of age standardization requires the initial selection of a standard population. There are three main ways to choose this standard population:

(1) A large population with a representative and relatively stable internal composition can be selected as the standard population. For example, the population in a national census can be used as the standard population.
(2) The sum of the numbers of the corresponding subgroups of the two groups of data to be compared can be used as the common standard population for the two groups.
(3) When the populations of the two groups to be compared are large enough, either group can be selected as the common standard population for the two groups.

In short, regardless of which method is used, the standard population for each subgroup is required to be large enough to ensure the stability of its structure.

Solution to Example 2.18 The detailed standardized calculation process is shown in Table 2.10.

The steps for this calculation are as follows:

(1) Determine the standard population. The standard population used in Table 2.10 was taken from the sum of the corresponding age groups in the two areas.
(2) The expected number of patients in this age group is given by the original prevalence p_k multiplied by the standard population N_k of the age group $k\ (k = 1, 2, \ldots, g)$. Adding the expected number of patients $N_k p_k$ in each subgroup yields the following:

Expected cases for area A: $\sum_k N_k p_k = 6900$

Expected cases for area B: $\sum_k N_k p_k = 7237$

(3) Divide the expected total number of cases by the standard total population N to get the standardized rates for area A and area B:

$$p'_A = \frac{\sum_k N_k p_k}{N} = \frac{6900}{26853} = 25.7\%,$$

$$p'_B = \frac{\sum_k N_k p_k}{N} = \frac{7237}{26853} = 27.0\%.$$

These results show that, after standardizing for age structure, the prevalence of hypertension is slightly lower in area A than in area B.

Table 2.10 Direct age standardization of the hypertension rate in the two areas.

Age group (years)	Standard population	Area *A*		Area *B*	
		Rate (%)	Expected cases	Rate (%)	Expected cases
k	N_k	p_k	$N_k p_k$	p_k	$N_k p_k$
18–	8923	9.6	857	9.9	883
25–	5563	14.8	823	17.7	985
35–	4249	25.8	1096	26.9	1143
45–	4085	41.8	1708	42.0	1716
55–	2322	55.2	1282	56.6	1314
65–	1226	64.4	790	68.2	836
75–	485	71.0	344	74.3	360
Total	26,853	26.8	6900	25.8	7237

The direct standardization method requires the rate of each subgroup to be relatively stable, so it is suitable for the comparison of high incidences and chronic diseases. Similarly, the direct standardization method can be extended to compare more than two sets of data.

2. Indirect Standardization

If the rate of each subgroup in the observed population is unknown or the number in any of the subgroups is too small for stable rates (as is the case with the incidence of tumors or rare diseases, for example), the indirect method shown in the following formula can be used for standardization:

$$p' = P \cdot \frac{r}{\sum_{k=1}^{g} n_k P_k}, \tag{2.20}$$

where p' denotes the standardized rate, P_k is the incidence of a disease in the age group $k\ (k = 1, 2, \ldots, g)$ of the standard population, P denotes the overall incidence in the standard population, n_k is the number of observations in the kth age group, and r denotes the total number of occurrences of a disease in the observed population.

The *standardized incidence ratio* (*SIR*) is the actual total number of occurrences of a certain disease r divided by the expected total number of occurrences of that disease, $\sum_k n_k P_k$. We multiply the SIR by the total incidence of the disease in the standard population and finally obtain the disease standardized rate for a certain population.

In fact, in Formula 2.20, compared with Formula 2.19, the incidence of the original subgroup has been replaced with the incidence of a certain disease in the standard population. The incidence of a certain disease in the standard population should be based on an official report or survey results with a large population.

Example 2.19 In an investigation of deaths from esophageal cancer in two counties of China in 2004, in county A, there were 2,694,627 subjects with 1162 esophageal cancer deaths (i.e., a mortality rate of 43.12/100,000); in county B, there were 2,622,826 subjects with 1035 esophageal cancer deaths (i.e., a mortality rate of 39.46/100,000). Table 2.11 presents the population size for each age group in counties A and B, along with the esophageal cancer mortality rate for each age group and the total esophageal cancer mortality rate in a large area as the standard mortality rate. Compare the mortality from esophageal cancer in countries A and B.

Solution

According to the results shown in Table 2.11, substituting into Formula 2.20, we have

County A: *standardized mortality ratio* (*SMR*): $\text{SMR} = \dfrac{1162}{170} = 6.835$

standardized mortality: $p'_A = \text{SMR} \times P = 6.835 \times 6.6 = 45.11/100{,}000;$

County B: standardized mortality ratio: $\text{SMR} = \dfrac{1035}{128} = 8.086$

standardized mortality: $p'_B = \text{SMR} \times P = 8.086 \times 6.6 = 53.37/100{,}000$

After indirect standardization, the death rate from esophageal cancer in county B was higher than that in county A, which is the opposite of the result of county A having a higher crude rate compared with county B.

3. Precautions for Using Standardized Rates

(1) Regardless of whether the direct or indirect method is used, the standardized rate cannot truly reflect the actual level of occurrence of a phenomenon; rather, this rate can only be used to compare relative levels between the groups being compared. Therefore, when reporting research results, it is recommended to include both the crude rate and the standardized rate.

(2) When calculating the standardized rate, the selection of a different "standard" can lead to a different standardized rate. Therefore, when comparing standardized rates, attention should be paid to whether the standards adopted are the same.

Table 2.11 Indirect standardization of esophageal cancer mortality in two counties.

Age group (years)	Standardized mortality (1/100,000)	County A		County B	
		Population	Expected deaths	Population	Expected deaths
k	P_k	n_k	n_kP_k	n_k	n_kP_k
0–	0.00	1,756,897	0	1,725,819	0
30–	0.50	244,942	1	289,298	1
40–	6.53	251,678	16	250,480	16
50–	17.41	206,947	36	191,204	33
60–	35.94	143,893	52	114,355	41
70–	71.85	90,270	65	51,670	37
Total	6.60	2,694,627	170	2,622,826	128

There is no basis for comparison between standardized rates using different standards.

(3) When there is an interaction between age groups and the groups being compared on rates – that is, when the trend in the rate of each subgroup in the groups being compared is inconsistent – the standardized method is not suitable.

(4) The standardized rate is still a sample rate. To compare the obtained standardized rates, hypothesis testing is required to draw a final conclusion (see Chapter 7 for more information on hypothesis testing).

2.4 Constructing Statistical Tables and Graphs

In descriptive statistics, statistical tables and graphics are common tools to intuitively display the basic characteristics of data. Certain criteria and requirements should be strictly followed in the process of creating statistical tables and graphs, but the specific method of presentation depends on factors such as the types of data used, the study objective, and specific professional requirements.

2.4.1 Statistical Tables

1. Elements of Statistical Tables

A *statistical table* is composed of a title, headings, lines, and numbers, as shown in Figure 2.5:

(1) Table number: In presenting results, statistical tables should be numbered and appear in order.

(2) Title: The title, one of the most important parts of the statistical table, is located above the table. The title concisely summarizes the basic contents of the table, including information such as attributes, sources, collection time, and location of the data presented.

(3) Row and column headings: Headings usually appear in the first row and the first column of the statistical table, displaying the data name and type, reflecting the attributes of the data presented in the rows and columns.

(4) Lines: Statistical tables only use horizontal lines – not vertical lines or slashes. Generally, horizontal lines usually appear only at the top and bottom of the table and under the vertical index (heading); thus, statistical tables are sometimes called

Table number. Title

	Heading 1		**Heading 2**	
	Subheading 1	**Subheading 2**	**Subheading 1**	**Subheading 2**
Heading 1				
Heading 2				
⋮				
Total				

Top line

Bottom line

Note: XXX

Figure 2.5 Illustration of the statistical table.

"three-line tables," although a few adjustments may be appropriate depending on the specific situation and table contents.

(5) Numbers: All data should be marked with a unified unit of measurement in the horizontal and vertical headings and expressed in Arabic numerals. Data on the same attribute should be presented with the same number of decimal places. If certain data do not exist or are not needed, this is usually indicated by "—" or "NA."

(6) Notes: If an explanation of the table content is needed, a footnote beginning with "Note": can be used. Alternatively, the content can be marked with a special symbol in the table and explained in a footnote that appears below the bottom line.

2. Types of Statistical Tables

(1) Simple tables

The contents of a simple table consist only of a group of horizontal headings or a group of vertical headings. The frequency distribution tables shown as Tables 2.2 to 2.4 are examples of this type of table. We now use an example to further illustrate the characteristics of the simple table.

Example 2.20 Referring to Example 2.3. In the same survey, data on the education level were obtained from 775 participants. The frequency distribution of the education level is given in Table 2.12. We see there is only one group of horizontal headings – the education level.

(2) Combinative tables

The combinative table is a combination of two or more horizontal and vertical headings that expresses the relationship between them. The content and form of statistical tables presenting categorical data and numerical data are generally slightly different. To reflect the central tendency and dispersion, tables presenting categorical data include frequencies and percentages for different groups, whereas tables presenting numerical data include frequencies, means, and standard deviations (or medians and interquartile ranges) for different groups. We further use an example to illustrate combinative tables for categorical data and numerical data.

Example 2.21 Referring to Example 2.20. In the same survey, the occupation and blood pressure (mmHg) of 775 adult men were obtained at the same time. Combinative

Table 2.12 Frequency distribution of education levels among 775 adult men.

Education level	Frequency	Relative frequency (%)	Cumulative relative frequency (%)
High school and above	158	20.4	20.4
Junior high school	378	48.8	69.2
Primary school	206	26.6	95.8
Illiteracy or little literacy	33	4.2	100.0
Total	775	100.0	—

Table 2.13 Frequency distribution of occupation among 775 adult men with different education levels.

Education level	Occupation			Total
	Herdsmen	Farmer	Worker	
High school and above	29	66	63	158
Junior high school	145	227	6	378
Primary school	109	96	1	206
Illiteracy or little literacy	15	18	0	33
Total	298	407	70	775

Table 2.14 Distribution of blood pressure (mmHg) among 775 adult men with different education levels.

Education level	Frequency	Systolic blood pressure		Diastolic blood pressure	
		$\bar{x}_1$	s_1	$\bar{x}_2$	s_2
High school and above	158	134.1	19.47	85.7	11.99
Junior high school	378	136.4	22.25	86.2	13.37
Primary school	206	139.5	19.44	87.2	12.22
Illiteracy or little literacy	33	150.8	28.36	89.7	20.03
Total	775	137.4	21.52	86.5	13.16

Note: For blood pressure values, $\bar{x}$ is the mean and s is the standard deviation.

tables for the frequency distribution of occupation and the distribution of blood pressure among the 775 adult men with different education levels are given in Tables 2.13 and 2.14. There are two groups of headings (education level and occupation) in Table 2.13 and three groups of headings (education level, systolic blood pressure, and diastolic blood pressure) in Table 2.14.

2.4.2 Statistical Graphs

Statistical graphs are used to describe the characteristics of data visually using points, lines, and planes. We only introduce commonly used graphics here, including graphics used to describe categorical data and those used to describe numerical data. These statistical graphs can be created with a variety of statistical software packages.

1. Statistical Graphs for Categorical Data

Bar charts or pie charts are commonly used to describe categorical data.

(1) Bar charts

Bar charts depict numerical values against distinct categories in a two-axis plot. The category levels are listed on one axis, one bar is drawn for each category, and the length of the bar along the other axis corresponds to the numerical value associated with the category. In Example 2.3, we used a bar chart to describe the distribution of hypertension status (Figure 2.3). We now continue with this example to illustrate the construction process of the bar chart.

(i) Perform the grouping: First, the blood pressure of Kazakh residents in a certain region of Xinjiang was divided into five groups according to the "Chinese Guidelines for the Prevention and Treatment of Hypertension": normal, high normal, and grades 1, 2, and 3 hypertension.
(ii) Construct a rectangle for each group: The height of the rectangle should be proportional to the frequency of the group (e.g., the unit height of the rectangle in Figure 2.3 corresponds to the frequency of 100), and the width of each group is the same.
(iii) Create equal intervals: The rectangles are generally separated by intervals of the same width.

There are two types of bar chart: single and compound. The type of bar chart is determined by the nature of the quantities presented in one chart. Figure 2.3 is a single bar chart, and we use an example to show a compound bar chart.

Example 2.22 From China's cancer registry data, we obtain the incidences of three types of cancer (lung, liver, and colorectal cancer) by gender in 2015. A compound bar is used to express the three quantities by gender, as shown in Figure 2.6. The factor of gender is added. Intuitively, it is easy to see that the incidence rates of the three cancers are higher in men than in women.

In the compound bar chart, it is important to ensure that the sequence of indicators presented is consistent for each group.

(2) Percentage bar charts and pie charts

Percentage bar charts and *pie charts* are used to show the composition of various components.

Example 2.23 From the data of a large surgical safety survey in 2015, we divide the ages of patients into three groups (<45, 45–64, and ≥65 years) and obtain age compo-

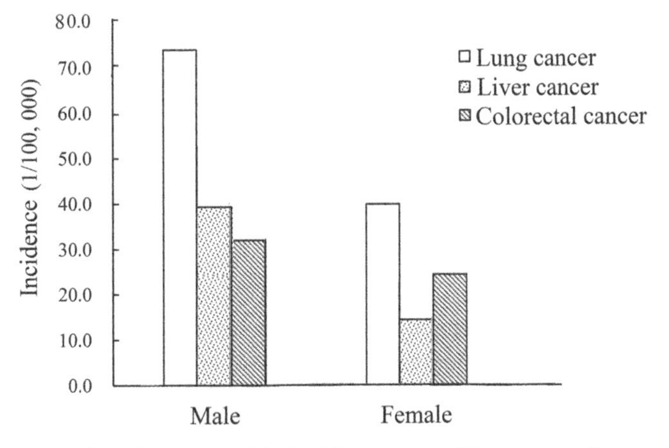

Figure 2.6 Bar chart of the incidence rates of three types of cancer by gender from China's cancer registry data for 2015.

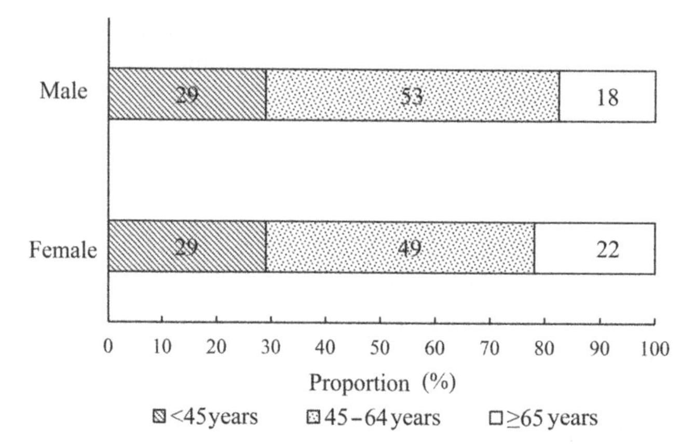

Figure 2.7 Percentage bar chart of the age compositions of patients of the two sexes in a large surgical safety survey in 2015.

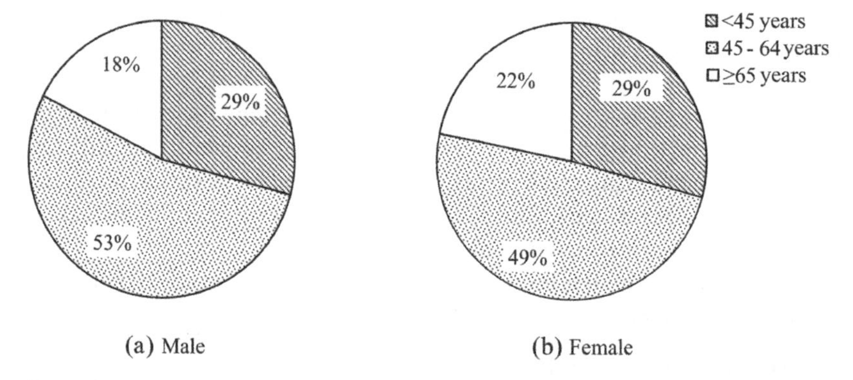

Figure 2.8 Pie chart of the age composition of both sexes using the same data displayed in Figure 2.7.

sitions of the two sexes. A percentage bar chart is used to express the age composition, as shown in Figure 2.7.

Pie charts use a circle (pie) to indicate 100%, and this circle is divided into multiple parts, each representing a category. The size of each part corresponds to each category's proportion of the total.

Example 2.24 Referring to Example 2.23. The same set of data presented in Figure 2.7 is expressed in a pie chart (Figure 2.8).

2. Statistical Graphs for Numerical Data

Graphical descriptions of numerical data commonly use histograms, stem-and-leaf plots, boxplots, scatterplots, and line graphs.

(1) Histograms

Histograms are drawn on the basis of the frequency distribution table, which divides the value range of the measurement indicator of interest into several intervals. These intervals are then used to form a horizontal axis scale to determine the relative frequency of observations in each group interval, and a series of rectangular graphs are plotted. Figures 2.1 and 2.2 are typical histograms.

It should be noted that the area rather than the height of the rectangle represents the frequency of the interval. This is especially important when there are unequal intervals.

(2) Stem-and-leaf plots

Histograms are characterized by two problems: (i) it is not suitable to construct a histogram when the sample size is small; and (ii) there may be missing sample points in some intervals. If you draw a histogram of the food poisoning incubation period data shown in Table 2.6, the effect would not be very good. In such cases, you can use a stem-and-leaf plot instead.

Example 2.25 Referring to Example 2.7. A stem-and-leaf plot (Figure 2.9) is used to describe the distribution of the incubation period (hour) for the 84 food poisoning patients.

The process of constructing a *stem-and-leaf plot* is explained as follows:

(i) Divide each observation into two parts: the stem and the leaf. We take the last digit of the number as the "leaf" and the other numbers as the "stem." For example, in Figure 2.9, the value 15 has a "stem" of 1 and a "leaf" of 5.
(ii) Arrange the "stems" in a column in order, starting with the smallest "stem" and ending with the largest "stem." For example, in this example, the "stems" start with the smallest number of 0 and end with the largest number of 3.
(iii) The "leaf" of each measurement value is placed on the row of the corresponding "stem," and "leaves" with observations on the same "stem" are arranged in ascending order horizontally from left to right, as shown in Figure 2.9, where the second row of observations all have the same "stem" of 0 and the "leaves" are arranged in sequence from 5 to 9. For example, there are three observations valued "5" and six observations valued "6."
(iv) Draw a vertical line to the right of the "stem" numbers, with all "leaves" appearing to the right of this line.
(v) The stem width is generally in the form of 10^m, where m represents the multiplier factor so that the stem-and-leaf plot can represent data with decimal points. For the multiplier factor m, the actual number is stem.leaf $\times 10^m$; specially, when $m = 0$, the figures shown are the actual values.

```
Frequency   Stem|Leaf
2              0|44
34             0|5556666667777778888888888899999999
18             1|000011122233334444
14             1|55666777788899
10             2|0011223344
2              2|56
1              3|1
3        Extremes (≥ 33)

Stem width:  10
```

Figure 2.9 Stem-and-leaf plot of the incubation period (hour) for the 84 food poisoning patients from Example 2.7. Extremes are points that have a distance from the upper or lower quartile exceeding 1.5 times the interquartile range.

In stem-and-leaf plots drawn by software packages, a frequency distribution column is given at the left end, indicating the number of "leaves" contained on each "stem."

The shape and function of the stem-and-leaf plot are very similar to that of the histogram, and both types of graphs can describe numerical data well. However, the scope of use of the two graphs is different. The histogram is very effective for generalizing and organizing large datasets but lacks details, whereas the stem-and-leaf plot completely retains the information in the original data. Obviously, this feature of the stem-and-leaf plot is useful only when describing small datasets. Rotating the "stems" and "leaves" in the stem-and-leaf plot by 90 degrees counterclockwise shows an approximate histogram.

(3) Boxplots

Boxplots are similar to histograms, and both types of graphs are used to describe the distribution of numerical data. The histogram is a detailed investigation of the distribution of continuous data, whereas the boxplot uses the mean, median, and upper and lower quartiles to describe the distribution; thus, the boxplot pays more attention to displaying important statistical information. These features make the boxplot more suitable for comparing the distributions of multiple groups of numerical data.

Example 2.26 In a study that investigated the imaging characteristics of patients with different types of lung cancer, dual-energy CT scans were performed for 26 patients with small-cell lung cancer (SCLC) and 80 patients with non-small-cell lung cancer (NSCLC). The iodine ratio as a quantitative measurement of the tumor characteristics was obtained. A boxplot was used to describe the distributions and to compare the two patient groups.

The boxplot in Figure 2.10 displays six basic statistics after the observation data are arranged from smallest to largest: the minimum, $X_{25\%}$, median, mean, $X_{75\%}$, and maximum. Additionally, outlier points are marked outside the two ends of the rectangular boxes. The boxplot mainly comprises a box with thin lines extending above and below the box. The height of the box represents the interquartile range of the data. The horizontal line in the box represents the median. The symbol "×" is generally used to represent the mean. The horizontal lines shown above the upper line of

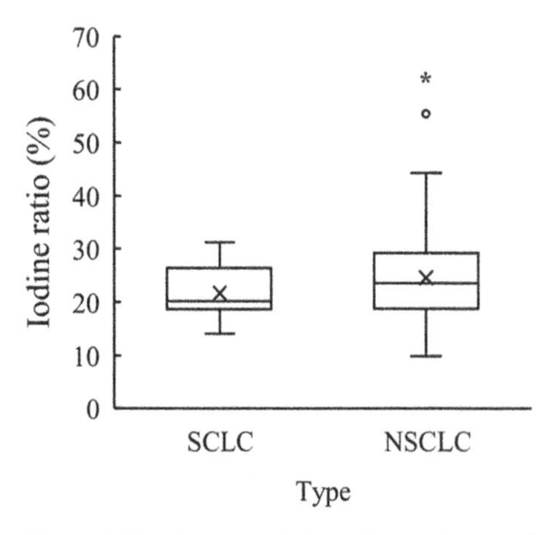

Figure 2.10 Boxplot of the iodine ratio in patients with SCLC and NSCLC.

the box and below the lower line of the box represent the maximum (upper) and minimum (lower) values after removing the outliers. Two symbols, "o" and "*," are used to represent outliers. The symbol "o" indicates that the distance of a point from the upper or lower quartile (the upper and lower boundaries of the box in the figure) exceeds 1.5 times the interquartile range, and "*" is used for points where this distance exceeds 3.0 times the interquartile range.

This graph shows that the NSCLC patients had a slightly higher average iodine ratio than SCLC patients and that the degree of variation was slightly greater for NSCLC than for SCLC. The boxplot in Figure 2.10 also shows that are two outliers in the NSCLC data that are worthy of special attention.

The boxplot examines the shape of the distribution of numerical data by comparing the relationship between the median and the mean across different groups. If the distribution is symmetric, the distances of the upper and lower quartiles from the median should be approximately equal, and the median and the mean should be approximately the same. If the upper quartile is more distant from the median than is the lower quartile, the distribution is positively skewed; if the converse is true, the distribution is negatively skewed.

(4) Scatterplots

Scatterplots are often used to identify a potential relationship between two measurement variables by presenting the distribution of data points in a Euclidean coordinate system. Especially when the observed values of numerical data are not in one-to-one correspondence and cannot be drawn with a line graph, using a scatterplot is effective. We use an example to illustrate the application of scatterplots.

Example 2.27 Referring to Example 2.3. In the same survey, we obtained data on the SBP and DBP of 229 Kazakh adult men at one of the study sites. A scatterplot is used to express the relationship between the SBP and DBP.

As shown in Figure 2.11, the value of one variable is taken as the x-axis, and the value of the other variable is taken as the as the y-axis. The position of each pair of observations is then drawn in a coordinate system. The scatterplot shows the general

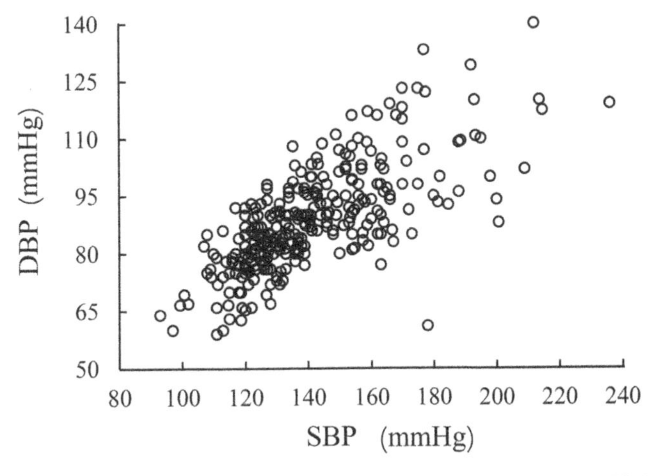

Figure 2.11 Scatterplot of the correlation between SBP and DBP for 229 Kazakh adult men in a survey in the Altay region of Xinjiang, China.

trend of correlation between two measurements. The starting points of the horizontal and vertical coordinates of the scatterplot depend on the data.

(5) Line graphs

Line graphs use the rise and fall of lines to indicate trends of correlation between two sets of numerical data (i.e., two variables).

One variable is plotted along the x-axis (horizontal), and the other variable is plotted along the y-axis. In the xy-plane, each observation point is determined by the horizontal and vertical coordinates of each observation, which must be in one-to-one correspondence; otherwise, the line graph cannot be connected. Depending on the shape of the line segments connecting the observation points, this type of graph can be categorized as a line graph or a curve graph. When multiple sets of data need to be compared, multiple line graphs can be drawn in the same coordinate system to allow for intuitive comparison.

Example 2.28 Referring to Example 2.22. From China's cancer registry data, we also obtain the incidence rates of three types of cancer among men from 2011 to 2015. The line graph in Figure 2.12 describes the incidence rates of three types of cancer among men in China from 2011 to 2015.

Method for drawing the line graph:

(i) Draw the horizontal and vertical axes: The horizontal axis represents time or variable groups, such as year or concentration. The labeled points on the vertical axis must be equidistant, representing the value of the variable of interest, such as frequency, relative frequency, or mean. The starting point of the horizontal and vertical coordinates of the line graph does not need to be 0.

(ii) There should not be too many lines in the same graph. If several lines are needed for comparison, they should be represented by different types (or colors) of lines, with figure labels.

(iii) To enhance the function of statistical graphic, the corresponding confidence interval of the mean is sometimes presented (see Chapter 6). This presentation is generally used in scientific research papers.

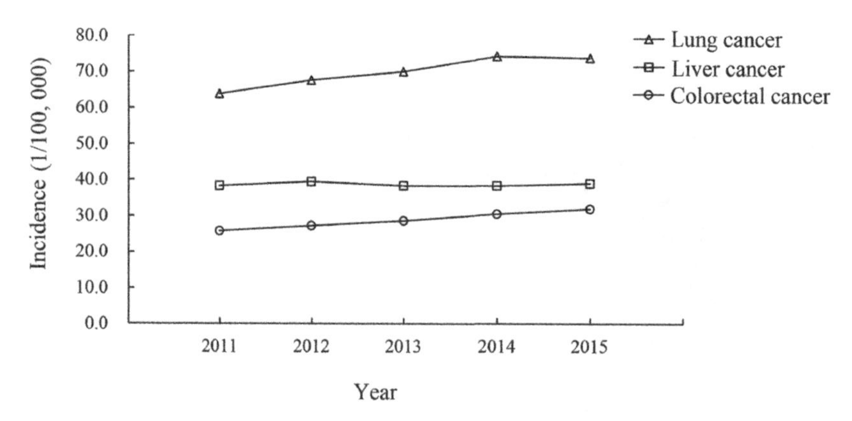

Figure 2.12 Line graph of the incidence rates of three types of cancer in men from China's cancer registry data from 2011 to 2015.

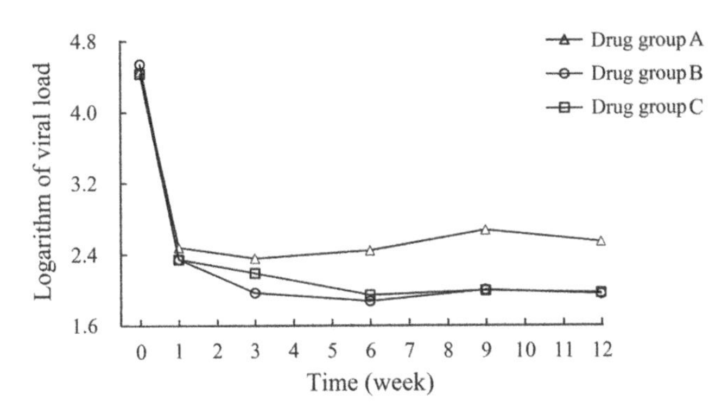

Figure 2.13 Semi-logarithmic line graph for the viral load over time among patients with AIDS after treatment with different drug combinations as part of a multicenter project on AIDS in 2015.

The *semi-logarithmic line graph* is a special example of the line graph. It is suitable for representing data in which the data have a skewed distribution. This type of graph is also used to compare the relative change speed of two or more datasets. Additionally, logarithmic graphs can be used when magnitude differences exist between different categories.

The semi-logarithmic line graph uses time as the x-axis and the logarithmically transformed indicator as the y-axis. Unlike ordinary line graphs that describe trends between datasets, semi-logarithmic line graphs are mainly used to reflect and compare the rate of change.

Example 2.29 In a multicenter project that investigated the therapeutic effects of different drugs on AIDS, the viral load over time among patients with AIDS after treatment with different drug combinations was obtained. Figure 2.13 shows the logarithm of the viral load for three groups of patients with AIDS treated with different drug combinations over time. The results show that the inhibitory trends of various drug combinations on viral load are roughly the same.

2.5 Summary

In this chapter, we introduced tabular and graphical methods for the statistical description of numerical data and categorical data. These methods are used to generate an intuitive presentation of the distributions of different types of data and thus inform the choice of statistical analysis methods.

For numerical data, central tendency and dispersion can be quantitatively described using descriptive indicators. To assess central tendency, we can choose from the arithmetic mean, median, and geometric mean. The indicators of dispersion include range, interquartile range/percentile, variance/standard deviation, and the coefficient of variation. This chapter has discussed the conditions for the application of each of these measures, emphasizing that an appropriate combination of measures of central tendency and dispersion should be selected, depending on the distribution type, to objectively describe the distribution characteristics of numerical data.

For categorical data, relative numbers are generally used for statistical description. Commonly used relative numbers include rates and ratios. It is important to pay attention to the difference between these two types of numbers when using them and to ensure that there are enough observations to make the selected relative number stable. When comparing rates across two or more groups, standardization is usually necessary before they are compared. The basic idea here is to adopt a unified standard to eliminate the influence of internal composition when making comparisons across groups.

We also briefly introduced the production and roles of statistical tables and statistical graphs, such as histograms, stem-and-leaf plots, boxplots, scatterplots, and line graphs, which are used for measurement data, as well as bar charts, percent bar charts, and pie charts, which are used for categorical data.

On the basis of the description of the sample data, the following chapters move forward to address questions on how to draw inferences about the population from which the sample was drawn. To do that, we need to understand the basics of probability and random variables, which will be introduced in Chapters 3–5. The basic knowledge and the content presented in this chapter can also provide a "material" basis for the statistical inference that will be discussed in Chapter 6 and in subsequent chapters.

2.6 Exercises

1. A survey was conducted among 100 adult men aged 30–40 years. The data on their body mass index (BMI) and serum triglyceride levels are summarized as histograms shown in Figure 2.14.
   - **(a)** Are histograms a proper choice for describing these data? Are there possible alternatives? How can you visualize the relationship between BMI and serum triglyceride levels? What are the advantages of graphic description in this sample?
   - **(b)** Can we replace the frequencies in the histograms with relative frequencies (%)? What are the similarities and difference between frequencies and relative frequencies?
   - **(c)** Which statistics do you plan to use to describe the distribution of BMI and serum triglyceride levels? Justify your choices.

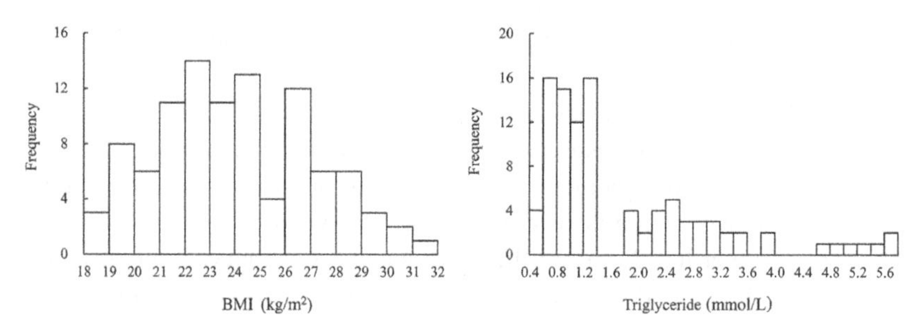

Figure 2.14 Histograms of BMI and serum triglyceride levels among adult men.

(d) What are the advantages of using descriptive statistics? What are the advantages of using both descriptive statistics and graphics?

(e) What are the roles of statistics in the description of central tendency and degree of dispersion? Is the joint use of these two types of statistics always necessary?

2. In a survey on the health status of preschool children, researchers conducted physical examinations of preschool children aged 4-5 years in a daycare center. Table 2.15 shows the numerical data on chest circumference for 120 healthy preschool boys.

Table 2.15 Chest circumference (cm) for 120 healthy preschool boys.

51.6	54.1	51.3	56.6	51.2	53.6	56.0	58.3
54.0	56.9	55.5	57.7	56.0	57.4	55.2	53.6
57.7	55.5	57.4	53.5	56.3	54.0	57.5	55.4
58.3	55.4	55.9	53.3	54.1	55.9	57.2	56.1
53.8	57.7	56.0	58.6	57.6	56.0	58.1	49.1
51.3	53.8	50.5	53.8	56.8	56.0	54.5	51.7
57.3	54.8	58.1	56.5	51.3	50.2	55.5	53.6
52.1	55.3	58.3	53.5	53.1	56.8	54.5	56.1
54.8	54.7	56.2	53.7	52.4	58.1	56.6	56.7
53.4	57.1	54.4	53.7	54.1	59.0	56.2	55.7
53.1	55.9	56.6	56.4	50.4	53.3	56.7	50.8
51.4	54.6	56.1	58.0	54.2	53.8	55.3	55.9
56.1	61.8	56.7	52.7	52.4	51.4	53.5	56.6
59.3	56.8	58.1	59.0	53.1	54.2	54.0	54.7
59.8	53.9	52.6	54.6	52.7	56.4	55.5	54.4

(a) Describe the data using graphics, and summarize the distribution characteristics using statistics. Justify your choices between the possible alternative methods.

(b) What is the difference between calculating the statistics using the direct method or the weighted method?

(c) Suppose that the unit of chest circumference was meters instead of centimeters; how would the distribution and the statistics change?

(d) Suppose that height and weight data for the 120 preschool boys were also available; how would you determine and compare the degree of dispersion across the measurements? Please state your suggestion.

3. In a multicenter surgical patient safety survey, a research team collected data on 200 patients with postoperative pulmonary infection. The gender and age distributions are shown in Table 2.16. For both male patients and female patients, the risk of post-operative pulmonary infection was highest for those aged 55–64 years, and female patients had a higher risk than male patients in this age group. Thus, the researchers argued that closer attention should be paid to female patients aged 55–64 years.

(a) Present the data using a graph.

(b) Is the researchers' statement that closer attention should be paid to female patients aged 55–64 years correct? If not, what is the correct interpretation of these data? What data would you need to support the researchers' statement?

(c) If the difference between male and female patients is of interest, how would you make a comparison between these groups? Why?

Table 2.16 Postoperative pulmonary infection among 200 surgical patients.

Age group (years)	Male patients		Female patients	
	Infection case	**Proportion (%)**	**Infection case**	**Proportion (%)**
14–29	21	19.1	11	12.2
30–54	29	26.4	15	16.7
55–64	35	31.8	39	43.3
65–	25	22.7	25	27.8
Total	110	100.0	90	100.0

4. Measles vaccination was performed among 62 children aged 1 year, and their hemagglutination inhibition antibody titers were measured 1 month later. Calculate the mean of the data presented in Table 2.17.

Table 2.17 Hemagglutination inhibition antibody titers of 62 children aged 1 year.

Antibody titer	1:4	1:8	1:16	1:32	1:64	1:128	1:256
Frequency	5	8	14	17	11	5	2

5. Table 2.18 shows the age-specific population number, deaths, and all deaths from cancer in a county in 2018. Answer the following questions:

(a) Calculate and report which age groups account for the highest proportions of the population, deaths, and deaths from cancer.

(b) Calculate and report which age groups have the highest rate of death and the highest rate of death from cancer.

(c) Illustrate the difference between a proportion and a rate using these data. What should a researcher pay attention to before using these figures?

Table 2.18 Population number, deaths, and all deaths from cancer in a county in 2018.

Age group (years)	Population	Death	Death owing to cancer
0–	82,920	138	4
20–	46,639	63	12
40–	28,161	172	52
60–	9370	342	42
Total	167,090	715	110

6. Table 2.19 details the incidence rates of influenza and bronchitis in a city during 2000–2008. Draw and compare a line graph and a semi-logarithmic line graph for the data. Are there any difference between the two graphs? When is a semi-logarithmic line graph preferred over an ordinary line graph?

Table 2.19 Incidence rates of influenza and bronchitis in a city during 2000–2008.

Year	Influenza (‰)	Bronchitis (‰)
2000	126.27	6.63
2001	92.19	6.37
2002	107.59	5.90
2003	101.93	5.69
2004	92.60	5.49
2005	73.20	4.32
2006	51.40	3.04
2007	42.39	2.42
2008	33.92	2.27

3

Fundamentals of Probability

CONTENTS

In Chapter 2, we outlined various techniques. These methods allow an investigator to summarize a set of data through either descriptive statistics or graphic representation. However, we typically want to do more with data than describe them only. In particular, we might want to draw specific inferences about the behavior of the data with respect to the population. In the vast majority of cases, data are collected to test hypotheses. Because of the variability of individuals in a population, the inferences based on sample data are also uncertain. The sample rarely provides an accurate description of the population, so the uncertainty of inference plays an important role in statistics. Probability theory is a mathematical discipline that may quantify this "uncertainty." To test hypotheses adequately, we must have an elementary knowledge of probability. Although a thorough discourse on probability is well beyond the scope and intent of this text, aspects of probability are of interest in biomedicine and considerations of probability theory underlie the many procedures for statistical hypothesis testing. Therefore, in this chapter, we introduce probability concepts and useful notation that are most pertinent to biomedicine and biostatistical analysis.

Applied Medical Statistics, First Edition. Jingmei Jiang.

Companion website: www.wiley.com\go\jiang\appliedmedicalstatistics

3.1 Sample Space and Random Events

In nature, people often encounter two types of phenomena: One is the *deterministic phenomenon*, which is characterized by conditions under which the results are completely predictable, that is, the same result is observed each time the experiment is conducted. For example, heavy objects thrown into the sky inevitably fall to the ground because of the earth's gravity, and water at 100°C under standard atmospheric pressure inevitably boils. The other is the *random phenomenon*, which is characterized by conditions under which the results are not predictable, that is, one of several possible outcomes is observed each time the experiment is conducted, for example, the outcome (heads or tails) of flipping a coin and the number of calls received by an emergency center in an hour. However, the actual appearance of the predicted result is accidental in a random phenomenon, such as predicting heads when we flip a coin. These occasional phenomena demonstrate a certain regularity after many repeated experiments and observations, which is regarded as a statistical law. In this section, we first introduce vocabulary terms and definitions to lay the foundation required to further describe and quantify this law.

3.1.1 Definitions of Sample Space and Random Events

The process of obtaining an observation or making a measurement for a random phenomenon is called a *random experiment* (briefly, an experiment), and is denoted by E.

Here are some examples of experiments:

$E1$: Flip a coin and observe whether it lands heads or tails.

$E2$: Flip two coins and observe all possible outcomes.

$E3$: Count the number of calls received by an emergency center in an hour.

$E4$: Calculate the average height (cm) of college freshmen boys in Beijing in 2020.

Each result of a random experiment is called a *sample point*, and is typically denoted by ω. All sample points constitute the *sample space* of an experiment, which is denoted by $\Omega = \{\omega\}$. Thus, the corresponding sample space of the experiments above can be represented in set notation:

$\Omega_1 = \{\omega_1, \omega_2\}$, where ω_1 denotes H and ω_2 denotes T (H: heads, T: tails).

$\Omega_2 = \{\omega_1, \omega_2, \omega_3, \omega_4\}$, where ω_1, ω_2, ω_3, ω_4 denote HH, HT, TH, TT, respectively (H: heads, T: tails).

$\Omega_3 = \{\omega_i;\ i = 0, 1, 2, \ldots\}$, where ω_i denotes that the emergency center received i calls in an hour.

$\Omega_4 = \{\omega_h;\ 0 < h < +\infty\}$, where ω_h denotes the average height of colleges freshman boys in Beijing in 2020 is h cm.

A set of sample points (a subset of Ω) is called a *random event*, or *event* for short, and is denoted by capital letters A, B, C, ...

The set of single sample point is called the *simple event*, they cannot be decomposed any further. For example, for $E1$, $A = \{\omega_1\}$ is a simple event.

Another type of event that is composed of several simple events is called a *composite event*. For example, in $E3$, the event we are interested in is "receiving no more than three calls". Then $B = \{0 \text{ times}, 1 \text{ time}, 2 \text{ times}, 3 \text{ times}\}$ is a composite event and is a subset of Ω_3.

For convenience, we also regard Ω as a *deterministic event* and null set $\varnothing$ as an *impossible event*. They can be regarded as special random events.

3.1.2 Operation of Events

The relationship between events is consistent with that between sets, and set theory and *Venn diagrams* are efficient approaches to organizing experimental scenarios that enable probability problems to be solved more easily. Therefore, we briefly introduce several basic operations of events using set language, and use Venn diagrams to express that relationship.

1. Containment of Events

For any two events A and B, we say "event A contains event B" if the following is satisfied: if event B occurs, then event A must occur. This is denoted by $A \supseteq B$ or $B \subseteq A$, where the symbols "$\supseteq$" and "$\subseteq$" represent "contain" and "be contained," respectively. The Venn diagram is shown in Figure 3.1.

Example 3.1 Let X denote the systolic blood pressure (SBP, mmHg) readings of a person, A be the event that the person has high SBP readings: $A = \{X \geq 140\}$, and B be the event that the person has SBP readings of grade 1 hypertension (we only consider SBP): $B = \{140 \leq X < 160\}$. Then, $B \subseteq A$.

2. Union of Events

For any two events A and B, "at least one of A and B occurs" is also an event. This event is called the union of A and B, and is denoted by $A \cup B$, which includes only A occurring, only B occurring, and A and B occurring simultaneously. The Venn diagrams are shown in Figure 3.2.

Clearly, $(A \cup B) \supseteq A$, and $(A \cup B) \supseteq B$.

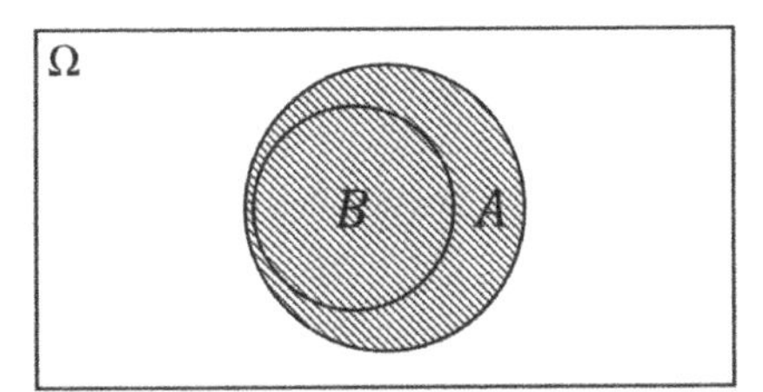

Figure 3.1 Venn diagram showing the containment of events A and B.

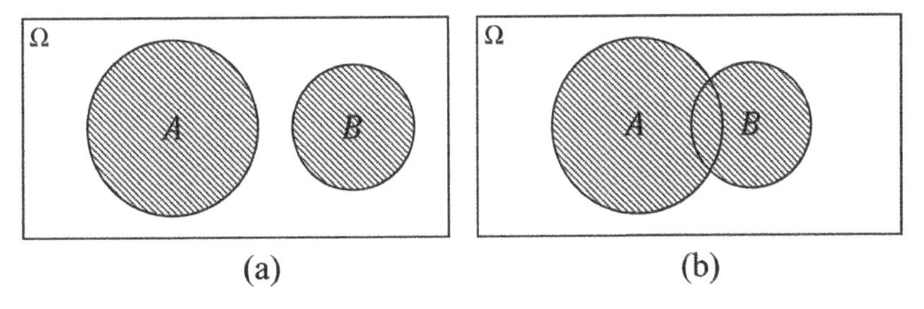

Figure 3.2 Venn diagrams showing the union of events A and B.

Example 3.2 Let A and B be defined as in Example 3.1, that is, $A=\{X\geq 140\}$ and $B=\{140\leq X<160\}$. Then $A\bigcup B=A=\{X\geq 140\}$.

The union of two events can be extended to several events. For n events $A_1, A_2,\ldots, A_n$, their union is defined as the event that "at least one of $A_1, A_2,\ldots, A_n$ occurs." Let B denote this event. Then $B=\bigcup\limits_{i=1}^{n}A_i$.

3. Intersection of Events

For any two events A and B, "A and B occur simultaneously" is also an event. This event is called the intersection of A and B, and is denoted by $A\bigcap B$. The Venn diagram is shown in Figure 3.3.

Clearly, $(A\bigcap B)\subseteq A$, and $(A\bigcap B)\subseteq B$.

Example 3.3 Let A and B be defined as in Example 3.1, that is, $A=\{X\geq 140\}$ and $B=\{140\leq X<160\}$. Then $A\bigcap B=B=\{140\leq X<160\}$.

The intersection of two events can be extended to several events. For n events $A_1, A_2,\ldots, A_n$, the intersection of them is defined as the event that "$A_1, A_2,\ldots, A_n$ occur simultaneously." Let B denote this event. Then $B=\bigcap\limits_{i=1}^{n}A_i$.

4. Inverse Events

For any event A, "event A does not occur" is also an event. This event is called the inverse of event A or the complement of A, and is denoted by $\bar{A}$. The Venn diagram is shown in Figure 3.4.

5. Difference of Events

For any two events A and B, "event A occurs and event B does not occur" is also an event. This event is called the difference of B from A, and is denoted by $A\bigcap\bar{B}$. The Venn diagrams are shown in Figure 3.5.

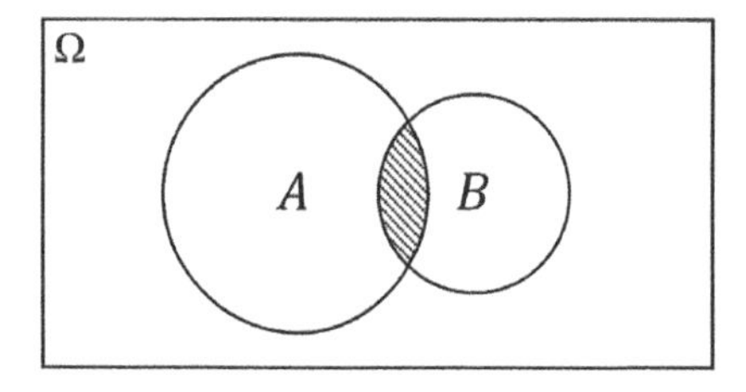

Figure 3.3 Venn diagram showing the intersection of events A and B.

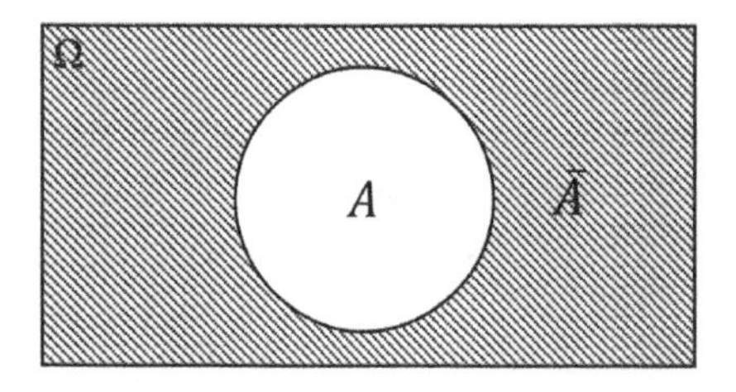

Figure 3.4 Venn diagram showing event A and its inverse event $\bar{A}$.

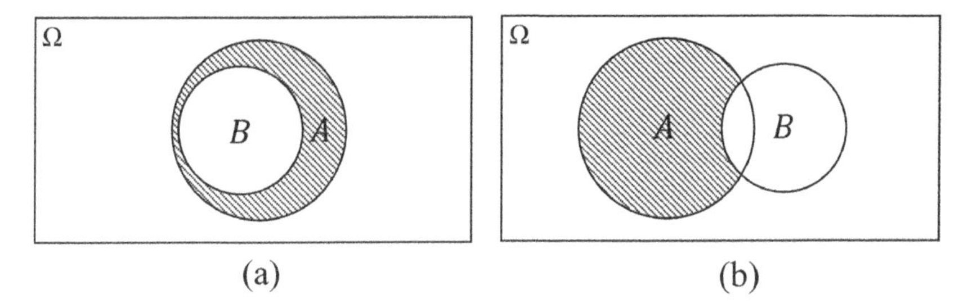

Figure 3.5 Venn diagrams showing the difference of event B from event A.

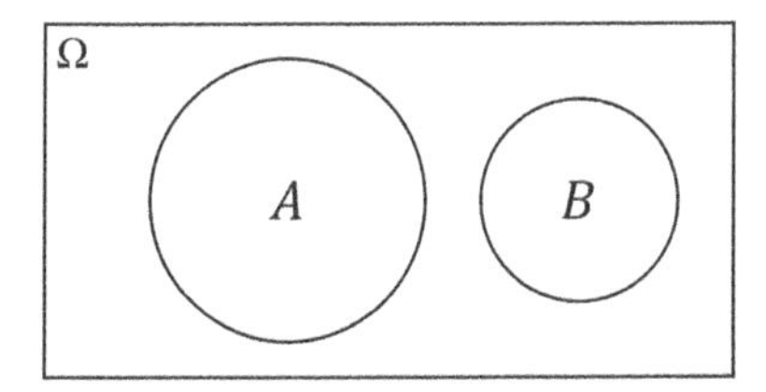

Figure 3.6 Venn diagram showing mutually exclusive events A and B.

Example 3.4 Let A and B be defined as in Example 3.1, that is, $A = \{X \geq 140\}$ and $B = \{140 \leq X < 160\}$. Then $A \cap \bar{B} = \{X \geq 160\}$.

6. Mutually Exclusive Events

For any two events A and B, if events A and B cannot occur simultaneously, that is, $A \cap B = \varnothing$, then A and B are called mutually exclusive events. The Venn diagram is shown in Figure 3.6.

"Mutually exclusive" is not only applicable to two events; it can also be extended to several events. For n events $A_1, A_2, \ldots, A_n$, we say that the n events are mutually exclusive if A_i and A_j are mutually exclusive for any i and j $(i, j \in \{1, 2, \ldots, n\}, i \neq j)$. By definition, all the simple events in any sample space Ω are mutually exclusive.

Example 3.5 Let event $A = \{X \geq 140\}$ and event $B = \{140 \leq X < 160\}$, as defined in Example 3.1, and let event C be the event that a person has normal SBP readings: $C = \{X < 120\}$. Then events A and C are mutually exclusive because they cannot both occur simultaneously; by contrast, events A and B are not mutually exclusive.

7. Complementary Events

Complementary events are a special type of mutually exclusive events. If "events A and B cannot occur simultaneously, and their sum constitutes the sample space," that is, $A \cap B = \varnothing$ and $A \cup B = \Omega$, then A and B are called complementary events.

Example 3.6 Let event $A = \{X \geq 140\}$, as defined in Example 3.1, and let event D be the event that a person's SBP readings are not considered high: $D = \{X < 140\}$. Then events A and D are called complementary events because $A \cap D = \varnothing$ and $A \cup D = \Omega$.

We summarize these terms and notation both in set theory and probability theory in Table 3.1.

Table 3.1 Meaning of symbols in set theory and probability theory.

Symbol	Sets theory	Probability theory
Ω	Space/Complete set	Sample space/Deterministic event
$\varnothing$	Empty set	Impossible event
ω	point	Sample point
$\{\omega\}$	Single point set	Simple event
$A \subseteq \Omega$	A is a subset of Ω	Event A
$A \subseteq B$	Set B contains set A	Event B contains event A
$A \cup B$	The union(sum) of sets A and B	The union(sum) of events A and B
$A \cap B$	The intersection of sets A and B	The intersection of events A and B
$\overline{A}$	The complementary set of A	The inverse event of A
$A \cap \overline{B}$	The difference of set B from set A	The difference of event B from event A
$A \cap B = \varnothing$	There are no elements in common in sets A and B	Events A and B are mutually exclusive

3.2 Relative Frequency and Probability

When investigating random phenomena, rather than merely determining all the possible events that might occur, we are more interested in how likely it is that a particular event would occur under certain conditions, which requires a quantitative measure that describes the likelihood of the occurrence of an event. Such a measure should meet at least two requirements:

(1) It should be an inherent objective measure that does not depend on the subjective will of a person, and it can be identified and tested by conducting a large number of repeated experiments under the same conditions.
(2) If event B contains event A, then event A is no more likely to occur than event B. The deterministic event should have the maximum value under this measure, and similarly, the impossible event should have the minimum value.

The quantitative measure that measures the likelihood of the occurrence of an event A is called the probability of the event A, denoted by $P(A)$, which could take any value between 0 and 1: $0 \leq P(A) \leq 1$.

Example 3.7 In an experiment involving flipping a coin, because of the impact of many random factors, such as the speed and angle when the coin is flipped, the elasticity and smoothness of the drop location, and the movement of airflow, we cannot predict the result of every experiment. However, as the number of experiments increases, some regularity will be demonstrated. In the past, many scholars conducted thousands of coin flipping experiments. Table 3.2 lists the experimental results of some scholars.

Table 3.2 Experimental results of flipping coins.

Experimenter	Number of flips (n)	Frequency of heads (m)	Relative frequency of heads (m/n)
A. De Morgan	4092	2048	0.5005
G. L. Lecterc	4040	2048	0.5069
W. Feller	10,000	4979	0.4979
K. Pearson	24,000	12,012	0.5005

Source: Küchenhoff (2008).

The results in Table 3.2 show that, although the relative frequency of heads is not exactly the same, it fluctuates around a fixed value (0.5), which demonstrates a certain degree of stability.

3.2.1 Definition of Probability

Relative frequency. Suppose E is a random experiment, A is one of the events, and E is repeated n times under the same conditions. Let m denote the number of times event A occurs in these n experiments. Then the ratio m/n is called the relative frequency of event A, and is denoted by

$$F(A)=\frac{m}{n} \tag{3.1}$$

Definition 3.1 Suppose that the experiment is repeated n times under the same conditions, and the random event A occurs m times. Suppose that the number of experiments n becomes infinite. The relative frequency m/n will fluctuate around a certain value p. Then p is called the *probability* of event A, and is denoted by

$$P(A)=p\approx\frac{m}{n} \tag{3.2}$$

Therefore, we may say that the probability of an event is the relative frequency of this set of outcomes over an indefinitely large (or infinite) number of experiments.

Definition 3.1 not only illustrates the objectivity of probability, but also highlights the approximate method of determining the probability value. It is very important to understand this because, in practice, the concept of relative frequency is simple and easy to understand. We often infer the properties of probability based on the properties of relative frequency. This is why we need to introduce them first.

3.2.2 Basic Properties of Probability

We now consider the axioms of probability that we use to develop certain general rules of probability. Let Ω be the sample space of an experiment and A be any subset of Ω. The probability of an event A, denoted by $P(A)$, satisfies the following three axioms (axioms are general truths that are offered without proof and are intuitively obvious):

(1) For any event $A \subseteq \Omega$, $0 \leq P(A) \leq 1$
(2) $P(\Omega) = 1$
(3) Let $A_1, A_2, A_3, \ldots$ be mutually exclusive events. Then $P(A_1 \cup A_2 \cup A_3 \cup \cdots) = P(A_1) + P(A_2) + P(A_3) + \cdots$

3.3 Conditional Probability and Independence of Events

In the previous section, we described events in general. In this section, we discuss the dependence and independence of events using conditional probability.

3.3.1 Conditional Probability

The probabilities discussed in Section 3.2 were defined based on random experiments without any special conditions attached, and are referred to as *unconditional probability*. However, the probability of an event may change when there are conditions that may affect the result. The probability in this case is called conditional probability.

Definition 3.2 For any events A and B, *conditional probability* refers to the probability that event B occurs given that event A occurs, and is denoted by $P(B \mid A)$. It equals the probability that both A and B occur divided by the probability that A occurs:

$$P(B \mid A) = \frac{P(A \cap B)}{P(A)}, \text{ assuming } P(A) > 0 \tag{3.3}$$

Definition 3.2 indicates that the probability of event B is related to whether event A occurs. Therefore, whether there is a correlation between two events can be studied through conditional probability.

3.3.2 Independence of Events

Definition 3.3 For any events A and B, if $P(B \mid A) = P(B)$ or $P(A) = 0$, then events A and B are called *independent*. Thus, Formula 3.3 can be written as

$$P(A \cap B) = P(A) \times P(B) \tag{3.4}$$

Example 3.8 Given that the proportion of men in the Chinese population is 51.1% and the proportion of blood type *AB* is 7.0%, estimate the proportion of men with blood type *AB* in the Chinese population.

Solution

Suppose that event A represents "man" and event B represents "blood type AB." Then $P(A)=0.511$ and $P(B)=0.070$. Because the ABO blood group system is not inherited in a sex-linked manner, the two events are independent of each other. Hence, based on Definition 3.3, the probability of men with blood type AB in the Chinese population is

$$P(A \cap B)=P(A)\times P(B)=0.511\times 0.070=0.036$$

Thus, the estimated proportion of men with blood type AB in the Chinese population is 3.6%.

From this example, we can see that, in biomedical research, the independence of events can be assessed based on experimental conditions and biological knowledge.

The concept of "independence" can also be extended to n events. For events $A_1, A_2, \ldots, A_n$, we say that the n events are independent if

$$P\left(A_{i_1} \cap A_{i_2} \cap \cdots \cap A_{i_m}\right)=P\left(A_{i_1}\right)\times P\left(A_{i_2}\right)\times \cdots \times P\left(A_{i_m}\right)$$

for any subset of these n events $\left(i_1, i_2, \ldots, i_m \in \{1,2,\ldots,n\}\ , m \le n\right)$. Clearly, if the events in a group are independent, then any pairs of events are also independent.

3.4 Multiplication Law of Probability

Based on Formula 3.3, the *multiplication law of probability* can be directly obtained as

$$P(A \cap B)=P(A)\times P(B \mid A), \text{ assuming } P(A)>0$$

or

$$P(A \cap B)=P(B)\times P(A \mid B), \text{ assuming } P(B)>0; \tag{3.5}$$

that is, the probability of the intersection of two events is equal to the probability of one event (its probability is not zero) multiplied by the conditional probability of the other event under the condition of the occurrence of the event.

Example 3.9 Suppose that the prevalence of hypertension in adult men in a rural area is 30% and the awareness rate of hypertension (among those who have hypertension) among adult men is 52%. An adult man is randomly selected. Calculate the probability that he is hypertensive and aware of it.

Solution

Suppose that event A represents "the adult man is hypertensive" and event B represents "he knows he is hypertensive." Then $P(A)=0.3$, and the probability of an adult man that is hypertensive being aware that he is hypertensive is $P(B \mid A)=0.52$. Then if an adult man is randomly selected, the probability that he is hypertensive and aware of it is

$$P(A \cap B)=P(A)\times P(B \mid A)=0.30\times 0.52=0.156$$

3.5 Addition Law of Probability

3.5.1 General Addition Law

If A and B are any events, the probability of the union of A and B is the sum of the probabilities of events A and B minus the probability of the intersection of events A and B, i.e.,

$$P(A \cup B) = P(A) + P(B) - P(A \cap B) \tag{3.6}$$

Example 3.10 Referring to Example 3.9, given that the prevalence of hypertension in adult men in a rural area is 30%, two adult men are randomly selected. Calculate the probability of at least one man being hypertensive.

Solution

Suppose that event A represents "the first man is hypertensive," event B represents "the second man is hypertensive," and event C represents "at least one of the two men is hypertensive." Then $C = A \cup B$. Because whether these two men are hypertensive does not affect either man, $P(A \cap B) = P(A) \times P(B)$.

Thus,

$$\begin{aligned} P(C) &= P(A \cup B) = P(A) + P(B) - P(A \cap B) \\ &= P(A) + P(B) - P(A) \times P(B) \\ &= 0.3 + 0.3 - 0.3 \times 0.3 \\ &= 0.51, \end{aligned}$$

so the probability of at least one adult man being hypertensive is 51%.

It is possible to extend the addition law (Formula 3.6) to more than two events. For example, if there are three events A, B, and C, then

$$P(A \cup B \cup C) = P(A) + P(B) + P(C) - P(A \cap B) - P(A \cap C) - P(B \cap C) + P(A \cap B \cap C)$$

This result can be generalized to any number of events, but this is beyond the scope of this text.

3.5.2 Addition Law of Mutually Exclusive Events

If A and B are two mutually exclusive events in sample space Ω, the probability of the union of the events is equal to the sum of the probabilities of the two events:

$$P(A \cup B) = P(A) + P(B) \tag{3.7}$$

Formula 3.7 is self-evident because events A and B are mutually exclusive. Thus, $P(A \cap B) = 0$. From this formula, the probability of a composite event can be decomposed into the sum of the probabilities of the mutually exclusive events using the interrelationship between events.

The probability of the inverse event $\bar{A}$ is $P(\bar{A})=1-P(A)$, and the addition law can be extended naturally to the case of many events.

Example 3.11 Twelve mice of similar size and weight are placed in a cage: four white mice, two piebald mice, and six black mice. One mouse is taken out of the cage randomly. Calculate the probability that the mouse is white or piebald.

Solution
If a mouse is taken out of the cage randomly, there are 12 possible results, and the probability of each is 1/12.

Suppose that event A represents "taking a white mouse" and event B represents "taking a piebald mouse." Then,

$$P(A)=\frac{4}{12}=\frac{1}{3},\ P(B)=\frac{2}{12}=\frac{1}{6}$$

Because A and B are mutually exclusive events, use Formula 3.7. Then

$$P(A\cup B)=P(A)+P(B)=\frac{1}{3}+\frac{1}{6}=\frac{1}{2}$$

Hence, the probability of taking a white or piebald mouse is 50%.

3.6 Total Probability Formula and Bayes' Rule

In practice, complex problems are often appropriately decomposed into several simple problems and solved separately. Similarly, when solving complex probability problems, we can decompose the composite events into several mutually exclusive events, calculate the probabilities of these events separately, and use the addition law and multiplication law to obtain the final result. Consider the following two formulas:

3.6.1 Total Probability Formula

For event group $A_1, A_2,\ldots, A_n$, if the following two conditions are satisfied:

(1) $A_1, A_2,\ldots, A_n$ are mutually exclusive, and $P(A_i)>0\ (i=1, 2,\ldots, n)$,
(2) $A_1\cup A_2\cup\cdots\cup A_n=\Omega$,
then for any event B,

$$P(B)=\sum_{i=1}^{n}P(A_i)P(B\mid A_i) \tag{3.8}$$

Formula 3.8 is called the *total probability formula*, which indicates that the probability of B can be represented as the weighted average of the conditional probabilities given the occurrence of A_i.

Example 3.12 A serum biomarker is used to screen for lung cancer in a certain population. Previous studies have shown that 90% of lung cancer patients are positive using this biomarker, but 3% in non-lung cancer participants. The proportion of lung cancer patients in this population is 0.3%. Calculate the probability that the biomarker is positive when screening for lung cancer in this population.

Solution
Suppose that event B represents "positive for this biomarker," event A_1 represents "lung cancer patients," and event A_2 represents "non-lung cancer patients."

Then $P(A_1)=0.003$, $P(A_2)=1-P(A_1)=0.997$, $P(B \mid A_1)=0.90$, and $P(B \mid A_2)=0.03$,

$$\begin{aligned} P(B) &= P(A_1)P(B \mid A_1)+P(A_2)P(B \mid A_2) \\ &= 0.003 \times 0.90 + 0.997 \times 0.03 \\ &= 0.033. \end{aligned}$$

Hence, the probability that the biomarker is positive when screening for lung cancer in this population is 3.3%.

3.6.2 Bayes' Rule

For n mutually exclusive events $A_1, A_2, \ldots, A_n$, their union is a deterministic event Ω. The conditional probability of event $A_k\ (k=1, 2, \ldots, n)$ given that event B has occurred is

$$P(A_k \mid B)=\frac{P(A_k)P(B \mid A_k)}{\sum_{i=1}^{n} P(A_i)P(B \mid A_i)} \quad (k=1, 2, \ldots, n), \text{ assuming } P(B)>0 \tag{3.9}$$

Formula 3.9 is called the *Bayes' rule* or *Inverse probability formula*. The significance of Bayes' rule is that it can change the direction of conditional probability, that is, it can infer the cause when the result is known. This is called the *posterior probability*, and is denoted by $P(A_k \mid B)$, where $P(A_k)$ represents the possibility of various causes. It is generally a summary of past experience and called the *prior probability*.

Example 3.13 Referring to Example 3.12, if a participant is screened with a positive result for this biomarker, calculate the probability that he/she has lung cancer.

Solution
We have $P(A_1)=0.003$, $P(A_2)=1-P(A_1)=0.997$, $P(B \mid A_1)=0.90$, and $P(B \mid A_2)=0.03$. According to Bayes' rule,

$$\begin{aligned} P(A_1 \mid B) &= \frac{P(A_1)P(B \mid A_1)}{P(A_1)P(B \mid A_1)+P(A_2)P(B \mid A_2)} \\ &= \frac{0.003 \times 0.90}{0.003 \times 0.90 + 0.997 \times 0.03} = 0.083. \end{aligned}$$

Therefore, when the biomarker result is positive, the probability that the participant has lung cancer is 8.3%.

From this example, we know that caution should be exercised regarding the cause-outcome direction when calculating conditional probability: although the positive rate of testing is high among lung cancer patients, the lung cancer probability is low among those who test positive. This is because the prevalence of lung cancer $P(A_1)$ is very low, thereby making the numerator, which is also the first additive term in the denominator, much smaller than the second additive term in the denominator.

Bayes' rule was proposed by T. Bayes (1702–1761). A set of theories and methods have developed from it, and have formed a school of probability and statistics, collectively called the Bayesians. Bayesian methods are also widely used in natural sciences and many other fields.

3.7 Summary

For a deterministic phenomenon, the results are always the same for each observation when an experiment is conducted under the same conditions. For a random phenomenon, one of several possible outcomes is observed each time the experiment is conducted under the same conditions.

Probability is a measure of the likelihood of the occurrence of an event, which is an inherent property of things. It can be approximated by relative frequency through a large number of repeated experiments under the same conditions, which makes probability easy to understand and calculate intuitively.

Probability can be calculated using the addition law and multiplication law when the events satisfy the corresponding conditions.

The basic idea of the total probability formula and Bayes' rule is to divide a composite event into several mutually exclusive events, calculate the probabilities of these events separately, and use the addition law and multiplication law of probability to obtain the final result. The total probability formula represents the probability of an event as the weighted average of the conditional probabilities of another mutually exclusive event group; and Bayes' rule infers the cause under the premise of knowing the result, and uses the prior probability to infer the posterior probability.

In the next two chapters, we use the general principles and models of probability in biomedical research. The most important models are the normal distribution, binomial distribution, and Poisson distribution. These models are widely used in statistical inference.

3.8 Exercises

1. Assume that A, B, and C represent three events in sample space Ω. Describe the following events using operations of A, B, and C:
   - **(a)** A does not occur.
   - **(b)** Only A occurs among A, B, and C.
   - **(c)** A, B, and C all occur.
   - **(d)** At least one of A, B, and C occurs.
   - **(e)** At most one of A, B, and C occurs.

2. In research aiming to investigate the clinical characteristics of familial aggregation of hypertension, a female patient with hypertension is selected as a hypertensive proband and hypertension information about her family members. Let A_1 = "her sister has hypertension," A_2 = "her brother has hypertension," A_3 = "her daughter has hypertension," and A_4 = "her son has hypertension."
Answer the following questions:
   (a) What does $A_1 \cup A_2$ mean?
   (b) What does $A_1 \cap A_2$ mean?
   (c) What is the relationship between $\bar{A}_1 \cap \bar{A}_2$ and $A_1 \cup A_2$?
   (d) What does $A_1 \cup A_2 \cup A_3 \cup A_4$ mean?

3. Suppose 10% of residents in a community have diabetes, 20% of the diabetes cases have obesity, and 10% of residents without diabetes have obesity. Suppose one resident in this community is randomly selected.
   (a) Given that this person has diabetes, what is the probability that this person has obesity?
   (b) What is the probability that this person has diabetes and obesity?
   (c) What is the probability that this person has obesity?
   (d) Is having diabetes independent of having obesity?
   (e) Given that this person does not have obesity, what is the probability that this person has diabetes?

4. A total of 1000 type 2 diabetes patients are registered at a community diabetes management center, and the age and sex composition are shown in the Table 3.3. Suppose that 100 of these patients develop diabetic nephropathy (70 men and 30 women).
Suppose one patient is randomly selected. Answer the following questions:
   (a) What is the probability that this patient is less than 40 years old?
   (b) What is the probability that this patient is a man and less than 40 years old?
   (c) Given that this patient is a woman, what is the probability that she is less than 60 years old?
   (d) What is the probability that this patient is a man and has diabetic nephropathy?
   (e) Given that this patient is a woman, what is the probability that she has diabetic nephropathy?

Table 3.3 Age (year) and sex composition of 1000 type 2 diabetes patients.

Sex	**Age group**		
	<40	**40–60**	**>60**
Men	70	310	170
Women	50	270	130

5. Suppose that the prevalence of smoking among men in a region is 20%, and 0.4% of men that smoke develop lung cancer. Answer the following questions:
   - **(a)** If two men are randomly selected, what is the probability that at least one of them is a smoker?
   - **(b)** If one man is randomly selected, what is the probability that he is a smoker and has lung cancer?
   - **(c)** If 0.1% of men in the region have lung cancer and one man is randomly selected, given that this man is a non-smoker, what is the probability that he has lung cancer?
   - **(d)** If one man is randomly selected, given that this man has lung cancer, what is the probability that he is a smoker?
   - **(e)** According to the definition of an independent event, demonstrate whether smoking and lung cancer are independent from each other using results obtained from the previous questions.

4

Discrete Random Variable

CONTENTS

4.1 Concept of the Random Variable

In Section 3.1, we observed that if random events in the sample space are not denoted by numeric values, this is very troublesome for notation. Recall $E1$ in Chapter 3. When we flip a coin, we use $\omega_1 = H$ and $\omega_2 = T$ to denote the events of heads and tails, respectively; hence, the sample space is expressed as $\Omega = \{H, T\}$. However, if we are interested in the number of "heads" events in 50 consecutive flips, it is clearly cumbersome to describe such a sample space using H. Instead, we use the letter X to denote the number of "heads," which is a variable that may take the value of $0, 1, \ldots, 50$. Similarly for $E3$ in Chapter 3, when we observe the number of calls received by an emergencycenterinanhour,thesamplespaceis $\Omega = \{0 \text{ times}, 1 \text{ time}, 2 \text{ times}, 3 \text{ times}, \ldots\}$. We use letter X to denote the number of calls, which is a variable that may take the values $0, 1, 2, 3, \ldots$.

The above example shows that we may use a variable X to represent all possible results of a random phenomenon, and different values indicate the occurrence of different events; however, the value it takes in one experiment is unknown in advance. We call X a random variable.

Applied Medical Statistics, First Edition. Jingmei Jiang.

Companion website: www.wiley.com\go\jiang\appliedmedicalstatistics

Definition 4.1 Assume that E is a random experiment with sample space $\Omega = \{\omega\}$. If for each $\omega \in \Omega$, there is one and only one numeric value $X(\omega)$ corresponding to it, then a function $X(\omega)$ defined on Ω is obtained, and $X(\omega)$ is called a random variable.

We typically use capital letters X, Y, Z,... to denote *random variables*.

For example, in the experiment of flipping one coin, the sample space is $\Omega = \{\omega_1, \omega_2\}$, where ω_1 denotes heads and ω_2 denotes tails. According to Definition 4.1, the random variable X is a function of ω defined on Ω:

$$X = X(\omega) = \begin{cases} 1, & \omega = \omega_1 \\ 0, & \omega = \omega_2 \end{cases}$$

For the experiment of flipping 50 coins and counting the number k of "heads" events, the sample space is $\Omega = \{\omega_i;\ i = 0, 1, 2, \ldots, 50\}$ and the random variable X can be expressed as

$$X = X(\omega_i) = i\ (i = 0, 1, \ldots, 50)$$

An important characteristic of random variables is that each value of the variable has a corresponding probability. Therefore, to fully understand a random variable, we need to know:

(1) every possible value, or the interval of values of the random variable.
(2) the probabilities corresponding to the values or value ranges.

Two classes of random variables exist: discrete and continuous. A *discrete random variable* can assume only certain values, either finite or countably infinite. A *continuous random variable* can assume values that cannot be enumerated or may be expressed within intervals of real numbers. In the following, we discuss the discrete random variable and continuous random variable separately because these two classes are handled somewhat differently. We first examine the pattern of behavior and predictability of discrete random variables in this chapter. Then we introduce the continuous random variable in Chapter 5.

4.2 Probability Distribution of the Discrete Random Variable

4.2.1 Probability Mass Function

In statistics, the pattern of behavior of a discrete random variable is described by the *probability mass function (pmf)*. We illustrate this concept using Example 4.1.

Example 4.1 From a survey on surgical safety status, we selected a total of 1238 surgical patients who developed one or more postoperative infections (e.g., surgical site infection, bloodstream infection, urinary infection, and lung infection) before discharge. Table 4.1 shows the number of specific infections in these patients and the corresponding relative frequency of each number.

Table 4.1 Relative frequency distribution of the number of specific infections in 1238 surgical patients.

X	1	2	3	4
Relative frequency $(X = x_k)$	0.807	0.105	0.056	0.032

Source: Yu et al. (2019).

Table 4.2 Probability distribution of the discrete random variable.

X	x_1	x_2	...	x_k	...
$P(X = x_k)$	p_1	p_2	...	p_k	...

Table 4.1 indicates that the value of the random variable x_k can be denoted by the value of $1, 2, 3, 4$, and the probability corresponding to each value is approximated by the relative frequency. This probability distribution is called the pmf, sometimes called the probability distribution column.

Table 4.2 presents the general relationship between x_k and the corresponding probability $P(X = x_k)$.

Definition 4.2 Let X be a discrete random variable. The pmf or *probability distribution column* of X is

$$P(X = x_k) = p_k \ (k = 1, 2, \ldots). \tag{4.1}$$

The pmf has two properties:

(1) $0 \leq p_k \leq 1 \ (k = 1, 2, \ldots)$.

(2) $\sum_{k=1}^{\infty} p_k = 1$.

The validity of property (1) is obvious. For property (2), because each simple event in the sample space has one and only one value corresponding to it, when all possible values are taken, the collection of all simple events is a deterministic event, so the validity of property (2) is also justified.

4.2.2 Cumulative Distribution Function

Definition 4.3 Let X be a discrete random variable with a pmf. The *cumulative distribution function* (*cdf*) for X is denoted by

$$F(x) = P(X \leq x) = \sum_{x_k \leq x} p_k, \tag{4.2}$$

where x is any real number.

Example 4.2 Referring to Example 4.1, calculate the cdf of the number of infections X based on the data in Table 4.1.

Solution

By Definitions 4.2 and 4.3, the cdf is easily obtained from the pmf of X. Simply add all the probabilities for the values of X less than or equal to x; that is

$$F(x) = P(X < 1) = 0, \ x < 1,$$

$$F(x) = P(X \leq 1) = P(X < 1) + P(X = 1) = 0 + 0.807 = 0.807, \ 1 \leq x < 2,$$

$$F(x) = P(X \leq 2) = P(X \leq 1) + P(X = 2) = 0.807 + 0.105 = 0.912, \ 2 \leq x < 3,$$

$$F(x) = P(X \leq 3) = P(X \leq 2) + P(X = 3) = 0.912 + 0.056 = 0.968, \ 3 \leq x < 4,$$

$$F(x) = P(X \leq 4) = P(X \leq 3) + P(X = 4) = 0.968 + 0.032 = 1.000, \ x \geq 4.$$

The corresponding distribution graph of the cdf is shown in Figure 4.1.

The graph of the cdf can be used to identify discrete random variables and continuous random variables. For discrete random variables, the distribution graph is a ladder-like function, whereas for continuous random variables, it is a smooth curve (see Chapter 5). When the number of possible values of a discrete random variable increases, the ladder-like graph of the variable gradually approximates a smooth curve, while the discrete random variable approaches a continuous random variable.

4.2.3 Association Between the Probability Distribution and Relative Frequency Distribution

In Chapter 2, we discussed the concept of a relative frequency distribution in the context of a sample. We described it as a list of each value in the dataset and a corresponding count of how frequently the value occurs. In this section, we introduce the *probability distribution* of the discrete random variable. The former is typically called the empirical distribution or statistical distribution, and the latter is called the theoretical distribution or overall distribution. In practice, to solve problems, we typically use the property that the empirical distribution is a good approximation to the probability distribution under the condition of large samples; that is, we replace probability by

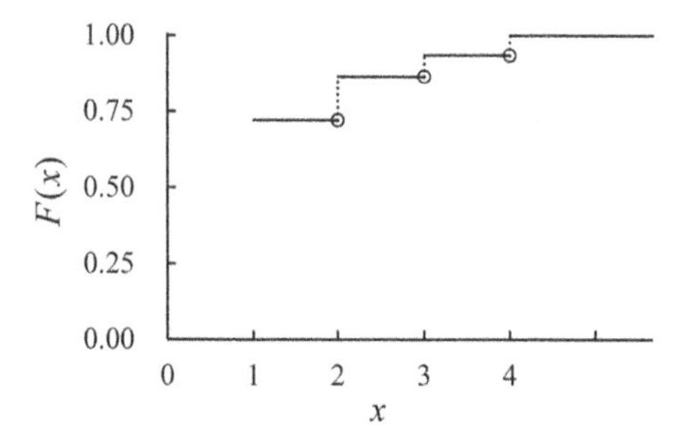

Figure 4.1 Cumulative distribution function of the nubmer of infections for Example 4.2.

relative frequency, as in the previous two subsections (Examples 4.1 and 4.2). The test of the applicability of the probability distribution is performed by comparing the difference between the probability distribution and the relative frequency distribution of the limited observation sample, which is called the goodness-of-fit test; see Chapter 11 for details.

4.3 Numerical Characteristics

An investigation of the characteristics of the random variable is the same as that of the characteristics of samples. It is often not necessary to describe the probability distribution of random variables in detail; instead, knowing some characteristic values of the variable is sufficient in solving problems. Generally, we can understand a random variable by knowing its central tendency and dispersion. Values that describe the characteristics of the probability distribution of random variables are called population characteristics, including the mathematical expected value (*expected value* for short), variance, and standard deviation. These characteristic values have an important effect in theory and practice.

4.3.1 Expected Value

Definition 4.4 If X is a discrete random variable, then the expected value (or population mean) of X, denoted by $E(X)$ or μ, is

$$E(X) \equiv \mu = \sum_k x_k p_k \; (k = 1, 2, \ldots). \tag{4.3}$$

The expected value represents a weighted "average" of the values of the random variable, where the weight p_k is the positive (i.e., nonzero) probability of $X = x_k$.

Note that the number of values of the random variable in the definition of μ may be either finite or infinite. In either case, the individual values must be distinct from each other.

Recall the formula of the mean of sample frequency data in Chapter 2 (Formula 2.4). We can rewrite it as

$$\bar{x} = \frac{\sum_{k=1}^{g} f_k x_{mk}}{n} = \sum_{k=1}^{g} \left(\frac{f_k}{n} \right) x_{mk}$$

When n is sufficiently large, the relative frequency of a certain event, which is f_k / n in the above formula, gradually stabilizes to the corresponding probability, as in Formula 4.3. The only difference is that the weight here is the observed relative frequency, whereas the weight in Formula 4.3 is the theoretical probability.

Example 4.3 Referring to the data in Table 4.1, find the expected value of the number of infections in patients.

Solution

From the given data, we cannot obtain the expected value according to Definition 4.4, but can only use the sample mean as an estimate of it. The estimated average number of infections is

$$\mu = \sum_k x_k p_k \approx \bar{x}$$
$$= 1 \times 0.807 + 2 \times 0.105 + 3 \times 0.056 + 4 \times 0.032 = 1.313 \,.$$

Thus, on average, a patient would be expected to have about 1.3 complications.

In Example 4.3, we use the sample relative frequency instead of probability to approximate the expected value, so the result of the mean is not unique. If we investigate another group of surgical patients, we can obtain another set of observations, so we can also obtain another average, which is often different from the first average. Despite this, because the relative frequency converges to the probability in a sample of sufficient size, the averages $\bar{x}$ are not substantially different from μ. In Chapter 6, we discuss the estimation of parameter μ using statistics $\bar{x}$ in detail.

4.3.2 Variance and Standard Deviation

The analog to the sample variance S^2, a variance of the random variable, or call population variance, is denoted by $Var(X)$ or σ^2. The variance represents the average degree of spread of all values relative to the expected value.

Definition 4.5 Suppose X is a discrete random variable. The population variance (variance for short) of X is defined as

$$Var(X) \equiv \sigma^2 = E(X - \mu)^2 . \tag{4.4}$$

A convenient way to calculate this quantity is

$$Var(X) = \sum_k x_k^2 p_k - \mu^2 . \tag{4.5}$$

The standard deviation is the arithmetic square root of the variance, denoted by σ:

$$\sigma = \sqrt{\sigma^2} . \tag{4.6}$$

Example 4.4 Referring to the data in Table 4.1, find the variance and standard deviation of the number of infections.

Solution

Similar to the expected value, we cannot obtain the population variance according to Definition 4.5, but can only calculate an estimate of it.

The estimated variance is

$$\sigma^2 = \sum_k x_k^2 p_k - \mu^2 \approx s^2$$
$$= \left(1^2 \times 0.807 + 2^2 \times 0.105 + 3^2 \times 0.056 + 4^2 \times 0.032\right) - 1.313^2 = 0.519.$$

The estimated standard deviation is

$$\sigma = \sqrt{\sigma^2} \approx s = \sqrt{0.519} = 0.720.$$

In this section, we use sample statistics to approximate the expected value and variance of the random variable (population), which is based on the property that the relative frequency and probability have a good approximation under the condition of large samples, so the corresponding distribution has a good approximation. Using this property, we can unify the theoretical distribution and practical applications. The subsequent statistical inferences that we learn later are based on quantitative methods to determine whether the differences in statistics and parameters are simply caused by sampling errors.

4.4 Commonly Used Discrete Probability Distributions

In this section, we introduce probability distributions of several commonly used discrete random variables. Among them, the binomial distribution and Poisson distribution are particularly important in biomedical research.

4.4.1 Binomial Distribution

1. Basic Concept

The *binomial distribution* is an important theoretical distribution with wide applications in biomedicine. Many biological phenomena can be described using a binomial distribution. We introduce the concept of the binomial distribution using an example.

Example 4.5 Toxicological research is commonly conducted using animals such as mice. Suppose the probability of the death of a mouse given a certain dose of poison is 0.8. There are four mice called A, B, C, and D. What is the probability of A, B, and C dying, and D remaining alive?

Solution

We use "ddda" to denote this event. Because the probabilities of dying and remaining alive are given by 0.8 and 0.2, respectively, and the outcomes for different mice are presumed to be independent, the probability of "ddda" is

$$0.8 \times 0.8 \times 0.8 \times 0.2 = 0.8^3 \times 0.2 = 0.1024$$

Now consider the more general question: What is the probability that any three mice out of four die?

The arrangement "ddda" is only one of four possible orderings that result in three deaths. Table 4.3 provides the four possible orderings.

The four scenarios shown in Table 4.3 are mutually exclusive events. The probability of any three mice dying and one remaining alive is calculated as

$$C_4^3 (0.8)^3 (0.2) = 4 \times (0.8)^3 \times 0.2 = 0.4096$$

Table 4.3 Possible orderings for the events of three deaths out of four mice and their corresponding probabilities.

A	*B*	*C*	*D*	**Probability**
Die	Die	Die	Alive	$0.8 \times 0.8 \times 0.8 \times 0.2$
Die	Die	Alive	Die	$0.8 \times 0.8 \times 0.2 \times 0.8$
Die	Alive	Die	Die	$0.8 \times 0.2 \times 0.8 \times 0.8$
Alive	Die	Die	Die	$0.2 \times 0.8 \times 0.8 \times 0.8$

C_4^3 is called a *combination*, where $C_4^3 = \frac{4!}{3!(4-3)!} = 4$, which indicates the number of ways of selecting three mice that die out of four mice, and $n!$ is called the n factorial and defined as $n! = n \times (n-1) \times \cdots \times 2 \times 1$.

The combination is an important topic for studying the binomial distribution. We provide general notation, that is, C_n^k, which represents the number of ways of selecting k objects from n without regard to order:

$$C_n^k = \frac{n!}{k!(n-k)!}. \tag{4.7}$$

Formula 4.7 may be simply expressed as "choose k from n."
Suppose the question is considered further: What is the probability of k deaths from four mice given poison (in a more formal way, k successes in 4 trials)?

Solution
The probability that k successes occur among the 4 trials and that the remaining $4-k$ trials are failures is

$$\pi^k (1-\pi)^{4-k}$$

Clearly, in this example, for four mice given poison, the number of deaths k may be 0, 1, 2, 3, or 4.

To compute the probability of k successes in any of the four trials, the probability must be multiplied by the number of ways in which k trials for the successes and $4-k$ trials for the failures can be selected, that is, C_4^k.

Table 4.4 shows all the probabilities of k successes in 4 trials.

This is a typical example of a binomial distribution. The trial results that can be fitted using a binomial distribution have a common structure: a sample of n (in our example, $n = 4$) independent trials, where each has only two possible outcomes: "success" or "failure." We designate the occurrence of death for a mouse as a "success," and hence, remaining alive as a "failure." Furthermore, the probability of success in each trial is assumed to be some constant π (in our example, $\pi = 0.8$); hence, the probability of failure in each trial is $1-\pi$ (in our example, $1-\pi = 0.2$). The term "success" is used in a general manner, without any specific contextual meaning.

We provide the formal definition of the binomial distribution.

Table 4.4 Probability distribution corresponding to k successes in four trials.

Number of successes k	Calculation formula	Probability p_k
0	$C_4^0(0.8)^0(0.2)^4$	0.0016
1	$C_4^1(0.8)^1(0.2)^3$	0.0256
2	$C_4^2(0.8)^2(0.2)^2$	0.1536
3	$C_4^3(0.8)^3(0.2)^1$	0.4096
4	$C_4^4(0.8)^4(0.2)^0$	0.4096

Definition 4.6 If the pmf of a discrete random variable X is

$$P(X=k)=p_k=C_n^k\pi^k(1-\pi)^{n-k}\ (k=0,1,\ldots,n), \tag{4.8}$$

then X follows a binomial distribution characterized by parameters (n,π), and is denoted by $X\sim B(n,\pi)$. X represents the number of "successes" that occur in n independent trials.

Clearly, this distribution satisfies two basic properties of the probability distribution:

(1) $0\le p_k\le 1\ (k=0,1,\ldots,n)$.

(2) $\sum_{k=0}^{n}p_k=\sum_{k=0}^{n}C_n^k\pi^k(1-\pi)^{n-k}=[\pi+(1-\pi)]^n=1.$

Model Assumption

(1) A fixed number n of trials are conducted.
(2) The trials are independent, and the outcome of each trial can be classified in precisely one of two mutually exclusive ways.
(3) The probability of success in each trial is assumed to be some constant π and the probability of failure is $1-\pi$.

2. Cumulative Probability

In the binomial distribution, we can calculate the probability of a possible value, and also the probability (*cumulative probability*) on an interval. For example, in a sample with n trials, the probability that at most k_0 results of the trials are "successes" is

$$P(X\le k_0)=\sum_{k=0}^{k_0}p_k, \tag{4.9}$$

and the probability that at least k_0 results of the trials are "successes" is

$$P(X\ge k_0)=\sum_{k=k_0}^{n}p_k. \tag{4.10}$$

Example 4.6 Following Example 4.5, for Table 4.4, the probability that at most three out of four mice die $(k_0 = 3)$ is

$$P(X \le 3) = \sum_{k=0}^{3} p_k = 0.0016 + 0.0256 + 0.1536 + 0.4096 = 0.5904$$

The probability of at least two deaths $(k_0 = 2)$ is

$$P(X \ge 2) = \sum_{k=2}^{4} p_k = 0.1536 + 0.4096 + 0.4096 = 0.9728$$

3. Distribution Characteristics

Because the binomial distribution is a family of distributions, each defined by its parameters n and π, we present a group of graphs to illustrate their characteristics.

Figure 4.2 shows the graphical characteristics of the binomial distribution. Figures 4.2(a)–(c) show the distribution characteristics of the graph when π changes while n remains unchanged. When $\pi = 0.5$, the figure is symmetrical, and when $\pi \ne 0.5$, the figure is asymmetrical. When $\pi > 0.5$, the graph is left skewed, and when $\pi < 0.5$, the graph is right skewed. Furthermore, as shown in Figures 4.2, when π is fixed and n increases, all the various distributions tend to be symmetrical. Hence, the shape of the binomial distribution is determined by the parameters n and π. We can prove that when $n\pi(1-\pi) \ge 5$, the binomial distribution is a good approximation to the normal distribution. We introduce the normal distribution in Chapter 5.

4. Numerical Characteristics

Let X denote the number of successes that follows a binomial distribution, that is, $X \sim B(n, \pi)$. Then the numerical characteristics of the distribution of X are:

The expected value is

$$\mu = E(X) = E(X_1 + X_2 + \cdots + X_n) = \sum_{i=1}^{n} E(X_i) = \sum_{i=1}^{n} \pi = n\pi. \tag{4.11}$$

The variance is

$$\sigma^2 = Var(X) = Var(X_1 + X_2 + \cdots + X_n) = \sum_{i=1}^{n} Var(X_i) = \sum_{i=1}^{n} \pi(1-\pi) = n\pi(1-\pi)$$

Note that

$$Var(X_i) = E(X_i^2) - \mu^2 = \left[1^2 \times \pi + 0^2 \times (1-\pi)\right] - \pi^2 = \pi(1-\pi) \tag{4.12}$$

The standard deviation is

$$\sigma = \sqrt{n\pi(1-\pi)}. \tag{4.13}$$

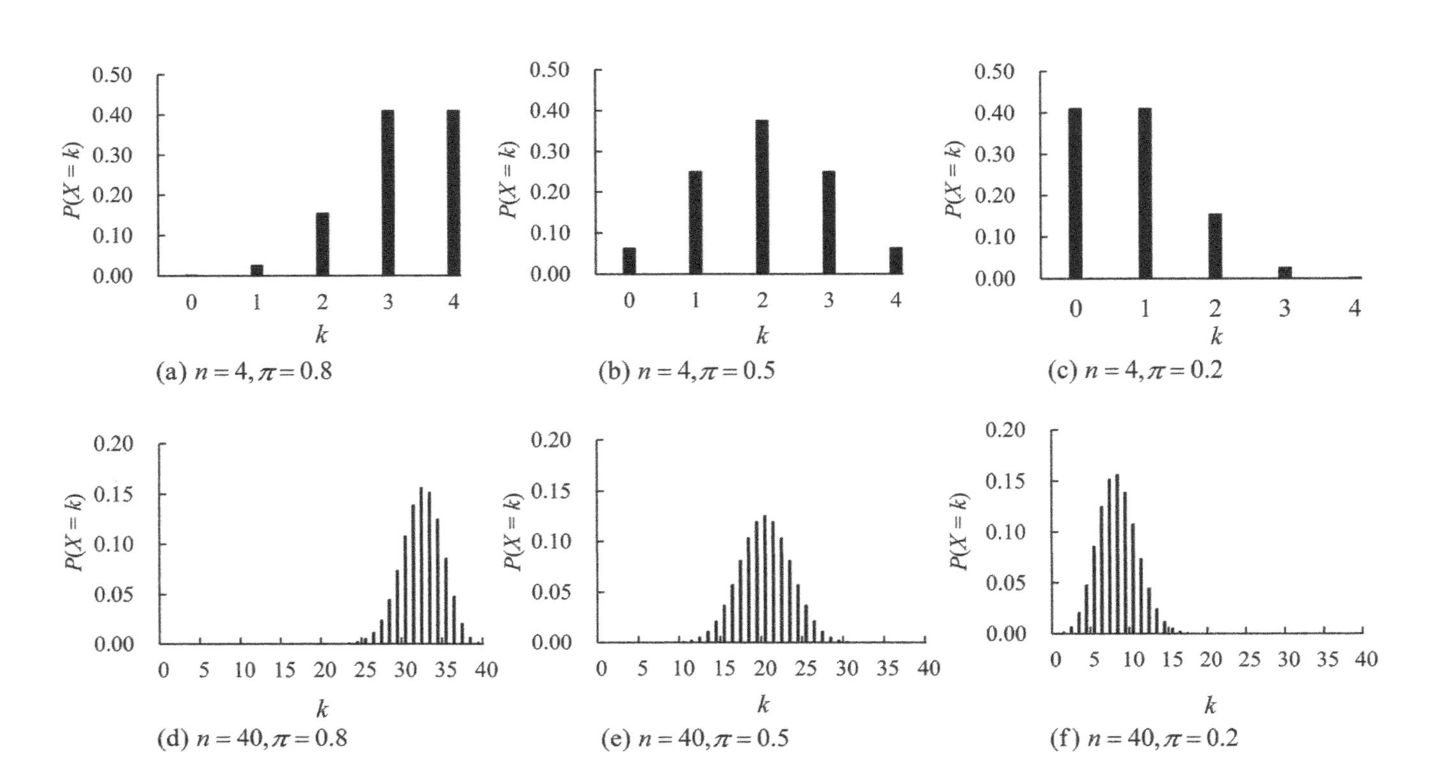

Figure 4.2 Graphical characteristics of the binomial distribution with different n and π.

Example 4.7 Refer to Example 4.5. Given that the number of mice deaths $X \sim B(4, 0.8)$, determine the expected value, variance, and standard deviation of the number of mice deaths.

Solution
We have $n=4,\ \pi=0.8$.
The expected value is $\mu=n\pi=4\times0.8=3.20$.
The variance is $\sigma^2=n\pi(1-\pi)=4\times0.8\times0.2=0.64$.
The standard deviation is $\sigma=\sqrt{\sigma^2}=\sqrt{0.64}=0.80$.

4.4.2 Multinomial Distribution

1. Basic Concept
Many types of trials result in observations on an unordered categorical variable with more than two possible outcomes, for example, the blood types (A, B, AB, O) of a group of patients with hematological diseases; different treatment methods (physical therapy, drug therapy, surgery) used for a certain disease; and surgical operation positions (supine position, lateral position, prone position). Clearly, the levels of these variables are not ordered. Similar to the binomial distribution, we define the *multinomial distribution*.

Definition 4.7 Assume that an experiment consists of n (sample size) independent and identical trials, and each trial has k mutually exclusive results $A_1,\ldots,A_i,\ldots,A_k$, which have corresponding probabilities $\pi_1,\ldots,\pi_i,\ldots,\pi_k$ that remain unchanged in each trial and satisfy $\sum_{i=1}^{k}\pi_i=1$. If the random variable $X=(X_1,\ldots,X_i,\ldots,X_k)$ represents the number of occurrences of $A_1,\ldots,A_i,\ldots,A_k$ in n independent trials, then the probability of the occurrence of various results with $n_1,\ldots,n_i,\ldots,n_k$ is

$$P(X_1=n_1,\ldots,X_i=n_i,\ldots,X_k=n_k)=\frac{n!}{n_1!\ldots n_i!\ldots n_k!}\pi_1^{n_1}\cdots\pi_i^{n_i}\cdots\pi_k^{n_k}, \tag{4.14}$$

where the random variable $X=(X_1,\ldots,X_i,\ldots,X_k)$ follows a multinomial distribution, which is denoted by $X\sim M(n,\ \pi_1,\ \pi_2,\ldots,\ \pi_k)$, and $n=n_1+\cdots+n_i+\cdots+n_k$ is the number of trials. Clearly, this represents an extension of the binomial distribution discussed in Section 4.4.1.

Example 4.8 Based on a large epidemiological survey that enrolled over 10 thousand study subjects (Zhu et al. 2009), the probabilities of adult women suffering from stress urinary incontinence, urge urinary incontinence, mixed urinary incontinence, and no urinary incontinence are $\pi_1=0.174,\ \pi_2=0.025,\ \pi_3=0.083,\ \pi_4=0.718$, respectively. Suppose 50 adult women are randomly selected from this population. Calculate the probability that the numbers of women suffering from stress urinary incontinence, urge urinary incontinence, mixed urinary incontinence, and no urinary incontinence are 8, 1, 4, and 37, respectively.

Analysis

This example is simply an extension of the binomial distribution and involves $k = 4$ possible outcomes – stress, urge, mixed, or none – for each trial. Thus, the properties of the multinomial distribution are satisfied, and we may apply Definition 4.7 to calculate the probability.

Solution

Let X_1 denote the number of women suffering from stress urinary incontinence, X_2 denote the number of women suffering from urge urinary incontinence, X_3 denote the number of women suffering from mixed urinary incontinence, and X_4 denote the number of women with no urinary incontinence. According to Formula 4.14,

$$\begin{aligned} &P(X_1 = 8, X_2 = 1, X_3 = 4, X_4 = 37) \\ &= \frac{50!}{8! \times 1! \times 4! \times 37!} \times 0.174^8 \times 0.025^1 \times 0.083^4 \times 0.718^{37} \\ &= 0.011, \end{aligned}$$

then, of 50 adult women, the probability of 8 women suffering from stress urinary incontinence, 1 woman suffering from urge urinary incontinence, 4 women suffering from mixed urinary incontinence, and 37 women with no urinary incontinence is 0.011.

2. Numerical Characteristics

The method for determining the numerical characteristics of the multinomial probability distribution is similar to that for the binomial distribution. We divide events $A_1, A_2, \ldots, A_k$ into two groups. For simplicity, we assume that the group of interest is called A_i $(i = 1, 2, \ldots, k)$ and has only one simple event, and we combine the remaining events as another group B_i. Thus, the possible results of multiple trials become two opposite results: A_i and B_i. According to the properties of the binomial distribution, the formulas for the expected value, variance, and standard deviation of A_i can be directly derived from those of the binomial distribution:

$$\mu_{A_i} = n\pi_{A_i}, \tag{4.15}$$

$$\sigma^2_{A_i} = n\pi_{A_i}(1 - \pi_{A_i}), \tag{4.16}$$

$$\sigma_{A_i} = \sqrt{n\pi_{A_i}(1 - \pi_{A_i})}, \tag{4.17}$$

where $i = 1, 2, \ldots, k$.

Example 4.9 Refer to Example 4.8. Calculate the expected value, variance, and standard deviation of the number of women suffering from stress urinary incontinence.

Solution

The probability of stress urinary incontinence is known, $\pi_1 = 0.174$, and $n = 50$. The expected value of the number of women suffering from stress urinary incontinence is

$$\mu_1 = n\pi_1 = 50 \times 0.174 = 8.70$$

The variance is

$$\sigma_1^2 = n\pi_1(1-\pi_1) = 50 \times 0.174 \times 0.826 = 7.186$$

The standard deviation is

$$\sigma_1 = \sqrt{\sigma_1^2} = 2.681.$$

The calculation for the numerical characteristics of the number of women suffering from urge incontinence and from mixed urinary incontinence is similar to the above process.

4.4.3 Poisson Distribution

1. Basic Concept

The *Poisson distribution*, proposed by S.D. Poisson (1781–1840), is perhaps the second most frequently used discrete distribution after the binomial distribution. The distribution is typically associated with "rare events" and provides a model for the probability of the number of rare events that occur in, for example, a unit of time, area, or volume. For example, the number of people who develop a certain malignant tumor in a certain time (such as 1 year) in an area, the number of fatal accidents on a highway per month, the number of genetic diseases caused by a genetic mutation, and the number of bacteria in a container.

Definition 4.8 Random variable X is called a Poisson distribution if the probability of the occurrence of k events in a unit of time/space is

$$P(X=k) = p_k = \frac{\lambda^k}{k!}e^{-\lambda} \; (\lambda>0;\; k=0,1,\ldots), \tag{4.18}$$

then, X is a Poisson distribution with parameter λ, denoted by $X \sim P(\lambda)$. The parameter λ denotes the expected value (mean) of rare events occurring in a unit time/space and e is the base of the natural logarithm: $e \approx 2.71828$.

The Poisson distribution also satisfies two basic properties of the probability distribution:

(1) $0 \le p_k \le 1, \; (k=0,1,\ldots)$.

(2) $\sum_{k=0}^{\infty} p_k = 1$.

These two properties are obvious. For all non-negative integers k, the Poisson probability function is $0 < \frac{\lambda^k}{k!}e^{-\lambda} \le 1$; hence, property (1) holds. Because $\sum_{k=0}^{\infty} \frac{\lambda^k}{k!}e^{-\lambda} = e^{-\lambda} \cdot e^{\lambda} = 1$, property (2) also holds.

Model Assumption

(1) The experimental result is the count, that is, the number of times that a particular (rare) event occurs during a given unit of time or in a given time/space.

(2) Stationarity: The probability of one event occurring in a given time/space unit is the same for all units.
(3) Independence: The number of events that occur in a time/space unit is independent of the number of events that occur in other units.

Note that the Poisson distribution is not suitable for communicable disease research because a new morbidity or death often affects the number of morbidities or deaths in the next period; thus, the assumption of the independence of events is violated.

Example 4.10 Given that the daily number of new cases of lung cancer in Beijing in 2007 follows a Poisson distribution with a mean of 11, determine the probability of at least 5 cases of lung cancer and the probability of at most 15 cases of lung cancer on a certain day in that year.

Solution

Suppose X is the daily number of new cases of lung cancer and $X \sim P(\lambda)$, where $\lambda = 11$. According to Definition 4.8, calculate the probability of $X = 0$ first:

$$P(X=0) = p_0 = \frac{11^0}{0!}e^{-11} = 0.00002$$

Similarly, all calculation results are shown in Table 4.5.

Then the probability of at least five cases of lung cancer on a certain day of the year is

$$\begin{aligned} P(X \geq 5) &= \sum_{k=5}^{\infty}\frac{11^k}{k!}e^{-11} = 1 - \sum_{k=0}^{4}\frac{11^k}{k!}e^{-11} \\ &= 1 - (0.00002 + 0.00018 + \cdots + 0.01019) \\ &= 1 - 0.01510 \\ &= 0.9849. \end{aligned}$$

Table 4.5 Probability distribution of daily number of new cases of lung cancer.

k	$P(X=k)$
0	0.00002
1	0.00018
2	0.00101
3	0.00370
4	0.01019
5	0.02242
6	0.04109
⋮	⋮
14	0.07275
15	0.05335
≥16	0.09260

The probability that the number of cases of lung cancer on a certain day of the year is at most 15 is

$$P(X \leq 15) = \sum_{k=0}^{15} \frac{11^k}{k!} e^{-11}$$
$$= 0.00002 + 0.00018 + \cdots + 0.07275 + 0.05335$$
$$= 0.9074.$$

2. Distribution Characteristics

We use Example 4.11 to show the graphic characteristics of the Poisson distribution.

Example 4.11 The average daily number of new cases of 4 malignant tumors in Beijing in 2007 was 2 cases of lymph cancer, 4 cases of gastric cancer, 7 cases of colorectal cancer, and 11 cases of lung cancer. Draw Poisson probability distribution diagrams for the corresponding parameters.

Solution

The daily numbers of the four tumors all follow the Poisson distribution, and the corresponding parameters are $\lambda_1 = 2, \lambda_2 = 4, \lambda_3 = 7$, and $\lambda_4 = 11$, respectively. The corresponding probability distributions are shown in Figure 4.3.

Figure 4.3 shows that the daily number of new cases of tumors, k, fluctuates around the parameter λ. The shape of the graph changes with different λ. The smaller λ, the more skewed the distribution, and the distribution gradually tends to be more symmetric as the value increases. As shown in Figure 4.3, when $\lambda = 11$, the distribution is a good approximation to normality (we introduce this in Chapter 5). Generally, the Poisson distribution can be approximated using the normal distribution when $\lambda \geq 10$.

3. Numerical Characteristics

By Formulas 4.3 to 4.6, for the Poisson distribution:

The expected value is

$$\mu = \sum_{k=0}^{\infty} k p_k = \lambda. \tag{4.19}$$

The variance is

$$\sigma^2 = E(X - \lambda)^2 = \sum_{k=0}^{\infty} k^2 p_k - \lambda^2 = \lambda. \tag{4.20}$$

The standard deviation is

$$\sigma = \sqrt{\sigma^2} = \sqrt{\lambda}. \tag{4.21}$$

Parameter λ in the Poisson distribution is both the mean and variance. This feature is very useful in practice because if the mean and variance of a sample are approximately equal, then we have reason to believe that the sample data may approximately follow a Poisson distribution.

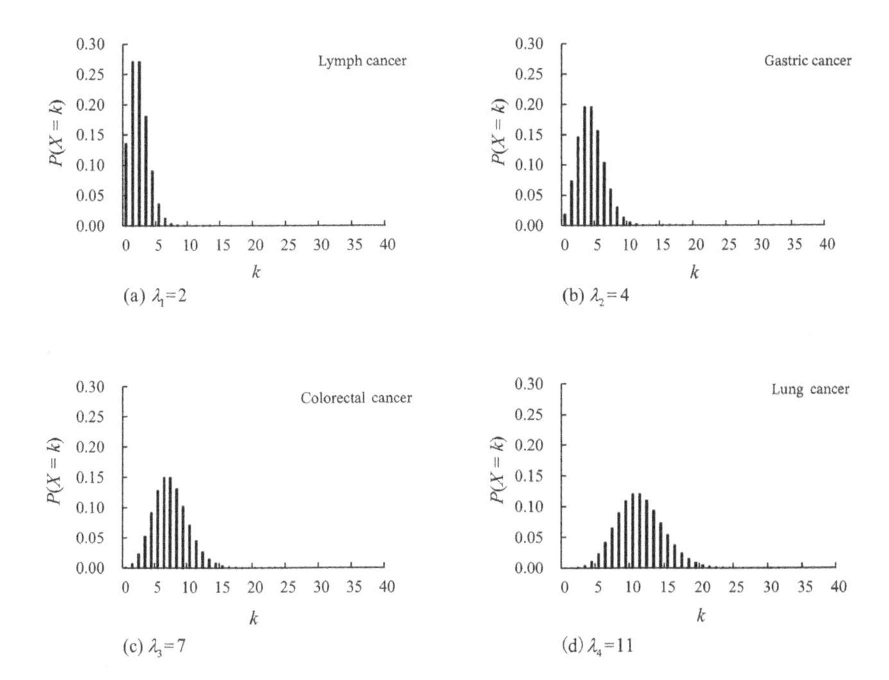

Figure 4.3 Graphical characteristics of the Poisson distribution with different parameters λ.

Example 4.12 Table 4.6 shows the number of new cases of four malignant tumors in a certain week in Beijing in 2007. Evaluate the applicability of the Poisson distribution of this data.

Solution

For lung cancer, the estimated mean of the number of incident cases is $\frac{1}{7}\times(14+9+\cdots+16)=11.29$, and the estimated variance is $\frac{1}{7-1}\times\left[(14-11.29)^2+(9-11.29)^2+\cdots+(16-11.29)^2\right]=11.24$. The calculations for other malignant tumors are the same and the results are shown in the last two columns in Table 4.6. The mean and variance of the daily number of new cases are approximately equal for each type of tumor, which indicates that the Poisson distribution was a good choice for the analysis of this data.

4. Approximation of the Poisson Distribution to the Binomial Distribution

Another important use of the Poisson distribution is as an approximation to the binomial distribution. Consider a binomial distribution with large n and small π. The mean of this distribution is $n\pi$, and the variance is $n\pi(1-\pi)$. When π is very small, $1-\pi\approx 1$, and then, $n\pi(1-\pi)\approx n\pi$. In this case, the mean and variance of the binomial distribution are approximately equal; that is, the binomial distribution at this time can be well approximated by the Poisson distribution with a parameter of $\lambda=n\pi$, and the approximate formula is

$$P(X=k)=C_n^k\pi^k(1-\pi)^{n-k}\approx\frac{\lambda^k}{k!}e^{-\lambda}. \tag{4.22}$$

Table 4.6 Daily number of new cases of four types of malignant tumor in a certain week in Beijing in 2007.

Tumors type	Monday	Tuesday	Wednesday	Thursday	Friday	Saturday	Sunday	Mean	Variance
Lung cancer	14	9	11	10	13	6	16	11.29	11.24
Colorectal cancer	5	6	7	8	12	7	4	7.00	6.67
Gastric cancer	3	4	2	5	7	4	1	3.71	3.90
Lymph cancer	1	4	2	2	0	1	3	1.86	1.81

Thus, we can avoid the trouble of calculating the binomial distribution and use the Poisson distribution to approximate the binomial distribution.

Then, how large should n be and how small should π be to make the above approximation appropriate? A conservative rule is $n \geq 100$ and $\pi \leq 0.01$.

Example 4.13 Referring to Example 4.5, when a mouse receives a certain dose of a certain poison, assume that the survival probability is $\pi = 0.01$. Determine the probability distribution of the number of mice that survive among 100 mice that received this dose of poison.

Solution

(1) Using the binomial distribution (Definition 4.6), for an exact calculation, where $n = 100$, $\pi = 0.01$,

$$P(X=0) = C_{100}^{0}(0.01)^{0}(0.99)^{100} = 0.3660;$$

$$P(X=1) = C_{100}^{1}(0.01)^{1}(0.99)^{99} = 0.3697;$$

......

$$P(X=6) = C_{100}^{6}(0.01)^{6}(0.99)^{94} = 0.0005;$$

$$P(X \geq 7) = 1 - \sum_{k=0}^{6} p_k = 1 - 0.3660 - \cdots - 0.0005 = 0.0001.$$

(2) Using the Poisson distribution (Definition 4.8) for an approximate calculation, where $\lambda = 100 \times 0.01 = 1$,

$$P(X=0) = \frac{1^0}{0!}e^{-1} = 0.3679$$

$$P(X=1) = \frac{1^1}{1!}e^{-1} = 0.3679$$

......

$$P(X=6) = \frac{1^6}{6!}e^{-1} = 0.0005$$

Table 4.7 Probability distribution of the number of mice that survive among 100 mice.

k	Binomial distribution	Poisson distribution	k	Binomial distribution	Poisson distribution
(1)	(2)	(3)	(1)	(2)	(3)
0	0.3660	0.3679	4	0.0149	0.0153
1	0.3697	0.3679	5	0.0029	0.0031
2	0.1849	0.1839	6	0.0005	0.0005
3	0.0610	0.0613	≥ 7	0.0001	0.0001

$$P(X \geq 7) = 1 - \sum_{k=0}^{6} p_k = 1 - 0.3679 - \cdots - 0.0005 = 0.0001$$

All results are listed in Table 4.7.

The results in Table 4.7 show that the values of the two distributions are very close. The calculation using the Poisson distribution is much simpler.

4.5 Summary

Based on an introduction to the definition of random variables, in this chapter, we discussed the probability mass function of discrete random variables and its distribution, expected value, variance, and standard deviation. These concepts are very similar to the corresponding concepts of samples in Chapter 2. In particular, the relative frequency distribution is the realization of the probability distribution in a sample. Additionally, the sample mean $\bar{x}$ and variance s^2 that we introduced in Chapter 2 are actually the sample versions of the population mean and population variance of random variables.

In this chapter, we also introduced several important probability distributions of discrete random variables, particularly the binomial distribution and Poisson distribution, both of which have important roles in biomedical research.

4.6 Exercises

1. To explore the establishment of a centralized appointment system for outpatients based on big data, the status of patients who applied for multiple examinations (number of examination items ≥ 2) in a large hospital outpatient department in one day is investigated. For eight common examinations (e.g., computerized tomography and pathology), the probability distribution of the number of examination items for the patients (pmf) is shown in Table 4.8.

Table 4.8 Distribution of the number of patient examination items for multiple examinations in the outpatient department.

X	2	3	4	5	6	7	8
$P(X = x_k)$	0.582	0.237	0.112	0.043	0.018	0.006	0.002

(a) Find the probability that the number of examination items for multiple examinations of a patient is less than six.

(b) Plot the cdf of the number of patient examination items for multiple examinations and describe its graphical characteristics.

(c) What is the difference between the pmf and cdf?

(d) Find the expected value, variance, and standard deviation of the number of patient examination items for multiple examinations.

(e) Describe the relationship between the probability distribution and relative frequency distribution.

2. Assume that the proportion of general people with blood type A is 30%.

(a) Suppose one person is randomly selected. Determine the probability that the person has blood type A, and calculate the expected value and variance.

(b) Suppose 20 persons are randomly selected. Determine the probability distribution of the number of persons with blood type A, and calculate the expected value and variance.

(c) What is the relationship between the distribution in (a) and the distribution in (b)?

3. For patients who wanted to use cephalosporin drugs in a hospital, the rapid allergy skin test was used for the cephalosporin drug allergy test. The results showed that the positive rate was 8%. Assume that 20 patients had the allergy test.

(a) What is the distribution of the number of positive patients? What are the parameters that determine its distribution?

(b) Determine the expected value and variance of the number of positive patients.

(c) Determine the pmf of the number of positive patients.

(d) What is the probability of two positive patients?

(e) Determine the cdf of the number of positive patients.

(f) What is the probability that at most one patient is positive?

(g) Describe the graphical characteristics of the probability distribution of the number of positive patients. Assume that the number of patients in the drug allergy test is changed to 100. How does the distribution graph change?

(h) Assume that another type of drug allergy test shows that 1% of patients are positive. After 100 patients have the allergy test, which distribution can be used to approximate the probability distribution of the number of positive patients? Explain the relationship between the two distributions.

4. About 85% of lung cancers are of non-small cell type, which includes adenocarcinoma, squamous cell carcinoma, large cell lung cancer, and other types of non-small cell lung cancer. Adenocarcinoma accounts for about 45%, squamous cell carcinoma accounts for about 30%, large cell carcinoma accounts for about 9%, and other types of non-small cell lung cancer account for about 1%.

(a) Given a patient who has non-small cell lung cancer, determine the probability of this patient suffering from adenocarcinoma, the probability of suffering from squamous cell carcinoma, the probability of suffering from large cell carcinoma, and the probability of suffering from other types of non-small cell lung cancer.

(b) Ten patients are randomly selected from the non-small cell lung cancer patients. Determine the probability that six patients have adenocarcinoma, three patients have squamous cell carcinoma, one patient has large cell carcinoma, and zero patients have other types of non-small cell lung cancer.

(c) Ten patients are randomly selected from the non-small cell lung cancer patients. Determine the probability that four patients have adenocarcinoma.

(d) What is the probability distribution of (b) and (c), and what is the relationship between these two distributions?

(e) Ten patients are randomly selected from the non-small cell lung cancer patients. Determine the expected value, variance, and standard deviation of the number of squamous cell carcinomas.

5. The incidence rate of leukemia in a certain place is 10/100,000, and a study randomly investigates 100,000 participants.

(a) What is the distribution of the number of incidence cases of leukemia? What are the parameters that determine this distribution?

(b) Determine the expected value and variance of the number of incidence cases of leukemia, and describe the relationship between the expected value and variance.

(c) Calculate the probability that no leukemia case is found.

(d) Calculate the probability that the number of incidence cases of leukemia is no more than two.

5

Continuous Random Variable

CONTENTS

We now consider another major class of random variables: the continuous variable. Unlike a count that is common in the discrete random variable, the continuous random variable can assume any value over an entire interval. Recall the example of the height of 10-year-old girls in Table 2.1, where the measurement value of height was kept to one decimal place so that the measured values were discrete. Assume that we improve the measurement precision to a theoretical maximum. The value of height can be any real number in a certain value range. Similarly, assume there is no measurement error, the measured values of physiological indices, for example, body weight, vital capacity, and serum test indices can be regarded as the collection of infinite points in a value range. These variables, in contrast to discrete random variables, are called continuous random variables. However, because all possible values of a continuous random variable fill an interval $[a,b]$, it is impossible to assign finite probabilities to uncountable points in the interval in this manner. Therefore, the probability distribution of a continuous random variable can no longer be presented in the form of a probability mass function. Instead, a probability density function should be used. We start to discuss this new concept using the example of girls' height.

Applied Medical Statistics, First Edition. Jingmei Jiang.

Companion website: www.wiley.com\go\jiang\appliedmedicalstatistics

5.1 Concept of Continuous Random Variable

In Example 2.1, the distribution characteristics of the height of 153 10-year-old girls were described by a frequency distribution. We consider the sample mean (142.3) and sample variance (6.82^2) obtained from this dataset as parameters of a normal population (see Section 5.3), from which 5000 height values are drawn and presented in the relative frequency histograms shown in Figure 5.1. The area of each rectangle is the relative frequency of a certain range in variable X, and because n is sufficiently large, the relative frequency can be used to approximate the probability P. Thus, the height of the rectangle = the probability/the width of the rectangle $= P / \Delta x$, which means that the ordinate of the graph is no longer the probability P, but $P / \Delta x$. Assume that we make Δx as small as possible (in Figure 5.1, (a) $\Delta x = 5$, (b) $\Delta x = 0.5$, and (c) $\Delta x \to 0$). The more rectangles that make up the probability histogram, the narrower the width and the smoother the line between the middle points of the top of the rectangles. When $\Delta x \to 0$, the line tends to be a smooth curve. We use $f(x)$ to denote the limiting form of $P / \Delta x$ when $\Delta x \to 0$, and this is called the *probability density function (pdf)* or *density function*; the corresponding curve (Figure 5.1(c)) is called the density curve. A pdf is a theoretical model for this distribution.

We have the following interpretations for the pdf: For any two values (a and b) of continuous random variable X, if $f(a) > f(b)$, there is a greater chance of X taking a value around a than around b; and the area under the pdf curve between the two points a and b is equal to the probability that the random variable X has a value in the range between a and b. Clearly, unlike the discrete random variable, which considers the probability of an event occurring at a certain point, the continuous random variable considers the probability of an event occurring in a value range $(a \le X \le b)$.

Definition 5.1 Assume that X is a random variable. If there is a non-negative integrable function $f(x)$ in the interval $(-\infty, +\infty)$, and for any real number a, $b\,(a<b)$ that satisfies

$$P(a \le X \le b) = \int_a^b f(x)dx, \tag{5.1}$$

then X is called a *continuous random variable*, and $f(x)$ is the pdf of X.

Clearly, in Formula 5.1, the probability of a certain point value in X is zero, and the area under the corresponding curve of the interval $(-\infty, +\infty)$ should be 1.

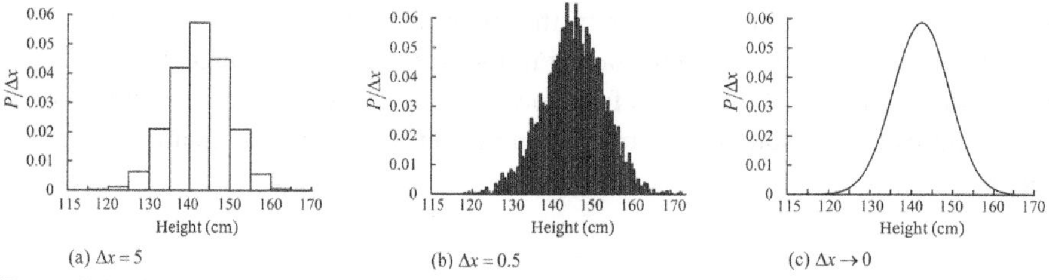

Figure 5.1 Simulated height distribution of 153 10-year-old girls.

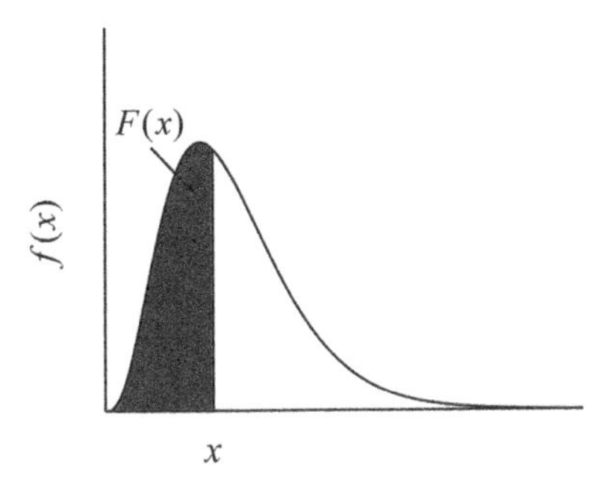

Figure 5.2 Illustration of the cdf for the continuous random variable X.

Definition 5.2 For any real number x, the *cumulative distribution function (cdf)* of the random variable X is defined as

$$F(x) = P(X \leq x) = \int_{-\infty}^{x} f(t)dt. \tag{5.2}$$

It is the probability of the event "$X \leq x$" occurring, that is, $F(x)$ denotes the cumulative area under the curve between $-\infty$ and x. The graph illustrating this is shown in Figure 5.2.

The cdf must satisfy the following three properties:

(1) $F(x)$ is a non-decreasing function. For any real numbers $x_1 < x_2$, $F(x_1) \leq F(x_2)$.

This is because $F(x_2) - F(x_1) = \int_{-\infty}^{x_2} f(t)dt - \int_{-\infty}^{x_1} f(t)dt = \int_{x_1}^{x_2} f(t)dt = P(x_1 \leq X \leq x_2) \geq 0$.

(2) $0 \leq F(x) \leq 1$, $F(-\infty) = \lim_{x \to -\infty} F(x) = 0$, $F(+\infty) = \lim_{x \to +\infty} F(x) = 1$.

(3) Right continuity: $F(x+0) = \lim_{\Delta x \to 0^+} F(x + \Delta x) = F(x)$.

In fact, both discrete and continuous random variables' cdfs have these three properties.

5.2 Numerical Characteristics

The definition and meaning of the numerical characteristics of the continuous random variable are similar to those of the discrete random variable, except that the density function $f(x)$ is used to replace the distribution column $\{p_k\}$ in the definition of the continuous random variable, and $F(x)$ substitutes the integration for the summation.

Suppose the pdf of a continuous random variable X is $f(x)$. Then, the expected value (or population mean) of X, denoted by $E(X)$ or μ, is the average value taken on by the random variable:

$$E(X) \equiv \mu = \int_{-\infty}^{+\infty} xf(x)dx. \tag{5.3}$$

The variance of a continuous random variable X, denoted by $Var(X)$ or σ^2, is the average squared distance of each value of the random variable from its expected value:

$$Var(X) \equiv \sigma^2 = E(X-\mu)^2 = \int_{-\infty}^{+\infty} (x-\mu)^2 f(x)dx. \tag{5.4}$$

To simplify the calculation, the variance is typically calculated as

$$\sigma^2 \equiv E(X^2) - \mu^2 = \int_{-\infty}^{+\infty} x^2 f(x)dx - \left[\int_{-\infty}^{+\infty} xf(x)dx\right]^2. \tag{5.5}$$

The standard deviation σ is the square root of the variance:

$$\sigma = \sqrt{\sigma^2}. \tag{5.6}$$

5.3 Normal Distribution

The normal (or Gaussian) pdf was proposed by C.F. Gauss (1777–1855) as a model for the relative frequency distribution of errors, such as measurement errors. The normal distribution provides an adequate model for the relative frequency distributions of data collected from many different biomedical areas, such as adult height, weight, vital capacity, and red blood cell count. Many other distributions that are not normal themselves can be made approximately normal by transforming the data into a different scale. The normal distribution is also the theoretical basis for learning statistics. Three well-known distributions that are commonly used in statistical inference, the χ^2 distribution, t distribution, and F distribution, are derived from the normal distribution; that is, the basic parts of probability theory and mathematical statistics are established and developed with the normal distribution as the core.

5.3.1 Concept of the Normal Distribution

Definition 5.3 If the pdf of a continuous random variable X satisfies

$$f(x) = \frac{1}{\sqrt{2\pi}\sigma} e^{-\frac{(x-\mu)^2}{2\sigma^2}} \quad (-\infty < x < +\infty), \tag{5.7}$$

then X follows the *normal distribution*, and is denoted by $X \sim N(\mu, \sigma^2)$.

In Formula 5.7, μ and σ^2 are two parameters of the normal distribution: μ is the population mean, also known as the location parameter, which determines the central location or average level of the distribution; and σ^2 is the population variance, also known as the scale parameter, which determines the dispersion of distribution.

The curve $f(x)$ has three characteristics (see Figure 5.3):

(1) The curve is symmetric with respect to $x = \mu$, and reaches the highest point at $x = \mu$, which indicates that the values of the variable concentrate toward μ.
(2) The curve has inflection points at $x = \mu \pm \sigma$. These are the points at which the concavity-convexity of the curve changes.
(3) The x-axis is the asymptote, that is, regardless of how far the curve goes in either the left or right direction, it approaches the x-axis but does not intersect it, and the total area encompassed by the curve and the x-axis is equal to one.

Figure 5.3 shows the rules of curve changes under various parameters μ and σ. In addition to μ as the symmetrical center of the distribution, the normal curve corresponding to a small σ value is "tall and thin" and the normal curve corresponding to a large σ value is "short and wide." However, regardless of the values of μ and σ, the graph of the normal distribution pdf always remains "bell-shaped."

Definition 5.4 The cumulative distribution function of the normal random variable X is

$$F(x) = P(X \le x) = \int_{-\infty}^{x} f(t)dt = \frac{1}{\sqrt{2\pi}\sigma}\int_{-\infty}^{x} e^{-\frac{(t-\mu)^2}{2\sigma^2}} dt \left(-\infty < x < +\infty\right). \quad (5.8)$$

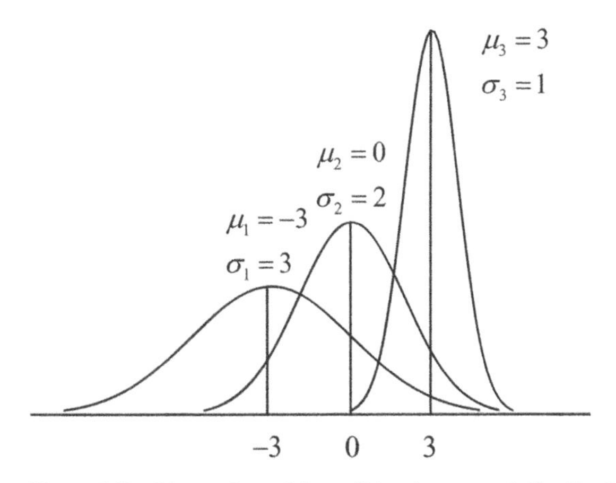

Figure 5.3 Illustration of the pdf for the normal distributions with various values of μ and σ.

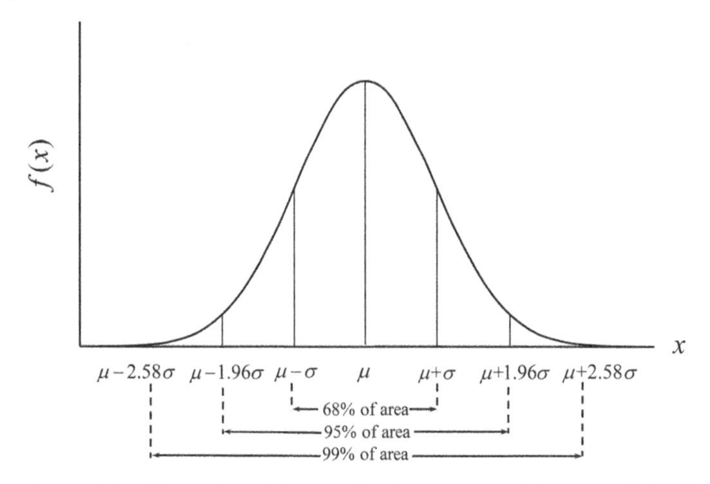

Figure 5.4 Illustration of the empirical properties of the normal distribution.

The probability that the variable X takes in any interval $[x_1, x_2]$ is equal to the corresponding area under the probability density curve. The three most commonly used empirical intervals are shown in Figure 5.4.

Approximately two-thirds (68%) of the area (probability) under the curve lies in $\mu - 1\sigma \leq X \leq \mu + 1\sigma$; approximately 95% of the area under the curve lies in $\mu - 1.96\sigma \leq X \leq \mu + 1.96\sigma$; and approximately 99% of the area under the curve lies in $\mu - 2.58\sigma \leq X \leq \mu + 2.58\sigma$.

In fact, according to different parameters μ and σ, there should be an infinite number of normal distributions, theoretically. However, how do we determine the area under the curve in any interval $[a, b]$? Fortunately, this family of curves can be converted into one curve called the standard normal curve whose mean is zero and variance is 1.

5.3.2 Standard Normal Distribution

Any normal random variable $X \sim N\left(\mu, \sigma^2\right)$ can be expressed as follows using a linear transformation (also called the standardization of X):

$$Z = \frac{X - \mu}{\sigma}. \tag{5.9}$$

We call Z the *standard normal random variable*, which follows a *standard normal distribution* with the mean of zero and variance of one, denoted by $Z \sim N(0, 1)$.

Correspondingly, the pdf of Z is

$$\varphi(z) = \frac{1}{\sqrt{2\pi}} e^{-\frac{z^2}{2}} \left(-\infty < z < +\infty\right). \tag{5.10}$$

Similarly to $f(x)$, $\varphi(z)$ also has three characteristics:

(1) The curve is symmetric about $z=0$, that is, $\varphi(z)=\varphi(-z)$, and at $z=0$, $\varphi(z)$ reaches its maximum value.
(2) The curve has inflection points at $z=\pm 1$.
(3) The total area between the curve and x-axis is equal to 1.

The cdf for a standard normal distribution is

$$\Phi(z)=P(Z\le z)=\int_{-\infty}^{z}\varphi(v)dv=\frac{1}{\sqrt{2\pi}}\int_{-\infty}^{z}e^{-\frac{v^2}{2}}dv\left(-\infty<z<+\infty\right). \tag{5.11}$$

$\Phi(z)$ is the basis for calculating the probability of a normal distribution. From the relationship between X and Z, for any normal random variable X, we could obtain $Z=(X-\mu)/\sigma$ after the standardized transformation, and Z follows the standard normal distribution. Thus, any information concerning the $N(\mu, \sigma^2)$ distribution can be obtained from appropriate manipulations of the $N(0,1)$ distribution. For example, in Figure 5.5, X_1 and X_2 are any random variables that follow normal distributions. After standardization, both $Z_1=(X_1-(-1))/2$ and $Z_2=(X_2-1)/0.5$ are transformed into random variables that follow the standard normal distribution $N(0,1)$.

Thus, the probability that the random variable X that follows the normal distribution falls into an arbitrary interval $[a, b]$ can be obtained by transforming the probability $P(a\le X\le b)$ into the probability $P(z_a\le Z\le z_b)$:

$$\begin{aligned}
&P(a\le X\le b)=P(z_a\le Z\le z_b)\\
&=P\left(\frac{a-\mu}{\sigma}\le Z\le\frac{b-\mu}{\sigma}\right)=\Phi\left(\frac{b-\mu}{\sigma}\right)-\Phi\left(\frac{a-\mu}{\sigma}\right)\\
&=\Phi(z_b)-\Phi(z_a).
\end{aligned} \tag{5.12}$$

As is shown in Figure 5.5,

$$P(-3\le X_1\le 3)=P\left(\frac{-3-(-1)}{2}\le Z\le\frac{3-(-1)}{2}\right)=\Phi(2)-\Phi(-1)$$

As we described previously, there is no closed-form algebraic expression for areas under the normal distribution. Hence, numerical methods must be used to calculate these areas, which are generally displayed in "normal tables." A distribution table was

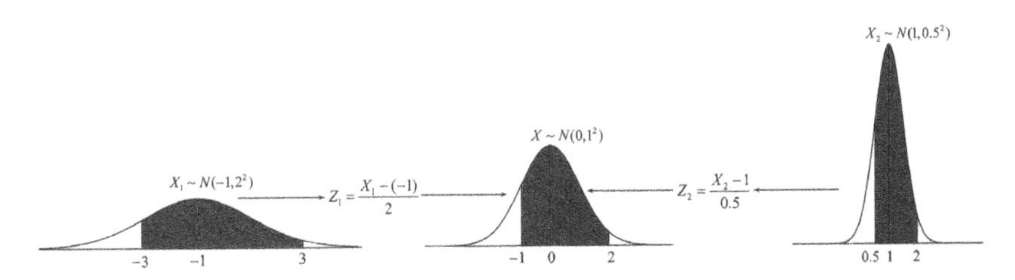

Figure 5.5 Illustration of the standardization of normal random variables.

prepared for $\Phi(z)$, and values for $z<0$ can be found in Appendix Table 3. The value of $z>0$ can be calculated as

$$\Phi(z)=1-\Phi(-z). \tag{5.13}$$

Example 5.1 Assume that the systolic blood pressure (SBP) X (mmHg) of Xinjiang adult Kazakh men (≥ 30 years old) follows the normal distribution $N(135.2, 19.2^2)$. Assume we only consider the SBP. Calculate the proportion of grade 1 $(140 \leq X < 160)$, grade 2 $(160 \leq X < 180)$, and grade 3 $(X \geq 180)$ hypertension in this population.

Solution

Given that $X \sim N(135.2, 19.2^2)$, the proportion of people who have grade 1 hypertension is the probability of the SBP X falling in the interval $[140, 160)$. According to Formula 5.12,

$$\begin{aligned}P(140 \leq X < 160) &= \Phi\left(\frac{160-135.2}{19.2}\right)-\Phi\left(\frac{140-135.2}{19.2}\right)\\ &= \Phi(1.29)-\Phi(0.25)\\ &= 1-\Phi(-1.29)-[1-\Phi(-0.25)]\\ &= (1-0.0985)-(1-0.4013)=0.3028,\end{aligned}$$

that is, the proportion of grade 1 hypertension among adult males in this population is 30.28%.

Similarly, the probability that the SBP X is in the interval $[160, 180)$ is equal to

$$\begin{aligned}P(160 \leq X < 180) &= \Phi\left(\frac{180-135.2}{19.2}\right)-\Phi\left(\frac{160-135.2}{19.2}\right)\\ &= \Phi(2.33)-\Phi(1.29)\\ &= 1-\Phi(-2.33)-[1-\Phi(-1.29)]\\ &= (1-0.0099)-(1-0.0985)=0.0886,\end{aligned}$$

that is, the proportion of grade 2 hypertension is 8.86%.

The probability of the SBP $X \geq 180$ is

$$\begin{aligned}P(X \geq 180) &= 1-P(X<180)=1-\Phi\left(\frac{180-135.2}{19.2}\right)\\ &= 1-\Phi(2.33)=\Phi(-2.33)=0.0099,\end{aligned}$$

that is, the proportion of grade 3 hypertension in this population is 0.99%.

Therefore, the probability distribution of Z in the three most commonly used intervals still applies, which are

$$P(-1 \leq Z \leq 1)=0.68$$

$$P(-1.96 \le Z \le 1.96) = 0.95$$

$$P(-2.58 \le Z \le 2.58) = 0.99$$

5.3.3 Descriptive Methods for Assessing Normality

In the following sections, we introduce methods to infer population characteristics based on sample information. Many of these methods are based on the assumption that the population is fully or approximately normally distributed. Therefore, before we discuss the methods, it is important to assess whether the distribution of a set of empirical data approximates the normal distribution. There are three simple and practical methods:

(1) **Histogram or Stem-and-Leaf Plot**
If the data are approximately normally distributed, the shapes of the histogram and stem-and-leaf plot are similar to the normal distribution curve.

(2) **Normal Probability Plot**
If the data are approximately normal, the scatter in the $P-P$ plot or $Q-Q$ plot approximately falls on a straight line. The $P-P$ plot is a scatterplot drawn with the cumulative relative frequency of actual observations on the x-axis and the cumulative probability of the theoretical distribution on the y-axis. The $Q-Q$ plot is a scatterplot drawn with the observed quantiles on the x-axis and the theoretical quantiles on the y-axis.

(3) **Moment Method**
According to the principle of moments, the skewness coefficient (denoted by g_1) and kurtosis coefficient (denoted by g_2) are derived, which are two special statistical indices for assessing the normal distribution.

The *skewness coefficient* g_1 is a statistic used to describe the distributional pattern of the variable. It reflects the direction and degree of distribution asymmetry. For n observations $x_1, x_2, \ldots, x_n$, $\bar{x}$ is the mean. The calculation formula for g_1 is

$$g_1 = \frac{\dfrac{n^2 m_3}{(n-1)(n-2)}}{\left(\dfrac{n}{n-1} m_2\right)^{3/2}} = \frac{n}{(n-1)(n-2)} \sum_{i=1}^{n} \left[\frac{(x_i - \bar{x})}{s}\right]^3, \tag{5.14}$$

where $m_3 = \sum_{i=1}^{n} (x_i - \bar{x})^3 / n$ is the third-order central moment; $m_2 = \sum_{i=1}^{n} (x_i - \bar{x})^2 / n$ is the second-order central moment (i.e., variance), and $s = \sqrt{\sum_{i=1}^{n} (x_i - \bar{x})^2 / (n-1)}$ is the sample standard deviation.

When $g_1 > 0$, the distribution is positive or right skewed; when $g_1 < 0$, the distribution is negative or left skewed; and when $g_1 = 0$, the distribution is symmetric.

The *kurtosis coefficient* g_2 is a statistic used to describe the steepness of the variable distribution. It reflects the sharpness or convexity of the distribution graph. The calculation formula for g_2 is

$$g_2 = \frac{\dfrac{n^2(n+1)m_4}{(n-1)(n-2)(n-3)}}{\left(\dfrac{n}{n-1}m_2\right)^2} - \frac{3(n-1)^2}{(n-2)(n-3)} \tag{5.15}$$
$$= \frac{n(n+1)}{(n-1)(n-2)(n-3)} \sum_{i=1}^{n} \left[\frac{(x_i - \bar{x})}{s}\right]^4 - \frac{3(n-1)^2}{(n-2)(n-3)},$$

where $m_4 = \sum_{i=1}^{n}(x_i - \bar{x})^4 / n$ is the fourth-order central moment.

When $g_2 > 0$, the distribution has a sharp peak that is steeper than the peak of the normal distribution; when $g_2 < 0$, the distribution is flatter than that of the normal distribution; and when $g_2 = 0$, the distribution has a normal peak.

Because both g_1 and g_2 are sample statistics, there are sampling errors. The calculation formulas for the standard errors are

$$\sigma_{g_1} = \sqrt{\frac{6n(n-1)}{(n-2)(n+1)(n+3)}}, \tag{5.16}$$

$$\sigma_{g_2} = \sqrt{\frac{24n(n-1)^2}{(n-3)(n-2)(n+3)(n+5)}}. \tag{5.17}$$

Standard errors can be used for statistical inference. It should be noted that data are considered approximately normally distributed only if both g_1 and g_2 do not significantly deviate from zero. We describe statistical inference methods in Chapter 7.

Estimates of the skewness coefficient and kurtosis coefficient, in addition to their results in a test for normality, can be obtained using statistical software.

Example 5.2 Determine the normality of the height data for the 153 10-year-old girls in Example 2.1.

Solution

For the first method, we can look at the histogram of the data (Figure 2.1). Clearly, the distribution of the height data is approximately bell-shaped, with a symmetric distribution centered on the mean of 142.3 cm.

For the second method, Figures 5.6(a) and (b) show the normal probability plots. The $P-P$ plot and $Q-Q$ plot have a linear trend, which indicates that the height data of 153 10-year-old girls are approximately normally distributed.

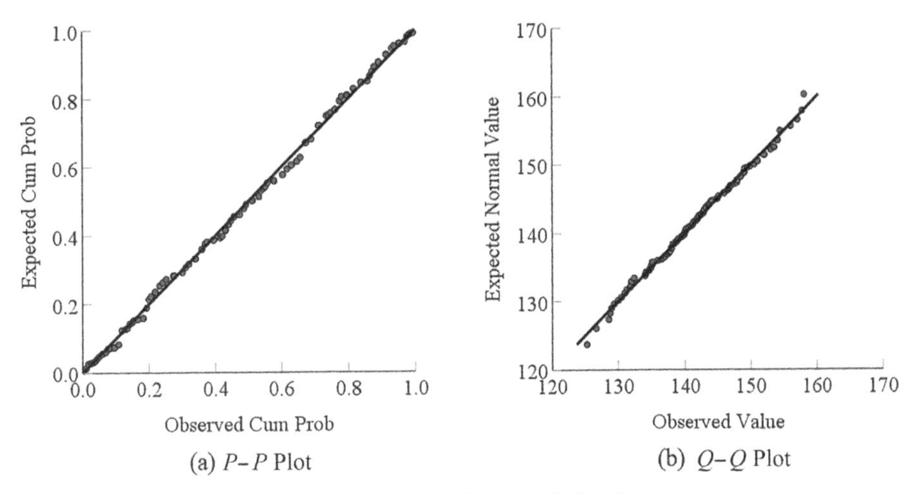

Figure 5.6 Normal probability plot of the height (cm) of 153 10-year-old girls.

For the third method for testing normality:
The skewness coefficient is

$$g_1 = \frac{n}{(n-1)(n-2)}\sum_{i=1}^{n}\left[\frac{(x_i - \bar{x})}{s}\right]^3 = \frac{153}{(153-1)(153-2)} \times 6.947 = 0.046,$$

and its standard error is

$$\sigma_{g_1} = \sqrt{\frac{6n(n-1)}{(n-2)(n+1)(n+3)}} = \sqrt{\frac{6 \times 153 \times (153-1)}{(153-2)(153+1)(153+3)}} = 0.196$$

The kurtosis coefficient is

$$\begin{aligned} g_2 &= \frac{n(n+1)}{(n-1)(n-2)(n-3)}\sum_{i=1}^{n}\left[\frac{(x_i - \bar{x})}{s}\right]^4 - \frac{3(n-1)^2}{(n-2)(n-3)} \\ &= \frac{153(153+1)}{(153-1)(153-2)(153-3)} \times 393.996 - \frac{3(153-1)^2}{(153-2)(153-3)} \\ &= -0.364, \end{aligned}$$

and its standard error is

$$\begin{aligned} \sigma_{g_2} &= \sqrt{\frac{24n(n-1)^2}{(n-3)(n-2)(n+3)(n+5)}} \\ &= \sqrt{\frac{24 \times 153 \times (153-1)^2}{(153-3)(153-2)(153+3)(153+5)}} = 0.390 \end{aligned}$$

The values of skewness g_1 and kurtosis g_2 are not far from zero, and the corresponding standard errors are small. Therefore, we could consider that the data approximately follow the normal distribution (see Section 9.4.1).

The conclusions using the three methods above are consistent in that the data are approximately normally distributed.

Even though, in practice, the methods are simple and effective, they are essentially descriptive. Hence, we must be careful in the interpretation of the results. Rather than overstating that the data essentially follow the normal distribution, it is better to say that there is no evidence to reject the claim that the data come from a normally distributed population.

5.4 Application of the Normal Distribution

Many statistical methods have been established on the basis of the normal distribution. Under the condition of a large sample, many distributions can be approximated by a normal distribution, and the normal approximation method can be used to solve a problem under this condition. Additionally, a wide range of applications of the normal distribution exist in methods for solving practical problems. We introduce some of the applications that are specific to the biomedical field.

5.4.1 Normal Approximation to the Binomial Distribution

Recall the binomial distribution introduced in Chapter 4. We are interested in the probability distribution of k successes in n independent trials, for which the parameters are n and π. We also know that when $n\pi(1-\pi)\geq 5$, the binomial distribution is approximately normal. As n increases, the calculation of probability p_k in the binomial distribution becomes very cumbersome, whereas the processing method for the normal distribution is relatively simple. Therefore, in practice, the approximate calculation of the normal distribution is often used instead of the calculation of the exact probability of the binomial distribution.

Example 5.3 Suppose there are 30 puerperae in a maternity ward, and the probability of delivering a female infant is 0.5. Let X be the number of female infants in the ward, which follows the binomial distribution, with parameters $n=30$ and $\pi=0.5$.

(1) Draw the probability p_k distribution graph and add the normal distribution curve.
(2) Use the binomial distribution to calculate $P(X\leq 10)$.
(3) Calculate the approximate value of $P(X\leq 10)$ using the normal approximation method.

Solution

According to the background of the problem, $X \sim B(30,\ 0.5)$. Because $n\pi(1-\pi)=30\times 0.5\times 0.5=7.5$ is greater than 5, the binomial distribution can be approximated by a normal distribution.

The mean and standard deviation of the binomial distribution are

$$\mu=n\pi=30\times 0.5=15,\ \sigma^2=n\pi(1-\pi)=30\times 0.5\times 0.5=7.5$$

Therefore, the binomial distribution can be approximated by the normal distribution $N(15, 7.5)$.

The specific solution process is as follows:

(1) Draw the graph
The binomial distribution is a discrete distribution, and the variable value can only be a positive integer. To approximate the probability using the normal distribution function, the binomial distribution needs to be continuous; hence, in Figure 5.7, the bar chart is replaced by a histogram, and the normal distribution curve is drawn with parameters $\mu = 15$ and $\sigma^2 = 7.5$.

(2) Calculate the exact $P(X \le 10)$ using the binomial distribution

$$\begin{aligned} P(X \le 10) &= \sum_{k=0}^{10} P(X = k) \\ &= C_{30}^{0} 0.5^{0} 0.5^{30} + C_{30}^{1} 0.5^{1} 0.5^{29} + \cdots + C_{30}^{10} 0.5^{10} 0.5^{20} \\ &= p_0 + p_1 + \cdots + p_{10} \\ &= 0.0000 + 0.0000 + \cdots + 0.0280 \\ &= 0.0494. \end{aligned}$$

(3) Calculate $P(X \le 10)$ using the normal approximation
Figure 5.7 shows that the probability $P(X \le 10)$ in the binomial distribution can be approximated by the probability $P(X \le 10.5)$ in a normal distribution. The value 0.5 is called the continuity correction factor of the normal approximation to the binomial distribution. Hence, the corresponding z value is

$$z = \frac{x - \mu}{\sigma} = \frac{10.5 - 15}{\sqrt{7.5}} = -1.64$$

From Appendix Table 3, $\Phi(-1.64) = 0.0505$. The result is very close to the result using the binomial distribution.

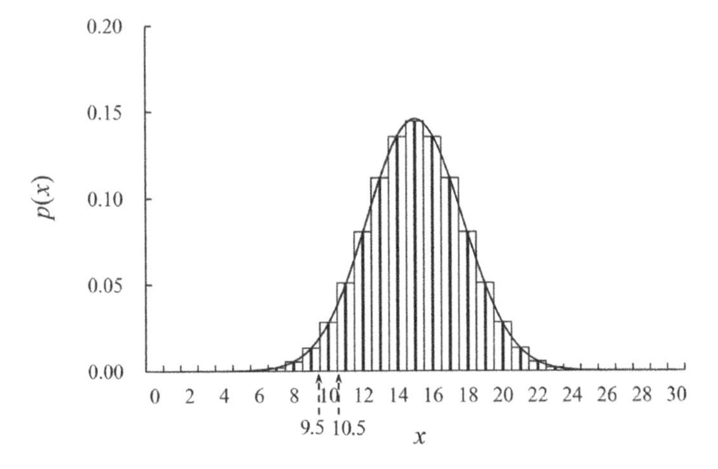

Figure 5.7 Diagram of the normal approximation $N(15, 7.5)$ to the binomial distribution $B(30, 0.5)$.

The general form of *continuity correction* is given as follows:

If $X \sim B(n,\pi)$ and $n\pi(1-\pi) \geq 5$, then the probability $P(a \leq X \leq b)$ can be approximated by the area from $a-0.5$ to $b+0.5$ under the normal distribution $N(n\pi,\ n\pi(1-\pi))$ curve. Suppose that Z is a random variable that follows a standard normal distribution. Then

$$P(X \leq b) \approx P\left(Z \leq \frac{(b+0.5)-n\pi}{\sqrt{n\pi(1-\pi)}}\right), \tag{5.18}$$

$$P(X \geq a) \approx P\left(Z \geq \frac{(a-0.5)-n\pi}{\sqrt{n\pi(1-\pi)}}\right), \tag{5.19}$$

$$P(a \leq X \leq b) \approx \Phi\left(\frac{(b+0.5)-n\pi}{\sqrt{n\pi(1-\pi)}}\right) - \Phi\left(\frac{(a-0.5)-n\pi}{\sqrt{n\pi(1-\pi)}}\right) \tag{5.20}$$

Furthermore, to understand the principle of approximation more visually, we give the following example.

Example 5.4 Refer to Example 5.3, compare the probabilities between the binomial distribution $B(30, 0.5)$ and normal approximation $N(15, 7.5)$.

Solution

Table 5.1 shows the probability calculated by the binomial distribution $B(30, 0.5)$ and the corresponding normal distribution $N(15, 7.5)$.

The scatterplot of the corresponding results in Table 5.1 is shown in Figure 5.8.

The results in Table 5.1 and Figure 5.8 show that, in this case where $\pi = 0.5$ and $n = 30$, the normality approximation can be used to estimate the number of female infants, which follows the binomial distribution.

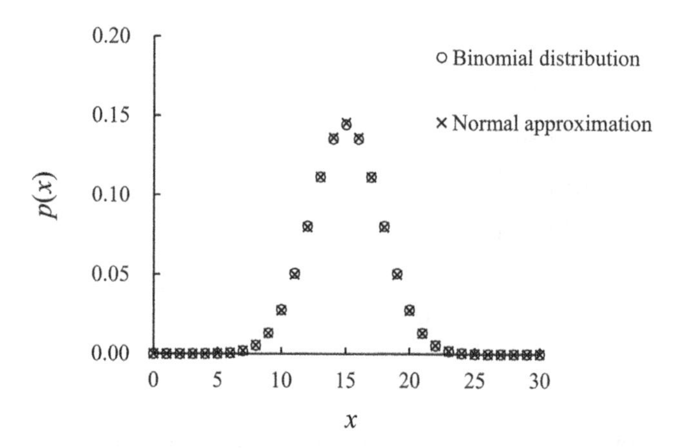

Figure 5.8 Normal approximation $N(15,\ 7.5)$ to the binomial distribution $B(30, 0.5)$.

Table 5.1 Probability calculation results of the binomial distribution $B(30, 0.5)$ and normal approximation $N(15, 7.5)$.

$X = k$	Binomial distribution p_k	Normal approximation $f(k)$	$X = k$	Binomial distribution p_k	Normal approximation $f(k)$
(1)	(2)	(3)	(1)	(2)	(3)
0	0.0000	0.0000	16	0.1354	0.1363
1	0.0000	0.0000	17	0.1115	0.1116
2	0.0000	0.0000	18	0.0806	0.0799
3	0.0000	0.0000	19	0.0509	0.0501
4	0.0000	0.0000	20	0.0280	0.0275
5	0.0001	0.0002	21	0.0133	0.0132
6	0.0006	0.0007	22	0.0055	0.0056
7	0.0019	0.0020	23	0.0019	0.0020
8	0.0055	0.0056	24	0.0006	0.0007
9	0.0133	0.0132	25	0.0001	0.0002
10	0.0280	0.0275	26	0.0000	0.0000
11	0.0509	0.0501	27	0.0000	0.0000
12	0.0806	0.0799	28	0.0000	0.0000
13	0.1115	0.1116	29	0.0000	0.0000
14	0.1354	0.1363	30	0.0000	0.0000
15	0.1445	0.1457			

5.4.2 Normal Approximation to the Poisson Distribution

When $\lambda \geq 10$, the normal distribution can approximate the Poisson distribution very well, and this characteristic can be used to simplify the calculation. In this case, the mean and variance of the Poisson distribution can be used as the mean and variance of the approximate normal distribution.

Example 5.5 The annual incidence rate of thyroid cancer in a city is 10/100,000. If 100,000 people in the city are followed up for 1 year, determine the probability that the number of new thyroid cancer cases is $0, 1, \ldots, 20$.

Solution

Let X be the annual number of new cases in the 100,000 people. X follows the Poisson distribution with parameter $\lambda = 10$.

(1) The Poisson distribution (Definition 4.8) is used for the exact calculation. Given that $\lambda = 10$,

$$P(X = 0) = \frac{10^0}{0!} e^{-10} = 0.0000$$

$$P(X=1)=\frac{10^1}{1!}e^{-10}=0.0005$$

……

$$P(X=20)=\frac{10^{20}}{20!}e^{-10}=0.0019.$$

(2) Approximate the calculation using the normal distribution (Definition 5.3). Given that $\mu=10$, $\sigma^2=10$,

$$f(0)=\frac{1}{\sqrt{10}\times\sqrt{2\pi}}e^{\frac{-(0-10)^2}{2\times10}}=0.0009$$

$$f(1)=\frac{1}{\sqrt{10}\times\sqrt{2\pi}}e^{\frac{-(1-10)^2}{2\times10}}=0.0022$$

……

$$f(20)=\frac{1}{\sqrt{10}\times\sqrt{2\pi}}e^{\frac{-(20-10)^2}{2\times10}}=0.0009$$

All the results are listed in Table 5.2 and shown in Figure 5.9.

The results show that the normal approximation to Poisson distribution can be used to estimate the probability of thyroid cancer in this city.

In the previous two sections, we showed that the normal approximations to both the binomial distribution and the Poisson distribution are applications of the central limit theorem under certain conditions. We will discuss the central limit theorem in Chapter 6. Understanding this will be very helpful for learning the subsequent statistical inference.

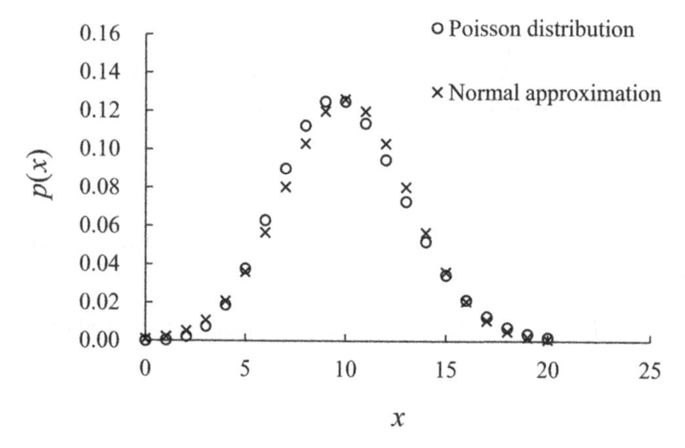

Figure 5.9 Normal approximation $N(10,10)$ to the Poisson distribution $P(10)$.

Table 5.2 Probability calculation results of the Poisson distribution $P(10)$ and normal approximation $N(10, 10)$.

$X = k$	Poisson distribution p_k	Normal approximation $f(k)$	$X = k$	Poisson distribution p_k	Normal approximation $f(k)$	$X = k$	Poisson distribution p_k	Normal approximation $f(k)$
(1)	(2)	(3)	(1)	(2)	(3)	(1)	(2)	(3)
0	0.0000	0.0009	7	0.0901	0.0804	14	0.0521	0.0567
1	0.0005	0.0022	8	0.1126	0.1033	15	0.0347	0.0361
2	0.0023	0.0051	9	0.1251	0.1200	16	0.0217	0.0209
3	0.0076	0.0109	10	0.1251	0.1262	17	0.0128	0.0109
4	0.0189	0.0209	11	0.1137	0.1200	18	0.0071	0.0051
5	0.0378	0.0361	12	0.0948	0.1033	19	0.0037	0.0022
6	0.0631	0.0567	13	0.0729	0.0804	20	0.0019	0.0009

5.4.3 Determining the Medical Reference Interval

An important application of the normal distribution in medical practice is to develop a medical reference interval.

1. Basic Concept

In medical practice, it is often necessary to know a range of values of anatomical, physiological, and biochemical indicators that is most likely for the majority of healthy individuals. This is called the *medical reference interval*, and also called (although incorrectly) the normal interval because it is based on a defined state of health rather than apparent health. A reference interval is very useful in medical practice because results of medical measurement indicators vary between individuals, and even for the same individual, the measurement indicators fluctuate because of changes in the internal and external environment. In practice, a 95% reference interval is frequently used.

2. Method

Once observation data for a sufficient number of subjects are obtained, one of the following two approaches can be selected according to the distribution type of the data.

(1) Normal distribution method

This method is applicable to normal or approximately normal distribution data.

The two-sided bound of $(1-\alpha)\times 100\%$ is

$$\bar{X} \pm z_{1-\alpha/2}S. \tag{5.21}$$

The one-sided bound of $(1-\alpha)\times 100\%$ is

$$\bar{X} - z_{1-\alpha}S \text{ or } \bar{X} + z_{1-\alpha}S, \tag{5.22}$$

where $\bar{X}$ and S are the mean and standard deviation of the observed data, respectively, and $z_{1-\alpha/2}$ and $z_{1-\alpha}$ are the two-sided and one-sided percentiles of the standard normal distribution, respectively (Appendix Table 3). In practice, α is typically set to 0.05; thus, the interval $(1-\alpha)\times 100\%$ becomes a 95% interval, which means that approximately 95% of the observed values lie within 1.96 $(z_{1-0.05/2} = 1.96)$ standard deviations of the mean.

Example 5.6 Refer to Example 2.1. Estimate the 95% reference interval of the height of 10-year-old girls in the region based on the mean 142.3 cm and standard deviation 6.82 cm.

Solution

According to medical knowledge, the height of 10-year-old girls follows a normal distribution, and if the height is too low or too high, it is regarded as abnormal. Therefore, the bound of the two-sided 95% medical reference interval of 10-year-old girls in the region is estimated according to the normal distribution method. Given that the mean $\bar{x} = 142.3$ and $s = 6.82$, from Appendix Table 3, $z_{1-0.05/2} = 1.96$; hence, the two-sided 95% reference interval is

lower bound: $\bar{x} - z_{1-0.05/2}s = 142.3 - 1.96 \times 6.82 = 128.9$

upper bound: $\bar{x} + z_{1-0.05/2}s = 142.3 + 1.96 \times 6.82 = 155.7$

that is, the two-sided 95% medical reference interval for the height of 10-year-old girls in the region is about [129, 156] cm.

(2) Percentile method
This approach does not make any assumptions about the distribution of the measurement; instead, it uses a central range that encompasses 95% of the data values. We sort our values in order of magnitude and use the 2.5th and 97.5th percentiles as our bounds (see Chapter 2):

The lower bound $X_{2.5\%}$ represents the value of X that has 2.5% of the observations in the ordered set lying below it and 97.5% of the observations lying above it.

Upper bound $X_{97.5\%}$ represents the value of X that has 97.5% of the observations in the ordered set lying below it and 2.5% of the observations lying above it.

Thus, this constitutes a two-sided 95% medical reference interval $\left[X_{2.5\%}, X_{97.5\%}\right]$.

Example 5.7 Following Example 2.2, estimate the 95% reference interval of triglycerides (mmol/L) based on the data of 153 10-year-old girls in the region (see Table 2.3).

Solution
Because the distribution of triglyceride in 153 10-year-old girls is right-skewed, according to Formula 2.10, the percentile method is used to calculate the bound of the two-sided 95% reference interval of triglyceride in the 10-year-old girls:

lower bound:

$$X_{2.5\%} = L + \frac{i}{f_{2.5\%}}\left(n \times 2.5\% - \sum f_L\right) = 0.3 + \frac{0.3}{22}\left(153 \times 2.5\% - 0\right) = 0.35$$

upper bound:

$$X_{97.5\%} = L + \frac{i}{f_{97.5\%}}\left(n \times 97.5\% - \sum f_L\right) = 1.8 + \frac{0.3}{4}\left(153 \times 97.5\% - 146\right) = 2.04$$

that is, the 95% reference interval of triglyceride in 10-year-old girls is [0.35, 2.04] mmol/L.

Note that the medical reference interval involves the use of one-sided or two-sided bounds, which are determined based on background medical knowledge. For example, as it is abnormal that the serum total cholesterol is either too low or too high, the upper and lower bound should be calculated using a two-sided reference interval. However, because only high serum lead is abnormal, the reference interval should be calculated using a single upper bound; and because only low vital capacity is abnormal, the reference interval should be calculated using a single lower bound. More attention should be paid to this in the specific application.

5.5 Summary

In this chapter, we mainly discussed the continuous random variable and introduced the concept of the probability density function, which corresponds to the probability mass function of discrete random variables. For the probability distribution of the continuous random variable, the central tendency can also be described by expected value, and the dispersion degree can be described by variance and standard deviation.

The normal distribution is the most important and commonly used distribution among continuous random variables because most phenomena in the biomedical field follow this distribution. In particular, the superposition of many independent random variables always approximates the normal distribution. The normal distribution is determined by the parameters μ and σ^2. Any probabilistic calculation problem for the normal distribution can be equivalently converted to the standard normal distribution, and then completed using the standard normal distribution table.

It is very important to assess whether the sample data approximately follow the normal distribution. There are three commonly used methods: histogram or stem-and-leaf plot; normal probability $P-P$ plot or $Q-Q$ plot; and moment method to calculate the skewness coefficient g_1 and kurtosis coefficient g_2, followed by hypothesis testing.

Because the normal distribution is easy to use, other distributions are typically calculated after approximating the normal distribution. In this chapter, we introduced the normal approximate calculation method of the binomial distribution and Poisson distribution. Under certain conditions (i.e., the binomial distribution when $n\pi(1-\pi)\geq 5$, and the Poisson distribution when $\lambda \geq 10$), both distributions can be considered approximately as the normal distribution. This is a special application of the central limit theorem (see Chapter 6).

Additionally, we discussed the important application of the normal distribution in medical practice to develop the medical reference interval, and as we discuss in subsequent chapters, the normal distribution is an important basis for statistical inference.

5.6 Exercises

1. Assume that the erythrocyte count of the normal male adult in a certain area is normally distributed, with a mean of 5.4×10^{12} / L and standard deviation of 0.43×10^{12} / L. Answer the following questions:
   (a) What is the probability of erythrocyte counts of less than 4.1×10^{12} / L?
   (b) What is the probability of erythrocyte counts of more than 6.7×10^{12} / L?
   (c) What is the probability of erythrocyte counts in $[4.1, 4.8]\times10^{12}$ / L?
2. Suppose that the weights of 5-year-old boys in a certain area are normally distributed, with a mean of 19.5 kg and a standard deviation of 2.3 kg. A 5-year-old boy is randomly selected from this area and his weight is measured. Answer the following questions:
   (a) What is the probability that his weight is less than 16.1 kg?
   (b) What is the probability that his weight is more than 22.9 kg?
   (c) What is the probability that his weight is between 16.1 kg and 22.9 kg?
   (d) Determine the smallest x such that the probability that his weight is more than x is ≤ 0.05.
   (e) If three 5-year-old boys are selected simultaneously, what is the probability that they all weigh less than 16.1 kg?

(f) Following (c), what is the probability of at least one in three 5-year-old boys weighing more than 22.9 kg?

(g) If two 5-year-old boys are selected successively and the first boy weighs less than 16.1 kg, what is the probability that the second boy also weighs less than 16.1 kg?

3. Suppose that 40% of students in a certain primary school are boys, and 10 students were involved in a survey at random. Answer the following questions:
   (a) What is the distribution of the number of boys in the survey? What are the parameters that determine its distribution?
   (b) What is the probability that there are 3 boys in the survey?
   (c) What is the probability that more than half of the students are boys?
   (d) If 100 students are randomly investigated, what are the results of (c)?
   (e) What are the approximate values of (d) using the normal approximation method?
4. A total of 300 healthy women are randomly selected from a city. The mean of the total protein level in blood serum is calculated as 77 g/L and the standard deviation is 5 g/L (assuming a normal distribution).
   (a) Estimate the number of healthy women whose total protein level is more than 90.
   (b) Estimate the number of healthy women whose total protein level is less than 70.
   (c) What is the meaning of the reference interval? Estimate the 95% reference interval for the total protein level of healthy women in this city.
5. The SBP of 120 healthy college girls is measured in a study, and the frequency table is compiled as shown in Table 5.3.
   (a) Determine the appropriate statistic to describe the distribution's characteristics.
   (b) Estimate the proportion of healthy college girls whose SBP is below 90 mmHg.
   (c) Estimate the 95% reference interval of SBP of healthy college girls.

Table 5.3 Frequency distribution of SBP (mmHg) of 120 college girls.

Group interval	Frequency	Relative frequency (%)	Cumulative frequency	Cumulative relative frequency (%)
80–	3	2.50	3	2.50
85–	7	5.83	10	8.33
90–	15	12.50	25	20.83
95–	19	15.83	44	36.67
100–	38	31.67	82	68.33
105–	16	13.33	98	81.67
110–	12	10.00	110	91.67
115–	7	5.83	117	97.50
120–125	3	2.50	120	100.00
Total	120	100.00	—	—

6

Sampling Distribution and Parameter Estimation

CONTENTS

In Chapters 4 to 5, we introduced the concept of random variables and their probability distributions. To understand a random variable well, it is important to capture its probability distribution or at least some numerical characteristics (parameters) of the distribution. In general, any attempt to obtain the exact information by studying the entire population would be impractical, if not impossible. Refer to Example 2.1. Suppose we want to characterize the distribution of heights of 10-year-old girls in a region. Let us assume that the underlying distribution of heights is normally distributed with an expected value μ and variance σ^2. Ideally, we want the exact values of μ and σ^2 using all the 10-year-old girls in this region. However, it is usually infeasible to collect all individual records. Instead, we draw a random sample of n girls to represent the population and use the heights $X_1, X_2, \ldots, X_n$ from the sample to estimate the parameters of interest.

Continuously, we know that the probability distribution of the random variable is derived approximately from its relative frequency distributions when the sample size is sufficiently large; therefore, population parameters (e.g., μ) can be estimated using a sample statistic (e.g., $\bar{x}$). Despite this, several questions remain: As we only have a random sample with limited size in practice, how can we address the randomness when drawing a conclusion? How do we measure the reliability of the estimation?

Applied Medical Statistics, First Edition. Jingmei Jiang.

Companion website: www.wiley.com\go\jiang\appliedmedicalstatistics

How large a sample should we collect? These questions essentially involve parameter estimation, which is based on several important "elements" such as the characteristics of the population and samples and the sampling distribution that connects them. In this chapter, we start with a discussion on the sample statistics and their sampling distributions, followed by the estimation of population parameters, including point estimation and interval estimation.

6.1 Samples and Statistics

From Chapters 1 and 2, we have a preliminary understanding of the concepts of random samples and statistics. We will extend the discussion on these topics before we proceed to parameter estimation.

Definition 6.1 If the random variables $X_1, X_2,..., X_n$ are independent and identically distributed with the unknown distribution of X or the unknown parameters of the distribution of X, then these random variables constitute a random sample of size n from the common distribution X.

When the sample is actually drawn, we use lowercase letters $x_1, x_2,..., x_n$ as the values or realizations of the sample.

We call random variable X the population; it is commonly referred to as the statistical or target population that we want to investigate. The random sample is a subset "selected" from the population. As the population is often infinite, and all possible subsets cannot be enumerated, no source can produce a truly random sample. Despite this, we assume that all samples behave as random samples in this text.

What happens once we have a random sample? Naturally, we would want a statistic derived from the given sample to summarize the information in a useful manner; a statistic is, formally, defined as follows:

Definition 6.2 Let $X_1, X_2,..., X_n$ denote a random sample from the population X. Let $\hat{\theta} = \hat{\theta}(X_1, X_2,..., X_n)$ be a function of a sample that does not depend on any unknown parameter θ of the population X. Then $\hat{\theta}$ is called a *statistic*.

For example, sample mean $\hat{\theta}_1 = \bar{X} = \sum_i X_i / n$ and sample variance $\hat{\theta}_2 = S^2 = \sum_i (X_i - \bar{X})^2 / (n-1)$ are statistics, whereas $\hat{\theta}_3 = \sum_i (X_i - \mu)^2 / n$ and $\hat{\theta}_4 = \sum_i [(X_i - \mu) / \sigma]$ are not statistics because both functions contain unknown parameters (μ or σ). Clearly, a statistic itself is a random variable.

On the basis of Definitions 6.1 and 6.2, we can easily imagine that a statistic represents certain information about a sample. When there is no information loss about the unknown parameter during the calculation of a statistic, we call it a *sufficient statistic*. For instance, the mean and variance of a random sample are sufficient statistics of the population mean and variance, respectively. However, the median of the sample is not a sufficient statistic because only part of the information is used in the calculation process.

6.2 Sampling Distribution of a Statistic

Let us recall the example in the opening remarks of this chapter: the heights of 10-year-old girls. Suppose we could repeatedly sample from the population X hundreds or even thousands of times to observe the changes of a statistic, e.g., the sample mean $\overline{X}$. The values of $\overline{X}$ derived from individual samples $\left(\overline{x} = \sum_i x_i / n\right)$ would differ, even though the difference may be trivial. The difference (or using the technical term, variability) is called the sampling variability, and the corresponding distribution is called the *sampling distribution* or the probability distribution of a statistic. As is the case for an original random variable, the mean of sampling distribution is the expected value of the statistic, and its standard deviation is called the standard error of the statistic.

In this section, we will discuss the sampling distributions of several commonly used statistics because they play an important role in statistical inference.

6.2.1 Sampling Distribution of the Mean

Assume that we have a population X with mean μ and variance σ^2, where $\overline{X}$ is the mean of a random sample drawn from the population.

Definition 6.3 The sampling distribution of $\overline{X}$ denotes the distribution of values of $\overline{x}$ over all possible samples of size n that could have been selected from the population X.

According to the distribution characteristics of the population and the sample size, the sampling distribution of $\overline{X}$, according to Definition 6.3, can be characterized by three scenarios:

Scenario 1. Normal Distribution with σ^2 Known

Example 6.1 Assume that the heights (cm) of the 10-year-old girls in a region follow a normal distribution with $\mu = 142.3$ and $\sigma^2 = 6.82^2$. Suppose 100 random samples are drawn from the population with a sample size of 30. The sample means and variances are calculated for each sample; some of the corresponding results are given in Table 6.1.

Table 6.1 Means and variances obtained for 100 simulated samples drawn randomly from a normal population $N\left(142.3, 6.82^2\right)$.

Sample ID (1)	Mean $\overline{x}$ (2)	Variance s^2 (3)	Sample ID (1)	Mean $\overline{x}$ (2)	Variance s^2 (3)
1	143.2	27.48	⋮	⋮	⋮
2	142.2	62.14	91	143.7	58.72
3	140.2	46.89	92	141.6	48.48
4	141.0	44.95	93	141.8	42.74
5	141.6	25.47	94	142.1	26.44
6	142.6	43.08	95	143.7	46.65
7	140.6	60.35	96	142.4	27.49
8	142.8	82.59	97	141.6	33.76
9	144.2	63.35	98	142.6	29.92
10	141.8	38.03	99	144.5	38.97
⋮	⋮	⋮	100	142.6	55.94

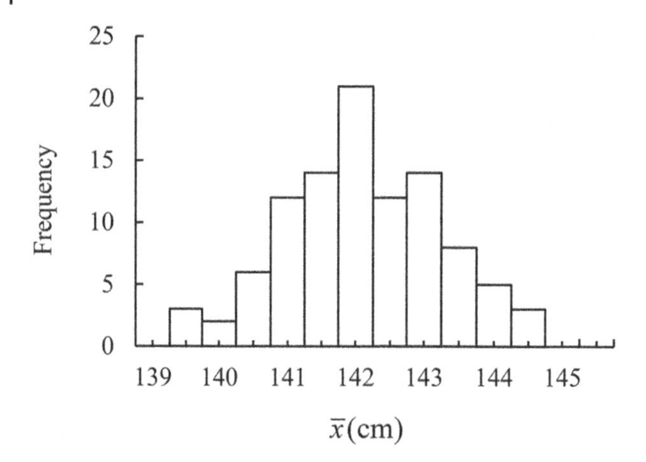

Figure 6.1 Sampling distribution of $\bar{X}$ obtained for 100 simulated samples drawn randomly from a normal population $N\left(142.3, 6.82^2\right)$.

In Table 6.1, the sample means are different from each other. Similar to the approach for describing the distribution of individual observation of height, a histogram (Figure 6.1) can be created according to the sample means $\left(\bar{x}'s\right)$.

Figure 6.1 shows an example of such a sampling distribution of $\bar{X}$; this is a frequency distribution of the sample mean from 100 randomly selected samples of size 30 drawn from the distribution of heights given in $N\left(142.3, 6.82^2\right)$. We see that the shape of the distribution of $\bar{X}$ is also symmetric (around 142.3) and is approximately distributed as normality. Just as with the original random variable X, this result represents a general rule for the sampling distribution of $\bar{X}$ from the normal population.

Normal Distribution of $\bar{X}$

If population X is normally distributed with mean μ and variance σ^2, and a random sample of size n is drawn, then the sample mean $\bar{X}$ follows a normal distribution with mean μ and variance σ^2/n:

$$\bar{X} \sim N\left(\mu, \frac{\sigma^2}{n}\right). \tag{6.1}$$

Similar to the original random variable X, when we standardize $\bar{X}$, thus creating a new random variable Z

$$Z = \frac{\bar{X} - \mu}{\sigma_{\bar{X}}} = \frac{\bar{X} - \mu}{\sigma / \sqrt{n}}, \tag{6.2}$$

then Z will be standard normally distributed.

$$Z \sim N(0,1)$$

Standard Error of the Mean

We see from Formula 6.1 that $E\left(\bar{X}\right) = \mu$; this is true for any sample size. The square root of the variance of $\bar{X}$ is called the standard deviation of the mean, or the *standard error* for short (see the denominator of Formula 6.2); i.e.,

$$\sigma_{\bar{X}} = \frac{\sigma}{\sqrt{n}}. \quad (6.3)$$

We can prove this using the properties of linear combinations of independent random variables, as

$$Var(\bar{X}) = \frac{1}{n^2}\sum_{i=1}^{n} Var(X_i)$$

For a normal population with σ^2 known, we have
$Var(X_i) = \sigma^2$ (i = 1, 2, . . , n), thus,

$$Var(\bar{X}) = \frac{1}{n^2}\sum_{i=1}^{n} Var(X_i) = \frac{1}{n^2}\sum_{i=1}^{n} \sigma_i^2 = \frac{n\sigma^2}{n^2} = \frac{\sigma^2}{n}$$

Therefore, the standard error $= \sqrt{Var(\bar{X})} = \sigma / \sqrt{n}$

In practice, σ^2 is rarely known. A reasonable estimator for σ^2 is the sample variance S^2. The estimator of the standard error can thus be obtained:

$$S_{\bar{X}} = \frac{S}{\sqrt{n}}. \quad (6.4)$$

The standard error is a quantitative measure of the variability of $\bar{X}$; it reflects the extent of the *sampling error*. In the sampling process, the larger the standard error, the greater the sampling error of $\bar{X}$, and the worse that the sample mean is a representation of the population parameter. Therefore, the standard error may be considered as representing the precision of estimating μ.

Scenario 2. Non-normal Distribution with Large Sample Size

We know from Scenario 1 that as long as the population is normally distributed, the principle introduced above works for any size n. However, in practice, a population with a non-normal distribution is likely. How do we characterize the distribution of $\bar{X}$ in such a case?

Central Limit Theorem

Let $X_1, X_2,\ldots, X_n$ be a random sample of size n from a population X with mean μ and finite variance σ^2. When the sample size is sufficiently large, the sampling distribution of $\bar{X}$ is approximately a normal distribution with mean μ and variance σ^2/n, even if the underlying distribution of the population is not normally distributed:

$$\bar{X} \mathrel{\dot{\sim}} N\left(\mu, \frac{\sigma^2}{n}\right), \quad (6.5)$$

where the symbol "$\dot{\sim}$" means "approximately distributed."

The *central limit theorem* is the mathematical theorem that gives the relationship between the sampling distribution of the sample mean and population mean. It is deemed one of the most important theorems in probability theory and statistics and generalizes the application of a normal distribution to a wider scope. To reinforce the understanding of this theorem, we visualize the sampling distribution for a series of non-normally distributed populations based on simulations.

Example 6.2 Simulation analysis: Four population distributions were assumed (A: uniform, B: triangulation, C: exponential, and D: bimodal). Random samples with different sizes (5, 10, and 30) were repeatedly drawn from these populations 2000 times per scenario. The sample mean was calculated for each scenario. Figure 6.2 shows the simulation results.

We see that regardless of the population distribution, the average of these sample means $\left(\overline{x}'s\right)$ approximates the population mean μ as the size of samples increases, while the variance of the $\left(\overline{x}'s\right)$ decreases. Notice that the shapes of the sampling distribution of $\overline{X}$ start to look approximately normal, and this trend is clear until $n = 30$.

Scenario 3. Normal Distribution with σ^2 Unknown

Because σ is unknown, it is reasonable to estimate σ using the sample standard deviation S. However, when the sample size is small, the error in estimating σ from S

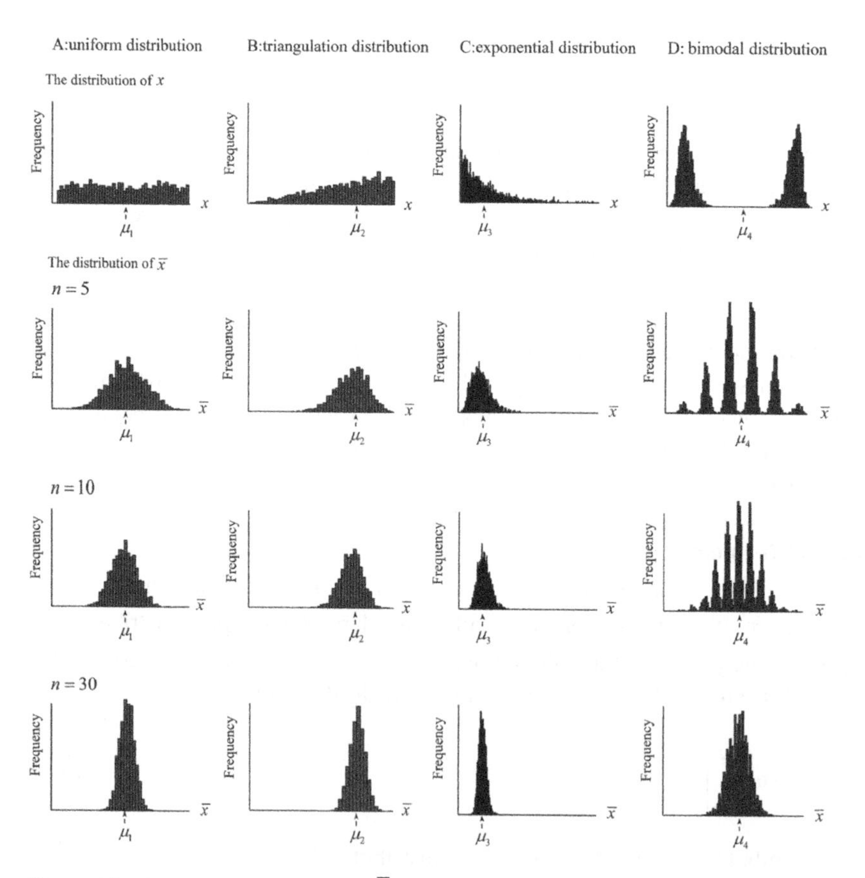

Figure 6.2 Sampling distribution of $\overline{X}$ obtained for 2000 simulated samples with different sample sizes drawn randomly from four population distributions.

becomes large. In this case, random variable $(\bar{X}-\mu)/(S/\sqrt{n})$ is no longer standard normally distributed. This problem can be addressed by a well-known distribution called the t *distribution*. The distribution, first proposed by statistician W.S. Gossett (Student, 1908), has a pattern that is very similar to the standard normal distribution.

t Distribution of $\bar{X}$

Let $X_1, X_2, \ldots, X_n$ be a random sample of size n from a normal population with mean μ and unknown variance σ^2. The random variable $(\bar{X}-\mu)/(S/\sqrt{n})$ then follows a t distribution with ν *degrees of freedom*, which is given as

$$t=\frac{\bar{X}-\mu}{S_{\bar{X}}}=\frac{\bar{X}-\mu}{S/\sqrt{n}}\sim t(\nu), \tag{6.6}$$

where $\nu=n-1$.

The pdf of the t distribution is

$$f_\nu(t)=\frac{\Gamma\left(\frac{\nu+1}{2}\right)}{\sqrt{\nu\pi}\,\Gamma\left(\frac{\nu}{2}\right)}\left(1+\frac{t^2}{\nu}\right)^{-\frac{\nu+1}{2}} \quad (-\infty<t<+\infty), \tag{6.7}$$

where $\Gamma(\nu)=\int_0^{+\infty} t^{\nu-1}e^{-t}dt \ (\nu>0)$.

Formula 6.7 shows that the pdf $f_\nu(t)$ is symmetric about zero, and the shape of the t distribution is entirely determined by the number of degrees of freedom ν. Thus, as shown in Figure 6.3, the t distribution is not a unique distribution but is instead a family of distributions indexed by a parameter referred to as the number of degrees of freedom of the distribution.

Despite its similarity with standard normal distribution $N(0,1)$, the t distribution is much more divergent. These differences, particularly in the tail areas, increase when

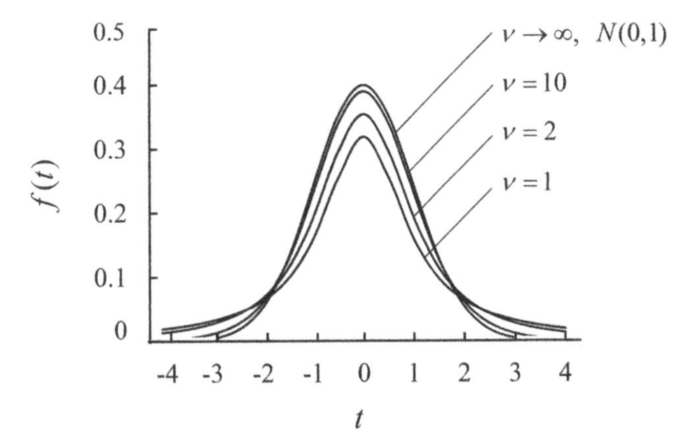

Figure 6.3 Comparison of the t distribution for different numbers of degrees of freedom with an $N(0, 1)$ distribution.

the number of degrees of freedom falls below 30. Conversely, as ν increases and eventually approaches infinity, the behavior of the t distribution tends toward the standard normal distribution. The underlying mechanism is self-evident; in a finite sample, the sample variance S^2 is only an approximation of the population variance σ^2, which yields variability for the random variable $\left(\bar{X}-\mu\right)/\left(S/\sqrt{n}\right)$ relative to $\left(\bar{X}-\mu\right)/\left(\sigma/\sqrt{n}\right)$. As ν increases (sample size increases), this approximation for σ^2 from S^2 greatly improves.

In the rest of this chapter and subsequent chapters, we will know that the sampling distributions of $\bar{X}$ described in the three scenarios are powerful tools for statistical inference.

6.2.2 Sampling Distribution of the Variance

As shown in Table 6.1, the sample variances S^2 are also different because of the sampling error. In this section, we will focus on the sampling distribution of the variance.

χ^2 Distribution

Let $X_1, X_2, \ldots, X_n$ be a random sample of size n from a normal population X with mean μ and variance σ^2. Suppose we could list all possible samples with a given size n from the population. For each sample, we compute the value $\left(n-1\right)S^2/\sigma^2$, which is a random variable as well. All these values form a sampling distribution called a χ^2 *(chi-square) distribution* with $\nu = n-1$ degrees of freedom, which is given as

$$\frac{\left(n-1\right)S^2}{\sigma^2} \sim \chi^2\left(\nu\right), \tag{6.8}$$

where $\nu = n-1$.

We see from Formula 6.8 that the sampling distribution of S^2 is built on its standardized form $\left(n-1\right)S^2/\sigma^2$ rather than its original form. The logic is the same as that for the sample mean $\bar{X}$, which depends on the standardized random variable Z or t.

The χ^2 distribution was originally introduced by F.R. Helmet in 1876. The pdf of the χ^2 distribution is

$$f_\nu(\chi^2) = \begin{cases} \dfrac{1}{2^{\frac{\nu}{2}}\Gamma\left(\dfrac{\nu}{2}\right)}\left(\chi^2\right)^{\frac{\nu}{2}-1} e^{-\frac{\chi^2}{2}}, \ \chi^2 > 0 \\ 0, \ \chi^2 \leq 0 \end{cases}. \tag{6.9}$$

The pattern of the pdf is shown in Figure 6.4.

The χ^2 distribution is also a family of distributions. Each distribution within the family is continuous, ranging from 0 to $+\infty$. As with the t distribution, the pattern of the χ^2 distribution is also determined by the number of degrees of freedom ν. For $\nu = 1$ and $\nu = 2$, the pdf is an L-shaped curve. When $\nu \geq 3$, the χ^2 distribution is right skewed and progressively approaches a normal distribution with $E\left(\chi^2\right) = \nu$ and $Var\left(\chi^2\right) = 2\nu$ as ν increases.

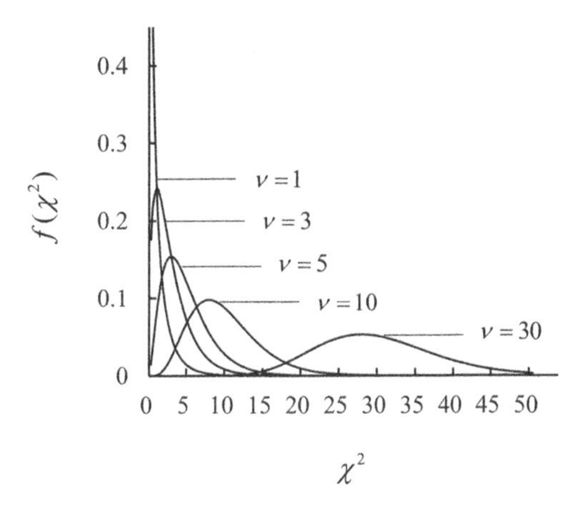

Figure 6.4 χ^2 distribution for different numbers of degrees of freedom.

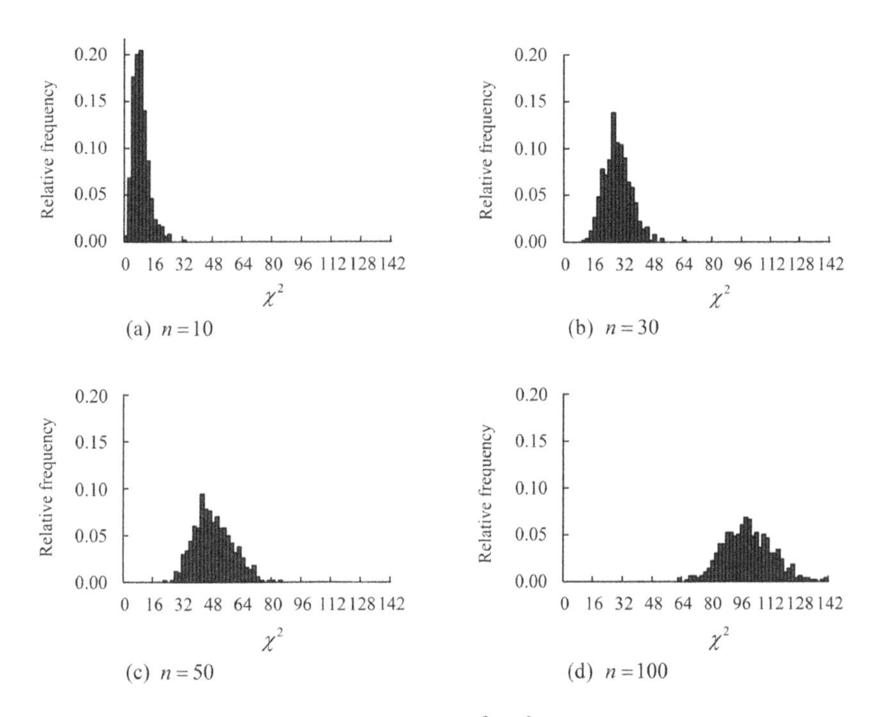

Figure 6.5 Frequency distribution of $(n-1)S^2/\sigma^2$ obtained for 500 simulated samples with different sample sizes drawn randomly from $N(142.3, 6.82^2)$.

The χ^2 distributions are considered a probability framework for the sample variance S^2. To develop an intuition, let us visualize the mechanism through simulation.

Referring to the normally distributed population $N(142.3, 6.82^2)$ in Example 6.1, random samples with different sizes (10, 30, 50, and 100) were drawn repeatedly (500 times per scenario). We calculated the sample variances S^2 and plotted the relative frequency of $(n-1)S^2/\sigma^2$; the corresponding results are shown in Figure 6.5.

We find that the relative frequency distribution of the χ^2 in Figure 6.5 and the pattern of the χ^2 distribution pdf in Figure 6.4 are consistent for any given sample size.

6.2.3 Sampling Distribution of the Rate (Normal Approximation)

In Sections 6.2.1 and 6.2.2, we demonstrated a method for characterizing the sampling distributions of the sample mean and variance for continuous variables. The method also applies to categorical data when the central limit theorem holds.

Example 6.3 Suppose mice have a probability of 0.6 of experiencing a toxicity event under a certain level of chemical exposure. We hypothetically (using statistical simulation) repeat the experiment 1000 times with a sample size of 50. Table 6.2 gives the frequency distribution for which each sample rate of toxicity is calculated as $p = x / n$.

Table 6.2 Frequency distribution of the sample rate of toxicity obtained for 1000 simulated samples of size 50 drawn randomly from a population with $\pi = 0.6$

Sample toxicity rate (1)	Frequency (2)	Relative frequency (3)
0.40	5	0.5
0.42	6	0.6
0.44	12	1.2
0.46	24	2.4
0.48	28	2.8
0.50	44	4.4
0.52	65	6.5
0.54	80	8.0
0.56	87	8.7
0.58	97	9.7
0.60	112	11.2
0.62	100	10.0
0.64	85	8.5
0.66	72	7.2
0.68	65	6.5
0.70	50	5.0
0.72	30	3.0
0.74	15	1.5
0.76	9	0.9
0.78	10	1.0
0.80	4	0.4
Total	1000	100.0

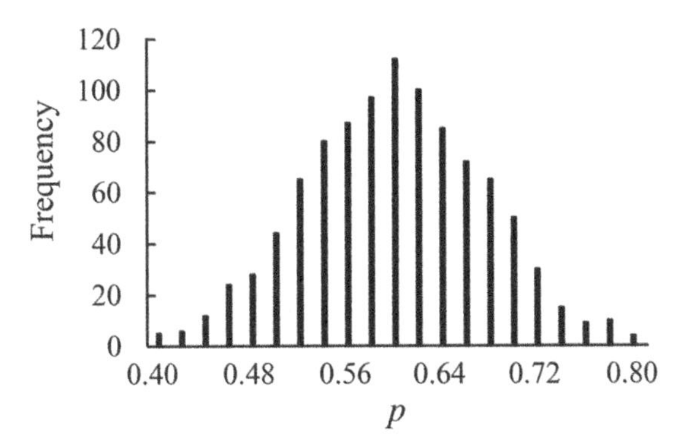

Figure 6.6 Frequency distribution of the sample rates of toxicity obtained for 1000 simulated samples of size 50 drawn randomly from a population with $\pi = 0.6$.

The frequency distribution in Figure 6.6 shows the sample rates using the data from Table 6.2. The heights of each bar represent the frequency of observed p. If the frequency is divided by the number of simulations (1000), it can be considered the approximate probability distribution of p.

The simulation exhibits the pattern of the sampling error, as shown in previous sections. Again, the distribution is symmetric about the population rate $\pi = 0.6$ and clusters along its symmetry axis.

Standard Error of *p*

Assume that a random variable X follows a binomial distribution with parameters n and π. It is easily obtained that $E(X) = n\pi$, $Var(X) = n\pi(1-\pi)$. As a statistic, the sample rate p is calculated as $p = X / n$. It follows that $E(p) = \pi$, $Var(p) = \pi(1-\pi)/n$ according to the central limit theorem.

The square root of $Var(p)$ is called the standard error of rate, which is given by

$$\sigma_p = \sqrt{\frac{\pi(1-\pi)}{n}}, \tag{6.10}$$

and is estimated using

$$S_p = \sqrt{\frac{p(1-p)}{n}}. \tag{6.11}$$

Again, the standard error represents the precision of estimating a population rate using a sampling measurement.

Furthermore, let us assume that the normal approximation to the binomial distribution is valid; we can obtain the sampling distribution of p.

Normal Approximation Method

Suppose a random sample is drawn from a population following a binomial distribution with parameters n and π. According to the central limit theorem, if n is moderately large and π is not too large or too small (i.e., satisfied $n\pi(1-\pi) \geq 5$), the sampling distribution of p is approximately normally distributed with mean π and variance $\pi(1-\pi)/n$, denoted as

$$p \dot{\sim} N\left(\pi, \frac{\pi(1-\pi)}{n}\right). \tag{6.12}$$

As π is usually unknown and estimated using the sample rate p, in practice, the requirement $np(1-p) \geq 5$ must be satisfied.

Thus far, we have discussed the concepts of common statistics and their sampling distributions. In subsequent sections, we will discuss parameter estimations.

6.3 Estimation of One Population Parameter

There are two types of estimation of population parameters: *point estimation* and *interval estimation*. A point estimate refers to the use of sample statistics to serve as the "best guess" for a population parameter. An interval estimate provides a range of plausible values for a population parameter associated with a confidence level (e.g., 95% confidence that the range or interval contains the unknown parameter). We discuss the interval estimation methods based on the sampling distribution of statistics.

6.3.1 Point Estimation and Its Quality Evaluation

In Section 6.2, we discussed the sampling distribution of three common statistics; i.e., the sample mean, sample variance, and sample rate. In fact, each of these statistics could be considered a point estimate of the corresponding population parameters. For example, the point estimate for the population mean μ is expressed as

$$\bar{X} = \sum_{i=1}^{n} X_i / n$$

Thus, as shown in Table 6.1, all 100 sample means obtained by repeated sampling can be considered as point estimates of the population mean μ. Theoretically, we may have countless $\bar{X}$, in this way, as point estimates of the population mean μ. We give the general definition of the point estimation.

Definition 6.4 Let θ denote a parameter of population X and $\hat{\theta} = \hat{\theta}(X_1, X_2, \ldots, X_n)$ denote a statistic that represents a numerical estimate of θ from the measurements contained in a sample. Any possible $\hat{\theta}$ is then called the *point estimator* of the parameter θ.

In fact, according to Definition 6.4, each $\bar{x}$ and s^2 shown in Table 6.1 is a point estimator of the population parameters.

Well, how "good" is the single-valued estimate for the population parameter? We partially addressed these questions in Section 6.1, where the concept of the sufficient statistic suggested that they can be considered as a good option. What then remains unanswered is how to evaluate the quality of these estimators. We introduce three criteria of point estimators for evaluating the quality of these statistics.

1. Unbiasedness

Definition 6.5 Let $X_1, X_2,\ldots,X_n$ be a random sample of size n from a population X with parameter θ, regardless of its underlying distribution. Let $\hat{\theta}=\hat{\theta}(X_1, X_2,\ldots,X_n)$ be an estimator of θ. An estimator $\hat{\theta}$ of parameter θ is unbiased if

$$E\left(\hat{\theta}\right)=\theta \tag{6.13}$$

Unbiasedness is a desirable property in a point estimate. Although the estimator $\hat{\theta}$ is unlikely to be exactly equal to parameter θ, the average value of $\hat{\theta}$ over a large number of random samples of size n is θ.

For example, because random variables $X_1, X_2,\ldots,X_n$ are independent and have an identical distribution to population X, we have $E(X_i)=\mu$, $Var(X_i)=\sigma^2\ (i=1,2,\ldots,n)$. The sample mean $\bar{X}$ is then an unbiased estimator of the population mean μ, according to Definition 6.5, because

$$E\left(\bar{X}\right)=\frac{1}{n}E\left(\sum_{i=1}^{n}X_i\right)=\frac{n\mu}{n}=\mu.$$

The estimator $S_n^2=\frac{1}{n}\sum_{i=1}^{n}\left(X_i-\bar{X}\right)^2$ of population variance σ^2 is biased, because

$$E(S_n^2)=E\left[\frac{1}{n}\sum_{i=1}^{n}\left(X_i-\bar{X}\right)^2\right]=\frac{n-1}{n}\sigma^2\neq\sigma^2,$$

while $S^2=\frac{1}{n-1}\sum_{i=1}^{n}\left(X_i-\bar{X}\right)^2$ is unbiased, because

$$E(S^2)=E\left(\frac{n}{n-1}S_n^2\right)=\frac{n}{n-1}E\left(S_n^2\right)=\frac{n}{n-1}\times\frac{n-1}{n}\sigma^2=\sigma^2$$

Therefore, in biostatistics, S^2 is often called the sample variance.

However, unbiasedness is only one of the preconditions of the estimator. For a symmetric distribution, there are many unbiased estimators of μ, for instance, mean $\bar{X}$ and median M. Despite the central tendency of these estimators, we prefer the estimate to have a minimal degree of variance. In particular, we want the spread of the sampling distribution of the estimator to be as small as possible so that estimates will tend to fall close to the μ.

2. Minimum Variance Unbiased Estimator

Definition 6.6 Let $X_1, X_2,\ldots, X_n$ be a random sample of size n from a population X with parameter θ. A statistic $\hat{\theta}$ is called a *minimum variance unbiased estimator* (*MVUE*) of parameter θ if $\hat{\theta}$ is unbiased and has minimum variance compared with other possible unbiased estimators.

For example, the sample mean $\bar{X}$ and the sample median M from a normal distribution are both unbiased estimators of μ, whereas the variance of $\bar{X}$ is $\sigma_{\bar{X}}^2 = \sigma^2 / n$ and that of M is $\sigma_M^2 = \pi\sigma^2 / 2n$ when n is sufficiently large. Clearly, the variance of M is $\pi / 2$ times that of $\bar{X}$. The sample mean, in this case, is more effective than the sample median M, and thus an MVUE according to Definition 6.6.

3. Consistency

Definition 6.7 Let $X_1, X_2, \ldots, X_n$ be a random sample of size n from a population X with parameter θ. Let $\hat{\theta}_n$ be an estimator of unknown population parameter θ. For any $\varepsilon > 0$, if

$$\lim_{n\to\infty} P\left(\left|\hat{\theta}_n - \theta\right| < \varepsilon\right) = 1, \tag{6.14}$$

then $\hat{\theta}_n$ is a consistent estimator of the population parameter θ.

The mathematical expression of *consistency* defined in terms of the limit (idea of closeness) may not be intuitive. In other words, consistency depicts activities in which estimates converge to the population parameter as the sample size increases to an arbitrarily large number. For example, $\bar{X}$ is used to estimate μ. As n approaches infinity, $\sigma_{\bar{X}}^2 = \sigma^2 / n$ approaches zero, for any $\varepsilon > 0$, and $\bar{X}$ satisfies

$$\lim_{n\to\infty} P\left(\left|\bar{X} - \mu\right| < \varepsilon\right) = 1$$

Therefore, according to Definition 6.7, we can say that the sample mean $\bar{X}$ is a consistent estimator of the population mean μ.

It is noteworthy that the three criteria are a theoretical presentation based on the mathematical description of the average effect of a large number of repeated experiments. In many contexts wherein only one sample can be observed, the accuracy and precision of the point estimate for the parameter cannot be directly evaluated because of the sampling error. Another way to estimate the value of a population parameter is to use an interval estimator.

6.3.2 Interval Estimation for the Mean

An interval estimator is a rule, usually expressed as a formula, for calculating two points from the sample data. The objective is to form an interval that contains θ with a high degree of confidence.

Definition 6.8 An interval estimator is a pair of random variables obtained from the sample data used to form an interval that estimates a population parameter.

We know from Section 6.2 that the sampling distribution of $\bar{X}$ can be explained according to three scenarios depending on the nature of the population distribution and the sample size. In this section, we provide the interval estimation for μ based on the same previous scenarios.

Scenario 1. Normal Distribution with σ^2 Known

Suppose $X_1, X_2, \ldots, X_n$ is a random sample from a normal distribution $N(\mu, \sigma^2)$, the sample mean $\bar{X}$, in this case, follows a normal distribution $N(\mu, \sigma^2/n)$ and its transformation $Z = (\bar{X} - \mu)/(\sigma/\sqrt{n})$ follows the standard normal distribution $N(0,1)$.

For the distribution of random variable Z, we specify a probability $\alpha(0<\alpha<1)$, which refers to the area under the curve in two tails (Figure 6.7). For any given α, we call $z_{\alpha/2}$ the *critical value* (percentile) corresponding to the lower $\alpha/2$, and $z_{1-\alpha/2}$ the critical value corresponding to the upper $\alpha/2$ of a Z distribution. As the Z distribution is symmetric, $z_{\alpha/2} = -z_{1-\alpha/2}$.

We may place the central area of size $1-\alpha$ in the Z distribution (see Figure 6.7): The probability $1-\alpha$ can also be presented as

$$\begin{aligned} 1-\alpha &= P\left(z_{\alpha/2} \le Z \le z_{1-\alpha/2}\right) \\ &= P\left(-z_{1-\alpha/2} \le \frac{\bar{X}-\mu}{\sigma/\sqrt{n}} \le z_{1-\alpha/2}\right) \\ &= P\left(-z_{1-\alpha/2}\frac{\sigma}{\sqrt{n}} \le \bar{X}-\mu \le z_{1-\alpha/2}\frac{\sigma}{\sqrt{n}}\right) \\ &= P\left(\bar{X}-z_{1-\alpha/2}\frac{\sigma}{\sqrt{n}} \le \mu \le \bar{X}+z_{1-\alpha/2}\frac{\sigma}{\sqrt{n}}\right). \end{aligned} \tag{6.15}$$

Formula 6.15 indicates that the probability that the interval includes μ is $1-\alpha$, which is called the *confidence level* of the interval estimation.

Thus, a $(1-\alpha)\times 100\%$ *confidence interval (CI)* for μ is given by

$$\left[\bar{X}-z_{1-\alpha/2}\frac{\sigma}{\sqrt{n}},\ \bar{X}+z_{1-\alpha/2}\frac{\sigma}{\sqrt{n}}\right]. \tag{6.16}$$

Formula 6.16 may be rewritten as

$$\bar{X} \pm z_{1-\alpha/2}\frac{\sigma}{\sqrt{n}}, \tag{6.17}$$

which is also called the $(1-\alpha)\times 100\%$ *confidence limit* of μ.

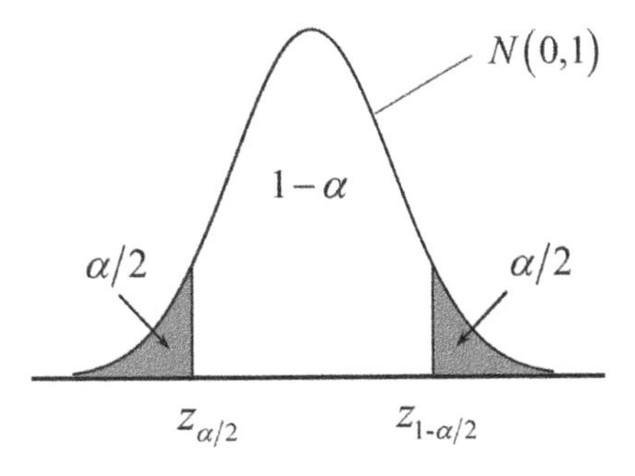

Figure 6.7 Illustration of critical values for the Z distribution.

The length of CI $\left(2 \times z_{1-\alpha/2}\sigma / \sqrt{n}\right)$ indicates the precision of the point estimate $\bar{X}$, which is determined by the standard error $\sigma / \sqrt{n}$ and α. Since σ is a constant, given fixed α as the sample size n increases, the length of the CI decreases, which means the estimate precision increases. Given fixed n the confidence level desired increases (α decreases), the length of the CI increases, which means the estimate precision decreases.

Scenario 2. Non-normal Distribution with a Large Sample Size

In this scenario, the sampling distribution of $\bar{X}$ is approximately normally distributed, and under the assumptions of central limit theorem, the distribution of $Z = \left(\bar{X} - \mu\right) / \left(S / \sqrt{n}\right)$ is approximately $N\left(0, 1\right)$. Hence, for given α,

$$1 - \alpha \approx P\left(-z_{1-\alpha/2} \le \frac{\bar{X} - \mu}{S / \sqrt{n}} \le z_{1-\alpha/2}\right). \tag{6.18}$$

Using the same algebraic derivation as that in Formula 6.15, an approximate $\left(1 - \alpha\right) \times 100\%$ CI for μ is given by

$$\left[\bar{X} - z_{1-\alpha/2}\frac{S}{\sqrt{n}},\ \bar{X} + z_{1-\alpha/2}\frac{S}{\sqrt{n}}\right], \tag{6.19}$$

which is also called a large sample CI for μ.

Example 6.4 The serum triglyceride (mmol/L) levels of the 153 10-year-old girls in Example 2.2 were measured. The sample mean was 1.02, with a standard deviation of 0.40. Construct the 95% CI.

Solution

Given $n = 153$, the sampling mean $\bar{X}$ is approximately normally distributed according to the central limit theorem. Here $\bar{x} = 1.02$, $s = 0.40$, and the estimate of standard error is

$$s_{\bar{x}} = \frac{s}{\sqrt{n}} = \frac{0.40}{\sqrt{153}} = 0.03$$

Let $z_{1-\alpha/2} = 1.96$ (Appendix Table 3). On the basis of Formula 6.19, the approximate 95% CI is

$$\begin{aligned}&\left[\bar{x} - z_{1-0.05/2}s / \sqrt{n},\ \bar{x} + z_{1-0.05/2}s / \sqrt{n}\right]\\ &= \left[1.02 - 1.96 \times 0.03, 1.02 + 1.96 \times 0.03\right]\\ &= \left[0.96, 1.08\right].\end{aligned}$$

Therefore, the 95% CI of mean serum triglyceride in the 10-year-old girls is $\left[0.96, 1.08\right]$ mmol/L. Under a confidence level of 95%, the maximum tolerance of the error for the population mean is $1.96 \times 0.03 = 0.06$ mmol/L.

Note that, in practice, we have limited understanding of whether the population is normally distributed. The central limit theorem plays an important role in constructing the CI.

Scenario 3. Normal Distribution with σ^2 Unknown

We know that if the population variance σ^2 is unknown, the statistic $t = \left(\bar{X} - \mu\right) / \left(S / \sqrt{n}\right)$ follows a t distribution with $v = n - 1$ degrees of freedom.

The procedure for constructing the $(1-\alpha)\times 100\%$ CI based on the t distribution is nearly identical to that for a normal distribution. For a given α, find $t_{v,\alpha/2}$ as the lower $\alpha / 2$ critical value (percentile) and $t_{v,1-\alpha/2}$ as the upper $\alpha / 2$ critical value of the t distribution with v degrees of freedom; the $(1-\alpha)\times 100\%$ CI is then derived according to

$$1-\alpha = P\left(t_{v,\alpha/2} \le \frac{\bar{X} - \mu}{S / \sqrt{n}} \le t_{v,1-\alpha/2}\right). \tag{6.20}$$

As $t_{\alpha/2} = -t_{1-\alpha/2}$, using a simple algebraic derivation, we get the $(1-\alpha)\times 100\%$ CI for μ as

$$\left[\bar{X} - t_{v,1-\alpha/2}\frac{S}{\sqrt{n}},\ \bar{X} + t_{v,1-\alpha/2}\frac{S}{\sqrt{n}}\right]. \tag{6.21}$$

For a given $\alpha = 0.05$ and ν, the probability that the interval includes μ is 95%.

Note that the accuracy and precision are contradictory aspects of the CI when measuring uncertainty. The higher the accuracy, the wider the CI; however, the higher the precision, the narrower the CI. For instance, when the sample size is fixed, a CI with a 99% confidence level is broader than a CI with a 95% confidence level; i.e., a 99% CI is more accurate than a 95% CI, but the precision of 95% CI is higher than that of 99% CI. Increasing the sample size is the most efficient strategy to improve accuracy and precision simultaneously.

Example 6.5 In a study on mariners' health status, a random sample was drawn with a size of 10. The sampling mean of the hemoglobin (g/L) level was 127.2, with a standard deviation of 20.8. Construct the 95% CI.

Solution Here, $n = 10$, $\bar{x} = 127.2$, and $s = 20.8$; then the estimator of standard error is

$$s_{\bar{x}} = \frac{s}{\sqrt{n}} = \frac{20.8}{\sqrt{10}} = 6.58.$$

Let $\alpha = 0.05$ and $v = 10 - 1 = 9$; we can find the critical value $t_{9,1-0.05/2} = 2.262$ according to the t_9 distribution (Appendix Table 4). Substitute these values into Formula 6.21:

$$\begin{aligned}&\left[\bar{x} - t_{9,1-0.05/2}s / \sqrt{n}, \bar{x} + t_{9,1-0.05/2}s / \sqrt{n}\right]\\ &= \left[127.2 - 2.262\times 6.58, 127.2 + 2.262\times 6.58\right]\\ &= \left[112.3, 142.1\right].\end{aligned}$$

Hence, the 95% CI of the mean hemoglobin in mariners is $[112.3, 142.1]$ g/L.

In practice, even if we sometimes know that the distribution of the population is normal, the variance σ^2 is often unavailable. A common approach is to substitute sampling variance S^2 for σ^2. The choice of z or t distribution should be justified according to the sample size. Generally, for a fixed probability α, the intervals based on $t_{v,1-\alpha/2}$ are wider than those based on $z_{1-\alpha/2}$. Hence, the interval in Formula 6.21 is considerably more conservative than that in Formula 6.19. We encourage the use of statistical software, which provides the exact computation of the t distribution and allows more options for the number of degrees of freedom that are not provided in Appendix Table 4.

6.3.3 Interval Estimation for the Variance

We also construct the CI for the estimate of the population variance σ^2.

Let $X_1, X_2, \ldots, X_n$ be a random sample from a normal distribution $N\left(\mu, \sigma^2\right)$. We know from Section 6.2.2 that the random variable $\left(n-1\right)S^2 / \sigma^2$ follows a χ^2 distribution with $v = n-1$ degrees of freedom. Because the χ^2 distribution is, in general, a skewed distribution, there is no simple relationship between the upper and lower percentiles. Under such circumstance, for a given α and v, we can locate the critical values ($\chi^2_{v,\alpha/2}$ and $\chi^2_{v,1-\alpha/2}$) corresponding to the tail areas $\alpha / 2$ from the lower and upper ends of the χ^2 distribution (Appendix Table 5), as shown in Figure 6.8.

The probability $1-\alpha$ is given as

$$1-\alpha = P\left(\chi^2_{v,\alpha/2} \le \frac{\left(n-1\right)S^2}{\sigma^2} \le \chi^2_{v,1-\alpha/2}\right). \tag{6.22}$$

This can be further manipulated as

$$1-\alpha = P\left(\frac{\left(n-1\right)S^2}{\chi^2_{v,1-\alpha/2}} \le \sigma^2 \le \frac{\left(n-1\right)S^2}{\chi^2_{v,\alpha/2}}\right). \tag{6.23}$$

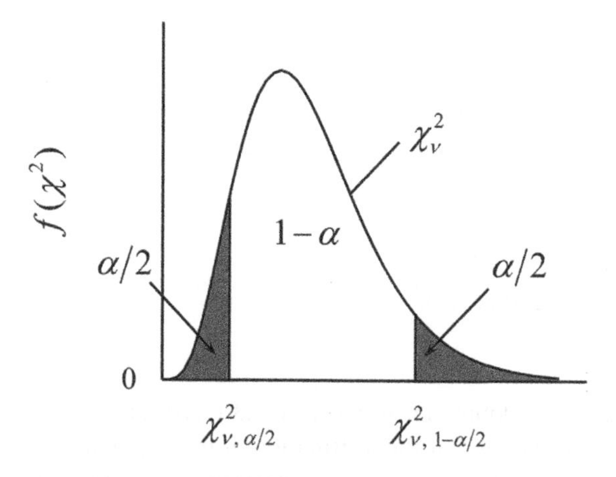

Figure 6.8 Illustration of critical values for the χ^2 distribution.

Thus, the $(1-\alpha)\times 100\%$ CI for σ^2 is finally given by

$$\left[\frac{(n-1)S^2}{\chi^2_{v,1-\alpha/2}}, \frac{(n-1)S^2}{\chi^2_{v,\alpha/2}}\right]. \quad (6.24)$$

Because σ is a monotonic function with σ^2 on $(0, \infty)$, to obtain a $(1-\alpha)\times 100\%$ CI for σ, we can simply take the square root of the confidence limits for σ^2:

$$\left[\frac{\sqrt{n-1}S}{\sqrt{\chi^2_{v,1-\alpha/2}}}, \frac{\sqrt{n-1}S}{\sqrt{\chi^2_{v,\alpha/2}}}\right]. \quad (6.25)$$

Note that the interval estimation for σ^2 is only valid for normally distributed samples. If the underlying distribution is not normal, then the confidence level for this interval may not be $1-\alpha$ even if the sample size is large.

Example 6.6 Referring to Table 6.1, the sample variance in sample No. 1 was $s^2 = 27.48$. Construct a 95% CI for the population variance σ^2.

Solution

Here, $v = 30 - 1 = 29$, $s^2 = 27.48$.

Given $\alpha = 0.05$ and $\nu = 29$, on the basis of the χ^2 distribution critical value table (Appendix Table 5), the critical values for the χ^2_{29} distribution are $\chi^2_{29,0.05/2} = 16.05$ and $\chi^2_{29,1-0.05/2} = 45.72$. Substituting these values into Formula 6.24, we have the 95% CI of variance.

lower limit: $(n-1)s^2 / \chi^2_{29,1-0.05/2} = 29 \times 27.48 / 45.72 = 17.43$

upper limit: $(n-1)s^2 / \chi^2_{29,0.05/2} = 29 \times 27.48 / 16.05 = 49.65$

Thus, the 95% CI for σ^2 is $[17.43, 49.65]$ cm^2.

There is a 95% probability that the CI includes the variance of height.

6.3.4 Interval Estimation for the Rate (Normal Approximation Method)

As discussed in Section 6.2, the sampling distribution of the sample means can be developed regardless of the population distribution, provided the central limit theorem holds. Therefore, a CI that is constructed based on the sampling distribution of p also complies with such a principle. In this section, we focus on the $(1-\alpha)\times 100\%$ CI for π, using the normal approximation method.

We know from Section 6.2.3 that, if $np(1-p) \geq 5$, the sampling distribution of p follows approximately normally distributed with mean π, and variance $\pi(1-\pi)/n$, the distribution of $Z = (p-\pi)/\sqrt{p(1-p)/n}$ is approximately $N(0,1)$.

Thus, for a given α, we have

$$1-\alpha \approx P\left(z_{\alpha/2} \leq \frac{p-\pi}{\sqrt{p(1-p)/n}} \leq z_{1-\alpha/2}\right), \quad (6.26)$$

where $z_{\alpha/2} = -z_{1-\alpha/2}$, we have

$$1-\alpha \approx P\left[p - z_{1-\alpha/2}\sqrt{\frac{p(1-p)}{n}} \le \pi \le p + z_{1-\alpha/2}\sqrt{\frac{p(1-p)}{n}}\right]. \tag{6.27}$$

Therefore, an approximate $(1-\alpha)\times 100\%$ CI for π is given by

$$\left[p - z_{1-\alpha/2}\sqrt{\frac{p(1-p)}{n}},\ p + z_{1-\alpha/2}\sqrt{\frac{p(1-p)}{n}}\right]. \tag{6.28}$$

Note again that this method of interval estimation should only be used when $np(1-p) \ge 5$.

Example 6.7 Take one of the results in Example 6.3, where the sample rate of toxicity p is 0.50 at a sample size 50. Construct the 95% CI for the π.

Solution
Here, $n = 50$ and $p = 0.50$, where $np(1-p) = 50 \times 0.50 \times 0.50 = 12.5 > 5$.

Based on Formula 6.11, the estimator of standard error of p is

$$s_p = \sqrt{\frac{p(1-p)}{n}} = \sqrt{\frac{0.50\times(1-0.50)}{50}} = 0.07$$

Thus, an approximate 95% CI for π is

$$\begin{aligned}&\left[p - z_{1-0.05/2}s_p,\ p + z_{1-0.05/2}s_p\right]\\&=\left[0.50 - 1.96\times 0.07, 0.50 + 1.96\times 0.07\right]\\&=\left[0.36, 0.64\right].\end{aligned}$$

We have 95% confidence that the interval $[0.36, 0.64]$ incorporates the population rate of toxicity π.

6.4 Estimation of Two Population Parameters

6.4.1 Estimation of the Difference in Means

In Section 6.3, we introduced the methods of parameter estimation for a single population. In this section, we will extend the context to the difference between two population means $\mu_1 - \mu_2$, i.e., use information from two separately collected random samples from two independent populations. The estimations also include point estimates and interval estimates.

6.4.1.1 Point Estimation

Let $\bar{X}_1$ be a mean of a random sample from the population X_1 with mean μ_1 and finite variance σ_1^2. Let $\bar{X}_2$ be a mean of a random sample from the population X_2 with mean μ_2 and finite variance σ_2^2. It can be proved (proof omitted) that

$$E(\bar{X}_1 - \bar{X}_2) = \mu_1 - \mu_2, \tag{6.29}$$

$$Var(\bar{X}_1 - \bar{X}_2) = \frac{\sigma_1^2}{n_1} + \frac{\sigma_2^2}{n_2}, \tag{6.30}$$

the statistic $\bar{X}_1 - \bar{X}_2$ is an MVUE of of $\mu_1 - \mu_2$.

6.4.1.2 Interval Estimation

The interval estimation method for the $\bar{X}_1 - \bar{X}_2$ is similar to that for estimating one population parameter. In this section, we will follow the same outlines, yet combine two types of utilizations (i.e., Scenario 1 and 2 in Section 6.3.2), considering their sampling distribution are similar (normal or approximately normal based on central limit theorem).

Scenario 1. Normal Distribution or the Central Limit Theorem Holds

We know from the simulation study in Section 6.2 that the sample mean tends toward a normal distribution for large n, regardless of the underlying distribution. This can easily be extended to two sample mean differences. For a large n (generally, $n_1 \geq 30$ and $n_2 \geq 30$), it can be proved that $\bar{X}_1 - \bar{X}_2$ approximately follows a normal distribution:

$$\bar{X}_1 - \bar{X}_2 \,\dot{\sim}\, N\left(\mu_1 - \mu_2, \frac{\sigma_1^2}{n_1} + \frac{\sigma_2^2}{n_2}\right). \tag{6.31}$$

Standardizing $\bar{X}_1 - \bar{X}_2$ into random variable Z, we have

$$Z = \frac{(\bar{X}_1 - \bar{X}_2) - (\mu_1 - \mu_2)}{\sqrt{\frac{\sigma_1^2}{n_1} + \frac{\sigma_2^2}{n_2}}} \,\dot{\sim}\, N(0,1). \tag{6.32}$$

In practice, σ_1 and σ_2 are usually taken as S_1 and S_2, respectively. Thus, similar to our previous result, an approximate $(1-\alpha)\times 100\%$ CI for $\mu_1 - \mu_2$ is given by

$$\left[\bar{X}_1 - \bar{X}_2 - z_{1-\alpha/2}\sqrt{\frac{S_1^2}{n_1} + \frac{S_2^2}{n_2}},\ \bar{X}_1 - \bar{X}_2 + z_{1-\alpha/2}\sqrt{\frac{S_1^2}{n_1} + \frac{S_2^2}{n_2}}\right], \tag{6.33}$$

where $\sqrt{(S_1^2 / n_1) + (S_2^2 / n_2)}$ is the estimator for the standard error of $\bar{X}_1 - \bar{X}_2$. Letting the lower confidence limit of the CI (LCL) and upper confidence limit of the CI (UCL) denote the $(1-\alpha)\times 100\%$ confidence limits, we can interpret the result of $(1-\alpha)\times 100\%$ CI for $\mu_1 - \mu_2$ as follows.

(1) If LCL > 0, then $\mu_1 > \mu_2$.
(2) If UCL < 0, then $\mu_1 < \mu_2$.
(3) If LCL ≤ 0 and UCL ≥ 0, then no evidence supports the statement that μ_1 and μ_2 are different.

Note that the CI estimation is exact when the population is normal and is only an approximation when the central limit theorem holds.

Scenario 2. Normal Distribution with Unknown but Equal σ^2

As stated above, let $\bar{X}_1$ be a random sample satisfying $\bar{X}_1 \sim N\left(\mu_1, \sigma_1^2 / n_1\right)$ and let $\bar{X}_2$ be a random sample satisfying $\bar{X}_2 \sim N\left(\mu_2, \sigma_2^2 / n_2\right)$. Assume $\bar{X}_1$ and $\bar{X}_2$ are independent, and $\sigma_1^2 = \sigma_2^2 = \sigma^2$. Similar to the sampling distribution of one sample mean, the mean difference $\bar{X}_1 - \bar{X}_2$ then follows a t distribution with v degrees of freedom:

$$t = \frac{\left(\bar{X}_1 - \bar{X}_2\right) - \left(\mu_1 - \mu_2\right)}{S_{\bar{X}_1 - \bar{X}_2}} \sim t(v), \tag{6.34}$$

where $v = n_1 + n_2 - 2$ and

$$S_{\bar{X}_1 - \bar{X}_2} = \sqrt{S_C^2 \left(\frac{1}{n_1} + \frac{1}{n_2}\right)}, \tag{6.35}$$

where $S_C^2 = \frac{(n_1 - 1)S_1^2 + (n_2 - 1)S_2^2}{n_1 + n_2 - 2}$ is a weighted average of S_1^2 and S_2^2, also called the pooled sample variance.

For a given α and ν, the critical value of the t_ν distribution corresponding to the two-sided tail areas of $\alpha / 2$ can be found (Appendix Table 4). We then have

$$1 - \alpha = P\left(t_{v,\alpha/2} \le \frac{\left(\bar{X}_1 - \bar{X}_2\right) - \left(\mu_1 - \mu_2\right)}{S_{\bar{X}_1 - \bar{X}_2}} \le t_{v,1-\alpha/2}\right). \tag{6.36}$$

Therefore, a $(1-\alpha) \times 100\%$ CI for $\mu_1 - \mu_2$ is

$$\left[\left(\bar{X}_1 - \bar{X}_2\right) - t_{v,1-\alpha/2} S_{\bar{X}_1 - \bar{X}_2}, \left(\bar{X}_1 - \bar{X}_2\right) + t_{v,1-\alpha/2} S_{\bar{X}_1 - \bar{X}_2}\right]. \tag{6.37}$$

Example 6.8 Suppose we are now interested in whether the mean heights of 10-year-old girls in two regions are different. Two samples were randomly selected from the two regions. The summary statistics are given in Table 6.3. Calculate the 95% CI for the difference (assume that the variances of the two populations are equal).

Solution

For region A, $n_1 = 15$, $\bar{x}_1 = 138.5$, $s_1 = 8.21$.

Table 6.3 Summary statistics of the height (cm) of 10-year-old girls in the two regions

Region	n	$\bar{x}$	s
A	15	138.5	8.21
B	15	140.3	7.82

For region B, $n_2 = 15$, $\bar{x}_2 = 140.3$, $s_2 = 7.82$.
The difference between the means of the two samples is $\bar{x}_1 - \bar{x}_2 = 138.5 - 140.3 = -1.8$.
The pooled sample variance is

$$s_C^2 = \frac{(n_1 - 1)s_1^2 + (n_2 - 1)s_2^2}{n_1 + n_2 - 2} = \frac{14 \times 8.21^2 + 14 \times 7.82^2}{15 + 15 - 2} = 64.28.$$

The estimator of standard error of $\bar{X}_1 - \bar{X}_2$ is

$$s_{\bar{x}_1 - \bar{x}_2} = \sqrt{s_C^2\left(\frac{1}{n_1} + \frac{1}{n_2}\right)} = \sqrt{64.28 \times (1/15 + 1/15)} = 2.93$$

For a given $\alpha = 0.05$ and $\nu = 15 + 15 - 2 = 28$, the critical value is $t_{28,1-0.05/2} = 2.048$, which can be found from the t_{28} distribution (Appendix Table 4). Substitute this into Formula 6.37. Then the 95% CI of the mean height difference between the two regions is obtained:

$$\begin{aligned}&\left[\bar{x}_1 - \bar{x}_2 - t_{28,1-0.05/2}s_{\bar{x}_1 - \bar{x}_2},\ \bar{x}_1 - \bar{x}_2 + t_{28,1-0.05/2}s_{\bar{x}_1 - \bar{x}_2}\right]\\ &= [-1.8 - 2.048 \times 2.93,\ -1.8 + 2.048 \times 2.93]\\ &= [-7.8, 4.2].\end{aligned}$$

The 95% CI of the difference of mean heights of 10-year-old girls between regions A and B is $[-7.8, 4.2]$ cm. $\text{LCL} = -7.8 < 0$, whereas $\text{UCL} = 4.2 > 0$. We conclude that with a confidence level of 95%, there is no evidence to support the statement that the mean heights of girls in regions A and B are different.

Scenario 3. Normal Distribution with Unknown and Unequal σ^2

In a scenario in which the unknown variances of the two normal distributions are not equal, in this case, we cannot assume a t distribution based on the pooled sample variance. We can use the *Satterthwaite method* to construct a statistic t' that approximately follows a t distribution:

$$t' = \frac{(\bar{X}_1 - \bar{X}_2) - (\mu_1 - \mu_2)}{\sqrt{\frac{S_1^2}{n_1} + \frac{S_2^2}{n_2}}} \dot{\sim} t(\nu'), \tag{6.38}$$

where

$$\nu' = \frac{\left(\frac{S_1^2}{n_1} + \frac{S_2^2}{n_2}\right)^2}{\frac{\left(\frac{S_1^2}{n_1}\right)^2}{n_1 - 1} + \frac{\left(\frac{S_2^2}{n_2}\right)^2}{n_2 - 1}} \text{(rounded to the nearest integer)} \tag{6.39}$$

denotes the adjusted number of degrees of freedom in terms of the original ν.

An approximate $(1-\alpha)\times 100\%$ CI for $\mu_1 - \mu_2$ is then given by

$$\left[\bar{X}_1 - \bar{X}_2 - t_{\nu',1-\alpha/2}\sqrt{\frac{S_1^2}{n_1}+\frac{S_2^2}{n_2}},\ \bar{X}_1 - \bar{X}_2 + t_{\nu',1-\alpha/2}\sqrt{\frac{S_1^2}{n_1}+\frac{S_2^2}{n_2}}\right]. \tag{6.40}$$

Example 6.9 In a community health survey that focuses on hyperlipidemia in women, 20 older women (age$\geq$ 65 years) and 30 younger women (age$\leq$ 40 years) were randomly sampled. Their serum total cholesterol (mmol/L) was measured with $\bar{x}_1 = 5.36$ and $s_1 = 1.44$ in the older group and $\bar{x}_2 = 3.25$ and $s_2 = 0.71$ in the younger group. Construct a 95% CI for the difference between the mean serum total cholesterol (assume that the population variances of the two samples are not equal).

Solution

For older women, $n_1 = 20$, $\bar{x}_1 = 5.36$, and $s_1 = 1.44$.

For younger women, $n_2 = 30$, $\bar{x}_2 = 3.25$, and $s_2 = 0.71$.

$$\nu' = \frac{\left(\frac{s_1^2}{n_1}+\frac{s_2^2}{n_2}\right)^2}{\frac{\left(\frac{s_1^2}{n_1}\right)^2}{n_1-1}+\frac{\left(\frac{s_2^2}{n_2}\right)^2}{n_2-1}} = \frac{\left(\frac{1.44^2}{20}+\frac{0.71^2}{30}\right)^2}{\frac{\left(\frac{1.44^2}{20}\right)^2}{19}+\frac{\left(\frac{0.71^2}{30}\right)^2}{29}} = 25.2 \approx 25.$$

Given $\alpha = 0.05$ and $\nu' = 25$, we can obtain the critical value $t_{25,\,1\text{-}0.05/2} = 2.060$ from the t_{25} distribution (Appendix Table 4). Substituting this into Formula 6.40, we obtain the approximate 95% CI for $\mu_1 - \mu_2$

$$\left[\bar{x}_1 - \bar{x}_2 - t_{25,1-0.05/2}\sqrt{\frac{s_1^2}{n_1}+\frac{s_2^2}{n_2}},\ \bar{x}_1 - \bar{x}_2 + t_{25,1-0.05/2}\sqrt{\frac{s_1^2}{n_1}+\frac{s_2^2}{n_2}}\right]$$
$$= \left[5.36 - 3.25 - 2.060\times\sqrt{\frac{1.44^2}{20}+\frac{0.71^2}{30}}, 5.36 - 3.25 + 2.060\times\sqrt{\frac{1.44^2}{20}+\frac{0.71^2}{30}}\right]$$
$$= [1.39, 2.83].$$

The 95% CI for the mean difference in serum total cholesterol between older and younger women in this community is $[1.39, 2.83]$ mmol/L. Because the LCL is greater than 0, we conclude that with a confidence level of 95%, there is evidence to show that the mean serum total cholesterol in the older women is higher than that in the younger women in the community.

6.4.2 Estimation of the Ratio of Variances

6.4.2.1 Point Estimation

Let S_1^2 and S_2^2 be sample variances of random samples from two independent normally distributed populations $X_1 \sim N(\mu_1, \sigma_1^2)$ and $X_2 \sim N(\mu_2, \sigma_2^2)$, respectively, it can be proved that the ratio of sample variances S_1^2 / S_2^2 is the MVUE of the parameter σ_1^2 / σ_2^2.

6.4.2.2 Interval Estimation

We know from Section 6.2.2 that the sampling distributions of S_1^2 and S_2^2 can be standardized into random variables $(n_1-1)S_1^2/\sigma_1^2$ and $(n_2-1)S_2^2/\sigma_2^2$, respectively. Thus, the sampling distribution of S_1^2/S_2^2 can be quantitated by a new random variable F:

$$F=\frac{\dfrac{(n_1-1)S_1^2}{\sigma_1^2}/(n_1-1)}{\dfrac{(n_2-1)S_2^2}{\sigma_2^2}/(n_2-1)}=\left(\frac{S_1^2}{S_2^2}\right)\left(\frac{\sigma_2^2}{\sigma_1^2}\right)\sim F(\nu_1,\nu_2), \tag{6.41}$$

where $\nu_1=n_1-1$ and $\nu_2=n_2-1$.

The F *distribution* is also a family of distributions, typically a positively skewed distribution toward the right with scale 0 to $+\infty$. The shape of the distribution is determined by the number of degrees of freedom $(\nu_1,\ \nu_2)$.

It is obvious from Figure 6.9 that the skewness weakens as the number of degrees of freedom increases. Additionally, the shape of the F distribution imitates a normal distribution with large ν_1 and ν_2.

To construct a $(1-\alpha)\times 100\%$ CI for σ_1^2/σ_2^2, the critical values corresponding to the two-sided tail areas of the F distribution need to be determined (Figure 6.10).

For a given α and $(\nu_1,\ \nu_2)$, the critical values $F_{(\nu_1,\nu_2),\alpha/2}$ and $F_{(\nu_1,\nu_2),1-\alpha/2}$ can be located from the $F_{(\nu_1,\nu_2)}$ distribution (see Figure 6.10 and Appendix Table 7). Note that $F_{(\nu_1,\nu_2),\alpha/2}=\dfrac{1}{F_{(\nu_2,\nu_1),1-\alpha/2}}$.

With simple algebraic manipulation, we obtain

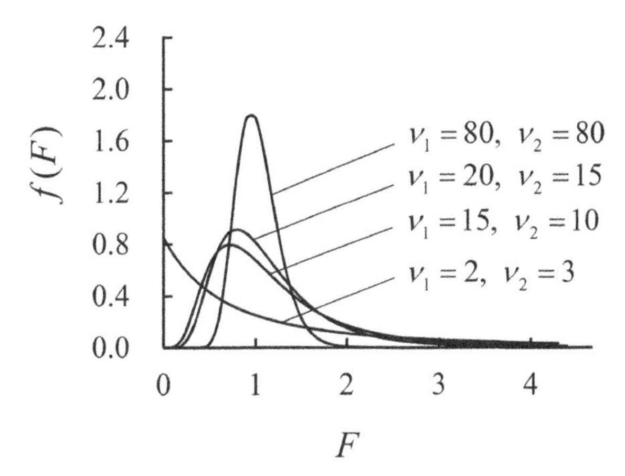

Figure 6.9 F distribution with different numbers of degrees of freedom.

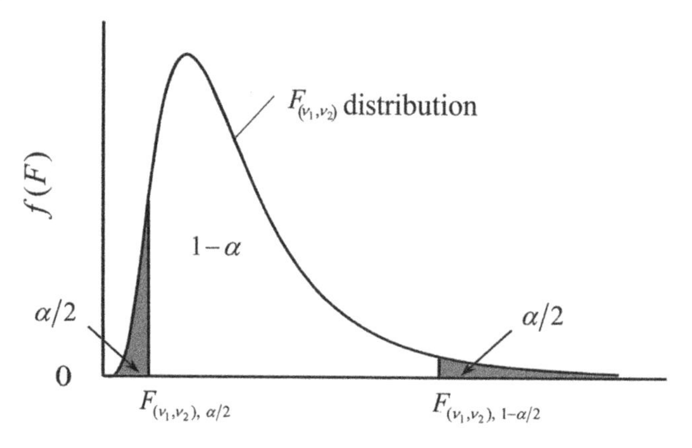

Figure 6.10 Illustration of critical values for the F distribution.

$$\begin{aligned}
1-\alpha &= P\left(F_{(\nu_1,\nu_2),\alpha/2} \le F \le F_{(\nu_1,\nu_2),1-\alpha/2}\right) \\
&= P\left(F_{(\nu_1,\nu_2),\alpha/2} \le \left(\frac{S_1^2}{S_2^2}\right)\left(\frac{\sigma_2^2}{\sigma_1^2}\right) \le F_{(\nu_1,\nu_2),1-\alpha/2}\right) \\
&= P\left(\frac{S_1^2}{S_2^2} \times \frac{1}{F_{(\nu_1,\nu_2),1-\alpha/2}} \le \frac{\sigma_1^2}{\sigma_2^2} \le \frac{S_1^2}{S_2^2} \times \frac{1}{F_{(\nu_1,\nu_2),\alpha/2}}\right).
\end{aligned} \tag{6.42}$$

Thus, the $(1-\alpha)\times 100\%$ CI for σ_1^2 / σ_2^2 is

$$\left[\frac{S_1^2}{S_2^2} \times \frac{1}{F_{(\nu_1,\nu_2),1-\alpha/2}},\ \frac{S_1^2}{S_2^2} \times \frac{1}{F_{(\nu_1,\nu_2),\alpha/2}}\right]. \tag{6.43}$$

We emphasize that the interval estimate introduced above is based on the assumption that two independent normally distributed populations hold regardless of the sizes of the two samples.

Example 6.10 Referring to Example 6.8, construct the 95% CI for the ratio of the population variances in the height between 10-year-old girls in the two regions.

Solution
We know $\nu_1 = 14,\ s_1 = 8.21,\ \nu_2 = 14,\ s_2 = 7.82$.

The critical value $F_{(14,14),1-0.05/2} = 2.98$ can be obtained according to the number of degrees of freedom $(\nu_1 = 14,\ \nu_2 = 14)$ from the critical value of the F distribution (Appendix Table 7), $F_{(14,14),0.05/2} = \dfrac{1}{F_{(14,14),1-0.05/2}} = \dfrac{1}{2.98} = 0.34$.

The 95% CI of σ_1^2 / σ_2^2 can be derived using Formula 6.43:

$$\text{LCL: } \frac{s_1^2}{s_2^2} \times \frac{1}{F_{(\nu_1,\nu_2),1-\alpha/2}} = \frac{8.21^2}{7.82^2} \times \frac{1}{2.98} = 0.37;$$

$$\text{UCL: } \frac{s_1^2}{s_2^2} \times \frac{1}{F_{(\nu_1,\nu_2),\alpha/2}} = \frac{s_1^2}{s_2^2} \times F_{(\nu_2,\nu_1),1-\alpha/2} = \frac{8.21^2}{7.82^2} \times 2.98 = 3.28.$$

Therefore, the 95% CI for σ_1^2 / σ_2^2 of 10-year-old girls' heights in regions A and B is $[0.37,\ 3.28]$.

6.4.3 Estimation of the Difference Between Rates (Normal Approximation Method)

In statistical terms, to compare two sets of data drawn from two binomial populations, we focus on the rates of success rather than the number of successes, unless the number of trials in each set is the same. Moreover, the difference between the rates is the most intuitive and straightforward measurement.

6.4.3.1 Point Estimation

Let p_1 and p_2 be sample rates from two binomial distributions that are independent of each other. According to the central limit theorem, we know that p_1 and p_2 approximately follow a normal distribution when $n_i p_i (1 - p_i) \geq 5$ $(i = 1,2)$. Then, the linear combination of p_1 and p_2 also approximately follows a normal distribution. It can be proved that the difference between $p_1 - p_2$ is an estimator of the difference $\pi_1 - \pi_2$, where

$$E(p_1 - p_2) = \pi_1 - \pi_2 \text{ and } Var(p_1 - p_2) = \frac{\pi_1(1-\pi_1)}{n_1} + \frac{\pi_2(1-\pi_2)}{n_2}.$$

Furthermore, it was verified that the difference between sample rates $p_1 - p_2$ is an MVUE of $\pi_1 - \pi_2$.

6.4.3.2 Interval Estimation

The interval estimation of the difference between rates has the same principles and procedure as the interval estimation of one sample rate. When $n_i p_i (1 - p_i) \geq 5$ $(i = 1,2)$, the sampling distribution of the difference $p_1 - p_2$ is approximately normally distributed with $\mu_{p_1 - p_2} = \pi_1 - \pi_2$ and $\sigma_{p_1 - p_2} = \sqrt{\pi_1(1-\pi_1)/n_1 + \pi_2(1-\pi_2)/n_2}$, given by

$$p_1 - p_2 \dot{\sim} N\left(\pi_1 - \pi_2, \frac{\pi_1(1-\pi_1)}{n_1} + \frac{\pi_2(1-\pi_2)}{n_2}\right). \tag{6.44}$$

Standardizing $p_1 - p_2$ into random variable Z, we have

$$Z = \frac{(p_1 - p_2) - (\pi_1 - \pi_2)}{S_{p_1 - p_2}} \dot{\sim} N(0,\ 1). \tag{6.45}$$

Thus, an approximate $(1-\alpha)\times 100\%$ CI for $\pi_1 - \pi_2$ is given by

$$\left[p_1 - p_2 - z_{1-\alpha/2}S_{p_1-p_2},\ p_1 - p_2 + z_{1-\alpha/2}S_{p_1-p_2}\right], \tag{6.46}$$

where $S_{p_1-p_2} = \sqrt{\frac{p_1(1-p_1)}{n_1} + \frac{p_2(1-p_2)}{n_2}}$ is the estimator of the standard error of $p_1 - p_2$.

Example 6.11 An occupational study was conducted to investigate the prevalence of hypertension in male workers. Among the participants, 299 were taxi drivers, with 162 having hypertension; furthermore, 408 participants were construction workers, with 195 having hypertension. Provide the 95% CI for the difference in the prevalence of hypertension between the two occupations.

Solution

Let n_1 and n_2 be the sample sizes and p_1 and p_2 be the prevalence of hypertension of the taxi drivers and construction workers, respectively:

$$p_1 = \frac{162}{299}\times 100\% = 54.2\%$$

$$p_2 = \frac{195}{408}\times 100\% = 47.8\%$$

We also have

$$n_1p_1(1-p_1) = 299\times 0.542\times(1-0.542) = 74.22 > 5$$

$$n_2p_2(1-p_2) = 408\times 0.478\times(1-0.478) = 101.80 > 5$$

which indicates the sampling distribution of difference $p_1 - p_2$ is approximately normally distributed, and we can use normal approximation method.

The estimator of the standard error of $p_1 - p_2$ is

$$S_{p_1-p_2} = \sqrt{\frac{p_1(1-p_1)}{n_1} + \frac{p_2(1-p_2)}{n_2}}$$
$$= \sqrt{\frac{54.2\%\times(1-54.2\%)}{299} + \frac{47.8\%\times(1-47.8\%)}{408}} = 0.038.$$

According to Formula 6.46, the approximate 95% CI of $\pi_1 - \pi_2$ is

$$\left[0.542 - 0.478 - 1.96\times 0.038, 0.542 - 0.478 + 1.96\times 0.038\right]$$
$$= \left[-0.010, 0.138\right].$$

The 95% CI for the difference in the prevalence of hypertension between taxi drivers and construction workers is $[-1.0\%, 13.8\%]$. Because $\text{LCL} = -0.010 < 0$,

$UCL = 0.138 > 0$. Under a 95% confidence level, there is no evidence to support the statement that the prevalence of hypertension is different between taxi drivers and construction workers.

6.5 Summary

In this chapter, we introduced several statistics with their sampling distributions. They are essential concepts that form the basis of parameter estimation and hypothesis testing, which we will discuss in the next chapter. In practice, although the sample we examined is only one of the possible random samples of a given size, the sample distribution can be found theoretically of good match to the probability distribution.

Several commonly used statistics (e.g., sample mean $\bar{X}$, sample variance S^2, and sample rate p) and their expansions (mean difference $\bar{X}_1 - \bar{X}_2$, variance ratio S_1^2 / S_2^2, and rate difference $p_1 - p_2$) are estimated by point estimation and interval estimation for the corresponding population parameters. A major topic of this chapter was interval estimation. CI establishes a range of values using sample statistics and its standard error, with a predefined confidence level to comprehensively support the parameter estimation.

Let us review the concepts and methods of point estimation and interval estimation.

(1) Scenarios for one population
   (i) The estimation of the population mean from a normal distribution or the central limit theorem holds,
   (ii) The estimation of the population variance from a normal distribution
   (iii) The estimation of parameter π from a binomial distribution when $np(1-p) > 5$ holds.

(2) Scenarios for two populations
   (i) The estimation of the mean difference $\mu_1 - \mu_2$ and rate difference $\pi_1 - \pi_2$
   (ii) The estimation of variance ratio σ_1^2 / σ_2^2.

The $(1-\alpha) \times 100\%$ CI estimation of the above parameters is based on the knowledge of random variables and their probability distributions. This highlights the importance of probability theory for statistics.

In Chapters 7 to 12, we continue our discussion on statistical inference, focusing on hypothesis testing. We see that to a certain extent, there is a coherent agreement between hypothesis testing and interval estimation.

6.6 Exercises

1. Concerning parameter estimation:
   (a) Are all statistics qualified to be estimators of the corresponding population parameters? Provide your justification.
   (b) What is the quality of "good" point estimation?

(c) How do we consider the precision of the estimation based on interval estimation? How can we improve the estimation precision?
(d) As discussed previously, the $(1-\alpha)\times 100\%$ CI can be classified into exact estimation and approximate estimation. What is the underlying rationale for such a classification?
(e) What is the role of the central limit theorem in parameter estimation?
(f) What is the interpretation of a 95% CI? Is the CI estimate with a higher level of confidence always preferred over a lower level of confidence? Suppose we set our confidence level at 99%, what would be the effect on the width of the CI?

2. The substance 3,4-dihydroxyphenylacetic acid (DOPAC, ng/ml) is a neuroactive metabolite in the tryptophan (TRP) pathway. A study was conducted to explore the differences in the concentration of DOPAC in the serum between male and female mice; the corresponding results are summarized in Table 6.4 (assuming the concentration of DOPAC is normally distributed and the population variances of male and female mice are equal).

Table 6.4 Concentration of DOPAC (ng/ml) in TRP pathways in the serum of male and female mice

Sex	n	$\bar{x}$	s
Male	32	11.43	2.87
Female	29	11.81	1.61

Source: Yao et al. (2018).

(a) Provide interval estimates of the mean and variance of the concentration of DOPAC of male mice.
(b) Which method would you use to construct the CI of the mean difference in the concentration of DOPAC in TRP pathways in the serum between male and female mice: Z or t? Justify your choice and estimate the mean difference.
(c) Estimate the ratio of variances between male and female mice.

3. A study was conducted to investigate whether elevated blood pressure is associated with maculopathy, and 100 people aged between 50 and 60 years with maculopathy were enrolled. The mean systolic blood pressure (SBP, mmHg) was 147 and the standard deviation was 27.
(a) Find the 95% CI for the population mean SBP in people with maculopathy.
(b) Find the 95% CI for the population variance of SBP in people with maculopathy.

4. In a health survey of preschool children aged 5–6 years, by stratified random sampling, the weight (kg) data of 133 boys and 162 girls were obtained. These weight data are summarized in Table 6.5 (assuming the weight is normally distributed, and its population variances of the boys and girls are equal).

Table 6.5 Summary statistics of weight (kg) of preschool children aged 5–6 years

Sex	n	$\bar{x}$	s
Boy	133	22.5	4.5
Girl	162	21.1	3.1

(a) Estimate the 90% and 95% CIs of the boys' weight. Compare and summarize the differences between these two CI estimates.
(b) Estimate the 95% CI of the mean differences between the boys' and girls' weights.
(c) Estimate the 95% CI of the ratio of variance between boys' and girls' weights.

5. In a randomized controlled trial conducted to evaluate the efficacy and safety of dopamine (DA) and norepinephrine (NE) as the initial vasopressor in septic shock, 134 and 118 septic shock patients underwent DA or NE therapy, respectively. The primary efficacy end point was all-cause 28-day mortality. The results are summarized in Table 6.6.

Table 6.6 Summary statistics of 28-day mortality following two therapies for septic shock

Treatment	n	Number of 28-day deaths	28-day mortality rate (%)
DA therapy	134	67	50.0
NE therapy	118	51	43.2

Source: Patel et al. (2010).

(a) Estimate the 95% CIs of the 28-day mortality rate following DA and NE therapy.
(b) Estimate the 95% CI of the 28-day mortality rate difference between DA and NE therapy.

6. It has been reported that the Kazakhs, a minority group in the Xinjiang area of China with agriculture and animal husbandry as their main employment, show a high rate of hypertension. Using a multistage sampling technique, a random sample of 1445 adult Kazakhs ($\geq$ 30 years old) living in Altay, Xingjiang region of China was obtained. Among them, 536 hypertensive individuals were identified; their daily salt intake was 18.7 ± 13.0 (g/day), whereas that for individuals with normal blood pressure was 12.2 ± 13.0 (g/day). Assume that daily salt intake is normally distributed, and its population variances for hypertensive and nonhypertensive Kazakh people are equal.

(a) Construct a 95% CI for the difference in the mean daily salt intake for hypertensive and nonhypertensive Kazakh people. What is the precision of the estimate?

(b) In this case, what conclusion can you draw based on the 95% CI?

(c) Describe the population about which an inference can be made.

7

Hypothesis Testing for One Parameter

CONTENTS

7.1 Overview

In Chapter 6, we introduced the sampling distributions of several common statistics and parameter estimation. We continue with this development in this chapter while introducing another primary tool of inference: *hypothesis testing*. Similar to parameter estimation, hypothesis testing is another utilization of sampling distribution of statistics to infer population parameters. However, the objectives of these two methods are different. Parameter estimation, as the name implies, is used to quantify the magnitude of unknown parameters of the population, whereas hypothesis testing is used to justify the assumptions and make the go/no-go decision on the population. For example, a pharmaceutical company wants to know whether the benefit–risk profile of a new therapy is more favorable than an existing treatment, or a health organization wants to determine whether the physiological indicators of newborns in rural areas are different from those in urban areas. Hypothesis testing can provide an

Applied Medical Statistics, First Edition. Jingmei Jiang.

Companion website: www.wiley.com\go\jiang\appliedmedicalstatistics

objective framework for making decisions using probabilistic methods rather than relying on subjective impressions. In other words, opinions can be different among individuals looking at the same data; however, a hypothesis test provides a uniform decision-making criterion regardless of the perceptions of the data.

7.1.1 Concepts and Procedures

In statistics, a hypothesis is a statement about characteristics of a population. A *hypothesis test (or significance test)* is a standard procedure for testing that statement. The usual procedure is as follows:

(1) State the hypotheses of interest as the null and alternative hypotheses.
(2) Select a significance level.
(3) Determine an appropriate method of hypothesis testing and calculate the test statistic.
(4) Determine the p value and draw a conclusion.

Let us discuss this procedure with an example.

Example 7.1 Suppose the mean pulse rate in healthy adults is 72 beats per min. Research was conducted to examine the pulse rate in patients with hyperthyroidism. Twenty patients were randomly enrolled with a mean of 80 and a standard deviation of 20. Assuming that the pulse rate follows a normal distribution, is the mean pulse rate in hyperthyroidism patients different from that in healthy adults?

This type of question can be formulated in a hypothesis testing framework by specifying two hypotheses: a null and an alternative hypothesis.

(1) State the hypotheses
The *null hypothesis*, denoted by H_0, is the hypothesis that is to be tested. The *alternative hypothesis*, denoted by H_1, is the hypothesis that, in some sense, contradicts the null hypothesis.

In Example 7.1, the null hypothesis H_0 is that the mean pulse rate in hyperthyroidism patients μ is the same as the mean pulse rate in healthy adults μ_0. Here μ_0 is known and μ is unknown; the alternative hypothesis H_1 is that the mean pulse rate in hyperthyroidism patients μ is not the same as the mean pulse rate in healthy adults μ_0. Note that H_1 may have multiple options (more than, less than, or not the same as).

These hypotheses can be written more succinctly in the following manner:

(i) $H_0 : \mu = \mu_0 = 72$,
(ii) $H_1 : \mu > \mu_0 = 72$,
(iii) $H_1 : \mu < \mu_0 = 72$, or
(iv) $H_1 : \mu \neq \mu_0 = 72$, including ($\mu > \mu_0$ or $\mu < \mu_0$).

Here, (ii) and (iii) are one-sided hypotheses and (iv) is a two-sided hypothesis (we will discuss them in Section 7.1.3). The three scenarios of H_1 cannot exist simultaneously. Usually, the null hypothesis H_0 is paired with one of three H_1 hypotheses, and the two-sided hypothesis is the most common selection in practice.

In Example 7.1, we state the two-sided hypothesis; i.e., assume that the mean pulse rate in hyperthyroidism patients may deviate from 72 in either direction. That is

$$H_0 : \mu = \mu_0 = 72 \text{ vs. } H_1 : \mu \neq \mu_0 = 72$$

Thus, we have generated two mutually exclusive and all-inclusive possibilities. Either H_0 or H_1 will be true, but not both. So is our decision when we compare the probabilities of obtaining the sample data under each of these hypotheses. In practice, the testing procedure usually starts with H_0, and when it is completed, the hypothesis testing will suggest either the rejection or non-rejection of H_0, indirectly also determining H_1.

(2) Select a significance level
After stating the hypotheses, a *significance level*, denoted as α, is specified. It is defined as the probability of making a mistake — rejecting H_0 when H_0 is true (i.e., Type I error, see Section 7.1.2). The selection of α is arbitrary although in practice, values of 0.01, 0.05, or 0.10 are commonly used. Because the significance level α reflects the probability of rejecting a true H_0, therefore this probability is deliberately selected.

In Example 7.1, we select $\alpha = 0.05$, indicating that a mistake having minor probabilities should not occur in a single trial. Thus, it is rational to reject H_0.

(3) Determine an appropriate test method and derive a test statistic
Once we set up the hypotheses and select significance level α, we need to determine a method of hypothesis testing. There are multiple aspects to be considered: research objective, type of data, and sample size.

Conventionally, the methods of hypothesis testing are named after the test statistics. For example, the t-test method, which we will discuss in this section, is built upon the t-test statistic. Here, we call a random variable t a *test statistic* under hypothesis H_0 because, as we will soon infer, procedures of the hypothesis testing are based on the distribution of the test statistics.

The test statistic is not a new concept in this text. For example, we know from Formula 6.6, for a random sample from a normal population, when σ is unknown, the sampling distribution of $\bar{X}$ follows a t distribution with ν degrees of freedom, that is

$$t = \frac{\bar{X} - \mu}{S / \sqrt{n}} \sim t(v),\ v = n - 1$$

Under $H_0: \mu = \mu_0$, we replace unknown parameter μ with known parameter μ_0. The random variable t, in this case, is called a test statistic

$$t = \frac{\bar{X} - \mu_0}{S / \sqrt{n}} \sim t(v),\ v = n - 1 \tag{7.1}$$

In Example 7.1, $H_0: \mu = \mu_0 = 72$, where σ is unknown, we have $\bar{x} = 80$, $s = 20$, and $\nu = n - 1 = 20 - 1 = 19$, the value of test statistic is

$$t = \frac{\bar{X} - \mu_0}{s / \sqrt{n}} = \frac{80 - 72}{20 / \sqrt{20}} = 1.79$$

We see from Formula 7.1 that it is more convenient to define the criterion for statistical inference in terms of standardized values rather than in terms of $\bar{X}$ (because $\bar{X}$ depends on the unit of measurement). The t-test statistic measures the standardized "distance" between $\bar{X}$ and μ_0. If $|t|$ is close to zero, which occurs when $\bar{X}$ is close to μ_0, H_0 is unlikely to be true. When $|t|$ is large, which occurs when $\bar{X}$ is far away from μ_0, H_0 is unlikely to be true. In hypothesis testing, we need to determine the point at which $|t|$ is "too large." This point is called the critical value of t in the t_ν distribution, which will be discussed in the next step.

(4) Determine the p value and draw a conclusion
The t-test statistic in Example 7.1 is a continuous random variable that ranges from negative to positive infinity. How can we make an explicit decision using this scale? With the density function of t-test statistic, we can locate the probability of its distribution, transforming the scale of the t-test statistic intuitively into a p value.

As we emphasized earlier, hypothesis testing is based on the test statistics where H_0 is assumed to be true. Hence the p value expresses the probability of given data if H_0 is true. Alternatively, a low p value indicates that the observed data are not consistent with the null hypothesis – they are unlikely to occur if H_0 is true. In this situation, we state that H_0 is not true or we reject H_0 and decide that H_1 is true.

How to obtain p value of the test statistic? Typically, there are two approaches:

(i) The critical-value method
The test is defined by its *critical region* (alternatively called the rejection region). A critical region defines the set of outcomes of a statistical test for which the null hypothesis is to be rejected. A visual description of this approach for one sample t-test is depicted in Figure 7.1, in which we compute a t-test statistic and determine the outcome of a test by comparing the t-test statistic with a critical value $t_{\nu,\alpha/2}$ or $t_{\nu,1-\alpha/2}$ according to the prespecified α in the Appendix Table 4.

In Figure 7.1, we can see that two critical values are essentially cut-offs dividing the area under the curve (probability) into three parts: lower-sided rejection, upper-sided rejection, and non-rejection regions in the center. If the value of the t-test statistic falls into the *rejection region* $\left(|t| > t_{\nu,1-\alpha/2}\right)$, corresponding to $p < \alpha$, we reject H_0 at the level α and accept H_1. We declare that μ and μ_0 are different. We can be confident that a correct decision has been made because the chance of committing a Type I error is minor (0.05). Otherwise, if the t value falls into the *non-rejection region* $\left(|t| \le t_{\nu,1-\alpha/2}\right)$, we do not reject H_0; we cannot confidently assume that a correct decision has been made (i.e., say accept H_0) because the probability of committing a Type II error is unknown (see Section 7.1.2 for further discussion). In such a case, a weaker statement is made at the conclusion of the test.

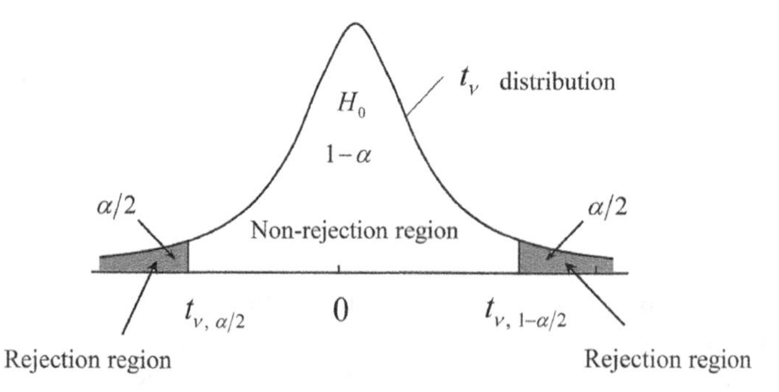

Figure 7.1 Illustration of the rejection and non-rejection regions for the one-sample t-test (two-sided alternative).

We use the following expression for a more formal representation of the critical-value method.

For a one-sample t-test, to test $H_0: \mu = \mu_0$ vs. $H_1: \mu \neq \mu_0$ with a significance level of α, the test statistic is $t = (\bar{X} - \mu_0)/(S/\sqrt{n})$, while $t_{\nu,\alpha/2}$ and $t_{\nu,1-\alpha/2}$ are critical values of the t_ν distribution.

If $|t| > t_{\nu,1-\alpha/2}$, then reject H_0;

If $|t| \leq t_{\nu,1-\alpha/2}$, then do not reject H_0.

In Example 7.1, the critical value is $t_{19,1-0.05/2} = 2.093$, whereas $t = 1.79$. Since $t = 1.79 < 2.093 = t_{19,1-0.05/2}$, $p > 0.05$. We do not reject H_0 at the $\alpha = 0.05$ level, and the evidence is insufficient to show that the mean pulse rate in hyperthyroidism patients is different from that in healthy adults.

(ii) The p-value method

The most popular decision method applied for hypothesis testing nowadays is to contrast the p value with a prespecified α. This is just a probabilistic presentation of the test statistic and critical value.

For example, the p value for the one-sample t-test for the mean of a normal distribution (two-sided alternative) is defined as

$$p = \begin{cases} 2 \times (\text{area to the left of } t) = 2 \times P(t_\nu < t), \text{ if } t \leq 0 \\ 2 \times (\text{area to the right of } t) = 2 \times P(t_\nu > t), \text{ if } t > 0 \end{cases}. \tag{7.2}$$

Thus, in plain language, if $t \leq 0$, then the p value equals twice the area under a t_ν distribution to the left of t; if $t > 0$, then the p value equals twice the area under a t_ν distribution to the right of t.

The p value is the probability under the null hypothesis of obtaining a test statistic (t_ν) as extreme as or more extreme than the observed test statistic (t value). As illustrated in Figure 7.2, the smaller the p value, the stronger the evidence against H_0. If the p value is less than the prespecified probability α, then H_0 is rejected; otherwise, it is not rejected.

In Example 7.1, $t = 1.79 > 0$, according to Formula 7.2, the p value (two-sided) is $p = 2 \times P(t_\nu > t) = 2 \times P(t_{19} > 1.79)$, using the TDIST function of Excel, the probability is given by $p = \text{TDIST}(1.79, 19, 2) = 0.0894 > 0.05$, where 19 is the number of degrees of freedom of the t distribution and the value 2 indicates a two-sided probability distribution. Again, we have insufficient evidence to reject H_0 (Note: the p value can also be calculated using other software).

Although the two approaches yield consistent results, the p-value method seems more favorable, particularly for research in which α is not prespecified. The p-value method can be used to evaluate the strength of the evidence. The following consensus provides the guidelines when interpreting the strength with p value:

If $0.01 \leq p < 0.05$, then the results are significant;

If $0.001 \leq p < 0.01$, then the results are highly significant;

If $p < 0.001$, then the results are strongly significant;

If $p \geq 0.05$, then the results are considered statistically nonsignificant (sometimes denoted by NS).

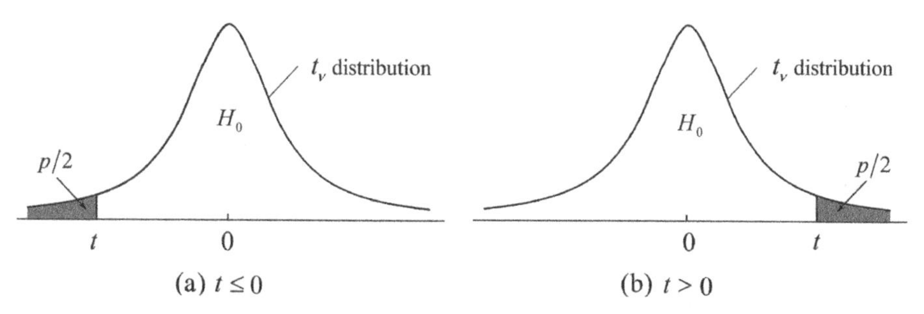

Figure 7.2 Illustration of the p-value method for the one-sample t-test (two-sided alternative).

It should be noted that regardless of whether the critical-value or the p-value methods are used, the decision about H_0 will always be the same if you use the same significance level. Observed significance levels (p value) are more easily obtained using a statistical software than probability tables or formulas.

At this point, we can summarize three crucial points for the process of hypothesis testing: (i) for a given null hypothesis, select the maximum value of α that we are willing to handle; (ii) determine a testing method (critical-value method or p-value method) of the test; and (iii) reject the null hypothesis if $p < \alpha$.

In addition, there are two major points to be noted. Shown in Example 7.1, the rejection of H_0 refers to the difference between population parameter μ and μ_0 rather than sample mean $\bar{X}$ and μ_0, although the test statistic is computed from sample data. As we explained at the beginning of this section, the purpose of hypothesis testing is to justify the assumption regarding the population parameter, where the sample mean $\bar{X}$ is only an estimate of μ. Furthermore, the results of hypothesis testing should be interpreted with caution. Despite a substantial difference between the two populations, the sample size has a strong effect when constructing the test statistic, and a larger sample size results in a smaller p value. Therefore, a proper power analysis or sample size calculation is crucial in research (we will discuss these in Section 7.2).

7.1.2 Type I and Type II Errors

There is always a probability of an error occurring when using hypothesis testing because uncertainty is part of any probability model. Even a statistically significant result cannot guarantee a conclusion having an accuracy of 100%. The mistakes, or errors, are mainly attributed to the following two sources:

(1) Hypothesis testing is typically performed using a random sample $X_1, X_2, \ldots, X_n$, although the conclusion is with regard to a population parameter.
(2) The decision to reject H_0 is based on the belief that events with low probabilities are unlikely to occur in a single trial. However, rare events will occur as long as the sample has a random property. Therefore, rejecting H_0 does not indicate that it is false because we can derive samples with a low probability of H_0 being true. Not rejecting H_0 does not imply that it is true because we can derive samples with a probability of H_1 being true and a small sample size can also contribute to the non-rejection of H_0. When we conduct hypothesis testing, there are four possible outcomes conditional on the unknown truth (see Table 7.1).

Table 7.1 The possible outcomes of testing H_0.

Results of test	True situation	
	H_0 **is true**	H_0 **is false**
Not reject H_0	Correct decision $(1-\alpha)$	Type II error (β)
Reject H_0	Type I error (α)	Correct decision $(1-\beta)$

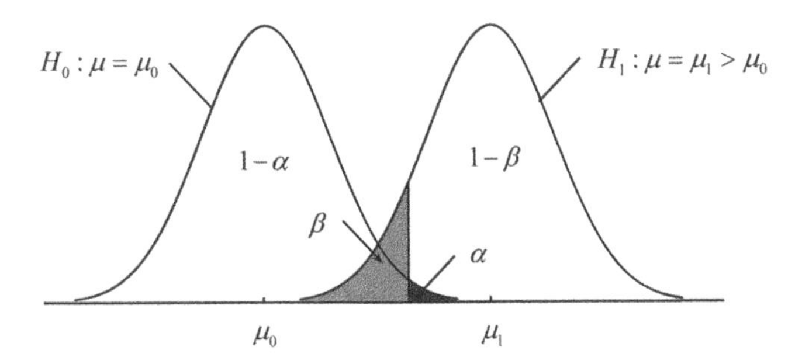

Figure 7.3 Illustration of the two types of errors of hypothesis testing (only $\mu_1 > \mu_0$ displayed).

In Table 7.1, apart from the correct decisions $1-\alpha$ and $1-\beta$, two errors can occur, and we label these as Type I and Type II errors, respectively.

The probability of *Type I error* (denoted by α) is the probability of rejecting H_0 when H_0 is true, i.e., $\alpha = P(\text{reject } H_0 \mid H_0 \text{ is true})$. We usually set a limit of 0.05 (5%) for a Type I error probability, which is equivalent to a 0.05 cut-off for statistical significance.

The probability of *Type II error* (denoted by β) is the probability of not rejecting H_0 when H_1 is true, i.e., $\beta = P(\text{not reject } H_0 \mid H_1 \text{ is true})$.

α is specified by the researcher and β regarding the truth of H_1 is difficult to calculate. Therefore, we attempt to reject H_0 based on sample data in favor of H_1 in hypothesis testing, and then we only need to focus on the level of α. It is widely accepted that the probability of a Type II error should be no more than 0.20 (20%).

We can further visualize the two types of error in a plot like that in Figure 7.3.

Then, what are the Type I and Type II errors for the data in Example 7.1?

Type I error occurs when deciding that patients with hyperthyroidism have a mean pulse rate not the same as 72 (μ_0), while their mean pulse rate is in fact the same as that level. Type II error occurs when deciding that patients with hyperthyroidism have a mean pulse rate the same as 72 (μ_0), while their mean pulse rate is in fact not the same as that level.

The chance of encountering two types of errors is inversely related when the sample size is fixed. Decreasing the risk of a Type I error will increase the risk of a Type II error. A proper decision should be made to minimize the probability of the error when conducting a hypothesis test. When H_0 is true, increasing the sample size is the only solution. It minimizes the sample variance, improving the robustness of the statistical inference.

7.1.3 One-sided and Two-sided Hypothesis

When conducting a hypothesis test, the choice of selecting a one-sided versus two-sided hypothesis is an important step. The selection may affect the conclusion. For example, in Example 7.1, we used a two-sided hypothesis, which suggests that the alternative hypothesis H_1 allows the difference to be in either direction. In other words, the patients with hyperthyroidism could have higher or lower pulse rates than the healthy adults.

In *two-sided hypothesis testing*, the significance level of 0.05 was split and 0.025 was allocated to each distribution tail. Conversely, *one-sided hypothesis testing* allots the significance level only in one direction to either the lower or upper tail. The probability of the other direction is thus completely ignored (see Figure 7.4).

In practice, selecting one-sided or two-sided testing depends on the research objective to be addressed. Sometimes in biological studies, any type of effect is of interest to researchers irrespective of whether it is either positive or negative, just like Example 7.1. In this case, the two-sided hypothesis is appropriate. Conversely, when the effect varies in only one direction, for instance, the average cholesterol level in an Asian population is usually lower than that in a European population, the one-sided hypothesis is appropriate. It does not distinguish between "no difference" and "higher cholesterol level."

Example 7.2 Let's continue with Example 7.1 and assume the investigator had a strong belief based on a clinical justification that the mean pulse rate in hyperthyroidism patients was higher than that in healthy adults. Conduct a one-sided hypothesis test.

Solution

(1) State the hypotheses and select a significance level

$$H_0: \mu = \mu_0 = 72$$

$$H_1: \mu > \mu_0 = 72$$

$$\alpha = 0.05$$

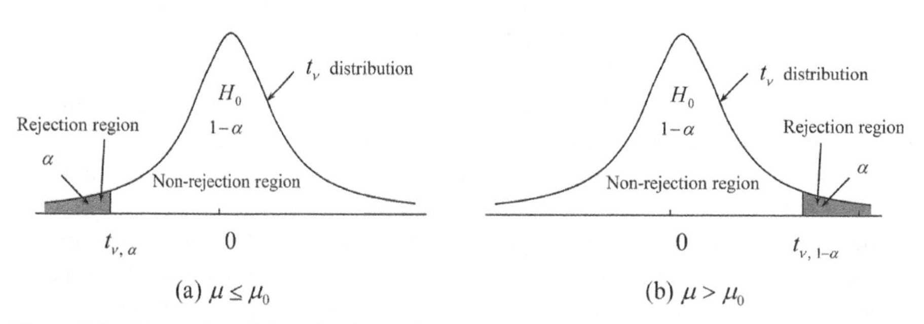

Figure 7.4 Illustration of the rejection and non-rejection regions for the one-sample t-test (one-sided alternative).

(2) Determine the test statistic

We know that $\bar{x}=80$, $s=20$, and $\nu=n-1=20-1=19$. The test statistic t value is

$$t=\frac{\bar{x}-\mu_0}{s/\sqrt{n}}=\frac{80-72}{20/\sqrt{20}}=1.79$$

(3) Draw a conclusion

(i) Critical-value method

For given $\alpha=0.05$, $\nu=19$, the critical value for one-sided testing is $t_{19,1-0.05}=1.729$. Since $t=1.79>1.729=t_{19,1-0.05}$, $p<0.05$, we reject H_0 and accept H_1 at the $\alpha=0.05$ level and declare that the mean pulse rate among patients with hyperthyroidism is significantly higher than that in healthy adults.

(ii) p-value method

Since $t=1.79>0$, we calculate the p value (one-sided) as $p=P(t_\nu>t)=P(t_{19}>1.79)$. Using the TDIST function of Excel, the probability is obtained as $p=\text{TDIST}(1.79,19,1)=0.0447<0.05$, where 19 is the number of degrees of freedom of the t distribution while the value 1 indicates a one-sided probability distribution. The obtained result is significant.

Comparing Examples 7.1 and 7.2, the same issue is investigated, and we may yield different conclusions with different types of hypothesis. The selection entirely depends on the research objective and expertise. There is a concrete rule about the testing process that states we must decide the type of hypothesis that would be used at the beginning of the research prior to looking at the data. Performing two-sided hypothesis testing, resulting in a nonsignificant conclusion, and subsequently switching to one-sided hypothesis testing, is not advocated.

7.1.4 Association Between Hypothesis Testing and Interval Estimation

We discussed the interval estimation in Chapter 6. Interval estimation is intuitively related to hypothesis testing. The conclusions based on the p value and CI agree with each other as the significance and confidence levels define the distance of variation in the same manner. Taking two-sided hypothesis testing ($H_0:\mu=\mu_0$, $H_1:\mu\neq\mu_0$) as an example, we can use the CI to determine whether to reject or to not reject H_0. Assuming that the two-sided significance level is α, the $(1-\alpha)\times 100\%$ CI of μ contains all values of μ_0 such that we do not reject H_0 using a two-sided test with significance level α. Conversely, the $(1-\alpha)\times 100\%$ CI does not contain any value μ_0 for which we can reject H_0 using a two-sided test with a significance level α. The proof is as follows:

We know that the $(1-\alpha)\times 100\%$ CI of μ is $[\bar{X}-t_{v,1-\alpha/2}S/\sqrt{n}, \bar{X}+t_{v,1-\alpha/2}S/\sqrt{n}]$; it translates to $t<t_{v,\alpha/2}$ or $t>t_{v,1-\alpha/2}$ when rejecting H_0 at significant level α.

If $t=\dfrac{\bar{X}-\mu_0}{S/\sqrt{n}}<t_{v,\alpha/2}$, then $\bar{X}<\mu_0+t_{v,\alpha/2}S/\sqrt{n}$, and we have

$$\mu_0>\bar{X}-t_{v,\alpha/2}S/\sqrt{n}\triangleq C_1$$

Otherwise, if $t > t_{\nu,1-\alpha/2}$, then $\bar{X} > \mu_0 + t_{\nu,1-\alpha/2} S / \sqrt{n}$, and we have

$$\mu_0 < \bar{X} - t_{\nu,1-\alpha/2} S / \sqrt{n} \triangleq C_2$$

where $\triangleq$ stands for "defined as."

When we reject H_0, either $\mu_0 > C_1$ or $\mu_0 < C_2$ must be true, suggesting that the $(1-\alpha)\times 100\%$ CI does not include μ_0. Conversely, if we fail to reject H_0, the $(1-\alpha)\times 100\%$ CI includes μ_0. Therefore, we can use $(1-\alpha)\times 100\%$ CI to determine the statistical significance.

Example 7.3 Recall Example 7.1. Construct the 95% CI for the mean pulse rate in hyperthyroidism patients and answer the same question: whether the mean pulse rate in patients with hyperthyroidism is different from the mean in healthy adults.

Solution

We have $\bar{x} = 80$, $s = 20$, and $n = 20$. Let $\alpha = 0.05$ and $\nu = 20 - 1 = 19$. We can determine the critical value $t_{19,1-0.05/2} = 2.093$ according to the t_{19} distribution. The 95% CI of μ is estimated as

$$\begin{aligned}&\left[\bar{x} - t_{19,1-0.05/2} s / \sqrt{n}, \bar{x} + t_{19,1-0.05/2} s / \sqrt{n}\right]\\ &= \left[80 - 2.093 \times 20 / \sqrt{20}, 80 + 2.093 \times 20 / \sqrt{20}\right]\\ &= \left[71, 89\right].\end{aligned}$$

The 95% CI $[71, 89]$ contains $\mu_0 = 72$, which is consistent with the conclusion for Example 7.1, where we do not reject $H_0 : \mu = \mu_0 = 72$ at the significance level $\alpha = 0.05$.

This example provides an empirical demonstration of the connection between the CI method and hypothesis testing. Let us illustrate this connection in a more formal manner using the probability presented.

Recalling Formula 6.21 on the $(1-\alpha)\times 100\%$ CI of the population mean, we have

$$P\left(-t_{\nu,1-\alpha/2} \le \frac{\bar{X} - \mu}{S / \sqrt{n}} \le t_{\nu,1-\alpha/2}\right) = 1 - \alpha. \tag{7.3}$$

Under $H_0 : \mu = \mu_0$ in hypothesis testing for one sample introduced in this chapter, we have the following:

If

$$P\left(-t_{\nu,1-\alpha/2} \le \frac{\bar{X} - \mu_0}{S / \sqrt{n}} \le t_{\nu,1-\alpha/2}\right) = 1 - \alpha, \tag{7.4}$$

then H_0 is not to be rejected.

If

$$P\left(\frac{\left|\bar{X} - \mu_0\right|}{S / \sqrt{n}} > t_{\nu,1-\alpha/2}\right) = \alpha, \tag{7.5}$$

then H_0 is to be rejected.

The probability $1-\alpha$ is identical in Formulas 7.3 and 7.4 yet intended for different purposes. Formula 7.3 quantifies the level of confidence in the interval estimation of the population parameter, whereas Formula 7.4 is for quantifying the probability that $H_0: \mu = \mu_0$ is true; otherwise, according to Formula 7.5, the hypothesis H_0 barely holds.

Here, we see that the sampling distribution of statistics is the common theoretical basis for interval estimation and hypothesis testing. What are the unique strengths of these two methods? In scientific research, there is a considerable focus on discovering statistically significant effects (typically, a p value less than 0.05). However, a statistically significant effect might not always translate to a practically meaningful finding. When the sample size is large, even a minor effect with no clinical meaning can be of statistical significance. Conversely, CI considers both the magnitude and precision of the observed effect. Ideally, we encourage the reporting of both p value and CI for statistical inference.

7.2 Hypothesis Testing for One Parameter

7.2.1 Hypothesis Tests for the Mean

Example 7.4 It is known from a large-scale survey that the mean birth weight (kg) of live births in a region is 3.12. A study was conducted to examine the birth weight of babies whose mothers have gestational diabetes (Chen et al. 2012). Twenty-five of the babies whose mothers have gestational diabetes were randomly selected in a hospital in this region. The mean birth weight was 3.22 and the standard deviation was 0.40. Assuming the birth weight follows a normal distribution, is there any difference between the mean birth weight of the babies whose mothers have gestational diabetes in this hospital and live births in the region?

Solution

(1) State the hypotheses and select a significance level

$$H_0: \mu = \mu_0 = 3.12$$

$$H_1: \mu \neq \mu_0 = 3.12$$

$$\alpha = 0.05$$

(2) Determine the test statistic

We know that $\mu_0 = 3.12$, $\bar{x} = 3.22$, $s = 0.40$, and $n = 25$. As σ is unknown and the sample size is small, and the t test statistic is selected and

$$t = \frac{\bar{x} - \mu_0}{s/\sqrt{n}} = \frac{3.22 - 3.12}{0.40/\sqrt{25}} = 1.25$$

(3) Draw a conclusion

(i) Critical-value method

For given $\alpha = 0.05$ and $\nu = n - 1 = 25 - 1 = 24$, the critical value for a two-sided test is $t_{24,1-0.05/2} = 2.064$ (Appendix Table 4). As $|t| = 1.25 < 2.064 = t_{24,1-0.05/2}$, then $p > 0.05$, and we do not reject H_0 at the $\alpha = 0.05$ level.

(ii) p-value method

Since $t = 1.25 > 0$, according to Formula 7.2, the p value (two-sided) is $p = 2 \times P(t_\nu > t) = 2 \times P(t_{24} > 1.25)$. Using the TDIST function of Excel, the probability is obtained as $p = \text{TDIST}(1.25, 24, 2) = 0.2234 > 0.05$, which shows no significant difference between the birth weight of the babies whose mothers have gestational diabetes in this hospital and live births in the region.

In Example 7.4, one assumption is that we do not know σ and the sample size is insufficient $(n < 30)$. In this case, the test statistic, often referred to as t, follows the t distribution with ν degrees of freedom. If the sample size is sufficiently large, an alternative test statistic $Z = (\bar{X} - \mu_0)/(S/\sqrt{n})$ based on the standard normal distribution may be used, and the results from these tests are virtually identical.

7.2.1.1 Power of the Test

The statistical power is an important quantity in hypothesis testing, which can be used as enrichment during the decision-making process. Unlike α, which is considered as a threshold for the p value, the statistical power provides a measurement of the ability to detect a specific effect if it exists. The reason we state "specific effect" is because the power against all possible values that negate to H_0 cannot be calculated unless their probabilities are known.

We generally denote *statistical power* as $1 - \beta$, which defines the probability of correctly rejecting H_0 (when a specific H_1 is true) under α.

$$\text{power} = 1 - \beta = P(\text{reject } H_0 | H_1 \text{ is true}). \tag{7.6}$$

In practice, the determination of power is used to plan a study before any data have been obtained. We also usually make a projection concerning the variances without having any data to estimate it. Therefore, we assume the variances are known and base power calculations on the one-sample Z-test as provided in the following calculation:

1. Two-sided Hypothesis

Suppose we wish to conduct the following test:

$H_0: \mu = \mu_0$, $H_1: \mu = \mu_1 \neq \mu_0$, assuming the population variances are known and equal, the sample mean $\bar{X}$ follows a normal distribution, i.e., $\bar{X} \sim N(\mu_0, \sigma^2/n)$ under H_0.

To reject H_0, the test statistic Z must satisfy

$$\begin{aligned} & P(Z < z_{\alpha/2} | \mu = \mu_1) \\ & = P\left(\frac{\bar{X} - \mu_0}{\sigma/\sqrt{n}} < z_{\alpha/2} \middle| \mu = \mu_1\right) \\ & = P\left(\bar{X} < \mu_0 + z_{\alpha/2}\sigma/\sqrt{n} \middle| \mu = \mu_1\right), \end{aligned} \tag{7.7}$$

or

$$\begin{aligned} & P(Z > z_{1-\alpha/2} | \mu = \mu_1) \\ & = P\left(\frac{\bar{X} - \mu_0}{\sigma/\sqrt{n}} > z_{1-\alpha/2} \middle| \mu = \mu_1\right) \\ & = P\left(\bar{X} > \mu_0 + z_{1-\alpha/2}\sigma/\sqrt{n} \middle| \mu = \mu_1\right). \end{aligned} \tag{7.8}$$

In addition, under H_1, the sample mean is $\bar{X} \sim N\left(\mu_1, \sigma^2 / n\right)$. By standardizing $\mu_0 + z_{\alpha/2}\sigma / \sqrt{n}$ and $\mu_0 + z_{1-\alpha/2}\sigma / \sqrt{n}$, the statistical power is obtained as

$$
\begin{aligned}
1-\beta &= \Phi\left(\frac{\mu_0 + z_{\alpha/2}\sigma / \sqrt{n} - \mu_1}{\sigma / \sqrt{n}}\right) + 1 - \Phi\left(\frac{\mu_0 + z_{1-\alpha/2}\sigma / \sqrt{n} - \mu_1}{\sigma / \sqrt{n}}\right) \\
&= \Phi\left(z_{\alpha/2} + \frac{(\mu_0 - \mu_1)}{\sigma}\sqrt{n}\right) + 1 - \Phi\left(z_{1-\alpha/2} + \frac{(\mu_0 - \mu_1)}{\sigma}\sqrt{n}\right) \\
&= \Phi\left(z_{\alpha/2} + \frac{(\mu_0 - \mu_1)}{\sigma}\sqrt{n}\right) + \Phi\left(z_{\alpha/2} + \frac{(\mu_1 - \mu_0)}{\sigma}\sqrt{n}\right).
\end{aligned}
\tag{7.9}
$$

Because one of the two additive terms on the right side of Formula 7.9 would approximate zero when H_1 is true, the power of the test can be approximated as

$$
1-\beta \approx \Phi\left(z_{\alpha/2} + \frac{|\mu_1 - \mu_0|}{\sigma}\sqrt{n}\right), \tag{7.10}
$$

where $|\mu_1 - \mu_0| / \sigma$ is defined as the *effect size*, denoted by ES, i.e.,

$$
\mathrm{ES} = \frac{|\mu_1 - \mu_0|}{\sigma}, \tag{7.11}
$$

which represents the standardized difference in means specified under H_0 and H_1.

Thus, Formula 7.10 can be rewritten as

$$
1-\beta \approx \Phi\left(z_{\alpha/2} + \mathrm{ES}\sqrt{n}\right). \tag{7.12}
$$

In practice, σ is rarely known, and we often use the sample standard deviation s to estimate it.

Figure 7.5 (a–b) provides an intuitive illustration. The area to the left of $\mu_0 + z_{\alpha/2}\sigma / \sqrt{n}$ and to the right of $\mu_0 + z_{1-\alpha/2}\sigma / \sqrt{n}$ under H_0 is the significance level α. The area defined by limit $\mu_0 + z_{\alpha/2}\sigma / \sqrt{n}$ and $\mu_0 + z_{1-\alpha/2}\sigma / \sqrt{n}$ under H_1 is the statistical power $1-\beta$.

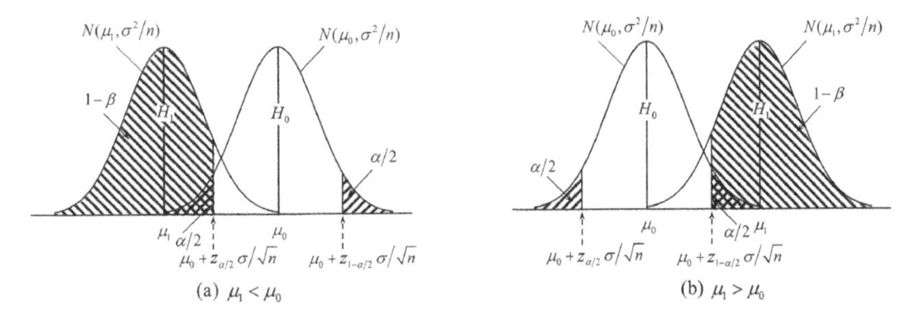

Figure 7.5 Illustration of power for the one-sample Z-test for the mean of a normal distribution with a known variance (two-sided alternative).

We infer from Formula 7.12 and Figure 7.5 that the statistical power $1-\beta$ is related to several factors:

(1) The larger the value of α, the closer the limits ($\mu_0 + z_{\alpha/2}\sigma/\sqrt{n}$ and $\mu_0 + z_{1-\alpha/2}\sigma/\sqrt{n}$) are toward μ_0 and the higher the power $1-\beta$.
(2) The larger the value of ES, the larger the standardized difference under H_0 and H_1 and the higher the power $1-\beta$.
(3) The larger the value of n, the narrower the shape of the distribution and the higher the power $1-\beta$.

Example 7.5 Following Example 7.4, calculate the statistical power for $\mu_1 \neq \mu_0$.

Solution
We know that $\mu_0 = 3.12$; assume that alternative mean $\mu_1 = 3.22$ (instead of $\bar{x} = 3.22$), $\sigma = 0.40$ (instead of $s = 0.40$), and $n = 25$, $z_{0.05/2} = -1.96$. Therefore, from Formula 7.12, the power is expressed as

$$
\begin{aligned}
1-\beta &\approx \Phi\left(z_{\alpha/2} + ES\sqrt{n}\right) \\
&= \Phi\left(-1.96 + \frac{|3.22 - 3.12|}{0.40} \times \sqrt{25}\right) \\
&= \Phi(-0.71) = 0.2389
\end{aligned}
$$

There is a probability of 23.89% to detect a significant difference using a two-sided test of a sample size of 25 at a significance level $\alpha = 0.05$. It is no accident that we fail to discover an effect from hypothesis testing in Example 7.4. One possible cause is an insufficient sample size.

2. One-sided Hypothesis
To test the hypothesis: $H_0 : \mu = \mu_0$, $H_1 : \mu = \mu_1 < \mu_0$, we have the power (Figure 7.6(a))

$$1-\beta = \Phi\left(z_\alpha + \frac{(\mu_0 - \mu_1)}{\sigma}\sqrt{n}\right). \tag{7.13}$$

Alternatively, for $H_1 : \mu_1 > \mu_0$, we can derive a similar function for power (Figure 7.6(b))

$$1-\beta = \Phi\left(z_\alpha + \frac{(\mu_1 - \mu_0)}{\sigma}\sqrt{n}\right). \tag{7.14}$$

Finally, the power of the test for a one-sided hypothesis can be denoted by the following:

$$1-\beta = \Phi\left(z_\alpha + \frac{|\mu_1 - \mu_0|}{\sigma}\sqrt{n}\right) = \Phi\left(z_\alpha + \mathrm{ES}\sqrt{n}\right), \tag{7.15}$$

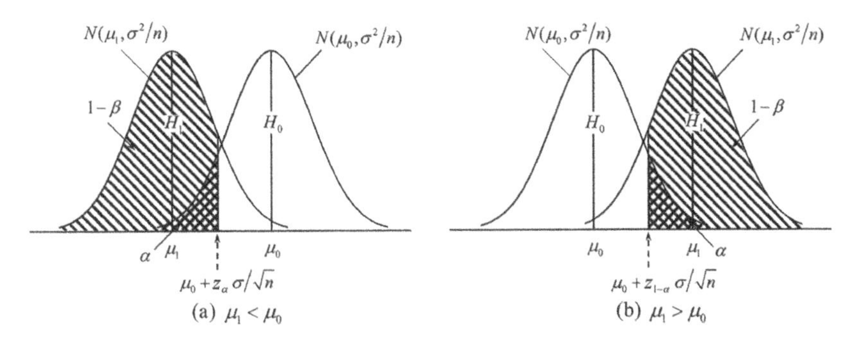

Figure 7.6 Illustration of power for the one-sample Z-test for the mean of a normal distribution with a known variance (one-sided alternative).

where $\text{ES}=|\mu_1-\mu_0|/\sigma$.

Formulas 7.12 and 7.15 are of the same form except that z_α used in the one-sided hypothesis replaces $z_{\alpha/2}$ in the two-sided hypothesis.

Similar to the two-sided hypothesis, we can see from Figure 7.6(a) that the area to the left of $\mu_0+z_\alpha\sigma/\sqrt{n}$ under H_0 happens to be the significance level α. The area to the left of limit defined by $\mu_0+z_\alpha\sigma/\sqrt{n}$ under H_1 is the statistical power $1-\beta$. A similar explanation is obtained for Figure 7.6(b).

Example 7.6 Following Example 7.4, the study also examined the birth weight (kg) of babies whose mothers are less than 20 years old. A total of 25 babies whose mothers are younger than 20 years old were randomly selected in this hospital in the region with a mean of 2.36 kg and a standard deviation of 1.02 kg. Assume that the investigator had a strong belief that the mean birth weight of these babies is lower than that of live births in the region, through clinical justification. Is there any difference between the mean birth weight of these babies and that of live births in the region? Construct a one-sided hypothesis and calculate the statistical power.

Solution

(1) One-sided hypothesis

$$H_0:\mu=\mu_0=3.12,\ H_1:\mu<\mu_0=3.12,\ \alpha=0.05.$$

We know that $\mu_0=3.12$, $\bar{x}=2.36$, $s=1.02$, and $n=25$. Because σ is unknown and the sample size is small, the t-test statistic is preferred and

$$t=\frac{\bar{x}-\mu_0}{s/\sqrt{n}}=\frac{2.36-3.12}{1.02/\sqrt{25}}=-3.73,\ \nu=n-1=25-1=24$$

The critical value for one-sided testing is $t_{24,1-0.05}=1.711$. As $t=-3.73<-1.711$, then $p<0.05$, and we reject H_0 and accept H_1 at the $\alpha=0.05$ level, and conclude that the mean birth weight of the babies whose mothers are younger than 20 years old in this hospital is significantly lower than that of live births in the region.

(2) Calculate the statistical power

We know that $\mu_0 = 3.12$, and assume that the alternative mean $\bar{x} = 2.36$, $s = 1.02$, $n = 25$, and $z_{0.05} = -1.645$, the statistical power is

$$\begin{aligned} 1-\beta &\approx \Phi\left(z_\alpha + \text{ES}\sqrt{n}\right) \\ &= \Phi\left(z_\alpha + \frac{|\mu_1 - \mu_0|}{\sigma}\sqrt{n}\right) \\ &= \Phi\left(-1.645 + \frac{|2.36 - 3.12|}{1.02} \times \sqrt{25}\right) \\ &= \Phi(2.08) = 0.9812. \end{aligned}$$

There is a 98.12% probability of detecting a statistically significant difference. Therefore, it is no surprise that we discover an effect from hypothesis testing.

7.2.1.2 Sample Size Determination

In biomedical research, reliable conclusions cannot be obtained with only a few cases. The accidental results obtained in limited cases cannot be regarded as reliable laws. There must be a sufficient number of observations to stabilize the results. An extremely small sample size will lead to large sampling errors and poor accuracy. However, it is not always "the larger, the better" with sample size. An excessive sample size could lead to poor feasibility, a waste of resource, and sometimes even system error (see Chapter 19). One should determine an appropriate sample size prior to starting the research.

1. Two-sided Hypothesis

Suppose we wish to conduct the following test: $H_0: \mu = \mu_0$, $H_1: \mu = \mu_1 \neq \mu_0$, $\alpha = 0.05$.

We know from Formula 7.12 that the power is $1-\beta \approx \Phi\left(z_{\alpha/2} + \text{ES}\sqrt{n}\right)$. To obtain the formula for calculating the sample size, we need to solve for n in terms of $\alpha/2$, β, and ES.

By definition of percentile and cumulative probability distribution of standard normal distribution, we know that $\Phi(z_{1-\beta}) = 1-\beta$; therefore,

$$z_{1-\beta} = z_{\alpha/2} + \text{ES}\sqrt{n}$$

Solve for n to obtain $n = \dfrac{(-z_{\alpha/2} + z_{1-\beta})^2}{\text{ES}^2}$

By replacing $-z_{\alpha/2}$ with $z_{1-\alpha/2}$, we obtain

$$n = \frac{(z_{1-\alpha/2} + z_{1-\beta})^2}{\text{ES}^2}. \tag{7.16}$$

According to Formula 7.16, we can determine that the sample size n is related to several factors:

(1) The smaller the value of α, the larger the value of n.
(2) The larger the value of $1-\beta$, the larger the value of n.
(3) The smaller the value of ES, the larger the value of n.

Example 7.7 Recall Example 7.4. If we desire the power $1-\beta$ to be 80% and we use a two-sided test with significance level $\alpha=0.05$, then we compute the appropriate sample size required to detect a significant difference.

Solution
We know that $\mu_0=3.12$, and we assume that $\mu_1=3.22$ (replaced by $\overline{x}$) and $\sigma=0.40$ (replaced by s). The critical value at $\alpha=0.05$ is $z_{1-0.05/2}=1.96$. $1-\beta=0.8$ and $z_{0.8}=0.84$. Thus, the sample size is

$$n=\frac{\left(z_{1-\alpha/2}+z_{1-\beta}\right)^2}{\mathrm{ES}^2}=\frac{\left(z_{1-0.05/2}+z_{0.8}\right)^2}{\left|\mu_1-\mu_0\right|^2/\sigma^2}=\frac{\left(1.96+0.84\right)^2}{\left|3.22-3.12\right|^2/0.40^2}\approx 126$$

Thus, a sample size of 126 is required to have an 80% chance of detecting a significant difference at the $\alpha=0.05$ level between the mean birth weight of the babies whose mothers have gestational diabetes in this hospital and that of live births in the region.

2. One-sided Hypothesis
Here, we extend the calculation of sample size to one-sided hypothesis testing $H_0:\mu=\mu_0$, $H_1:\mu=\mu_1<\mu_0$, or $H_1:\mu=\mu_1>\mu_0$. The sample size n is

$$n=\frac{\left(z_{1-\alpha}+z_{1-\beta}\right)^2}{\mathrm{ES}^2}. \tag{7.17}$$

Formulas 7.17 and 7.16 have the same form except that $z_{1-\alpha}$ used in the one-sided hypothesis replaces $z_{1-\alpha/2}$ in the two-sided hypothesis.

Example 7.8 Recall Example 7.6. If we simply desire the power $1-\beta$ to be 80% and we still use a one-sided test with significance level $\alpha=0.05$, then we compute the appropriate sample size required to detect a significant difference.

Solution
We know that $\mu_0=3.12$, and we assume $\mu_1=2.36$ (replaced by $\overline{x}$), $\sigma=1.02$ (replaced by s). The critical value at given $\alpha=0.05$ is $z_{1-0.05}=1.645$. $1-\beta=0.8$, and $z_{0.8}=0.84$. Thus, the sample size is

$$n=\frac{\left(z_{1-\alpha}+z_{1-\beta}\right)^2}{\mathrm{ES}^2}=\frac{\left(z_{1-0.05}+z_{0.8}\right)^2}{\left|\mu_1-\mu_0\right|^2/\sigma^2}=\frac{\left(1.645+0.84\right)^2}{\left|2.36-3.12\right|^2/1.02^2}\approx 12$$

Thus, we only need a sample size of 12 to have an 80% probability of detecting a significant difference at the $\alpha=0.05$ level if the alternative mean is 2.36 and a one-sided test is used.

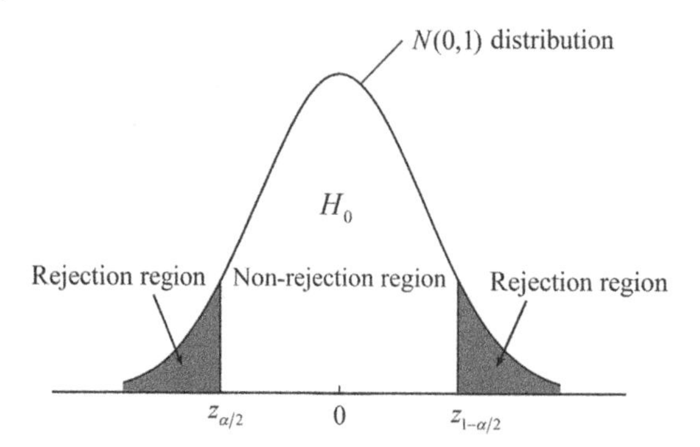

Figure 7.7 Illustration of rejection and non-rejection regions for the one-sample rate test (two-sided alternative).

7.2.2 Hypothesis Tests for the Rate (Normal Approximation Methods)

In Chapter 6, we learned that the sampling distribution of sample rate p when $np(1-p)\geq 5$ approximately follows a normal distribution with mean π and variance $\pi(1-\pi)/n$.

Under $H_0{:}\pi=\pi_0$, the test statistic

$$Z=\frac{p-\pi_0}{\sqrt{\pi_0(1-\pi_0)/n}} \tag{7.18}$$

follows a standard normal distribution $N(0,1)$. The rejection and non-rejection regions are illustrated in Figure 7.7.

If we use a continuity-corrected version of the test statistic, there will be a better approximation of the standard normal distribution. Specifically,

$$Z_{\text{corr}}=\frac{|p-\pi_0|-1/(2n)}{\sqrt{\pi_0(1-\pi_0)/n}}. \tag{7.19}$$

Notice that we can see in Formula 7.19 that when n is sufficiently large, we may ignore this correction.

Example 7.9 According to a national survey in 2018, the smoking prevalence among men aged 15 years and over was 50.5%. A study is conducted using stratified multistage sampling in a specific area. The smoking prevalence rate is 47.3% in 3113 men aged 15 years and over. Does the smoking prevalence in this area differ from the national average?

Solution

(1) State the hypotheses and select a significance level

$$H_0:\pi=\pi_0=0.505$$

$$H_1:\pi\neq\pi_0=0.505$$

$$\alpha=0.05$$

(2) Determine the test statistic
Here n is 3113, $n\pi_0(1-\pi_0)=3113\times0.505\times(1-0.505)=778.17\geq5$; therefore, we calculate the test statistic using Formula 7.18 as

$$z=\frac{p-\pi_0}{\sqrt{\frac{\pi_0(1-\pi_0)}{n}}}=\frac{0.473-0.505}{\sqrt{\frac{0.505\times(1-0.505)}{3113}}}=-3.57$$

(3) Draw a conclusion

(i) Critical-value method
Since $|z|=3.57>z_{1-\alpha/2}=1.96$, $p<0.05$. We reject H_0 and accept H_1 at the $\alpha=0.05$ level. We may declare that the smoking prevalence in this area is significantly lower than the national average.

(ii) p-value method
We also compute the p value, which is twice the area to the left of the z distribution under the $N(0,1)$ curve.
Thus, the p value (two-sided) is $p=2\times P(Z<z)=2\times\Phi(z)=2\times\Phi(-3.57)$, and using the NORMDIST function of Excel, $\Phi(-3.57)=$ NORMDIST $(-3.57,0,1,1)=0.0002$, where 0 and 1 represent the mean and standard deviation of the standard normal distribution, respectively, wherein 1 is a logical value meaning that the outcome is a cumulative distribution function. Then $p=2\times0.0002=0.0004<0.001$. These results are strongly significant.

7.2.2.1 Power of the Test

We can also calculate the power of the one-sample test for rate using normal approximation methods.

Suppose we use a two-sided test with a significance level $\alpha=0.05$ for the hypothesis of one-sample test for rate: $H_0:\pi=\pi_0$, $H_1:\pi=\pi_1\neq\pi_0$, the power is expressed as

$$1-\beta\approx\Phi\left(\sqrt{\frac{\pi_0(1-\pi_0)}{\pi_1(1-\pi_1)}}\left(z_{\alpha/2}+\frac{|\pi_1-\pi_0|\sqrt{n}}{\sqrt{\pi_0(1-\pi_0)}}\right)\right). \tag{7.20}$$

Note that Formula 7.20 can only be used when n is moderately large and π_0 is not considerably large or small (i.e., $n\pi_0(1-\pi_0)\geq5$).

Example 7.10 Calculate the statistical power in Example 7.9.

Solution
Knowing that $z_{0.05/2}=-1.96$, $\pi_0=0.505$, $n=3113$, and $\pi_1=0.473$(replaced by p), the statistical power is

$$\begin{aligned}1-\beta&\approx\Phi\left(\sqrt{\frac{\pi_0(1-\pi_0)}{\pi_1(1-\pi_1)}}\left(z_{\alpha/2}+\frac{|\pi_1-\pi_0|\sqrt{n}}{\sqrt{\pi_0(1-\pi_0)}}\right)\right)\\&=\Phi\left(\sqrt{\frac{0.505\times(1-0.505)}{0.473\times(1-0.473)}}\left(-1.96+\frac{|0.473-0.505|\times\sqrt{3113}}{\sqrt{0.505\times(1-0.505)}}\right)\right)\\&=\Phi(1.61)=0.9463\end{aligned}$$

With a sample size of 3113, there is a probability of 94.63% to detect a statistically significant difference between the specific area and the national average in terms of the smoking prevalence rate.

7.2.2.2 Sample Size Determination

Suppose we use a two-sided test with significance level $\alpha = 0.05$ and power $1-\beta$ for the hypothesis of one-sample test for rate: $H_0: \pi = \pi_0$, $H_1: \pi = \pi_1 \neq \pi_0$, the sample size is

$$n = \frac{\pi_0(1-\pi_0)}{(\pi_1-\pi_0)^2}\left(z_{1-\alpha/2} + z_{1-\beta}\sqrt{\frac{\pi_1(1-\pi_1)}{\pi_0(1-\pi_0)}}\right)^2. \tag{7.21}$$

Example 7.11 Recall Example 7.9. If we simply desire the power $1-\beta$ to be 80% and we use a two-sided test with significance level $\alpha = 0.05$, then we compute the appropriate sample size required to detect a significant difference.

Solution

We know that $\pi_0 = 0.505$ and $\pi_1 = 0.473$ (replaced by p). The critical value at given $\alpha = 0.05$ is $z_{1-0.05/2} = 1.96$. $1-\beta = 0.8$, and $z_{0.8} = 0.84$. Thus, the sample size is

$$\begin{aligned} n &= \frac{\pi_0(1-\pi_0)}{(\pi_1-\pi_0)^2}\left(z_{1-\alpha/2} + z_{1-\beta}\sqrt{\frac{\pi_1(1-\pi_1)}{\pi_0(1-\pi_0)}}\right)^2 \\ &= \frac{0.505\times(1-0.505)}{(0.473-0.505)^2}\left(1.96 + 0.84\times\sqrt{\frac{0.473\times(1-0.473)}{0.505\times(1-0.505)}}\right)^2 \\ &\approx 1913 \end{aligned}$$

Thus, a sample size of 1913 is required to have an 80% probability of detecting a significant difference at the 0.05 level if the alternative rate is 0.473, and a two-sided test is used.

Similarly, for the determination of the sample size for the one-sided test, we only change $z_{1-\alpha/2}$ into $z_{1-\alpha}$ in Formula 7.21, and the others remain unchanged.

The estimation of sample size is based on different research objectives and data types. At the same time, attention should be paid to clinical significance. In addition, when practical issues such as nonresponse and loss to follow-up are taken into account, it is necessary to increase the estimated minimum sample size by 10%–20% to ensure that a sufficient number of valid samples are obtained.

7.3 Further Considerations on Hypothesis Testing

7.3.1 About the Significance Level

The scientific community has determined statistical significance from various data typically assessed by comparing the p value with 0.05 or 0.01. Scientific journals favor publishing statistically significant results. However, there is no single concrete cut-off that defines what significance is. A p value of 0.049 is almost the same as 0.051, although it might lead to the opposite conclusion regarding significance. The proposal of 0.05 can be traced back to the research of R.A. Fisher in the early 1920s. It was impractical for the intensive computation of an exact p value at that time, and 0.05, which locates 1.96 (approximately 2) under the $N(0,1)$ distribution, is convenient for a quick justification. The statistical society continues to consider 0.05 as having a special status nowadays. Nevertheless, it is important to remember that hypothesis testing is a context rather than a single index. We should interpret hypothesis testing results carefully to avoid misuse, particularly when the p value is at the borderline significance level.

7.3.2 Statistical Significance and Clinical Significance

It should be borne in mind that the p value is determined by multiple factors such as:

(1) Effect size of the population.
(2) Sample size.
(3) Sample variance.

Therefore, statistical significance does not imply practical significance. Small p values are not equivalent to large effects. It might be the large sample sizes that magnify the effects numerically. Conversely, large p values also do not indicate a lack of important effect.

Clinical significance is a clinical adjudication rather than a mathematical quantity. We have learned from many examples that the effect size suggests a meaningful difference even if it is not statistically significant. A confirmatory interpretation may not be justified in such circumstances; however, it serves as an evidence to guide future research.

It is important to look at the effect size, confidence interval, and p value collectively. Isolating the statistical inference from clinical importance may lead to incorrect interpretation. Scientific conclusions or clinical decisions should be justified based not only on statistical significance but also contextual expertise.

Finally, hypothesis testing provides a framework to decide whether or not the observed effect can be attributed to random errors. It does not address any causal relationship. Good statistical practice should emphasize the principles of study design, understanding the modality, and complete reporting of context.

7.4 Summary

So far, we have covered the most popular methods for statistical inference – parameter estimation and hypothesis testing. Both are built upon sampling distribution of statistics but focus on the population parameters beyond the sample. As we demonstrated in these two chapters, they utilize probability as inference criteria rather than relying on subjective judgments. We also proved that the results from interval estimation and hypothesis testing are generally consistent.

Let us quickly summarise this chapter. We introduced the procedures of hypothesis testing involving null hypothesis and alternative hypothesis, significance level, test statistics, critical value, and p value. We discussed the concept of errors (Type I and

Table 7.2 t-test for a population mean μ.

	One-sided test	Two-sided test
H_0	$\mu = \mu_0$	$\mu = \mu_0$
H_1	$\mu > \mu_0$ or $\mu < \mu_0$	$\mu \neq \mu_0$
Test statistic	$t = \dfrac{\overline{X} - \mu_0}{S / \sqrt{n}}$	$t = \dfrac{\overline{X} - \mu_0}{S / \sqrt{n}}$
Rejection region	$t > t_{\nu,1-\alpha}$ or $t < -t_{\nu,1-\alpha}$	$\lvert t \rvert > t_{\nu,1-\alpha/2}$
p value	$p = P(t_\nu > t)$ or $p = P(t_\nu < t)$	$p = \begin{cases} 2 \times P(t_\nu < t), \text{ if } t \leq 0 \\ 2 \times P(t_\nu > t), \text{ if } t > 0 \end{cases}$

Type II), one-sided and two-sided hypothesis, statistical power, and sample size determination.

Critical value is calculated based on the prespecified significance level α; the p value is calculated through the distribution of test statistics using statistical software. Both approaches lead to the same conclusion; however, the p-value method is more precise than the critical-value method. Once again, we present a concise workflow of one-sample inference using a t-test for a population mean as an example (Table 7.2).

In the following chapters, we will introduce various hypothesis testing methods in different study designs. We will only focus on the methodology aspects because the principles remain the same as discussed in this chapter.

7.5 Exercises

1. Explain the following briefly with an example.
   - **(a)** Null hypothesis H_0 and alternative hypothesis H_1.
   - **(b)** Non-rejection and rejection of the null hypothesis H_0.
   - **(c)** One-sided and two-sided tests.
   - **(d)** Test statistic.
   - **(e)** Type I and Type II errors.
   - **(f)** Critical value.
   - **(g)** p value.
   - **(h)** Significance level α.
   - **(i)** Power of a test $(1 - \beta)$.

2. Suppose that it is known from a national survey that the length of newborns (cm) follows a normal distribution with $\mu = 50$. Answer the following questions.
   - **(a)** If you repeatedly draw samples from this population with a fixed sample of size, where should the sampling distribution of the sample means be centered around? Why?
   - **(b)** Suppose that you are interested in whether maternal anemia has an impact on the length of newborns and randomly draw 50 newborns whose mothers have

anemia; the sample $\bar{x} = 45$, $s = 3$. State your hypothesis and perform two-sided significance tests at significance level $\alpha = 0.05$.

3. A researcher hypothesizes that the lowering of cholesterol is associated with dieting. To test this, the researcher recruited 20 men aged 40–50 years and measured their cholesterol levels before and after dieting for 3 weeks (assuming the difference follows the normal distribution). The difference is calculated, which is non-significant $(p = 0.09)$ compared to zero in a two-sided test at the $\alpha = 0.05$ level.
   (a) Can you figure out how to perform a significance test using what you have learnt in this chapter? State H_0 and H_1 for this test.
   (b) Interpret in your own words what the p value and α level means in this case. What are their differences?
   (c) Can the researcher claim that the probability that H_0 is true is 0.09? Why?
   (d) Can the researcher claim that diet has no effect?
   (e) What is the advantage of a one-sided test? Is it appropriate if the researcher decides to select the critical value of a one-sided test after a two-sided value $p = 0.09$ has been obtained? Why?
   (f) Is it appropriate to select a more liberal α (say, 0.1) after the researcher found a p value of 0.09 if it was nonsignificant at a significance level of 0.05.

4. Suppose that a sample of 200 children aged 5–12 years is randomly drawn from a certain area. Let the proportion of obese children estimated in this sample be 0.13. For a significant test of $H_0: \pi = 0.2$ vs. $H_1: \pi \neq 0.2$, $\alpha = 0.05$:
   (a) Interpret and carry out the significance test.
   (b) What is the probability that a Type I error would be encountered given that H_0 is true?
   (c) What is the probability that a Type II error would be encountered given that H_0 is false?

5. A sample of 118 patients admitted to a hospital with a diagnosis of biliary cirrhosis had a mean IgM level (unit/ml) of 160.6. The sample standard deviation was 50.0. Do these data provide sufficient evidence to indicate that the population mean is greater than 150 when $\alpha = 0.05$?

   (a) List and explain the essential hypothesis testing procedure in this study.
   (b) Determine the p value.
   (c) Please interpret the test result.

8

Hypothesis Testing for Two Population Parameters

CONTENTS

In Chapter 7, we introduced the concepts of hypothesis testing and their application to one sample inference. The usage of one sample hypothesis testing, however, is limited in practice, as prespecified knowledge of the parameter is needed to establish the null and alternative hypotheses. Two sample inference is more common, regarding which underlying parameters of two populations are both unknown, and we are interested in whether the parameters are equal or not. Although the methods might differ based on the research design and the type of data, the principles and procedures are similar to those discussed in the previous chapter. We start with hypothesis testing for sample data from two populations of normal distribution or when the central limit theorem holds, and then, under this theorem, we discuss hypothesis testing for binominal data.

Imagine that a researcher is planning a pilot experiment on the effect of a new anticancer drug using S180 tumor-bearing mice. He has two options for the research design:

Design 1: The anticancer drug will be administrated to a group of mice, and their serum acid phosphatase (ACP, U/100 ml) will be measured and recorded at baseline

Applied Medical Statistics, First Edition. Jingmei Jiang.

Companion website: www.wiley.com\go\jiang\appliedmedicalstatistics

before administration and 10 days afterward. The change in serum ACP from baseline 10 days later will be considered the primary endpoint for evaluation.

Design 2: The mice will be randomly allocated to an experimental group and a control group. Only the experimental group will be administered the anticancer drug. The serum ACP will only be measured and recorded 10 days after the drug administration and will be considered the primary endpoint for evaluating the difference between groups.

The major difference between the two designs is that Design 1 uses a *paired samples design*, where each mouse is used as its own control. Therefore, the measurements at baseline and 10 days later are not independent. Design 2 uses a *completely randomized design*, where each mouse only contributes an independent measurement. In the following sections, we will show how to conduct a hypothesis test for paired samples and completely randomized designs.

8.1 Testing the Difference Between Two Population Means: Paired Samples

The paired samples design is frequently used in biomedical research. Depending on the research purpose, study subjects with similar characteristics (such as sex and strains) can be matched by self-pairing or non-self-pairing. For example, Design 1 uses self-pairing; a comparison is made within each subject. If two mice with similar characteristics (such as mice from the same litter) are treated differently, the two mice can be a pair; this is an example of non-self-pairing. Because the two subjects in a pair are in very similar circumstances (nontreatment factors) other than the studied factor (treatment factors), the systematic error within the pairs can be eliminated by calculating the difference between the data of the pair. Therefore, the paired samples design can effectively reduce the effect of nontreatment factors and improve the efficiency of the experiment.

Example 8.1 Using Design 1, the researcher studied the anticancer effect of the drug with 14 mice. The values of serum ACP (U/100 ml) are given in Table 8.1, recorded at baseline and 10 days later. Assume that serum ACP follows a normal distribution; is there any difference in the population mean serum ACP between baseline and 10 days later?

In Table 8.1, the measurements at baseline and 10 days later for each mouse $\left(x_{i1}, x_{i2}\right)\left(i=1,2,\ldots,14\right)$ are shown in the rows, and the paired data at two time points are not independent. In such a situation, we can address this issue by calculating the difference within the pairs and just focusing on the difference: it can be seen that the serum ACP of all 14 mice has (more or less) increased 10 days later compared with the baseline $\left(d_i > 0\right)$; this is suggestive of the efficacy of the anticancer drug. However, if the anticancer drug is ineffective, the changes in serum ACP would be simply due to a random factor effect, and the d_i would be expected to randomly allot around zero. Then we can state the research question in a statistical manner—whether $\mu_{\bar{d}} = \mu_1 - \mu_2 = 0$—and address it with the *paired samples t-test* as follows:

(1) State the hypotheses and select a significance level

$$H_0 : \mu_{\bar{d}} = 0$$

$$H_1 : \mu_{\bar{d}} \neq 0$$

Usually, let $\alpha = 0.05$ as the significance level.

Table 8.1 Serum ACP (U/100 ml) at baseline and 10 days later.

ID i (1)	Baseline x_{i1} (2)	10 days later x_{i2} (3)	Difference d_i (4)=(3)−(2)
1	58.27	120.61	62.34
2	59.51	126.33	66.82
3	53.84	108.35	54.51
4	54.70	139.99	85.29
5	54.03	115.29	61.26
6	61.29	146.96	85.67
7	54.72	115.64	60.92
8	70.43	124.62	54.19
9	66.45	121.40	54.95
10	59.31	134.81	75.50
11	63.48	130.73	67.25
12	67.19	118.37	51.18
13	52.92	129.28	76.36
14	71.99	117.40	45.41
Total	—	—	901.65

(2) Determine the test statistic
Similar to the hypothesis testing of one sample mean discussed in Chapter 7, when σ is unknown and the sample size is not sufficiently large, the standardized mean follows a t distribution with $\nu = n-1$ degrees of freedom, i.e.,

$$t = \frac{\bar{d} - \mu_{\bar{d}}}{S_{\bar{d}}} \sim t(\nu). \tag{8.1}$$

Under H_0, the test statistic is

$$t = \frac{\bar{d}}{S_{\bar{d}}}, \tag{8.2}$$

where $S_{\bar{d}} = S_d / \sqrt{n}$ is the estimate of standard error and n is the number of pairs.

(3) Draw a conclusion
Either of the two following methods can be used:

(i) Critical-value method
For a given α and $\nu = n-1$, we can obtain the critical values $t_{\nu,\alpha/2}$ and $t_{\nu,1-\alpha/2}$ from a t_ν distribution (Appendix Table 4).

If $t < t_{\nu,\alpha/2}$ or $t > t_{\nu,1-\alpha/2}$, then reject H_0;

If $t_{\nu,\alpha/2} \le t \le t_{\nu,1-\alpha/2}$, then do not reject H_0.

(ii) p-value method
Compute the p value for the paired samples t-test under a t_ν distribution.
If $t \le 0$, $p = 2\times$ (area to the left of t) $= 2\times P(t_\nu < t)$;
If $t > 0$, $p = 2\times$ (area to the right of t) $= 2\times P(t_\nu > t)$.

Solution to Example 8.1

(1) State the hypotheses and select a significance level

$$H_0 : \mu_{\bar{d}} = 0$$
$$H_1 : \mu_{\bar{d}} \ne 0$$

$$\alpha = 0.05$$

(2) Determine the test statistic
The summary statistics on the difference d are

$$\bar{d} = \frac{\sum_i d_i}{n} = \frac{901.65}{14} = 64.40,$$

$$s_d = \sqrt{\frac{\sum_i d_i^2 - \left(\sum_i d_i\right)^2 / n}{n-1}} = \sqrt{\frac{60091.4763 - \frac{901.65^2}{14}}{14-1}} = 12.47,$$

$$s_{\bar{d}} = \frac{s_d}{\sqrt{n}} = \frac{12.47}{\sqrt{14}} = 3.33.$$

The test statistic is

$$t = \frac{\bar{d}}{s_d / \sqrt{n}} = \frac{64.40}{3.33} = 19.34$$

(3) Draw a conclusion

(i) Critical-value method
For a given $\alpha = 0.05$, $\nu = 14 - 1 = 13$, the critical value is $t_{13,1-0.05/2} = 2.160$ (Appendix Table 4). Since $t = 19.34 > t_{13,1-0.05/2} = 2.160$, $p < 0.05$. We reject H_0 and accept H_1 at the $\alpha = 0.05$ level, that is, the difference between the mean serum ACP is statistically significant, and we conclude that the increase in serum ACP after administration is statistically significant.

(ii) p-value method
Since test statistic $t = 19.34 > 0$, the p value is $p = 2\times P(t_\nu > t) = 2\times P(t_{13} > 19.34)$; using the TDIST function of Microsoft Excel, the probability is given by $p = \text{TDIST}(19.34, 13, 2) = 5.7982\times 10^{-11} < 0.001$, which is strongly significant. Similarly, we have significant evidence to reject H_0, which suggests the new anti-cancer drug may have an effect on serum ACP level, i.e., it can increase serum ACP level.

Notice that, if the sample size is large enough $(n \geq 30)$ for the central limit theorem to hold, we can use test statistic $z = \bar{d} / (S_d / \sqrt{n})$ for statistical inference. These two test methods are approximately equivalent in this situation.

8.2 Testing the Difference Between Two Population Means: Independent Samples

8.2.1 *t*-Test for Means with Equal Variances

In practice, the application of the paired samples design may be limited by the availability of subjects that could be appropriate matches, especially in a complex scenario in which the matching should be based on many factors. The completely randomized design (independent samples) would be a good alternative in such scenarios.

Example 8.2 Using Design 2, 26 mice were randomly allocated to an experimental group $(n_1 = 14)$ that received the anticancer drug and a blank control group $(n_2 = 12)$. The serum ACP (U/100 ml) was measured and recorded 10 days later; the results are given in Table 8.2. Assume that the baseline levels of serum ACP were similar in the two groups. Is there any difference in serum ACP after administration of the two different treatment? (Assume that ACP levels are normally distributed with equal variances.)

Analysis
In this example, the serum ACP levels of 26 mice in both the experimental and control groups are independently measured at the same time point (10 days after treatment). We say the two samples are mutually independent.

Assume that serum ACP is normally distributed in the experimental group with mean μ_1 and variance σ_1^2 and in the control group with mean μ_2 and variance σ_2^2. We wish to test the hypothesis $H_0: \mu_1 = \mu_2$ vs. $H_1: \mu_1 \neq \mu_2$ and assume that variances are equal although unknown (i.e., $\sigma_1^2 = \sigma_2^2 = \sigma^2$); it seems reasonable to base the significance tests on the difference between the two sample means, $\bar{X}_1 - \bar{X}_2$. In Chapter 6, we learned that the sampling distribution of $\bar{X}_1 - \bar{X}_2$ follows a t distribution with $\nu = \nu_1 + \nu_2 = n_1 + n_2 - 2$ degrees of freedom.

Table 8.2 Serum ACP (U/100 ml) of mice in experimental and control groups.

Experimental group	120.61	126.33	108.35	139.99	115.29	146.96	115.64
	124.62	121.40	134.81	130.73	118.37	129.28	117.45
Control group	58.23	54.50	59.47	59.64	53.77	43.48	54.63
	71.91	53.97	49.72	61.26	78.17		

Under $H_0: \mu_1 = \mu_2$ or $\mu_1 - \mu_2 = 0$, the test statistic is

$$t = \frac{\bar{X}_1 - \bar{X}_2}{S_C\sqrt{\frac{1}{n_1} + \frac{1}{n_2}}}, \tag{8.3}$$

where S_C is the estimate of the pooled standard deviation of $\bar{X}_1 - \bar{X}_2$:

$$S_C = \sqrt{\frac{(n_1 - 1)S_1^2 + (n_2 - 1)S_2^2}{n_1 + n_2 - 2}}. \tag{8.4}$$

Here, we use S_C as the estimate of σ, which is the square root of the weighted average of two sample variances. This weighted estimation by degrees of freedom (ν) is rationalized by the fact that both S_1^2 and S_2^2 can be considered optimal estimators of σ^2 and that the larger the sample size, the more precise the estimate of σ^2.

Again, we introduce two methods for drawing a conclusion:

(i) Critical-value method

For a given α and $\nu = \nu_1 + \nu_2 = n_1 + n_2 - 2$ degrees of freedom, we can obtain the critical values $t_{\nu_1+\nu_2,\alpha/2}$ and $t_{\nu_1+\nu_2,1-\alpha/2}$ from a $t_{\nu_1+\nu_2}$ distribution (Appendix Table 4).

If $t < t_{\nu_1+\nu_2,\alpha/2}$ or $t > t_{\nu_1+\nu_2,1-\alpha/2}$, then reject H_0;

If $t_{\nu_1+\nu_2,\alpha/2} \le t \le t_{\nu_1+\nu_2,1-\alpha/2}$, then do not reject H_0.

The illustration of the rejection and non-rejection regions for the two independent samples t-test with equal variances is shown in Figure 8.1.

(ii) p-value method

Compute the p value for the two independent samples t-test with equal variances under a $t_{\nu_1+\nu_2}$ distribution.

If $t \le 0$, $p = 2\times$ (area to the left of t) $= 2 \times P\left(t_{\nu_1+\nu_2} < t\right)$;

If $t > 0$, $p = 2\times$ (area to the right of t) $= 2 \times P\left(t_{\nu_1+\nu_2} > t\right)$.

For an illustration of the p-value method, see Figure 8.2.

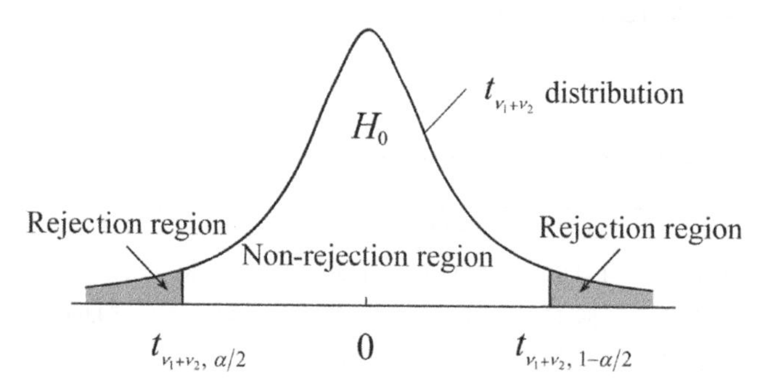

Figure 8.1 Illustration of the rejection and non-rejection regions for the two independent samples t-test with equal variances.

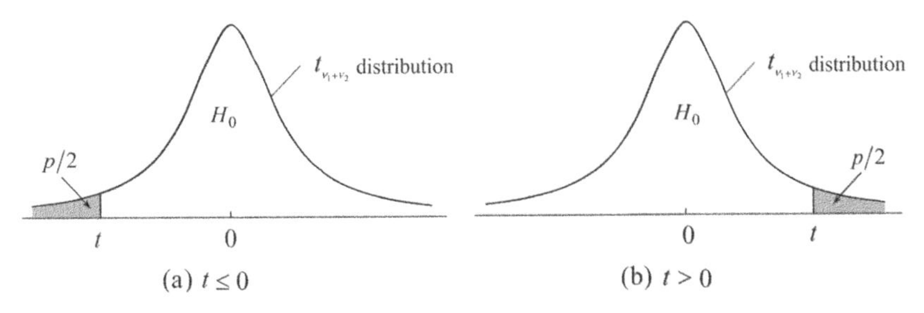

Figure 8.2 Illustration of the p-value method for the two independent samples t-test with equal variances.

Solution

(1) State the hypotheses and select a significance level

$H_0: \mu_1 = \mu_2$
$H_1: \mu_1 \neq \mu_2$

$\alpha = 0.05$

(2) Determine the test statistic
The summary statistics of the two groups are calculated

For the experimental group: $\bar{x}_1 = 124.99$, $s_1 = 10.56$, $n_1 = 14$.
For the control group: $\bar{x}_2 = 58.23$, $s_2 = 9.30$, $n_2 = 12$.

The pooled variance is $s_C^2 = \dfrac{13 \times 10.56^2 + 11 \times 9.30^2}{14 + 12 - 2} = 100.04$.

The test statistic is

$$t = \frac{\bar{x}_1 - \bar{x}_2}{s_C \sqrt{\dfrac{1}{n_1} + \dfrac{1}{n_2}}} = \frac{124.99 - 58.23}{10.00 \times \sqrt{\dfrac{1}{14} + \dfrac{1}{12}}} = \frac{66.76}{3.93} = 16.99.$$

(3) Draw a conclusion

(i) Critical-value method
For a given $\alpha = 0.05$ and $\nu = n_1 + n_2 - 2 = 24$, the critical value is $t_{24,1-0.05/2} = 2.064$ (Appendix Table 4). Since $t = 16.99 > t_{24,1-0.05/2} = 2.064$, $p < 0.05$. We reject H_0 and accept H_1 at the $\alpha = 0.05$ level, the population mean serum ACP between the two groups is not the same, and the evidence shows that the anticancer drug can increase the serum ACP in mice after treatment.

(ii) p-value method
The test statistic is $t = 16.99 > 0$, and the p value is $p = 2 \times P(t_\nu > t) = 2 \times P(t_{24} > 16.99)$; using the TDIST function of Microsoft Excel, the probability is given by $p = \text{TDIST}(16.99, 24, 2) = 6.9975 \times 10^{-15} < 0.001$, which is strongly significant. Similarly, we reject H_0 and accept H_1 at the $\alpha = 0.05$ level and reach the same conclusion.

Two designs (paired samples and completely randomized designs) are adopted to address the same question; the conclusions are consistent, but the sample size required for the completely randomized design is larger. The credibility of a conclusion is enhanced if it is consistent under different designs for the same research question.

8.2.2 F-Test for the Equality of Two Variances

The application of the two independent samples t-test requires that the variances of two populations should be equal. In this section, we discuss how to test the *equality of variances* with the F-test.

Assume that we have two independent samples randomly drawn from two normally distributed populations. The hypotheses for testing the equality of variances are

$$H_0 : \sigma_1^2 = \sigma_2^2 \text{ vs. } H_1 : \sigma_1^2 \neq \sigma_2^2.$$

We learned in Chapter 6 that the sample variances S_1^2 and S_2^2 are the optimal estimates of σ_1^2 and σ_2^2, respectively. Because the sampling distribution of variance is asymmetric, we need to construct a test statistic in the form of the ratio of sample variances rather than their differences. The hypothesis can be then expressed as

$$H_0 : \frac{\sigma_1^2}{\sigma_2^2} = 1 \text{ vs. } H_1 : \frac{\sigma_1^2}{\sigma_2^2} \neq 1.$$

The test statistic, proposed by R.A. Fisher and G.W. Snedecor, follows an F distribution with $\nu_1 = n_1 - 1$ (numerator) and $\nu_2 = n_2 - 1$ (denominator) degrees of freedom.

$$F = \frac{S_1^2}{S_2^2} \sim F(\nu_1, \nu_2). \tag{8.5}$$

Draw a conclusion:

(i) Critical-value method

For a given α and (ν_1, ν_2), we can obtain the critical values $F_{(\nu_1,\nu_2),1-\alpha/2}$ from distribution $F_{(\nu_1,\nu_2)}$ (Appendix Table 7).

If $F > F_{(\nu_1,\nu_2),1-\alpha/2}$, then reject H_0;

If $F \leq F_{(\nu_1,\nu_2),1-\alpha/2}$, then do not reject H_0.

The rejection and non-rejection regions in the F-test for equality of variances are illustrated in Figure 8.3.

Notice that the F-test of the equality of variances is always a two-sided test. However, for efficiency, we commonly put the higher value as numerator and the lower value as denominator to constrain $F \geq 1$. In this way, only the right critical value of the distribution needs to be considered.

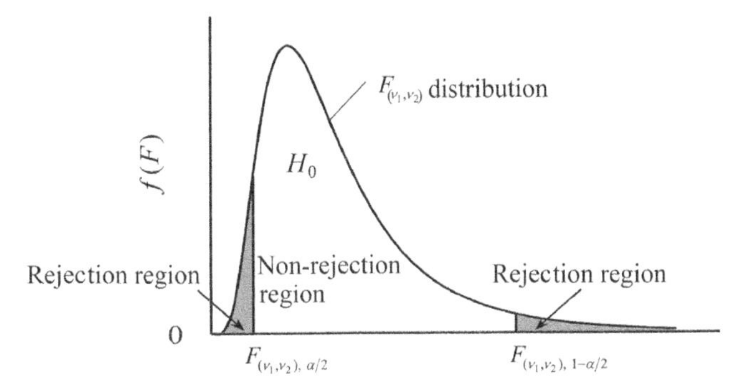

Figure 8.3 Illustration of the rejection and non-rejection regions for the *F*-test for equality of variances.

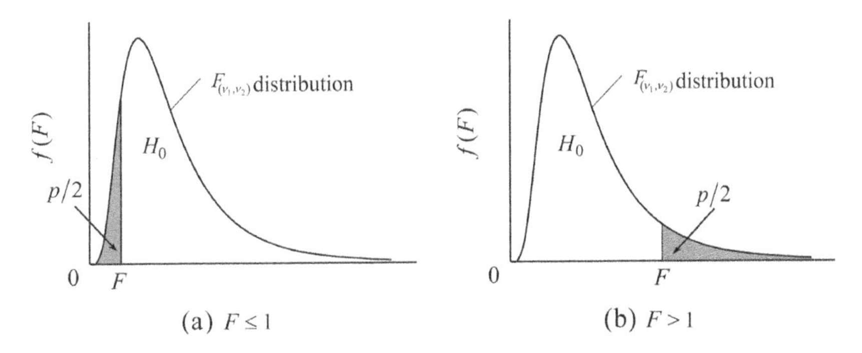

Figure 8.4 Illustration of the *p* value for the *F*-test for equality of variances.

(ii) p-value method

We continue computing the p value for the two-sided test.

If $F \le 1$, $p = 2 \times$ (area to the left of F under $F_{(\nu_1,\nu_2)}$ distribution) $= 2 \times P(F_{(\nu_1,\nu_2)} < F)$;

If $F > 1$, $p = 2 \times$ (area to the right of F under $F_{(\nu_1,\nu_2)}$ distribution) $= 2 \times P(F_{(\nu_1,\nu_2)} > F)$.

The computation of the p value is illustrated in Figure 8.4.

Example 8.3 Test the equality of variances for Example 8.2.

Solution

(1) State the hypotheses and select a significance level

$H_0: \sigma_1^2 = \sigma_2^2$, the population variances of the serum ACP are equal in the two groups

$H_1: \sigma_1^2 \ne \sigma_2^2$, the population variances of the serum ACP are not equal in the two groups

$\alpha = 0.05$

(2) Determine the test statistic

$$F = \frac{s_1^2}{s_2^2} = \frac{10.56^2}{9.30^2} = 1.29$$

(3) Draw a conclusion

(i) Critical-value method

For a given α and $v_1 = 13$ and $v_2 = 11$, the critical value is $F_{(13,11),1-0.05/2} = 3.39$ (Appendix Table 7). Since $F = 1.29 < F_{(13,11),1-0.05/2}$, $p > 0.05$. We do not reject H_0 at the $\alpha = 0.05$ level.

(ii) p-value method

Since the test statistic $F = 1.29 > 1$, the p value is $p = 2 \times P\left(F_{(\nu_1,\nu_2)} > F\right) = 2 \times P\left(F_{(13,11)} > 1.29\right)$; using the FDIST function of Microsoft Excel, the probability is given by $p = 2 \times \text{FDIST}(1.29, 13, 11) = 0.6803 > 0.05$, which is considered not statistically significant.

In conclusion, we do not have sufficient evidence to show that the population variances of the serum ACP of the experimental and control groups are unequal, so it is reasonable to apply the two independent samples t-test for means under equal variance in Example 8.2.

8.2.3 Approximation t-Test for Means with Unequal Variances

In this section, we will introduce an approximated t-test to address the heterogeneity of variances, denoted as the t'-test.

Considering hypothesis testing with $H_0: \mu_1 = \mu_2$ vs. $H_1: \mu_1 \neq \mu_2$, the t'-test statistic under H_0 is

$$t' = \frac{\bar{X}_1 - \bar{X}_2}{\sqrt{\frac{S_1^2}{n_1} + \frac{S_2^2}{n_2}}}. \tag{8.6}$$

Describing the exact distribution of the t' statistic is difficult. However, under appropriate significance level α, approximated alternatives are available.

1. Cochran & Cox Approximation t-Test

Here we introduce the Cochran & Cox approximation t-test, also known as the Cochran & Cox method. Because t' follows neither a t distribution nor a normal distribution, a specific calculation method for the critical values of t' is required, and the calculation formulas are

$$t'_{\alpha/2} = \frac{S_{\bar{X}_1}^2 t_{\nu_1,\alpha/2} + S_{\bar{X}_2}^2 t_{\nu_2,\alpha/2}}{S_{\bar{X}_1}^2 + S_{\bar{X}_2}^2}, \tag{8.7}$$

$$t'_{1-\alpha/2} = \frac{S_{\bar{X}_1}^2 t_{\nu_1,1-\alpha/2} + S_{\bar{X}_2}^2 t_{\nu_2,1-\alpha/2}}{S_{\bar{X}_1}^2 + S_{\bar{X}_2}^2}, \tag{8.8}$$

where $\nu_1 = n_1 - 1$, $\nu_2 = n_2 - 1$; $t_{\nu_1,1-\alpha/2}$, and $t_{\nu_2,1-\alpha/2}$ are critical values of the t_{ν_1} and t_{ν_2} distributions, respectively.

Formulas 8.7 and 8.8 show that the adjusted critical values are calculated as the sum of the individual critical values of the two samples weighted by their corresponding squared standard errors.

Because of the symmetry of the t distribution, we have $t_{\nu_1,\alpha/2} = -t_{\nu_1,1-\alpha/2}$; so, from Formulas 8.7 and 8.8, we know that $t'_{\alpha/2} = -t'_{1-\alpha/2}$.

Similar to the t-test, we reject H_0 if $t' < t'_{\alpha/2}$ or $t' > t'_{1-\alpha/2}$; otherwise, we do not reject H_0.

Example 8.4 In a study on 25 healthy subjects and 25 patients diagnosed with squamous cell carcinoma (SCC) of the lung, serum ferritin (μg/L) was measured, and the data are summarized in Table 8.3. Assume that serum ferritin follows a normal distribution; is the serum ferritin different between the healthy subjects and patients with SCC?

Solution

We have $s_1^2 = 38.60^2 = 1489.96$ and $s_2^2 = 63.80^2 = 4070.44$; then the F-test for equality of variances is $F = 2.73$. The corresponding $p = 0.0170$, which suggests that the population variances of the serum ferritin in the two groups are not equal. Therefore, the Cochran & Cox approximated t-test is applied.

(1) State the hypotheses and select a significance level

$H_0 : \mu_1 = \mu_2$, the population mean of serum ferritin is the same between the two groups
$H_1 : \mu_1 \neq \mu_2$, the population mean of serum ferritin is not the same between the two groups

$\alpha = 0.05$

(2) Determine the test statistic

We know that $n_1 = 25$, $\bar{x}_1 = 89.6$, $s_1 = 38.60$; $n_2 = 25$, $\bar{x}_2 = 286.0$, $s_2 = 63.80$. Then the test statistic is

$$t' = \frac{89.6 - 286.0}{\sqrt{\dfrac{38.60^2}{25} + \dfrac{63.80^2}{25}}} = -13.17.$$

Table 8.3 Summary statistics of serum ferritin (μg/L) in healthy subjects and patients with SCC of the lung

Group	n	$\bar{x}$	s
Health subjects	25	89.6	38.60
Patients with SCC	25	286.0	63.80

(3) Draw a conclusion

For a given α and $\nu_1 = \nu_2 = 24$ degrees of freedom, we obtain critical value $t_{24,1-0.05/2} = 2.064$ from distribution t_{24} (Appendix Table 4). The critical value of t' according to Formula 8.8 is

$$t'_{1-0.05/2} = \frac{\frac{38.60^2}{25} \times 2.064 + \frac{63.80^2}{25} \times 2.064}{\frac{38.60^2}{25} + \frac{63.80^2}{25}} = 2.064.$$

Since $t' = -13.17 < t'_{0.05/2} = -2.064$, $p < 0.05$. We reject H_0 and accept H_1 at the $\alpha = 0.05$ level and conclude that the population mean of serum ferritin is significantly different between the two groups. In particular, the serum ferritin in the patients with SCC of the lung is significantly higher than that in the healthy subjects.

2. Satterthwaite Approximation *t*-Test

As we demonstrated, the Cochran & Cox method adjusts critical values to address heterogeneity of variance. Another approach is the Satterthwaite method, which adjusts the degrees of freedom, denoted as ν' and calculated by Formula 6.39.

Under H_0, the t' statistic approximately follows a t distribution with ν' degrees of freedom. The test can then be completed by obtaining the critical value.

If $t' < t_{\nu',\alpha/2}$ or $t' > t_{\nu',1-\alpha/2}$, then reject H_0;

If $t_{\nu',\alpha/2} \le t' \le t_{\nu',1-\alpha/2}$, then do not reject H_0.

Example 8.5 Repeat Example 8.4 using the Satterthwaite method.

Solution

We first compute the adjustment ν':

$$\nu' = \frac{\left(\frac{S_1^2}{n_1} + \frac{S_2^2}{n_2}\right)^2}{\frac{\left(\frac{S_1^2}{n_1}\right)^2}{n_1 - 1} + \frac{\left(\frac{S_2^2}{n_2}\right)^2}{n_2 - 1}} = \frac{\left(\frac{38.60^2}{25} + \frac{63.80^2}{25}\right)^2}{\frac{\left(\frac{38.60^2}{25}\right)^2}{25 - 1} + \frac{\left(\frac{63.80^2}{25}\right)^2}{25 - 1}}$$
$$= 39.49 \approx 39.$$

Under H_0, the t' statistic approximately follows a t distribution with $\nu' \approx 39$ degrees of freedom; the critical value is $t_{39,1-0.05/2} = 2.023$ (Appendix Table 4). Since $t' = -13.17 < t_{39,0.05/2} = -2.023$, $p < 0.05$. We reject H_0 and accept H_1 at the $\alpha = 0.05$ level. The conclusion is the same as the one we reached with the Cochran & Cox method.

8.2.4 Z-Test for Means with Large-Sample Sizes

According to the central limit theorem, when the sample size is large enough $(n \geq 30)$, the sampling distributions of the two independent sample means approximately follow normal distributions, denoted as $\bar{X}_1 \dot{\sim} N\left(\mu_1, \frac{\sigma_1^2}{n_1}\right)$ and $\bar{X}_2 \dot{\sim} N\left(\mu_2, \frac{\sigma_2^2}{n_2}\right)$.

Considering hypothesis testing with $H_0: \mu_1 = \mu_2$, the test statistic Z under H_0 is

$$Z = \frac{\bar{X}_1 - \bar{X}_2}{\sqrt{\frac{S_1^2}{n_1} + \frac{S_2^2}{n_2}}}, \tag{8.9}$$

which approximately follows a standard normal distribution $N(0,1)$. In the calculation, Formula 8.9 directly uses the sample variances S_1^2 and S_2^2 as substitutes for the population variances σ_1^2 and σ_2^2.

(i) Critical-value method
For given α,
If $Z < z_{\alpha/2}$ or $Z > z_{1-\alpha/2}$, then reject H_0;
If $z_{\alpha/2} \leq Z \leq z_{1-\alpha/2}$, then do not reject H_0.

(ii) p-value method
If $Z \leq 0$, $p = 2\times$ (area to the left of Z under a standard normal Z distribution);
If $Z > 0$, $p = 2\times$ (area to the right of Z under a standard normal Z distribution).

Example 8.6 A pilot study was conducted to investigate systolic blood pressure (SBP) in a certain area. A group comprising 60 office workers was randomly sampled. Their mean SBP was 132.86 mmHg with a standard deviation of 15.34 mmHg. A group of 50 manual laborers was also sampled. The mean SBP was 127.44 mmHg with a standard deviation of 18.23 mmHg. Assume that SBP has a normal distribution; is the SBP different for the populations of office workers and manual laborers?

Solution
(1) State the hypotheses and select a significance level

$H_0: \mu_1 = \mu_2$
$H_1: \mu_1 \neq \mu_2$

$\alpha = 0.05$

(2) Determine the test statistic

We know that $n_1 = 60$, $\bar{x}_1 = 132.86$, $s_1 = 15.34$; $n_2 = 50$, $\bar{x}_2 = 127.44$, $s_2 = 18.23$. Here, n_1 and n_2 are both sufficiently large, then the test statistic is

$$z = \frac{\bar{x}_1 - \bar{x}_2}{\sqrt{\frac{s_1^2}{n_1} + \frac{s_2^2}{n_2}}} = \frac{132.86 - 127.44}{\sqrt{\frac{15.34^2}{60} + \frac{18.23^2}{50}}} = 1.67.$$

(3) Draw a conclusion

(i) Critical-value method

For a given $\alpha = 0.05$, since $z = 1.67 < z_{1-0.05/2} = 1.96$, $p > 0.05$. We do not reject H_0 at the $\alpha = 0.05$ level. That means there is nonsufficient evidence to show that the mean SBP of office workers is not the same compared to that of manual laborers.

(ii) p-value method

The test statistic is $z = 1.67 > 0$, and the p value is $p = 2 \times P(Z > z) = 2 \times [1 - P(Z \le z)] = 2 \times [1 - \Phi(z)] = 2 \times [1 - \Phi(1.67)]$; using the NORMDIST function of Microsoft Excel, $\Phi(1.67) = \text{NORMDIST}(1.67,0,1,1) = 0.9525$. Then $p = 2 \times (1 - 0.9525) = 0.0950 > 0.05$; therefore, the same conclusion is reached.

8.2.5 Power for Comparing Two Means

A researcher may often worry about a deficient sample size, possibly because of the unavailability of subjects or simply a failure to plan properly. The question to be answered is whether the study is powerful enough to detect a real difference. We discussed the power of a test for one sample in Section 7.2.1.1; in this section, we will discuss the same issue when comparing two independent sample means.

Assume that σ_1^2 and σ_2^2 are known; the approximated estimate of power using a two-sided test at the significance level α is given by

$$1 - \beta \approx \Phi\left(-z_{1-\alpha/2} + \frac{|\mu_1 - \mu_2|}{\sqrt{\sigma_1^2 / n_1 + \sigma_2^2 / n_2}}\right), \tag{8.10}$$

where μ_1, μ_2, σ_1^2, and σ_2^2 are the means and variances of the two groups and n_1 and n_2 are the sample sizes of the two groups, respectively.

To calculate the power for a one-sided rather than a two-sided test, simply substitute $z_{1-\alpha}$ for $z_{1-\alpha/2}$ in Formula 8.10.

Example 8.7 Referring to Example 8.6, how much power would such a pilot study have, using a two-sided test at a significance level of $\alpha = 0.05$?

Solution

From Example 8.6, the sample statistics $(\bar{x}_1, s_1^2, \bar{x}_2, s_2^2)$ are used as estimates of the population parameters $(\mu_1, \sigma_1^2, \mu_2, \sigma_2^2)$. Thus, we have $|\mu_1 - \mu_2| = |132.86 - 127.44| = 5.42$, $\sigma_1 = 15.34$, $\sigma_2 = 18.23$, $n_1 = 60$, $n_2 = 50$, and $\alpha = 0.05$.

Therefore, from Formula 8.10,

$$\begin{aligned} 1 - \beta &\approx \Phi\left(-z_{1-0.05/2} + \frac{|\mu_1 - \mu_2|}{\sqrt{\sigma_1^2 / n_1 + \sigma_2^2 / n_2}}\right) \\ &= \Phi\left(-1.96 + \frac{5.42}{\sqrt{15.34^2 / 60 + 18.23^2 / 50}}\right) \\ &= 0.385. \end{aligned}$$

Thus, there is a 38.5% chance of detecting a significant difference in the SBPs of the office workers and manual laborers using a two-sided test at the $\alpha = 0.05$ level. The power is low, primarily because of the small sample size.

8.2.6 Sample Size Determination

Given the low power calculated in Example 8.7, how do we determine the minimum sample size required for detecting a real difference between the means of two populations with sufficient power (usually 80%)?

Example 8.8 Consider the SBP data in Example 8.6 as a pilot study to obtain parameter estimates to plan for a larger study. Suppose the SBP distributions of office workers and manual laborers follow $N\left(\mu_1, \sigma_1^2\right)$ and $N\left(\mu_2, \sigma_2^2\right)$, respectively. We wish to test the hypothesis $H_0: \mu_1 = \mu_2$ vs. $H_1: \mu_1 \neq \mu_2$; how large a sample size is needed using a two-sided test with a significance level of 0.05 and a power of 0.80?

1. Equal Sample Sizes in the Two Groups

Suppose σ_1^2 and σ_2^2 are known and we plan to have equal sample sizes in the two groups. To conduct a two-sided test with a significance level of α and power of $1-\beta$, the appropriate sample size for each group is determined as follows:

$$n = \frac{\left(\sigma_1^2 + \sigma_2^2\right)\left(z_{1-\alpha/2} + z_{1-\beta}\right)^2}{\left(\mu_1 - \mu_2\right)^2}. \tag{8.11}$$

In other words, the estimated n is the appropriate sample size in each group to achieve a probability of $1-\beta$ for detecting a real difference based on a two-sided test with a significance level of α.

Solution to Example 8.8

In the pilot study, $\bar{x}_1 = 132.86$, $s_1 = 15.34$ and $\bar{x}_2 = 127.44$, $s_2 = 18.23$.

Ensuring an 80% chance of finding a real difference using a two-sided significance test with $\alpha = 0.05$, the sample statistics $\left(\bar{x}_1, s_1^2, \bar{x}_2, s_2^2\right)$ are used as estimates of the population parameters $\left(\mu_1, \sigma_1^2, \mu_2, \sigma_2^2\right)$, and the appropriate sample size for each group is as follows:

$$\begin{aligned} n &= \frac{\left(\sigma_1^2 + \sigma_2^2\right)\left(z_{1-0.05/2} + z_{0.8}\right)^2}{\left(\mu_1 - \mu_2\right)^2} \\ &= \frac{\left(15.34^2 + 18.23^2\right) \times \left(1.96 + 0.84\right)^2}{\left(132.86 - 127.44\right)^2} \\ &\approx 152. \end{aligned}$$

Therefore, 152 participants are needed in each group to achieve a power of 80% for detecting a real difference.

2. Unequal Sample Sizes in the Two Groups

Balanced sample sizes between groups ensure maximum statistical power at a fixed total sample size. However, in practice, the sample sizes do not necessarily need to be equal. Suppose $n_2 = kn_1$, i.e., the sample size of group 2 is k times that of group 1. The sample sizes required for a two-sided test to achieve a power of $1-\beta$ at a significance level of α are given by the following formulas:

$$n_1 = \frac{\left(\sigma_1^2 + \sigma_2^2 / k\right)\left(z_{1-\alpha/2} + z_{1-\beta}\right)^2}{\left(\mu_1 - \mu_2\right)^2}, \tag{8.12}$$

$$n_2 = \frac{\left(k\sigma_1^2 + \sigma_2^2\right)\left(z_{1-\alpha/2} + z_{1-\beta}\right)^2}{\left(\mu_1 - \mu_2\right)^2}, \tag{8.13}$$

where μ_1, μ_2, σ_1^2, and σ_2^2 are the means and variances of the two groups and $k = n_2 / n_1$ is the projected ratio of the two sample sizes.

To perform a one-sided rather than a two-sided test, simply substitute $z_{1-\alpha}$ for $z_{1-\alpha/2}$ in Formulas 8.11, 8.12, and 8.13.

Example 8.9 Referring to Example 8.8. Suppose we anticipate twice as many manual labor participants as office workers to be enrolled in the study to compare their SBP levels according to their compositions in the labor population. Determine the required sample size if a two-sided test is used with a 5% significance level and 80% power is desired.

Solution

If Formula 8.12 is used with $\mu_1 = 132.86$, $\sigma_1 = 15.34$, $\mu_2 = 127.44$, $\sigma_2 = 18.23$, and $k = 2$, then to achieve 80% power in the study using a two-sided significance test with $\alpha = 0.05$, the sample size of the office workers is

$$n_1 = \frac{\left(\sigma_1^2 + \sigma_2^2 / k\right)\left(z_{1-0.05/2} + z_{0.8}\right)^2}{\left(\mu_1 - \mu_2\right)^2} = \frac{\left(15.34^2 + 18.23^2 / 2\right) \times \left(1.96 + 0.84\right)^2}{\left(132.86 - 127.44\right)^2} \approx 108.$$

The sample size required of the participants who are manual laborers is $n_2 = 2 \times 108 = 216$.

If the population variances of the two groups are equal, then for a given α and β, the minimum sample size required is achieved by the equal-sample-size allocation rule in Formula 8.11. Thus, in the case of equal variances, the sample sizes of the two groups should be as nearly equal as possible.

8.3 Testing the Difference Between Two Population Rates (Normal Approximation Method)

The Z-test can easily be extended to binary data when the central limit theorem holds. As we discussed in Chapter 6, if the sample sizes n_1 and n_2 are moderately large (in the meantime, $n_1 p_1 (1-p_1) \geq 5$ and $n_2 p_2 (1-p_2) \geq 5$), then the sampling distribution of $p_1 - p_2$ should be approximately normally distributed.

Considering hypothesis testing $H_0 : \pi_1 = \pi_2$, or $\pi_1 - \pi_2 = 0$, the test statistic Z under H_0 approximately follows a standard normal distribution $N(0,1)$,

$$Z = \frac{p_1 - p_2}{S_{p_1 - p_2}} = \frac{p_1 - p_2}{\sqrt{p_C(1-p_C)\left(\frac{1}{n_1} + \frac{1}{n_2}\right)}}, \tag{8.14}$$

where

$$p_C = \frac{n_1 p_1 + n_2 p_2}{n_1 + n_2}. \tag{8.15}$$

Draw a conclusion

(i) Critical-value method
For a given α,
If $Z < z_{\alpha/2}$ or $Z > z_{1-\alpha/2}$, then reject H_0;
If $z_{\alpha/2} \leq Z \leq z_{1-\alpha/2}$, then do not reject H_0.

(ii) p-value method
If $Z \leq 0$, $p = 2 \times$ (area to the left of Z under a standard normal Z distribution);
If $Z > 0$, $p = 2 \times$ (area to the right of Z under a standard normal Z distribution).

Example 8.10 Referring to Example 8.6, a large-scale survey was conducted as an expansion of the pilot study. As a result, 161 of 338 (47.6%) and 174 of 428 (40.7%) participants were diagnosed as hypertensive in the office worker and manual labor groups, respectively. Is there any difference between the two types of occupations in terms of the rate of hypertension?

Solution
(1) State the hypotheses and select a significance level

$H_0 : \pi_1 = \pi_2$, the rates of hypertension of office workers and manual laborers are the same for the two groups
$H_1 : \pi_1 \neq \pi_2$, the rates of hypertension are not the same

$\alpha = 0.05$

(2) Determine the test statistic
If Formulas 8.14 and 8.15 are used, we know that $n_1 = 338$, $p_1 = 0.476$; $n_2 = 428$, $p_2 = 0.407$, then

$$p_C = \frac{n_1 p_1 + n_2 p_2}{n_1 + n_2} = \frac{161+174}{338+428} = 0.437.$$

$$S_{p_1-p_2} = \sqrt{p_C(1-p_C)\left(\frac{1}{n_1}+\frac{1}{n_2}\right)} = \sqrt{0.437(1-0.437)\left(\frac{1}{338}+\frac{1}{428}\right)} = 0.036.$$

Because $n_1 p_1(1-p_1) = 338 \times 0.476 \times 0.524 = 84.3 > 5$ and $n_2 p_2(1-p_2) = 428 \times 0.407 \times 0.593 = 103.3 > 5$, z-test can be used, and the test statistic is

$$z = \frac{0.476 - 0.407}{\sqrt{0.437 \times 0.563 \times \left(\frac{1}{338}+\frac{1}{428}\right)}} = 1.91.$$

(3) Draw a conclusion

(i) Critical-value method

For $\alpha = 0.05$, since $z = 1.91 < z_{1-0.05/2} = 1.96$, $p > 0.05$. Therefore, we do not reject H_0 at the $\alpha = 0.05$ level, which means we do not have significant evidence to show that the rates of hypertension for the two types of occupations are different.

(ii) p-value method

Since the test statistic $z = 1.91 > 0$, the p value is $p = 2 \times P(Z > z) = 2 \times [1 - P(Z \leq z)]$ $= 2 \times [1 - \Phi(z)] = 2 \times [1 - \Phi(1.91)]$. Using the NORMDIST function of Microsoft Excel $\Phi(1.91) = \text{NORMDIST}(1.91,0,1,1)$, then $p = 2 \times [1 - \Phi(1.91)] = 0.0561 > 0.05$, which is considered not statistically significant. The conclusion is therefore the same.

8.3.1 Power for Comparing Two Rates

Usually, the sample size required for a comparison of rates is greater than that for comparing means. Therefore, the exact statistical power with a constrained sample size for the comparison of rates requires greater attention. When $n_1\pi_1(1-\pi_1) \geq 5$, $n_2\pi_2(1-\pi_2) \geq 5$. The power of a hypothesis test for two rates is provided to test the hypothesis $H_0: \pi_1 = \pi_2$ vs. $H_1: \pi_1 \neq \pi_2$, with a significance level of α and sample sizes of n_1 and n_2 in the two groups.

$$1-\beta \approx \Phi\left(\frac{\frac{|\pi_1-\pi_2|}{\sqrt{\pi_1(1-\pi_1)/n_1+\pi_2(1-\pi_2)/n_2}} - z_{1-\alpha/2}}{\frac{\sqrt{\pi_C(1-\pi_C)(1/n_1+1/n_2)}}{\sqrt{\pi_1(1-\pi_1)/n_1+\pi_2(1-\pi_2)/n_2}}}\right), \tag{8.16}$$

where $\pi_C = \frac{n_1\pi_1 + n_2\pi_2}{n_1 + n_2}$ is the pooled rate of two populations.

Formula 8.16 can be used for a one-sided test after replacing $z_{1-\alpha/2}$ with $z_{1-\alpha}$.

Example 8.11 Referring to Example 8.10, how much power does such a study have in detecting a real difference if a two-sided test with an α level of 0.05 is used?

Solution

We have $\pi_1 = 0.476$ (replaced by p_1), $\pi_2 = 0.407$ (replaced by p_2), $n_1 = 338$, $n_2 = 428$, $|\pi_1 - \pi_2| = 0.069$, $\pi_C = 0.437$, $\alpha = 0.05$, and $z_{1-0.05/2} = 1.96$. Thus, from Formula 8.16, the power can be computed as follows:

$$1-\beta \approx \Phi\left(\frac{|\pi_1-\pi_2|}{\sqrt{\pi_1(1-\pi_1)/n_1+\pi_2(1-\pi_2)/n_2}} - z_{1-0.05/2}\frac{\sqrt{\pi_C(1-\pi_C)(1/n_1+1/n_2)}}{\sqrt{\pi_1(1-\pi_1)/n_1+\pi_2(1-\pi_2)/n_2}}\right)$$

$$=\Phi\left(\frac{0.069}{\sqrt{0.476\times0.524/338+0.407\times0.593/428}} - 1.96\times\frac{\sqrt{0.437\times0.563\times(1/338+1/428)}}{\sqrt{0.476\times0.524/338+0.407\times0.593/428}}\right)$$

$$=0.481$$

Thus, there is a 48.1% chance of finding a real difference given the available sample sizes.

8.3.2 Sample Size Determination

In Section 8.2.6, we discussed the methods for estimating the sample size needed to compare means from two normally distributed populations. This section covers similar methods for estimating the sample size required to compare two rates.

Suppose we wish to plan a hypothesis test for $H_0: \pi_1 = \pi_2$ vs. $H_1: \pi_1 \neq \pi_2$ at a significance level of α with a predetermined condition $n_2 = kn_1$; the sample sizes required in the two groups for a power of $1-\beta$ are provided by the following formulas:

$$n_1 = \frac{\left[\sqrt{\pi_C(1-\pi_C)\left(1+\frac{1}{k}\right)}z_{1-\alpha/2} + \sqrt{\pi_1(1-\pi_1)+\frac{\pi_2(1-\pi_2)}{k}}z_{1-\beta}\right]^2}{(\pi_1-\pi_2)^2}, \tag{8.17}$$

$$n_2 = kn_1, \tag{8.18}$$

where $\pi_C = \frac{\pi_1 + k\pi_2}{1+k}$ is the pooled rate of two populations.

To perform a one-sided test, simply substitute $z_{1-\alpha}$ for $z_{1-\alpha/2}$ in Formula 8.17.

Example 8.12 Consider the study proposed in Example 8.10. How large a sample size is needed for the larger study if an equal sample size is anticipated in each group? A two-sided test with a significance level of 0.05 is used and a power of 80% is desired.

Solution

Knowing that $\pi_1 = 0.476$ (replaced by p_1), $\pi_2 = 0.407$ (replaced by p_2), $|\pi_1 - \pi_2| = 0.069$, and $k = 1$, to achieve 80% power in the study using a two-sided test with $\alpha = 0.05$, we compute that

$$\pi_C = \frac{\pi_1 + k\pi_2}{1+k} = 0.442$$

Thus, referring to Formula 8.17,

$$\begin{aligned} n_1 &= n_2 \\ &= \left[\sqrt{\pi_C\left(1-\pi_C\right)\left(1+\frac{1}{k}\right)}z_{1-0.05/2} + \sqrt{\pi_1\left(1-\pi_1\right)+\frac{\pi_2\left(1-\pi_2\right)}{k}}z_{0.8}\right]^2 \Big/ \left(\pi_1 - \pi_2\right)^2 \\ &= \frac{\left[\sqrt{0.442\times 0.558\times\left(1+\frac{1}{1}\right)}\times 1.96 + \sqrt{0.476\times 0.524 + \frac{0.407\times 0.593}{1}}\times 0.84\right]^2}{0.069^2} \\ &\approx 812. \end{aligned}$$

Therefore, 812 participants are needed in each group.

8.4 Summary

We have discussed some methods for two-sample hypothesis testing in this chapter, including a paired samples t-test for means, two sample t-test for the means of independent samples, F-test for equality of variances, and two sample Z-test for large-sample means and rates. All these methods assume that either the samples come from normally distributed populations or the central limit theorem holds.

The choice of method depends on the research design and type of data. Essentially, we need to construct a proper test statistic, where the hypotheses are justified based on the sampling distribution. This echoes the earlier statement that hypothesis testing and parameter estimation in Chapter 6 have the same origin.

The power and sample size determination methods were introduced for detecting a real difference between two means and rates. These are important considerations for research design, and it is strongly recommended that these methods be applied before collecting data.

The two sample hypothesis testing follows the same principle we discussed in Chapter 7. We recommend revisiting Section 7.1.

In the next two chapters, we will extend the discussion of hypothesis testing from two populations to multiple normal populations using ANOVA methods under different experimental designs.

8.5 Exercises

1. A study aimed to investigate the relationship between chronic bronchitis and serum cholinesterase activity by comparing the serum cholinesterase activities of rats with chronic bronchitis and healthy rats. Sixteen Wistar rats were matched into eight pairs by litter, sex, and body weight. The rats in each pair were then randomly allocated to either the experimental or control group. The rats in the experimental group were supplied air containing 0.3 mg/m^2 formaldehyde (chronic bronchitis rat model with inhalation of formaldehyde), and the control group was supplied clean air. The serum cholinesterase activity (μmol/ml) was measured after 8 weeks; the results are given in Table 8.4.
   Please answer the following questions:
   (a) What is the design of this study? What is the advantage of this design?
   (b) Which method could be employed for testing the two population means in such a design? What are the necessary assumptions for applying the test?
   (c) Is it appropriate to employ two independent samples t-test in this study? If not, what is the consequence of misusing a paired samples t-test with a two independent samples t-test?
2. To investigate the anti-inflammatory effect of buckwheat flavonoid, 20 mice injected with 0.2 ml 2% agar solution to form an agar granuloma were randomly divided into an experimental group and a control group. The 10 mice in the experimental group received buckwheat flavonoid, and the remaining 10 mice in the control group were injected with 0.5 ml 65% ethanol. The weight of the granulomas

Table 8.4 The serum cholinesterase activity (μmol/ml) of rats in the two groups.

Pair ID	Experimental group	Control group
1	3.28	2.36
2	2.60	2.40
3	3.32	2.40
4	2.72	2.52
5	2.38	3.04
6	3.64	2.64
7	2.98	2.56
8	4.40	2.40

(mg) was measured after 10 days (assuming normal distributions in both groups). Table 8.5 displays the results.

Table 8.5 Weight of granuloma (mg) for the 20 mice after 10 days of treatment.

Experimental group	108.0	74.8	31.2	132.0	147.6	98.5	82.2	93.3	85.5	110.4
Control group	94.8	122.5	144.1	151.2	189.3	204.2	155.6	160.3	178.3	165.4

Please answer the following questions:

(a) What is the type of design? What are the advantage and disadvantage of this design?

(b) Which testing methods are appropriate for this design, and what assumption other than normality should be made for conducting the hypothesis testing? Check this assumption.

(c) Perform a test to investigate whether buckwheat flavonoid has an inhibitory effect on agar granuloma in mice and draw a conclusion.

(d) Calculate the 95% CI for the mean of difference. Would the conclusion based on the confidence interval agree with the result of hypothesis testing? What are the inherent relationships between the hypothesis testing and CI results?

(e) Using a two-sided test at a significance level of $\alpha = 0.05$, what is the power of the test in (c)?

3. To investigate the difference in $\alpha 1$ antitrypsin levels between healthy subjects and patients with grade III emphysema, 15 healthy subjects and 13 patients with grade III emphysema were randomly sampled. The $\alpha 1$ antitrypsin levels (g/L) in their sputum were measured and are displayed in Table 8.6.

Table 8.6 $\alpha 1$ antitrypsin levels (g/L) in healthy people and patients with grade III emphysema.

Healthy subjects	Patients with grade III emphysema
1.7	1.6
2.2	2.4
3.1	3.7
3.3	5.4
2.6	3.6
1.9	6.8
2.7	4.7
0.9	2.9
3.9	4.8
2.3	6.6
1.5	4.1
1.7	3.3
2.3	6.3
3.4	
1.9	

Source: Guojonsdottir et al. (2015).

Please answer the following questions:

(a) Assuming that normality has been satisfied, is it appropriate to apply the two independent samples t-test for testing the difference of the mean $\alpha 1$ antitrypsin levels between the two groups? What other assumptions should be considered, and why should such assumptions be satisfied?

(b) Which statistic can be calculated in testing the assumption in (a)? Please carry out the test.

(c) Based on (b), what methods can be used to address this issue?

4. A study aims to compare the body mass index (BMI, kg/m^2) of women aged ≥ 45 years residing within and outside the capital area. The mean and standard deviation for each group of individuals is presented in Table 8.7.

Table 8.7 BMI (kg/m^2) of women aged ≥ 45 years residing within and outside the capital area.

Within capital area ($n_1 = 208$)		Outside capital area ($n_2 = 138$)	
$\bar{x}$	s	$\bar{x}$	s
25.7	4.8	28.4	4.0

Please answer the following questions:

(a) Which tests could be employed for testing the population mean differences in BMI? Please give your reasons.

(b) hat do you think about the relationship between the t-test and Z-test? Under what conditions could the Z-test be used as a substitute for the t-test, and which theorem is needed to guarantee such a substitution?

(c) Please conduct the hypothesis tests and interpret the results with a summary report.

5. In the toxicological study of a new anticancer drug, 78 rats were randomly divided into two groups of 39. One group received a low-dose injection and the other a high-dose injection of the drug. Eighteen rats in the high-dose group and nine rats in the low-dose group died.

(a) What is the design of this study?

(b) Which type of statistical test could be used to deal with this type of data, and what theorem should hold when applying the test method?

(c) Conduct hypothesis testing to determine whether there is a difference in population rates of death between the two groups.

(d) Compute and interpret the 95% CI for the difference in population rates of death between the two groups.

(e) Using a one-sided test at a significance level of $\alpha = 0.05$, what is the power of this test?

(f) How large a sample size is needed if an equal sample size is assigned in each group, for a one-sided and two-sided test, respectively, with a significance level of 0.05 and a power of 80%. Is the sample size requirement higher in the one-sided test or the two-sided test, explain your answer?

6. To explore the efficacy of a combination of antihypertensive agents, 16 hypertensive patients were enrolled and randomly divided into a monotherapy regime group and a combination therapy regime group (eight patients in each group). Their systolic blood pressure (mmHg) before and after treatment was measured, as given in Table 8.8. The researcher first compared the baseline level of systolic blood pressure between the two groups using the two independent samples t-test. After failing to reject H_0 $(p = 0.407)$, the researcher claimed that there was no statistical difference at baseline. Then, by conducting another independent t-test in comparing the post-treatment systolic blood pressures, the researcher concluded that there is no difference in efficacy between the monotherapy and combination therapy owing to an insignificant p value of 0.088.

Table 8.8 Systolic blood pressure (mmHg) before and after treatment in two groups of hypertensive patients.

ID	Monotherapy regime ($n_1 = 8$)		ID	Combination therapy regime ($n_2 = 8$)	
	Pre-treatment	Post-treatment		Pre-treatment	Post-treatment
1	146	134	9	148	120
2	158	136	10	159	121
3	175	150	11	178	148
4	144	134	12	169	130
5	138	126	13	149	126
6	143	124	14	145	114
7	144	128	15	150	118
8	172	168	16	167	129

Please answer the following questions:

(a) Is this analytical method appropriate? If not, please give reasons and use the appropriate method to compare the efficacy of the two therapeutic regimes. What assumptions should be made when conducting this analysis?

(b) What is the 95% CI for the difference in efficacy between the monotherapy and combination therapy?

9

One-way Analysis of Variance

CONTENTS

In Chapter 7, we introduced the concept and methods of hypothesis testing and one-sample testing. Chapter 8 extended the ability to make statistical inferences from two sample situations. In this chapter, we introduce the use of *analysis of variance* (*ANOVA*) for hypothesis testing of more than two sample means with normal distributions. ANOVA was first introduced by the statistician R.A. Fisher in 1921 and is now widely applied in the biomedical and other research fields. ANOVA is a family of hypothesis testing methods for dealing with data obtained from different experimental designs. The basic principles of ANOVA methods are similar despite using different calculation ways with different designs. We focus on one-way ANOVA in this chapter and continue discussing ANOVA in different experimental designs in the next chapter. Further discussion of experimental designs can be found in Chapter 20.

9.1 Overview

One-way ANOVA refers to the analysis of variance for a completely randomized design under which all subjects are mutually independent. The experimental subjects are randomly assigned to k groups, and each group is assigned to a specific

Applied Medical Statistics, First Edition. Jingmei Jiang.

Companion website: www.wiley.com\go\jiang\appliedmedicalstatistics

treatment. The effect of experimental factors is inferred based on the hypothesis testing of the differences between the means of the treatment groups. The term "one-way" is used because the subjects are separated into groups by one factor (e.g., treatment).

9.1.1 Concept of ANOVA

Example 9.1 To investigate the effect of exercise-induced fatigue on pain response, 15 rats were randomly assigned to 3 groups of 5 and were subjected to low-, medium-, or high-intensity exercise. The rats were injected with formalin immediately after exercise to induce pain. Behavioral observation was started 10 min after injection, lasting for 300 s. The paw-licking durations (s) of the rats were recorded. The results are given in Table 9.1(a). Are the mean paw-licking durations different among the rats subjected to different exercise intensities?

Suppose another experiment was conducted under the same experimental conditions, and the paw-licking durations of the rats were recorded 20 min after the formalin injection. The results are given in Table 9.1(b). Are the mean paw-licking durations different among the rats subjected to different exercise intensities? (Assume that the paw-licking durations in each group follow a normal distribution.)

In Table 9.1, only one factor (exercise intensity) was considered. The rats were randomly divided into three groups according to exercise intensity. We say that this treatment factor has three levels and the exercise intensity at each level is a type of treatment. For example, low-intensity exercise was a type of treatment.

The mean paw-licking durations of the rats in the three groups were the same at two independent observation time points $\left(\bar{x}_1 = 50\text{s}, \bar{x}_2 = 30\text{s}, \bar{x}_3 = 15\text{s}\right)$. Then, the question arises as to how we should assess the differences between the mean paw-licking durations. For a better understanding, the data are displayed in the following plots.

Table 9.1(a) Paw-licking durations (s). (10 min after the formalin injection)

	Exercise intensity		
	Low	Medium	High
	53.5	33.2	11.5
	43.7	30.6	21.9
	46.5	23.9	18.6
	50.3	26.4	13.6
	56.1	35.9	9.5
$\bar{x}_{\cdot j}$	50.0	30.0	15.0

j represents the jth column, $j = 1, 2, 3$.

Table 9.1(b) Paw-licking durations (s). (20 min after the formalin injection)

	Exercise intensity		
	Low	Medium	High
	27.4	13.7	16.7
	42.9	27.1	9.1
	59.1	21.2	3.5
	66.6	35.8	39.6
	54.0	52.2	6.1
$\bar{x}_{\cdot j}$	50.0	30.0	15.0

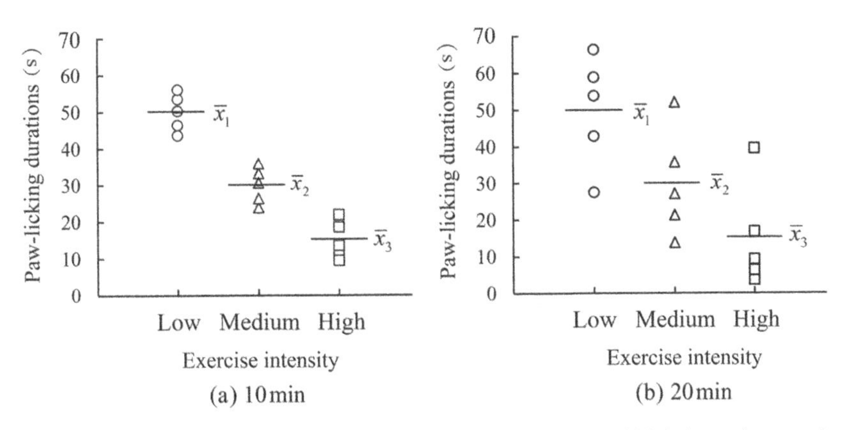

Figure 9.1 Paw-licking durations (s) of rats in low, medium, and high-intensity exercise groups 10 and 20 min after the formalin injection.

As shown in Figure 9.1, the sample means corresponding to each exercise intensity level between the three groups were the same at two independent observation time points. However, the variation of the sample means between the three groups was larger than that of the individual observations within each group in Figure 9.1(a). Therefore, a true difference in population means is more likely. Conversely, we can see in Figure 9.1(b) that there is a substantial variation within each group and large overlaps between groups, so a true difference in population means is less likely. Therefore, the variation of observations within groups played an important role in identifying the differences between means when hypothesis testing was performed to compare multiple population means.

This example suggests that when testing the differences between population means, we can analyze the problem from the aspect of source of variability and separate the "variances" into variance across groups (between groups) and in the same groups (within group). Then we can test whether the variability in the data comes mostly from the variability within each group or can truly be attributed to the variability between groups. This is the basic idea of ANOVA.

9.1.2 Data Layout and Modeling Assumption

The data layout for one-way ANOVA is usually presented in the form given in Table 9.2.

Suppose each data element of the experiment results is denoted by X_{ij}, we can structure the following model:

$$X_{ij} = \mu + \alpha_j + \varepsilon_{ij} \left(i = 1, 2, \ldots, n_j;\, j = 1, 2, \ldots, k\right), \tag{9.1}$$

where μ is an expected mean, which is usually estimated from the overall mean of observations in all groups, $\bar{X}_{..} = \left(\sum_{j=1}^{k} \sum_{i=1}^{n_j} X_{ij} \Big/ n \right)$.

$\alpha_j = \mu_j - \mu$ ($\mu = \frac{1}{k}\sum_{j=1}^{k}\mu_j$) is the effect of the jth treatment, where μ_j is the expected mean of observations of the jth treatment.

ε_{ij} is an *error term*, which is normally distributed with mean 0 and variance σ^2.

Thus, a typical observation X_{ij} from the jth group is normally distributed with mean $\mu + \alpha_j$ and variance σ^2.

Model Assumptions

1. The k samples represent independent random samples drawn from k specific populations.
2. Each sampled population is normally distributed.
3. Each sampled population has equal variance (i.e., $\sigma_1^2 = \sigma_2^2 = \cdots = \sigma_k^2 = \sigma^2$).
4. The model should satisfy $\sum_{j=1}^{k}\alpha_j = 0$.

9.2 Procedures of ANOVA

A more common way to interpret ANOVA is that it partitions the variation into different components, that is, the essence of ANOVA is the partitioning of variances.

Table 9.2 Data layout of one-way ANOVA.

Levels of treatment factor A	A_1	A_2	$\cdots$	A_k	
Observation X_{ij}	X_{11}	X_{12}	$\cdots$	X_{1k}	
	X_{21}	X_{22}	$\cdots$	X_{2k}	
	$\vdots$	$\vdots$	$\vdots$	$\vdots$	
	X_{i1}	X_{i2}	$\cdots$	X_{ik}	
	$\vdots$	$\vdots$	$\vdots$	$\vdots$	
	$X_{n_1 1}$	$X_{n_2 2}$	$\cdots$	$X_{n_k k}$	
n_j	n_1	n_2	$\cdots$	n_k	$n = \sum_{j=1}^{k} n_j$
$\sum_{i=1}^{n_j} X_{ij}$	$\sum_{i=1}^{n_1} X_{i1}$	$\sum_{i=1}^{n_2} X_{i2}$	$\cdots$	$\sum_{i=1}^{n_k} X_{ik}$	$\sum_{j=1}^{k}\sum_{i=1}^{n_j} X_{ij}$
$\bar{X}_{\cdot j}$	$\bar{X}_{\cdot 1}$	$\bar{X}_{\cdot 2}$	$\cdots$	$\bar{X}_{\cdot k}$	$\bar{X}_{\cdot\cdot} = \frac{\sum_{j=1}^{k}\sum_{i=1}^{n_j} X_{ij}}{n}$

From Chapter 2, we know that sample variance can be used to describe the average variation of the observational data with sample size n.

$$s^2 = \frac{\sum_i (x_i - \bar{x})^2}{n-1}$$

The sample variance is difficult for direct partitioning. Instead, in the ANOVA procedure, we analyze this relative quantity by portioning its numerator (sum of squares of deviations from the mean) and denominator (degrees of freedom) first and then calculating the "variance" of different sources (called mean square), and finally completing the hypothesis testing. The steps of one-way ANOVA are as follows:

1. Partitioning the Sum of Squares of Deviations
The deviation of any individual observation X_{ij} from the overall mean $\bar{X}_{..}$ can be represented as the following identical equation:

$$X_{ij} - \bar{X}_{..} = \left(\bar{X}_{.j} - \bar{X}_{..}\right) + \left(X_{ij} - \bar{X}_{.j}\right). \tag{9.2}$$

The first term on the right-hand side $\left(\bar{X}_{.j} - \bar{X}_{..}\right)$ represents the deviation of a jth group mean from the overall mean and indicates between-group variability. The second term on the right-hand side $\left(X_{ij} - \bar{X}_{.j}\right)$ represents the deviation of an individual observation from the group mean and indicates within-group variability. Square the left and right terms of the formula and summing together (note that the cross product is proved to be zero) gives the following relationship:

$$\sum_j \sum_i \left(X_{ij} - \bar{X}_{..}\right)^2 = \sum_j n_j \left(\bar{X}_{.j} - \bar{X}_{..}\right)^2 + \sum_j \sum_i \left(X_{ij} - \bar{X}_{.j}\right)^2, \tag{9.3}$$

where $\sum_j n_j \left(\bar{X}_{.j} - \bar{X}_{..}\right)^2 = \sum_j \sum_i \left(X_{.j} - \bar{X}_{..}\right)^2$.

Formula 9.3 displays the partitioning of the *sum of squares* (SS), which has been described and is named as follows:

The *total sum of squares*, denoted by SS_T, measures the *total variation* of all observations.

$$SS_T = \sum_j \sum_i \left(X_{ij} - \bar{X}_{..}\right)^2. \tag{9.4}$$

The calculation of SS_T can be simplified using

$$SS_T = \sum_j \sum_i X_{ij}^2 - \frac{\left(\sum_j \sum_i X_{ij}\right)^2}{n}, \tag{9.5}$$

where $\left(\sum_j \sum_i X_{ij}\right)^2 \Big/ n$ is a correction term and is usually expressed as C.

The *between groups sum of squares*, denoted by SS_A, measures the variation between group means at various levels of the treatment factor A, that is, the *between-group variation*

$$SS_A = \sum_j n_j \left(\bar{X}_{.j} - \bar{X}_{..}\right)^2. \tag{9.6}$$

The calculation of SS_A can be simplified as

$$SS_A = \sum_j \frac{\left(\sum_i X_{ij}\right)^2}{n_j} - C. \tag{9.7}$$

The *within groups sum of squares*, denoted by SS_E, measures the variation of observations within treatment groups, that is, the *within-group variation.*

$$SS_E = \sum_j \sum_i \left(X_{ij} - \bar{X}_{.j}\right)^2. \tag{9.8}$$

This reflects the random error of an experiment not related to the treatment factor.

Thus, the relationship in Formula 9.3 can be simply written as

$$SS_T = SS_A + SS_E. \tag{9.9}$$

2. Partitioning Degrees of Freedom

The degrees of freedom for the sums of squares can be partitioned similar to the sum of squares of deviations. The degrees of freedom of SS_T are $\nu_T = n - 1$, because all observations have one common overall mean. The treatment factor A has k levels, so the associated degrees of freedom of SS_A are $\nu_A = k - 1$. The degrees of freedom of SS_E are $n - k$, specifically, because the degrees of freedom within each treatment group are $n_j - 1$ and there are k treatment groups; thus, $\nu_E = \sum_j (n_j - 1) = n - k$.

The relationship among the degrees of freedom can be presented as follows:

$$\nu_T = \nu_A + \nu_E. \tag{9.10}$$

3. Formulation of Variances from Different Sources

As mentioned above, variance is equal to the ratio of the sum of squares to the degrees of freedom, which is called the *mean square* (MS) in the ANOVA.

Between groups mean square (or *treatment mean square*)

$$MS_A = \frac{SS_A}{k - 1}, \tag{9.11}$$

which reflects the variation between the treatment group means. It contains both the *treatment effect* and *random error effect.*

Within groups mean square (or *error mean square*)

$$\mathrm{MS}_E = \frac{\mathrm{SS}_E}{n-k}, \tag{9.12}$$

which reflects the variation within each treatment group caused by the random error effect.

4. Hypothesis Testing for the Means

(1) State the hypotheses and select a significance level

$H_0 : \mu_1 = \mu_2 = \cdots = \mu_k$; k population means are the same

This null hypothesis is equal to testing $\alpha_1 = \alpha_2 = \cdots = \alpha_k = 0$

$H_1 : \mu_1, \mu_2, \ldots, \mu_k$ are not all the same

Let α be the significance level

(2) Determine a test statistic

Under H_0, all observations can be viewed as random samples from the same normally distributed population $N(\mu, \sigma^2)$. As $\mathrm{SS}_T / (n-1)$ is an unbiased estimate of σ^2, according to Formula 6.8, we have

$$\frac{\mathrm{SS}_T}{\sigma^2} \sim \chi^2(\nu), \quad \nu = \nu_T = n-1$$

Similarly,

$$\frac{\mathrm{SS}_E}{\sigma^2} \sim \chi^2(\nu), \quad \nu = \nu_E = n-k$$

According to the independent additivity of the χ^2 distribution, we have

$$\frac{\mathrm{SS}_A}{\sigma^2} = \frac{\mathrm{SS}_T}{\sigma^2} - \frac{\mathrm{SS}_E}{\sigma^2} \sim \chi^2(\nu), \; \nu = \nu_A = k-1$$

Then, test statistic

$$F = \frac{\dfrac{\mathrm{SS}_A}{(k-1)\sigma^2}}{\dfrac{\mathrm{SS}_E}{(n-k)\sigma^2}} = \frac{\dfrac{\mathrm{SS}_A}{k-1}}{\dfrac{\mathrm{SS}_E}{n-k}} = \frac{\mathrm{MS}_A}{\mathrm{MS}_E} \tag{9.13}$$

follows an F distribution with a pair of degrees of freedom $\nu_A = k-1$ (numerator) $\nu_E = n-k$ (denominator).

(3) Draw a conclusion

(i) Critical-value method

For a given α and (ν_A, ν_E), we can obtain the critical value $F_{(\nu_A,\nu_E),1-\alpha}$ from the $F_{(\nu_A,\nu_E)}$ distribution (Appendix Table 6).

If $F > F_{(\nu_A,\nu_E),1-\alpha}$, then reject H_0;

If $F \le F_{(\nu_A,\nu_E),1-\alpha}$, then do not reject H_0.

Notice that ν_A and ν_E denote ν_1 and ν_2, respectively, in Appendix Table 6.

The rejection and non-rejection regions for the one-way ANOVA F-test are given in Figure 9.2.

(ii) p-value method

The p value (Figure 9.3) is given by the area to the right of F under an $F_{(\nu_A,\nu_E)}$ distribution, that is,

$$p = P\left(F_{(\nu_A,\nu_E)} > F\right). \tag{9.14}$$

The results of one-way ANOVA are typically displayed in an ANOVA table (Table 9.3).

The F-test done in conjunction with the ANOVA table is often called the global F-test. It tells us whether there are any differences worth examining further. If H_0 is not rejected, then the analysis is complete, and the conclusion is that there are no significant differences among the treatment groups analyzed. Multiple comparisons are required if the global F-test indicates that H_0 is rejected (see Section 9.3).

From the entire ANOVA procedure, we can understand that the F distribution can be used to test the null hypothesis of no difference between the treatment group means. The additive property of the sums of squares led early researchers to view this analysis as a partitioning of variation into sources corresponding to the factors included in the experiment and error. The simple formulas for computing the sums of squares,

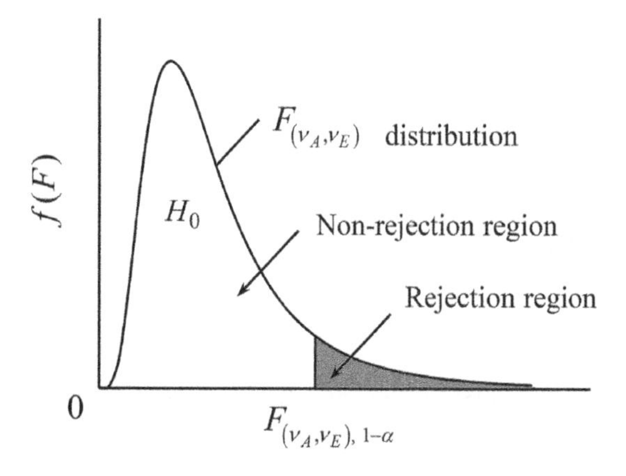

Figure 9.2 Illustration of rejection and non-rejection regions for the F-test for one-way ANOVA.

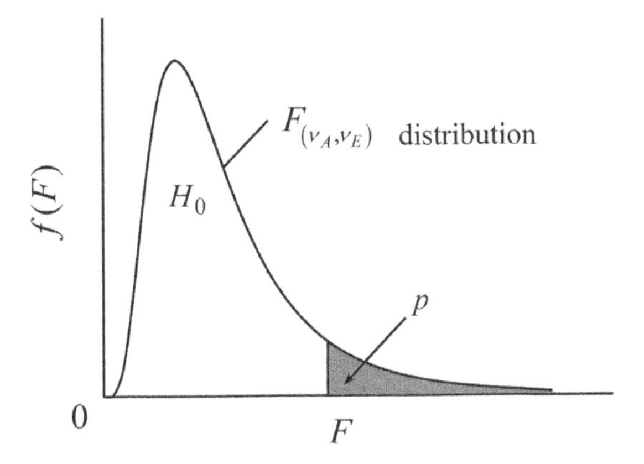

Figure 9.3 Illustration of p value for the F-test for one-way ANOVA.

Table 9.3 General format of the ANOVA table for one-way ANOVA.

Source of variation	SS	ν	MS	F	p value
Between groups	SS_A	$k-1$	$SS_A/(k-1)$	MS_A/MS_E	*
Within groups	SS_E	$n-k$	$SS_E/(n-k)$		
Total	SS_T	$n-1$			

Note: Unless otherwise specified in this test, p value(s) are given in the ANOVA result tables and are determined from the statistical software. The conclusion will be drawn according to the predetermined significance level.

their additive property, and form of the test statistic made it natural for this procedure to be called analysis of variance.

Solution to Example 9.1 In Table 9.4, we present the sample data and summary statistics for Example 9.1 (10 min).

(1) State the hypotheses and select a significance level
$H_0: \mu_1 = \mu_2 = \mu_3$, the population mean paw-licking durations of rats subjected to each exercise intensity are the same
$H_1: \mu_1, \mu_2, \mu_3$ are not all the same

$$\alpha = 0.05$$

(2) Calculate the test statistic and construct the ANOVA table
First, performing basic calculations based on the data in Table 9.4, we have

$$\sum_j \sum_i x_{ij} = 475.2$$

$$\sum_j \sum_i x_{ij}^2 = 53.5^2 + 43.7^2 + \cdots + 9.5^2 = 18440.10$$

Table 9.4 Calculation of Example 9.1 (10 min).

Exercise-intensity group	Low	Medium	High	
Observation x_{ij}	53.5	33.2	11.5	
	43.7	30.6	21.9	
	46.5	23.9	18.6	
	50.3	26.4	13.6	
	56.1	35.9	9.5	
n_j	5	5	5	$n=15$
$\sum_i x_{ij}$	250.1	150.0	75.1	$\sum_j \sum_i x_{ij} = 475.2$
$\bar{x}_j$	50.0	30.0	15.0	$\bar{x} = 31.7$
s_j^2	25.4	23.9	26.3	

$$C = \left(\sum_j \sum_i x_{ij}\right)^2 \bigg/ n = 475.20^2 / 15 = 15054.34$$

The sum of squares and corresponding degrees of freedom are as follows:
Total

$$SS_T = \sum_j \sum_i x_{ij}^2 - C = 18440.10 - 15054.34 = 3385.76,$$
$$\nu_T = n - 1 = 14.$$

Between groups

$$SS_A = \sum_j n_j \left(\bar{x}_j - \bar{x}\right)^2 = \sum_j \frac{\left(\sum_i x_{ij}\right)^2}{n_j} - C$$
$$= \frac{250.10^2}{5} + \frac{150.00^2}{5} + \frac{75.10^2}{5} - 15054.34 = 3083.66,$$
$$\nu_A = k - 1 = 2.$$

Within groups

$$SS_E = SS_T - SS_A$$
$$= 3385.76 - 3083.66 = 302.10,$$
$$\nu_E = n - k = 12.$$

The mean squares and test statistic are as follows:

$$MS_A = \frac{SS_A}{\nu_A} = \frac{3083.66}{2} = 1541.83,$$

Table 9.5 ANOVA table for Example 9.1 (10 min).

Source of variation	SS	ν	MS	F	p value
Between groups	3083.66	2	1541.83	61.23	<0.0001
Within groups	302.10	12	25.18		
Total	3385.76	14			

Table 9.6 ANOVA table for Example 9.1 (20 min).

Source of variation	SS	ν	MS	F	p value
Between groups	3083.33	2	1541.67	6.93	0.0100
Within groups	2667.88	12	222.32		
Total	5751.21	14			

$$MS_E = \frac{SS_E}{\nu_E} = \frac{302.10}{12} = 25.18,$$

$$F = \frac{MS_A}{MS_E} = \frac{1541.83}{25.18} = 61.23.$$

The ANOVA results (10 min) are given in Table 9.5.

(3) Draw a conclusion

Given $\alpha = 0.05$ and $\nu_A = 2, \nu_E = 12$, the critical value $F_{(2,12),1-0.05} = 3.89$ can be obtained from the $F_{(2,12)}$ distribution (Appendix Table 6). It can be seen that $F = 61.23 > 3.89$ and $p < 0.05$. We reject H_0 and accept H_1 at the $\alpha = 0.05$ level and conclude that the population means of the paw-licking durations of rats subjected to low-, medium-, and high-intensity exercises are not all the same 10 min after the formalin injection.

The ANOVA results (20 min) are given in Table 9.6.

This shows that H_0 is rejected at the $\alpha = 0.05$ level for the 20-min data, and the conclusion is consistent with that of the 10-min data. However, the MS_E in the 20-min data was markedly greater than that in the 10-min data, resulting in the smaller test statistic F value.

Regarding the relationship with the two independent samples t-test, the one-way ANOVA gives exactly the same results as the t-test when there are only two groups. The F statistic (with 1 and $n-2$ degrees of freedom) exactly equals the square of the corresponding t statistic (with $n-2$ degrees of freedom), $F = t^2$, and the corresponding p values are identical.

Points of note: (i) Do not be misled by the word variance in ANOVA. Variance here refers to the statistical method being used, not the subject for the hypothesis being tested. ANOVA is concerned with differences among population means; it does not test whether the variances of the groups are different. Contrarily, ANOVA assumes that the population variances are all the same and uses that assumption as part of its comparison of means. (ii) When the treatment factor has more than two levels, the natural order of the levels (such as low, medium, and high intensity in Example 9.1) is not relevant in ANOVA. Even if some experimental time points have a trend or a dose–response relationship, you will get the same ANOVA results if you randomly disorganize the time points or doses. The regression model (see Chapter 13) is often a better choice in such situations.

9.3 Multiple Comparisons of Means

As mentioned in the previous section, once we reject H_0 in ANOVA, it does not imply that all k population means are different from one another. It is often of interest to further examine which of the means of the treatment levels are statistically significantly different and which are not. In this case, it is invalid to employ multiple two independent samples t-test to examine the difference among more than two means. We know that when $k(k \geq 3)$ sample means are compared, the number of pairwise comparisons N will increase rapidly as the number of comparison groups k increases, where $N = k!/[2!(k-2)!]$, this will inevitably lead to a rapid increase in the probability of Type I errors, which will be $\left[1-(1-\alpha)^N\right]$ after N comparisons.

In Example 9.1, when $k=3$, $N=3$, $\alpha=0.05$, than the probability of type I errors is $\left[1-(1-0.05)^3\right]=0.14$.

Multiple comparison procedures (*MCP*) represent a method to solve this kind of problem. Although there are many methods for multiple comparisons, their main principle is the same. In particular, all observations are used to calculate the within groups mean square MS_E to avoid the inflation of the probability of Type I errors and keep it at a fixed significance level α when rejecting H_0 in the pairwise comparisons between any two groups.

To choose a multiple comparison test, you must articulate the goals of the study, as different MCPs are used for different sets of comparisons. In this section, we will present three commonly used and highly regarded tests used for a variety of purposes: Tukey's test, Dunnett's test, and the LSD-t test.

9.3.1 Tukey's Test

Tukey's test, also called Tukey's honestly significant difference (Tukey's HSD) test, is widely applied for multiple comparisons in practice. It has good computational efficiency because not all pairwise comparisons have to be made during the procedure.

Tukey's test involves several steps. First, the k means need to be ordered from largest to smallest. Next, for comparisons between any two groups, the convenient way we use is to compare the largest mean with the smallest, then the largest with the next smallest, and so on until the largest mean has been compared with all means. Then we compare the second largest mean with all means in the same way. In the case of equal sample sizes across groups, if no significant difference is found between two means, then it is concluded that no significant difference exists between any means enclosed by those two, and the differences between the enclosed means are no longer tested.

Tukey's test is based on the studentized range statistic

$$q = \frac{\bar{X}_{\max} - \bar{X}_{\min}}{S_{\bar{X}_{\max} - \bar{X}_{\min}}}, \tag{9.15}$$

where

$$S_{\bar{X}_{\max} - \bar{X}_{\min}} = \sqrt{MS_E / n} \tag{9.16}$$

is the standard error for the difference between $\bar{X}_{\max}$ and $\bar{X}_{\min}$, which are the largest and smallest sample means out of k means in an experiment, respectively. MS_E is the within groups mean square in one-way ANOVA, and n is the sample size of each treatment group.

For a group of k treatment means, we can calculate Tukey's HSD as follows:

$$\text{HSD} = q_{(k,\nu_E),1-\alpha} \times S_{\bar{X}_{\max} - \bar{X}_{\min}}, \tag{9.17}$$

where $q_{(k,\nu_E),1-\alpha}$ is the critical value of the studentized range, that is, the $(1-\alpha)\times 100$ th percentile of $q_{(k,\nu_E)}$ distribution given in Appendix Table 9. $q_{(k,\nu_E),1-\alpha}$ depends on the significance level α, the number of treatment groups k involved in the analysis, and the error degrees of freedom $\nu_E = k(n-1)$.

For any two of k treatment groups i and j to be compared, with means $\bar{X}_i$ and $\bar{X}_j$ (ordered with $\bar{X}_i > \bar{X}_j$), if

$$\bar{X}_i - \bar{X}_j > \text{HSD}, \tag{9.18}$$

then Tukey's test declares that the two means are significantly different.

Example 9.2 The ANOVA results (10 min) in Example 9.1 show that the differences between the means are statistically significant. Use Tukey's test to compare the means of any two from three treatment levels.

Solution

(1) State the hypotheses and select a significance level

Once for each pair of treatment levels i and j $(i \neq j)$,

$$H_0: \mu_i = \mu_j$$

$$H_1: \mu_i \neq \mu_j$$

$$\alpha = 0.05$$

(2) Determine the test statistic

First, sort the sample means from largest to smallest; the results are given in Table 9.7.

According to $\alpha = 0.05$, $\nu_E = 12$, and three treatment groups involved, we find critical value $q_{(3,12),1-0.05} = 3.77$ from Appendix Table 9. Thus,

$$\text{HSD} = q_{(3,12),1-0.05} \times s_{\bar{x}_{\max} - \bar{x}_{\min}} = q_{(3,12),1-0.05} \times \sqrt{MS_E / n} = 3.77 \times \sqrt{25.18 / 5} = 8.46$$

Table 9.7 Means of exercise-intensity groups in descending order (10 min).

Exercise-intensity group	Low	Medium	High
Mean	$\bar{x}_1 = 50.0$	$\bar{x}_2 = 30.0$	$\bar{x}_3 = 15.0$
Order	1	2	3

Table 9.8 Tukey's test for pairwise comparisons of three means of paw-licking durations in three exercise-intensity groups (10 min).

Comparison of ordered groups $(\bar{x}_i > \bar{x}_j)$	Difference $(\bar{x}_i - \bar{x}_j)$	HSD	p value
1 vs 3	50.0−15.0=35.0	8.46	<0.05
1 vs 2	50.0−30.0=20.0	8.46	<0.05
2 vs 3	30.0−15.0=15.0	8.46	<0.05

(3) Draw a conclusion

Calculate the difference of the means between two comparison groups $d_{(i,j)} = \bar{x}_i - \bar{x}_j$ and compare with HSD. If $d_{(i,j)} > \text{HSD}$, then reject H_0; otherwise do not reject H_0. The results are given in Table 9.8.

From Table 9.8, as the differences among all three comparison groups are greater than HSD, it follows that $p < 0.05$ for all the comparisons. We reject all H_0 at the $\alpha = 0.05$ level. The differences between any two exercise intensities were statistically significant. We conclude that the population means of the paw-licking durations are different among rats subjected to exercises with different intensities. Higher exercise intensity can induce higher fatigue, resulting in a lower pain response.

Tukey's test is only suitable for equal sample sizes in each compared group. If the sample sizes of the k treatment groups are not equal, we should substitute $S_{\bar{X}_{\max}-\bar{X}_{\min}} = \sqrt{\text{MS}_E / n}$ in Formula 9.16 with

$$S_{\bar{X}_{\max}-\bar{X}_{\min}} = \sqrt{\frac{\text{MS}_E}{2}\left(\frac{1}{n_i} + \frac{1}{n_j}\right)}, \tag{9.19}$$

where n_i and n_j are the sample sizes of two compared groups. This is called a *Tukey–Kramer test*. It maintains the probability of a Type I error near α and can operate with good power for data of unbalanced designs.

However, when Tukey–Kramer tests are performed on sample means with unequal sample sizes, it is advisable to complete all comparisons because the differing sample sizes affect the magnitude of the standard error in the denominator in the q statistics. This can subsequently affect the significance of the various mean comparisons.

9.3.2 Dunnett's Test

In practice, it is sometimes necessary to compare the mean of a common control level (denoted by C) with that of each other level (usually, treatment levels of interest, denoted by T), and there is no need to compare the means of all treatment levels. In this case, we may use the *Dunnett's test* (also call the q'-test). The Dunnett's test was introduced by C.W. Dunnett in 1955. It is an amendment to the two independent samples t-test.

The Dunnett's test procedure is outlined as follows:

(1) State the hypotheses and select a significance level

$$H_0: \mu_T = \mu_C$$

$$H_1: \mu_T \neq \mu_C$$

Let α be the significance level

(2) Determine the test statistic

$$q' = \frac{\bar{X}_T - \bar{X}_C}{\sqrt{\text{MS}_E\left(\frac{1}{n_T} + \frac{1}{n_C}\right)}} \sim q'(\nu, a), \tag{9.20}$$

where

MS_E is the within groups mean square in ANOVA.

$\nu = \nu_E$ denotes the degrees of freedom associated with MS_E.

a denotes the number of groups (including treatment group and control group).

n_T and n_C are the sample sizes of one experimental group and the control group, respectively.

(3) Draw a conclusion

The Dunnett's test statistic q' has a special critical-value table (Appendix Table 10). The critical value obtained depends on the degrees of freedom $\nu = \nu_E$, the number of groups a, and significance level α.

For given α, a, and ν_E, we can find the common critical value $q'_{(a,\nu_E),1-\alpha/2}$ for each of the compared groups in the q' distribution.

If $|q'| > q'_{(a,\nu_E),1-\alpha/2}$, then reject H_0;

If $|q'| \leq q'_{(a,\nu_E),1-\alpha/2}$, then do not reject H_0.

Example 9.3 Refer to Example 9.1 (10 min). Suppose we define the low-intensity exercise group as the control group (denoted by C). We wish to compare whether the mean paw-licking duration of rats in the medium- (denoted by M) and high-intensity (denoted by H) exercise groups are different from that of rats in C. The Dunnett's test is used to compare their means in pairs.

Solution

(1) State the hypotheses and select a significance level

For M vs. C and H vs. C (M and H are represented by T), that is,

$$H_0: \mu_T = \mu_C$$

$$H_1: \mu_T \neq \mu_C$$

$$\alpha = 0.05$$

(2) Determine the test statistic

We know that $n_T = n_C = 5$, $\text{MS}_E = 25.18$.

Calculate the estimated standard error

$$s_{\bar{x}_T - \bar{x}_C} = \sqrt{\text{MS}_E\left(\frac{1}{n_T} + \frac{1}{n_C}\right)} = \sqrt{25.18 \times \left(\frac{1}{5} + \frac{1}{5}\right)} = 3.17$$

The test statistic comparing the M and C group is

$$q'_{M-C} = \frac{\bar{x}_M - \bar{x}_C}{s_{\bar{x}_M - \bar{x}_C}} = \frac{30 - 50}{3.17} = -6.31$$

The test statistic comparing the H and C group is

$$q'_{H-C} = \frac{\bar{x}_H - \bar{x}_C}{s_{\bar{x}_H - \bar{x}_C}} = \frac{15 - 50}{3.17} = -11.04$$

(3) Draw a conclusion

Given $\alpha = 0.05$, $a = 3$, and $\nu_E = 12$, for each hypothesis test, the common critical value $q'_{(3,12),1-0.05/2} = 2.50$ can be obtained from the q' distribution (Appendix Table 10). For M and C exercise groups, we have $\left|q'_{M-C}\right| = 6.31 > q'_{(3,12),1-0.05/2} = 2.50$ and $p < 0.05$. Therefore, we reject H_0 and accept H_1 at the $\alpha = 0.05$ level. We conclude that the rats' mean paw-licking duration after medium-intensity exercise was significantly shorter than that after low-intensity exercise. Similar results can be found between the means of high- and low-intensity exercises $(p < 0.05)$.

The results of the Dunnett's test are given in Table 9.9.

Results should be interpreted with caution when the test statistics of ANOVA are close to the critical value. Rarely, one may find under such circumstances that the F-test does not reject H_0, while Tukey's test or Dunnett's test shows a significant difference in the population means of the two groups, or the F test rejects H_0, while Tukey's test or Dunnett's test shows no difference in the population means of any two groups. It is recommended that attention be paid to the Tukey's test or Dunnett's test results in such a case. However, the best solution is to repeat the experiment with a larger sample size. This will avoid such contradictions to a certain extent. The decision to use the Dunnett's test should be part of the experimental design. Switching to the Dunnett's test after a Tukey's test to get more power should be avoided.

Table 9.9 Dunnett's test for the comparisons of the means in the paw-licking durations of rats in the experimental and control groups (10 min).

Comparison group	$\bar{x}_T - \bar{x}_C$	$\left\|q'_{T-C}\right\|$	$q'_{(3,12),1-0.05/2}$	p value
M vs C	−20	6.31	2.50	<0.05
H vs C	−35	11.04	2.50	<0.05

9.3.3 Least Significant Difference (LSD) Test

The *least significant difference method*, also known as the LSD-t test, was first introduced by R.A. Fisher in 1935. It is applied when a decision has been made at the design stage that there is no need for multiple comparisons of the means; in view of the research objectives or professional knowledge, only the means of one or several pairwise comparison groups of interest need to be tested.

The LSD-t test procedure is outlined as follows:

(1) State the hypotheses and select a significance level

$$H_0: \mu_i = \mu_j$$

$$H_1: \mu_i \neq \mu_j$$

i and j $(i \neq j)$ denote the specific groups to be compared,
Let α be the significance level.

(2) Determine the test statistic

$$\text{LSD-}t = \frac{\bar{X}_i - \bar{X}_j}{S_{\bar{X}_i - \bar{X}_j}} = \frac{\bar{X}_i - \bar{X}_j}{\sqrt{\text{MS}_E\left(\dfrac{1}{n_i} + \dfrac{1}{n_j}\right)}}, \quad \nu = \nu_E, \tag{9.21}$$

where MS_E is the within groups mean square of ANOVA; ν_E denotes the degrees of freedom associated with MS_E.

Under H_0, the test statistic follows the t distribution with degrees of freedom $\nu_E = n - k$.

(3) Draw a conclusion

For a given α and $\nu_E = n - k$, we find the critical value $t_{\nu_E, 1-\alpha/2}$ from the t_{ν_E} distribution (two-sided, Appendix Table 4).

If LSD-$t < t_{\nu_E, \alpha/2}$ or LSD-$t > t_{\nu_E, 1-\alpha/2}$, then reject H_0;

If $t_{\nu_E, \alpha/2} \leq$ LSD-$t \leq t_{\nu_E, 1-\alpha/2}$, then do not reject H_0.

The rejection and non-rejection regions for this test are shown in Figure 9.4.

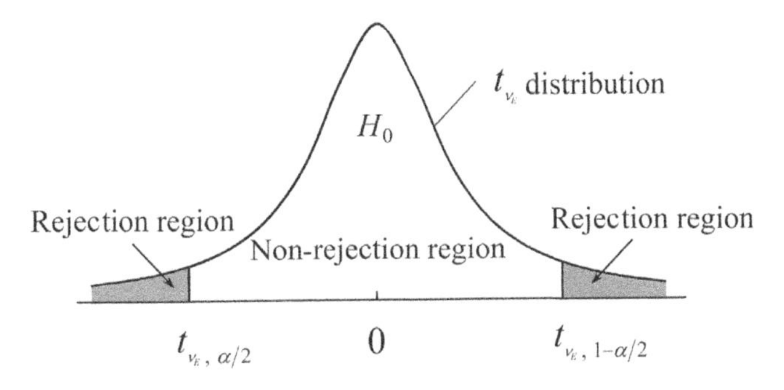

Figure 9.4 Illustration of rejection and non-rejection regions for LSD-t test for the comparison of pairs of groups for one-way ANOVA.

Example 9.4 Refer to Example 9.1 (10 min). If we have decided to investigate the difference in the mean paw-licking durations of rats with medium- (denoted by M) and high-intensity (denoted by H) exercises in the design stage, use the LSD-t test method for hypothesis testing.

Solution

(1) State the hypotheses and select a significance level

$H_0: \mu_M = \mu_H$, the population means of paw-licking durations of the rats between M and H are the same.

$H_1: \mu_M \neq \mu_H$, the population means of paw-licking durations of the rats between M and H are not the same.

$$\alpha = 0.05$$

(2) Determine the test statistic

For $n_1 = n_2 = 5$, $\text{MS}_E = 25.18$, $v = v_E = 12$, by Formula 9.21, we have

$$s_{\bar{x}_1 - \bar{x}_2} = \sqrt{\text{MS}_E\left(\frac{1}{n_1} + \frac{1}{n_2}\right)} = \sqrt{25.18 \times \left(\frac{1}{5} + \frac{1}{5}\right)} = 3.17$$

$$LSD\text{-}t = \frac{30.0 - 15.0}{3.17} = 4.73$$

(3) Draw a conclusion

For a given α and $\nu_E = 12$, we find the critical value $t_{12,1-0.05/2} = 2.179$ from the t_{12} distribution (Appendix Table 4). As $LSD\text{-}t = 4.73 > 2.179$, $p < 0.05$. We reject H_0 and accept H_1 at the $\alpha = 0.05$ level; we conclude that the mean paw-licking durations of rats after high-intensity exercise is significantly shorter than that after medium-intensity exercise.

Points of note: (i) The LSD-t method is suitable for cases in which the populations being compared have equal variances. ANOVA and the multiple comparison test method is no longer applicable for cases of unequal variances, and the t-test or t'-test has to be applied in such a circumstance. (ii) The LSD-t method cannot effectively control the Type I error probability; therefore, this method is often used to compare a pair or several pairs of means in several treatment levels that have particular meanings in domain knowledge.

In addition to the three test methods, a considerable number of methods has been proposed for multiple-comparison tests with various objectives. The output of many statistical computer packages enhances the application of MCP. However, using the mean square MS_E of ANOVA to construct a test statistic is the only constant criterion.

9.4 Checking ANOVA Assumptions

Section 9.1 introduced three assumptions of ANOVA: *independence, normality,* and *homogeneity of variances.* The requirement for independence is strict. However, in practice, this condition can be met by experimental design. Here we introduce ways to verify the assumptions of normality and homogeneity of variances.

9.4.1 Check for Normality

We have the following methods to check the normality of data:

1. For each treatment group, construct a histogram, stem-and-leaf plot, or normal probability plot for the response $X_{ij}\left(i=1,2,\ldots,\ n_j;\ j=1,2,\ldots,\ k\right)$ to check whether the data from each group follows a normal distribution. Slight departures from normality will have little impact on the validity of the inferences. If the sample size for each treatment is small, these graphs will probably be of limited use. In this case, the data of each treatment group can be merged and plotted. This practice does not violate the basic idea of the null hypothesis.
2. To test whether kurtosis and skewness are equal to zero (see Chapter 5 for the corresponding calculation methods and their standard errors).
3. There are formal statistical tests of normality, such as the *Shapiro–Wilk test* or *Kolmogorov–Smirnov test.* Generally, the Shapiro–Wilk and Kolmogorov–Smirnov tests (Lilliefors correction) are suitable for small and large samples, respectively. Because both tests are based on the assumption of normality, they are sensitive to slight departures from normality. Therefore, in scientific applications, normality assumption should be assessed through a combination of these methods. In addition, the tests use order statistics; the calculations are relatively complicated and are generally performed using software.

Example 9.5 Refer to Example 5.2, for the height data for the 153 10-year-old girls, the skewness coefficient $g_1=0.046$ and its standard error $\sigma_{g_1}=0.196$, the kurtosis coefficient $g_2=-0.364$ and its standard error $\sigma_{g_2}=0.390$. Perform hypothesis testing for skewness coefficient and kurtosis coefficient.

Solution

Assume that skewness and kurtosis coefficients both follow a normal distribution. For the population skewness coefficient γ_1,

(1) State the hypotheses and select a significance level

$H_0:\gamma_1=0$

$H_1:\gamma_1\neq 0$

$$\alpha=0.05$$

(2) Determine the test statistic

We have $g_1 = 0.046$ and $\sigma_{g_1} = 0.196$, thus

$$z_1 = \frac{g_1 - 0}{\sigma_{g_1}} = \frac{0.046}{0.196} = 0.235$$

(3) Draw a conclusion

For $\alpha = 0.05$, the critical value $z_{1-0.05/2} = 1.96$, we have $|z_1| < 1.96$ and $p > 0.05$, there is no significant evidence to show that skewness coefficient is not equal to zero.

Similarly, for the population kurtosis coefficient, we have $z_2 = \frac{g_2 - 0}{\sigma_{g_2}} = \frac{-0.364}{0.390} = -0.933$, $|z_2| < 1.96$, and $p > 0.05$, there is no significant evidence to show that population kurtosis coefficient is not equal to zero. We can then conclude that there is no significant evidence to show that the data deviates from normality.

Example 9.6 Refer to Example 9.1 (10 min). Test the normality of the paw-licking durations of rats subjected to exercises of different intensities.

Solution

In this example, there were too few (only five) observations in each treatment group to plot separately. Therefore, the observations of the three groups were combined and plotted (Figure 9.5). The scattered points are approximately on a straight line. In addition, the result of the test using the *Shapiro–Wilk test* for normality calculated using software is $W = 0.945589$, $p > 0.05$. The assumption of normality is therefore not rejected at a significance level of $\alpha = 0.05$, that is, the data approximately follow a normal distribution.

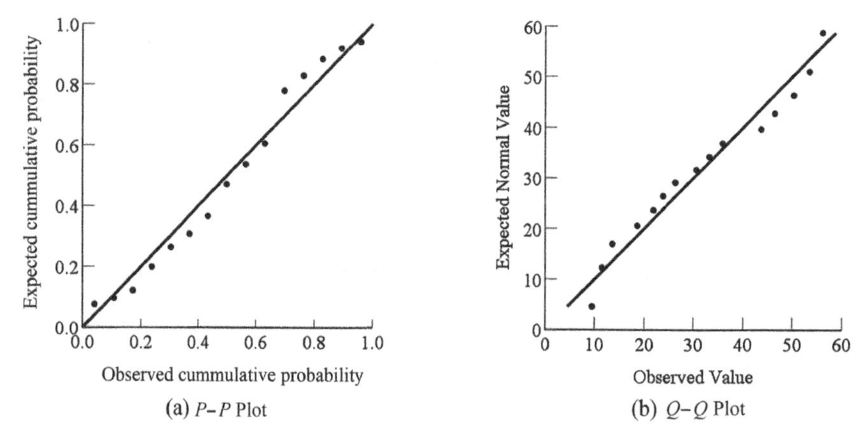

Figure 9.5 $P-P$ plot and $Q-Q$ plot of the data in Example 9.1 (10 min).

Points of note: (i) ANOVA is robust with respect to the normality assumption when sample size is relatively large. Simulation studies have shown that when the data distribution slightly deviates from the normal distribution, the results of ANOVA will not be significantly affected. (ii) The use of a normality test with small samples (three or four values) is not advocated; in this case, it is impossible to make valid inferences about the distribution of the population.

9.4.2 Test for Homogeneity of Variances

Compared to normality assumption, the assumption of homogeneity of variances has a greater influence on the results. A balanced design (equal sample size across treatment groups) can reduce but not eliminate the influence of unequal variances. The test for the homogeneity of variances should be done before the ANOVA. Bartlett's and Levene's tests are widely used to test for the homogeneity of variances of multiple samples. We introduce these two methods in this section.

9.4.2.1 Bartlett's Test

The basic idea of *Bartlett's test* is to compare the weighted arithmetic and geometric means of the variance of each group. If the difference between the two is too large, the variances between the groups are considered unequal. When sample size ≥ 5 in each group, the test statistic approximately follows the χ^2 distribution with $k-1$ degrees of freedom.

The procedure for Bartlett's test is outlined as follows:

(1) State the hypotheses and select a significance level

$$H_0: \sigma_1^2 = \sigma_2^2 = \cdots = \sigma_k^2$$

$H_1: \sigma_1^2, \sigma_2^2, \ldots, \sigma_k^2$ are not all equal

Let α be the significance level

(2) Determine the test statistic

The test statistic (equal sample sizes) is

$$B = \frac{(n-1)\left[k \ln \overline{S}^2 - \sum_{j=1}^{k} \ln S_j^2\right]}{1 + \frac{k+1}{3k(n-1)}} \sim \chi^2(v), \ v = k-1, \tag{9.22}$$

where n denotes the sample size of each group, S_j^2 denotes the sample variance of the jth treatment group, and $\overline{S}^2$ is the average of the k sample variances.

The test statistic (unequal sample sizes) is

$$B = \frac{\sum_{j=1}^{k}(n_j - 1)\ln\frac{\overline{S}^2}{S_j^2}}{1 + \frac{1}{3(k-1)}\left(\sum_{j=1}^{k}\frac{1}{n_j - 1} - \frac{1}{\sum_{j=1}^{k}(n_j - 1)}\right)} \sim \chi^2(v), \quad v = k - 1, \tag{9.23}$$

where n_j denotes the sample size of the jth treatment group and $\overline{S}^2$ is the weighted average of the k sample variances, $\overline{S}^2 = \left(\sum_{j=1}^{k}(n_j - 1)S_j^2\right) \Big/ \sum_{j=1}^{k}(n_j - 1)$.

For a given α and ν, the critical value $\chi^2_{\nu,1-\alpha}$ can be obtained from the χ^2_ν distribution (Appendix Table 5).

If $B > \chi^2_{\nu,1-\alpha}$, then reject H_0, which indicates that not all the samples come from populations with equal variances.

If $B \le \chi^2_{\nu,1-\alpha}$, then do not reject H_0. The evidence is not significant to show that the variances of the populations are unequal.

The application of Bartlett's test requires that the samples of k normal populations are independent and drawn randomly. Bartlett's test cannot be used when the normality assumption is not met.

Example 9.7 Refer to Example 9.1 (10 min). Test the assumption of homogeneity of variances in the paw-licking durations among rats of the three exercise intensity levels.

The paw-licking durations of rats in the three exercise intensity groups met the normality assumption. Therefore, Bartlett's test can be used to test the homogeneity of variances in this case.

Solution

(1) State the hypotheses and select a significance level
$H_0 : \sigma_1^2 = \sigma_2^2 = \sigma_3^2$. The population variances of the paw-licking durations of rats with three exercise intensities are equal
$H_1 : \sigma_1^2, \sigma_2^2, \sigma_3^2$ are not all equal

$$\alpha = 0.05$$

(2) Determine the test statistic
We have $n_1 = n_2 = n_3 = 5$, $k = 3$.

Table 9.4 shows the s_j^2 of paw-licking durations in the three exercise intensity groups. $\ln s_j^2$ were calculated (Table 9.10).

Calculate $\overline{s}^2$

$$\overline{s}^2 = \frac{(5-1)\times(25.4 + 23.9 + 26.3)}{3\times(5-1)} = 25.2$$

Table 9.10 Statistics used for Bartlett's test for equality of variances in Example 9.1.

Exercise-intensity group	s_j^2	$\ln s_j^2$
Low	25.4	3.23
Medium	23.9	3.17
High	26.3	3.27

The test statistic is

$$B = \frac{(n-1)\left(k\ln \bar{s}^2 - \sum_j \ln s_j^2\right)}{1+\frac{k+1}{3k(n-1)}}$$
$$= \frac{(5-1)\times(3\times\ln 25.2-(3.23+3.17+3.27))}{1+\frac{3+1}{3\times3\times(5-1)}}$$
$$= 0.038.$$

(3) Draw a conclusion

For a given α and $v=3-1=2$, the critical value $\chi^2_{2,1-0.05}=5.99$ can be obtained from the χ^2_2 distribution (Appendix Table 5). As $B=0.038<5.99$, $p>0.05$, we do not reject H_0 at the $\alpha=0.05$ level. The assumption of equal variance of paw-licking durations among rats subjected to three exercise intensity levels is not violated.

9.4.2.2 Levene's Test

Bartlett's test works well when the data come from normal distributions. The results, however, can be misleading for non-normal data. In cases in which the response is not normally distributed, Levene's test is more appropriate. *Levene's test* can be used to test for the homogeneity of variances for observations with arbitrary distribution in two or multiple groups. The method involves performing the Levene transformation on the original data, that is, calculating the absolute value Z_{ij} of the deviation of each original observation X_{ij} from group means within each group. Then, one-way ANOVA is performed on the transformed data Z_{ij} and a conclusion is drawn.

First, perform the Levene transformation

$$Z_{ij} = \left|X_{ij} - \bar{X}_{.j}\right| (i=1,2,\dots,n_j;\ j=1,2,\dots,k). \tag{9.24}$$

The test statistic W (based on the statistic F calculated after the transformation) is

$$W = \frac{MS_A}{MS_E} = \frac{\sum_j n_j\left(\bar{Z}_{.j}-\bar{Z}_{..}\right)^2/(k-1)}{\sum_j\sum_i\left(Z_{ij}-\bar{Z}_{.j}\right)^2/(n-k)} \sim F(\nu_1,\nu_2), \tag{9.25}$$

where $\nu_1 = k-1$, $\nu_2 = n-k$.

The assumptions of the Levene's test are as follows.

(1) Samples of k populations are independent and randomly drawn.

(2) Random variable X is continuous.

Example 9.8 Refer to Example 9.1 (10 min); test the assumption of homogeneity of variances in the paw-licking durations among rats subjected to three exercise intensity levels via the Levene method.

Solution

Perform the Levene transformation on the original data in Example 9.1. z_{ij} are obtained and given in Table 9.11.

Calculate the test statistic W

$$W = \frac{(n-k)\sum_j n_j\left(\bar{z}_{.j} - \bar{z}_{..}\right)^2}{(k-1)\sum_j\sum_i\left(z_{ij} - \bar{z}_{.j}\right)^2}$$

$$= \frac{(15-3)\times\left[5\times(3.9-4.0)^2 + 5\times(3.9-4.0)^2 + 5\times(4.2-4.0)^2\right]}{(3-1)\times\left[(3.5-3.9)^2 + (6.3-3.9)^2 + \cdots + (5.5-4.2)^2\right]}$$

$$= 0.0291,$$

where $v_1 = k-1 = 2, v_2 = n-k = 12$.

As the test statistic $W < 1$, $p > 0.05$, we do not reject H_0 at the $\alpha = 0.05$ level. The assumption of equal variance of paw-licking duration among rats subjected to three exercise intensity levels is not violated.

Points of note: The test for normality and homogeneity of variances can be performed using statistical software. However, in practice, professional knowledge is valuable for making a judgment. In specific applications, it is generally believed that when the sample size difference between groups is not too large, a slight violation of the assumption of homogeneity of variance has limited influence on the conclusion of ANOVA. Empirically, if the maximum/minimum variance ratio is less than 3, the results are relatively robust.

Table 9.11 z_{ij} after transformation in the Levene's test.

Exercise-intensity group	Low	Medium	High	
	3.5	3.2	3.5	
	6.3	0.6	6.9	
	3.5	6.1	3.6	
	0.3	3.6	1.4	
	6.1	5.9	5.5	
$\bar{z}_{.j}$	3.9	3.9	4.2	$\bar{z}_{..} = 4.0$

9.5 Data Transformations

When the assumptions of ANOVA are grossly violated, such as data that deviate from the normal distribution or widely different variances of each group, the following methods can often be used: (i) Data transformation method. (ii) Use of a nonparametric method (see Chapter 12). The former is used to change the distribution of the original data through variable transformation to more closely satisfy the assumptions. Meanwhile, for some types of data, it is known, on theoretical grounds, that a transformation will yield data more amenable to the intended statistical analysis. In this section, we will concentrate on three common transformations: square-root transformation, logarithmic transformation, and arcsine transformation.

1. Square-root Transformation
This transformation is suitable when the group variances are directly proportional to the means, that is, when the variances increase as the means increase. This most often occurs in biological data, especially when samples are taken from a Poisson distribution.

Make a transformation

$$Y = \sqrt{X}. \tag{9.26}$$

When there are zero or extremely small values in the original data, the following transformation can be used:

$$Y = \sqrt{X + a}, \tag{9.27}$$

generally, we may take a as 0.5 or 0.1.

2. Logarithmic Transformation
This transformation is applicable when there is heterogeneity of variances among groups and the group standard deviations are directly proportional to the means. This transformation can also convert a positively skewed distribution into a symmetrical one.

Use logarithm for transformation:

$$Y = \log X \text{ (usually using } e \text{ or 10 as the base of the logarithm)} \tag{9.28}$$

When zero or negative values exist in the original data, the following transformation values can be used

$$Y = \log(X + a) \tag{9.29}$$

to keep $X + a > 0$ (a is a real number).
Logarithmic transformation can be applied to natural or common logarithms according to the nature of the data, and the conclusions are consistent. The function "pulls" the observations in the tail toward the mean, and the heterogeneity of variances is simultaneously improved.

3. Arcsine Transformation (Also Called Arcsine Square-root Transformation)
Many indicators in medicine are expressed in terms of rate, e.g., prevalence, mortality, and turnover rate of lymphocytes. They follow a binomial (rather than a normal) distribution. The deviation from normality is greater when rates are large or small (0%–30% or 70%–100%). If the square root of each rate, π, in a binomial distribution is transformed into its arcsine (i.e., the angle whose sine is $\sqrt{\pi}$), this transformation is

$$Y = \arcsin\sqrt{\pi}. \tag{9.30}$$

Points of note: (i) The results of ANOVA on the above-mentioned transformed variables can only be used to compare the difference between the mean in the hypothesis testing. For a meaningful interpretation, the original (untransformed) data must be used. (ii) Data transformation will not compensate for the absence of random sampling. As with untransformed data, analysis of transformed data can be adversely affected by outliers.

9.6 Summary

One-way ANOVA is used to compare multiple-sample means. The basic idea is to partition the total variation of all observations into two parts (between group and within group) according to the principle of the partitioning of the sum of squares and degrees of freedom. Then, the variances (mean squares) from different sources are obtained, and the corresponding statistical inference is made based on the ratio of the between groups mean square to the within groups mean square.

The assumptions of ANOVA are the independence, normality, and homogeneity of variances.

When the results of ANOVA show that the difference is statistically significant, multiple comparisons between the means are further needed. This chapter introduced three common methods: Tukey's test, Dunnett's test, and LSD-t test.

Bartlett's and Levene's tests are widely used to test for the homogeneity of variances of multiple samples. In practice, the method used will depend on the distribution of the data.

When the assumptions of the ANOVA are grossly violated, data transformation methods can be used to change the distribution of the original data, for instance, square-root transformation, logarithmic transformation, and arcsine square-root transformation.

9.7 Exercises

1. To investigate the change of nitric oxide levels (μmol/L) due to renal ischemia-reperfusion, 24 male Sprague–Dawley rats were randomly divided into three groups: renal ischemia group, renal ischemia-reperfusion group, and control group.

Table 9.12 gives the nitric oxide levels in each group (assuming the normality and homogeneity of variance assumptions are satisfied).

Table 9.12 Nitric oxide level (μmol/L) of the Sprague–Dawley rats.

Renal ischemia	372.74	464.50	322.24	282.52	319.44	320.27	269.50	210.20
Renal ischemia-reperfusion	209.10	274.20	268.40	289.40	290.30	291.50	267.10	245.20
Control	437.98	285.75	369.93	344.53	378.96	350.92	299.70	282.45

(a) What is the experimental design of this study? What is the treatment factor?
(b) Draw plots to describe the data and inspect the between groups and within groups variations of the nitric oxide levels.
(c) Complete the following ANOVA table. Draw a conclusion.

Source of variation	SS	ν	MS	F	p value
Between groups					
Within groups	65122.767				
Total	89937.508				

2. To investigate whether epinephrine concentrations (ng/ml) differ between types of anesthesia, 40 laboratory mice were randomly divided into four groups $(A, B, C, \text{and } D)$. Each group received a different type of anesthesia. The arterial plasma epinephrine concentrations were measured. The results are given in Table 9.13. Conduct ANOVA using these data.

Table 9.13 Arterial plasma epinephrine concentrations (ng/ml) of 40 laboratory mice.

A	0.29	0.51	0.59	0.28	0.32	0.45	0.47	0.36	0.39	0.35
B	0.21	0.40	0.52	0.27	0.63	0.44	0.88	0.88	0.38	0.44
C	0.45	0.48	0.59	0.37	0.33	0.34	0.98	0.78	0.43	0.59
D	1.22	1.45	0.99	0.87	0.44	0.58	0.82	0.87	0.44	0.89

(a) State H_0 and H_1.
(b) State the assumptions of this ANOVA model and check whether the assumptions are satisfied in this study.
(c) Perform ANOVA and interpret the results obtained.
(d) If the overall F-test rejects H_0, how do you choose an appropriate method to further compare the population means of the different groups? Calculate the Type I error if the independent samples t-test was employed for multiple comparisons in this case?

3. To explore whether iodine uptakes on lung computerized tomography (CT) functional imaging differ between different lung cancer types, 19 patients with different types of lung cancer were enrolled. The patients' iodine uptake (Hounsfield unit: HU) on CT functional imaging was measured and is given in Table 9.14.

Table 9.14 Iodine uptake (HU) in patients with different types of lung cancer.

Small cell lung cancer	Squamous cell carcinomas	Adenocarcinoma
24.0	34.1	34.3
31.8	36.6	39.8
29.1	52.3	21.5
27.1	48.1	23.1
37.5	32.7	15.0
30.2	41.5	28.4
33.6		

(a) Compare the iodine uptake of the three groups using an appropriate method and interpret the results.

(b) If necessary, conduct Tukey's, Dunnett's, and LSD-t tests and discuss the differences in the results obtained using these methods. What are their advantages over independent samples t-tests?

4. In a study, 38 ovariectomized rats were randomly allocated to a control, low-dose, medium-dose, or high-dose group. The groups were fed different amounts of total isoflavones from Pueraria. One of the outcomes examined was the bone mineral density (g/cm^2) at the end of the femur. The data are given in Table 9.15.

Table 9.15 Bone mineral density (g/cm^2) of different dose groups.

Control	Low dose	Medium dose	High dose
0.215	0.237	0.265	0.293
0.179	0.249	0.274	0.299
0.177	0.248	0.292	0.284
0.193	0.243	0.275	0.263
0.199	0.250	0.262	0.296
0.195	0.233	0.280	0.284
0.176	0.261	0.289	0.311
0.196	0.241	0.272	0.289
0.222	0.239	0.270	
0.196	0.241	0.257	

(a) Examine the assumptions for ANOVA. Perform ANOVA and interpret the results.

(b) Note that there is an order in the treatment levels; can the ANOVA explore the impact of the order (dose–response)? Why?

10

Analysis of Variance in Different Experimental Designs

CONTENTS

We have discussed one-way ANOVA in Chapter 9. In this chapter, we will introduce ANOVA for various experimental designs, where an outcome variable is measured in several categories (levels) of one or more factors. Hypothesis testing asks whether the population mean of the variable differs among the levels of each factor. Although the designs differ depending on the research objectives, the analyses of variance follow a single logical step similar to one-way ANOVA. All such analyses are termed *univariate analyses of variance* because they examine the effect of the factor(s) on only one outcome variable.

10.1 ANOVA for Randomized Block Design

With one-way ANOVA for a completely randomized design, there are no restrictions in the randomized grouping process. Therefore, experimental results are easily affected by various factors that could lead to excess error within each treatment group. When such an error is treated as part of the estimate for random error, the testing efficiency is often low. ANOVA for randomized block design can be used to address such a

Applied Medical Statistics, First Edition. Jingmei Jiang.

Companion website: www.wiley.com\go\jiang\appliedmedicalstatistics

deficiency. The *randomized block design* is a commonly used noise-reducing design that employs groups (or blocks) of homogeneous experimental units to compare the population means associated with k levels of treatments. It can be considered an extension of the paired samples t-test (Section 8.1).

Example 10.1 To investigate the effect of different feeds on the weight gain of rats, six litters of rats of the same strain were selected. Three rats were randomly selected from each litter, and each was fed with feed A, B, or C. The experimental conditions other than the feeds were kept consistent. After 4 weeks, the weight gain (g) of all rats was recorded (Table 10.1). Are there differences in the rats' weight gain according to their feed? Are there differences in the weight gain of rats in different litters? (Assume that the rats' weights at the beginning of the experiment had no significant difference and the weight gain follows a normal distribution.)

Unlike one-way ANOVA, which considers only one factor (treatment), two factors are simultaneously considered in this example (Table 10.1). The treatment factor (feeds) and block factor (litters) may both affect the weight gain of rats. The last row in the table shows the mean weight gain of different treatment groups, and the variation between them is called the treatment effect. The last column in the table shows the mean weight gain of different blocks, and the variation between them is called the block effect. Thus, we can simultaneously analyze the effects of feeds and litters on the weight gain of rats.

In a randomized block design, the subjects are first grouped into b blocks based on the principle that the subjects within the same block have the same or similar conditions and traits (such as litter and weight) that may affect the results of experiments. Then, subjects in the same block are randomly assigned to k different treatment groups. In this way, the subjects are cross-grouped according to the block and treatment levels and form $n = b \times k$ cells, with only one datum in each cell. As two factors must be simultaneously considered in the analysis and there is only one datum in each cell, the ANOVA for randomized block design is also called *two-way ANOVA without replication*.

Table 10.1 Weight gain (g) of the rats with three types of feed after four weeks.

Litter	Feed			$\sum_j x_{ij}$	$\bar{x}_{i\cdot}$
	A	B	C		
1	48.6	54.4	78.3	181.3	60.4
2	55.0	69.5	85.9	210.4	70.1
3	76.2	74.5	92.3	243.0	81.0
4	57.3	62.1	99.5	218.9	73.0
5	72.7	86.6	100.3	259.6	86.5
6	76.9	66.6	101.2	244.7	81.6
$\sum_i x_{ij}$	386.7	413.7	557.5	1357.9	—
$\bar{x}_{\cdot j}$	64.5	69.0	92.9	—	75.4

10.1.1 Data Layout and Model Assumptions

The data layout of a randomized block design is given in Table 10.2, where

$$\bar{X}_{i\cdot} = \sum_{j=1}^{k} X_{ij} \Big/ k,\ \bar{X}_{\cdot j} = \sum_{i=1}^{b} X_{ij} \Big/ b,\ \bar{X}_{\cdot\cdot} = \sum_{i=1}^{b}\sum_{j=1}^{k} X_{ij} \Big/ bk\ (i = 1, 2, \ldots, b; j = 1, 2, \ldots, k)$$

The ANOVA model for a randomized block design is given as follows:

$$X_{ij} = \mu + \alpha_j + \beta_i + \varepsilon_{ij}, \tag{10.1}$$

where

X_{ij} is the observation of the ith block and the jth treatment group.

μ is an expected mean and is usually estimated from the overall mean of all observations.

α_j is an expected mean that represents the effect of the jth treatment group, $\alpha_j = \mu_j - \mu$.

β_i is an expected mean that represents the effect of the ith block group, $\beta_i = \mu_i - \mu$ (μ_j and μ_i are the expected means of the jth treatment group and ith block group, respectively).

ε_{ij} is an error term that reflects the random error of the observations $(\varepsilon_{ij} = X_{ij} - \mu_{ij})$ and follows a normal distribution $N(0, \sigma^2)$, where μ_{ij} is the expected mean for the combination of the ith block and jth treatment.

Model Assumptions

(1) Each observation is a random, independent sample from a population with mean μ_{ij} $(i = 1, 2, \ldots, b; j = 1, 2, \ldots, k)$; $b \times k$ of these populations are sampled.

Table 10.2 Data layout of a randomized block design.

Block factor B	Treatment factor A				$\sum_j X_{ij}$	$\bar{X}_{i\cdot}$
	1	2	...	k		
1	X_{11}	X_{12}	...	X_{1k}	$\sum_j X_{1j}$	$\bar{X}_{1\cdot}$
2	X_{21}	X_{22}	...	X_{2k}	$\sum_j X_{2j}$	$\bar{X}_{2\cdot}$
⋮	⋮	⋮	...	⋮	⋮	⋮
b	X_{b1}	X_{b2}	...	X_{bk}	$\sum_j X_{bj}$	$\bar{X}_{b\cdot}$
$\sum_i X_{ij}$	$\sum_i X_{i1}$	$\sum_i X_{i2}$	...	$\sum_i X_{ik}$	$\sum_j\sum_i X_{ij}$	—
$\bar{X}_{\cdot j}$	$\bar{X}_{\cdot 1}$	$\bar{X}_{\cdot 2}$	...	$\bar{X}_{\cdot k}$	—	$\bar{X}_{\cdot\cdot}$

(2) Each of the $b \times k$ populations is normally distributed with the same variance σ^2.

(3) The treatment and block effects are additive; the model should satisfy $\sum_{j=1}^{k} \alpha_j = 0$ and $\sum_{i=1}^{b} \beta_i = 0$.

As there is only one datum in a crossed cell in the randomized block design, it is impossible to check its normality and homogeneity of variance. We have two options regarding this issue: (i) Inspect a residual plot (see Chapter 13, which illustrates a similar principle) after fitting the ANOVA model. (ii) Check for extreme values across the cells, because as a simple rule, the normality and homogeneity of variance conditions could be approximately satisfied if there are no outliers (see Chapter 2).

10.1.2 Procedure of ANOVA

1. Partitioning Sum of Squares of Deviations

In Formula 10.1, the deviation between any individual observation X_{ij} and the expected mean μ can be theoretically partitioned as the following identical equation:

$$X_{ij} - \mu = (\mu_{.j} - \mu) + (\mu_{i.} - \mu) + (X_{ij} - \mu_{ij}). \tag{10.2}$$

The additivity condition above implies that $\mu_{ij} = \mu + (\mu_{.j} - \mu) + (\mu_{i.} - \mu)$.

Replacing the various μ with their unbiased estimators from the data, we have

$$X_{ij} - \bar{X}_{..} = (\bar{X}_{.j} - \bar{X}_{..}) + (\bar{X}_{i.} - \bar{X}_{..}) + (X_{ij} - \bar{X}_{.j} - \bar{X}_{i.} + \bar{X}_{..}). \tag{10.3}$$

If we square both sides of Formula 10.3 and sum the squared deviations for all observations, we can generate a very useful relationship (because the sum of all cross-product terms on the right side of the formula is zero):

$$\begin{aligned} &\sum_j \sum_i (X_{ij} - \bar{X}_{..})^2 \\ &= \sum_j \sum_i (\bar{X}_{.j} - \bar{X}_{..})^2 + \sum_i \sum_j (\bar{X}_{i.} - \bar{X}_{..})^2 + \sum_j \sum_i (X_{ij} - \bar{X}_{.j} - \bar{X}_{i.} + \bar{X}_{..})^2 \\ &= \sum_j b(\bar{X}_{.j} - \bar{X}_{..})^2 + \sum_i k(\bar{X}_{i.} - \bar{X}_{..})^2 + \sum_j \sum_i (X_{ij} - \bar{X}_{.j} - \bar{X}_{i.} + \bar{X}_{..})^2. \end{aligned} \tag{10.4}$$

We term each component in Formula 10.4 as follows:

The total sum of squares, denoted by SS_T, measures the total variation of all observations:

$$\mathrm{SS}_T = \sum_j \sum_i (X_{ij} - \bar{X}_{..})^2 = \sum_j \sum_i X_{ij}^2 - C, \tag{10.5}$$

where $C = \left(\sum_j \sum_i X_{ij} \right)^2 \Big/ bk$ is the correction term.

Treatment sum of squares, denoted by SS_A, measures the variation between group means of treatment factor A:

$$SS_A = \sum_j b\left(\bar{X}_{.j} - \bar{X}_{..}\right)^2 = \frac{\sum_j \left(\sum_i X_{ij}\right)^2}{b} - C. \tag{10.6}$$

Block sum of squares, denoted by SS_B, measures the variation between block means of block factor B:

$$SS_B = \sum_i k\left(\bar{X}_{i.} - \bar{X}_{..}\right)^2 = \frac{\sum_i \left(\sum_j X_{ij}\right)^2}{k} - C. \tag{10.7}$$

Error sum of squares, denoted by SS_E, measures the random error other than that between treatments and between blocks:

$$SS_E = SS_T - SS_A - SS_B. \tag{10.8}$$

It can be seen from the above relationship that the between-block variation is a part of the partitioning of the within-group variation in one-way ANOVA, and the error term at this time is affected neither by the treatment factor nor block factor, which is the true source of random error.

2. Partitioning Degrees of Freedom
The degrees of freedom can be partitioned in the same way.

The degrees of freedom associated with SS_T are $\nu_T = n - 1$.

The degrees of freedom associated with SS_A are $\nu_A = k - 1$ because there are k levels of treatment factor A.

The degrees of freedom associated with SS_B are $\nu_B = b - 1$, because there are b levels of block factor B.

The degrees of freedom of the error term are $\nu_E = (k-1)(b-1)$.

Thus, the partitioning relationship of the degrees of freedom is obtained as follows:

$$\nu_T = \nu_A + \nu_B + \nu_E. \tag{10.9}$$

3. Formulation of Variance from Different Sources
The variances (mean squares) of different sources are formulated similar to the method used in one-way ANOVA.

Treatment mean square, denoted by MS_A,

$$MS_A = SS_A / (k-1) \tag{10.10}$$

is the variance of treatment factor A and reflects the effect of the treatment factor.
Block mean square, denoted by MS_B,

$$MS_B = SS_B / (b-1) \tag{10.11}$$

is the variance of block factor B and reflects the effect of the block factor.
Error mean square, denoted by MS_E,

$$MS_E = SS_E / [(k-1)(b-1)] \tag{10.12}$$

reflects the effect of the random error after removing the effects of treatment and block.

4. Hypothesis Testing for the Means
In a randomized block design, both treatment and block effects require hypothesis testing; therefore, there are two sets of hypotheses.
Between treatment groups:

$H_{0A}: \mu_1^{(A)} = \mu_2^{(A)} = \cdots = \mu_k^{(A)}$

$H_{1A}: \mu_1^{(A)}, \mu_2^{(A)}, \ldots, \mu_k^{(A)}$ are not all the same

Determine a significance level

Between blocks:

$H_{0B}: \mu_1^{(B)} = \mu_2^{(B)} = \cdots = \mu_b^{(B)}$

$H_{1B}: \mu_1^{(B)}, \mu_2^{(B)}, \ldots, \mu_b^{(B)}$ are not all the same

Determine a significance level

Under H_{0A}, the test statistic for testing the treatment effect A is

$$F_A = \frac{MS_A}{MS_E}, \tag{10.13}$$

which follows F distribution with $\nu_A = k-1$ and $\nu_E = (k-1)(b-1)$ degrees of freedom.

Similarly, the test statistic for testing the *block effect B* is

$$F_B = \frac{MS_B}{MS_E}, \tag{10.14}$$

which follows an F distribution with $\nu_B = b-1$ and $\nu_E = (k-1)(b-1)$ degrees of freedom.

For a given significance level α and degrees of freedom (ν_A, ν_E), the critical value $F_{(\nu_A,\nu_E),1-\alpha}$ can be obtained from the $F_{(\nu_A,\nu_E)}$ distribution (Appendix Table 6).

If $F_A > F_{(\nu_A,\nu_E),1-\alpha}$, then reject H_{0A}; otherwise, do not reject H_{0A};

If $F_B > F_{(\nu_B,\nu_E),1-\alpha}$, then reject H_{0B}; otherwise, do not reject H_{0B}.

Table 10.3 ANOVA table for a randomized block design.

Source of variation	SS	ν	MS	F	p value
Treatment	SS_A	$k-1$	SS_A / ν_A	MS_A / MS_E	*
Block	SS_B	$b-1$	SS_B / ν_B	MS_B / MS_E	*
Error	SS_E	$(k-1)(b-1)$	SS_E / ν_E		
Total	SS_T	$n-1$			

The results of ANOVA for randomized block design are usually summarized in the form of Table 10.3.

Solution to Example 10.1

(1) State the hypotheses and select a significance level

Between treatment groups:

$H_{0A}: \mu_A = \mu_B = \mu_C$, that is, the population mean weight gains of the rats fed with the three types of feed are the same

$H_{1A}: \mu_A, \mu_B, \mu_C$ are not all the same

$$\alpha = 0.05$$

Between blocks:

$H_{0B}: \mu_1 = \mu_2 = \cdots = \mu_6$, that is, the population mean weight gains of the rats in the six litters are the same

$H_{1B}: \mu_1, \mu_2, \ldots, \mu_6$ are not all the same

$$\alpha = 0.05$$

(2) Calculate the test statistic and construct the ANOVA table

From the data in Table 10.1,

$$\sum_j \sum_i x_{ij} = 1357.9, \sum_j \sum_i x_{ij}^2 = 107037.75,$$

$$C = \left(\sum_j \sum_i x_{ij} \right)^2 \bigg/ bk = 1357.9^2 / 18 = 102438.47$$

SS_T and ν_T are

$$SS_T = \sum_j \sum_i x_{ij}^2 - C = 107037.75 - 102438.47 = 4599.28,$$

$$\nu_T = n - 1 = 18 - 1 = 17.$$

SS_A, ν_A, and MS_A are

$$\begin{aligned}
\mathrm{SS}_A &= \frac{\sum_j\left(\sum_i x_{ij}\right)^2}{b} - C = \frac{386.7^2}{6} + \frac{413.7^2}{6} + \frac{557.5^2}{6} - 102438.47 \\
&= 2810.00, \\
\nu_A &= k-1 = 3-1 = 2, \\
\mathrm{MS}_A &= \frac{\mathrm{SS}_A}{\nu_A} = \frac{2810.00}{2} = 1405.00.
\end{aligned}$$

SS_B, ν_B, and MS_B are

$$\begin{aligned}
\mathrm{SS}_B &= \frac{\sum_i\left(\sum_j x_{ij}\right)^2}{k} - C \\
&= \frac{181.3^2}{3} + \frac{210.4^2}{3} + \frac{243.0^2}{3} + \frac{218.9^2}{3} + \frac{259.6^2}{3} + \frac{244.7^2}{3} - 102438.47 \\
&= 1352.97, \\
\nu_B &= b-1 = 6-1 = 5, \\
\mathrm{MS}_B &= \frac{\mathrm{SS}_B}{\nu_B} = \frac{1352.97}{5} = 270.59.
\end{aligned}$$

SS_E, ν_E, and MS_E are

$$\begin{aligned}
\mathrm{SS}_E &= \mathrm{SS}_T - \mathrm{SS}_A - \mathrm{SS}_B = 4599.28 - 2810.00 - 1352.97 \\
&= 436.31, \\
\nu_E &= (k-1)(b-1) = (3-1)(6-1) = 10, \\
\mathrm{MS}_E &= \frac{\mathrm{SS}_E}{\nu_E} = \frac{436.31}{10} = 43.63.
\end{aligned}$$

Calculate the test statistic F

$$\text{Between feeds: } F_A = \frac{\mathrm{MS}_A}{\mathrm{MS}_E} = \frac{1405.00}{43.63} = 32.20$$

$$\text{Between litters: } F_B = \frac{\mathrm{MS}_B}{\mathrm{MS}_E} = \frac{270.59}{43.63} = 6.20$$

The results of the ANOVA are given in Table 10.4.

(3) Draw a conclusion

Under H_{0A}: $\alpha = 0.05$, $\nu_A = 2$, and $\nu_E = 10$, the critical value is $F_{(2,10),1-0.05} = 4.10$ (Appendix Table 6). As $F_A = 32.20 > F_{(2,10),1-0.05}$, $p < 0.05$, we reject H_{0A} and accept H_{1A} at the $\alpha = 0.05$ level. We have significant evidence to show that the effects of the three types of feed on the rats' weight gain are not all the same.

Under H_{0B}: similarly, at the $\alpha = 0.05$ level, we conclude that the weight gains of rats in different litters are not all the same (see Table 10.4).

Table 10.4 ANOVA table for Example 10.1.

Source of variation	SS	ν	MS	F	p value
Feed	2810.00	2	1405.00	32.20	< 0.0001
Litter	1352.97	5	270.59	6.20	0.0072
Error	436.31	10	43.63		
Total	4599.28	17			

Example 10.1 illustrates the advantage of randomized block design in improving the experiment's efficiency by controlling between-block variation. The blocking removes the large amount of litter variation from SS_E, 1789.28 to 436.31, and the degrees of freedom for the error sum of squares have been reduced from 15 to 10. The test statistic F has subsequently increased, which demonstrates that there was significantly different weight gain in the rats, at least between two of the feeds.

However, the results should be interpreted with caution if there is no significant difference between block means because we do not know the probability of a Type II error. At present, this issue is controversial: on the one hand, it is believed that because of the loss of information from grouping into blocks, the block should be combined with the random error when there is no significant difference in the test of block. Thus, the ANOVA for randomized block design should be simplified to a one-way ANOVA. On the other hand, if the researcher is convinced that within block is more homogeneous than between block, the ANOVA for randomized block design can still be used even though the block effect is nonsignificant. This design should be preserved in future experiments.

10.2 ANOVA for Two-factor Factorial Design

Although the ANOVA approach for randomized block design is a two-factor design, the real interest is only in the effect of the treatment factor. We often wish to know the effect of two or more treatment factors and any interaction effects between them. *Factorial design* for testing the effect of interactions plays an important role in ANOVA. Factorial design is often named according to the number of levels of each factor. For example, the 2×2 factorial design has two factors, and each factor has two levels; the $2 \times 3 \times 4$ factorial design has three factors, and the factors have two, three, and four levels, respectively. The ANOVA for factorial design analyzes "interaction effect" through the crossed combination of multiple factors at each level. Thus, each factor in the research needs less times of experiment and can provide more information, thereby improving the efficiency of the experiment.

In this section, we focus on the ANOVA for two-factor factorial design experiments. This is also called *two-way ANOVA with replication*. It provides a basis for learning ANOVA for multifactor factorial experimental design.

Example 10.2 To investigate the hypoglycemic effect of two drugs with different dose levels on streptozotocin-induced diabetic male rats, a factorial design was adopted. The experimental data showing the decrease in fasting blood glucose (mmol/L) are given in Table 10.5. Analyze whether the hypoglycemic effect of the drugs on rats is significant and whether there is an interaction effect between the drugs.

We can see from Table 10.5 that in the four crossed combinations of different dose levels of drugs A and B, there are four replications for each combination. These observations are affected by both drugs A and B. Then, a natural question arises: is there an interaction effect between the two drugs? Before answering this question, we should understand the practical meaning of the tests for factor interaction and factor main effects. We illustrate these concepts in Section 10.2.1.

10.2.1 Concept of Factorial Design

There are several basic concepts in a two-way factorial design: simple effect, main effect, and interaction effect. These effects are all reflected by changes in the corresponding mean. To explain these concepts, we first calculate the mean of the observations for the four crossed combinations in Table 10.5; the results are given in Table 10.6.

(1) *Simple effect*: This refers to the effect in the mean between different levels of one factor when another factor is fixed at a certain level. As in this example, when drug A is fixed at level A_1, the difference between levels B_1 and B_2 is

$$A_1B_1 - A_1B_2 = 1.67 - 1.31 = 0.36$$

that is, the simple effect of drug B at level A_1 is 0.36.
Similarly, the simple effect of drug B at level A_2 is

$$A_2B_1 - A_2B_2 = 1.27 - 1.24 = 0.03$$

Table 10.5 Decrease in fasting blood glucose (mmol/L) in rats treated with two drugs.

		Drug *B*		**Total by levels of drug *A***
		B_1	B_2	
Drug *A*	A_1	1.56	1.24	11.90
		1.69	1.30	
		1.64	1.41	
		1.79	1.27	
	A_2	1.16	0.98	10.03
		1.23	1.17	
		1.37	1.32	
		1.33	1.47	
	Total by levels of drug *B*	11.77	10.16	21.93

(2) *Main effect*: This refers to the average of the simple effects of one factor at different levels of another factor.
As in this example, the main effect of drug B is

$$B = \frac{A_1B_1 - A_1B_2}{2} + \frac{A_2B_1 - A_2B_2}{2} = \frac{1.67 - 1.31}{2} + \frac{1.27 - 1.24}{2} = 0.20$$

Similarly, the main effect of drug A is

$$A = \frac{A_1B_1 - A_2B_1}{2} + \frac{A_1B_2 - A_2B_2}{2} = \frac{1.67 - 1.27}{2} + \frac{1.31 - 1.24}{2} = 0.24$$

(3) *Interaction effect*: This refers to the difference in the mean at different levels of one factor depending on the different levels of another factor.
As in this example, interaction effect between drug A and drug B is

$$A \times B = \frac{A_1B_1 - A_2B_1}{2} - \frac{A_1B_2 - A_2B_2}{2} = \frac{1.67 - 1.27}{2} - \frac{1.31 - 1.24}{2} = 0.17$$

and $A \times B = B \times A$.

In this example, the interaction effect estimate is 0.17, not equal to 0, which suggests that there might be a true interaction effect between the two drugs. The calculation results of simple effects, main effects, and interaction effects are given in Table 10.7.

The relationship between the main effect and interaction effect of factors A and B can be intuitively illustrated through Figure 10.1.

Table 10.6 Means of the crossed combinations of drugs A and B.

	B_1	B_2
A_1	1.67	1.31
A_2	1.27	1.24

Table 10.7 Three types of effects in Example 10.2.

	B_1	B_2	$B_1 - B_2$ (simple effect)	B (main effect)
A_1	1.67	1.31	0.36	0.20
A_2	1.27	1.24	0.03	
$A_1 - A_2$ (simple effect)	0.40	0.07		
A (main effect)	0.24			0.17 (interaction effect)

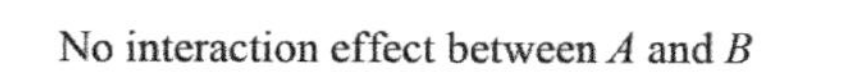

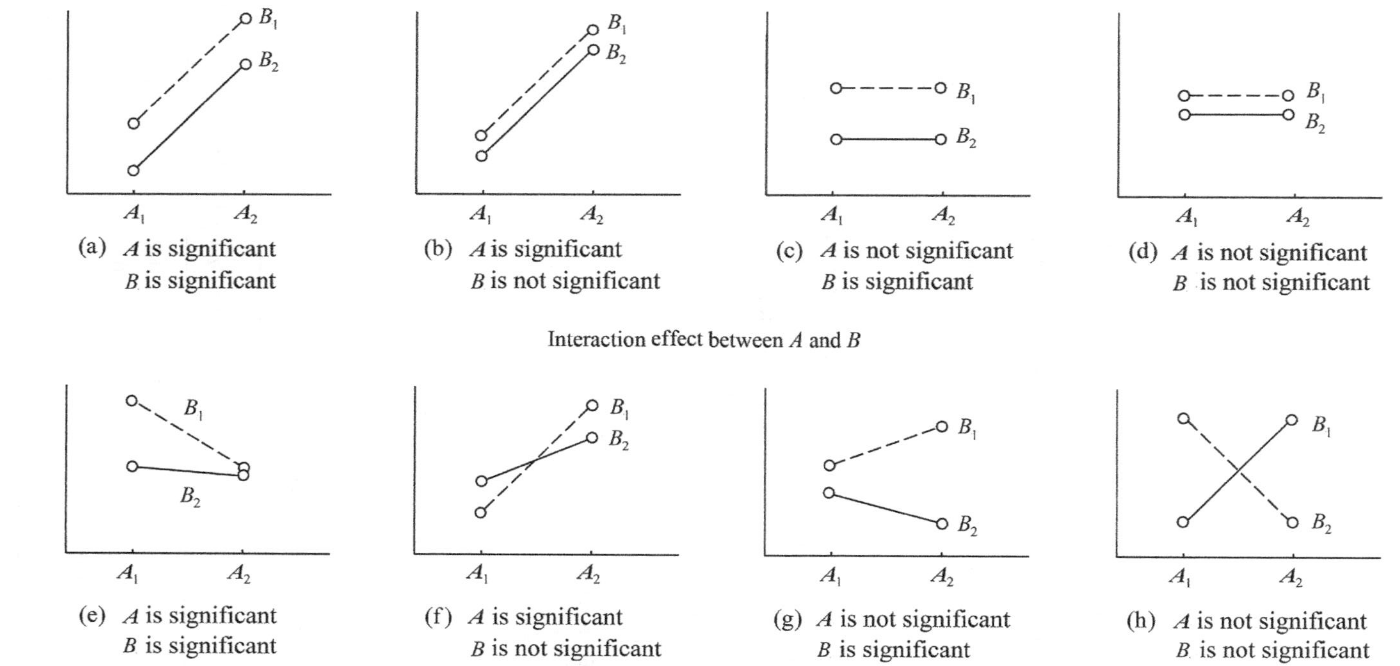

Figure 10.1 Illustration of main effect and interaction effect.

10.2.2 Data Layout and Model Assumptions

Extending from the simple 2×2 factorial design, let us formulate a two-factor factorial experimental design in a more general form. Suppose there are a levels of treatment factor A, b levels of treatment factor B, and a total of $a \times b$ crossed combinations (cells), each with n observations (balanced design). The data layout in an $a \times b$ factorial design is given in Table 10.8.

The model of ANOVA for two-factor factorial design is

$$X_{ijk} = \mu + \alpha_i + \beta_i + (\alpha\beta)_{ij} + \varepsilon_{ijk}, \qquad (10.15)$$

where

X_{ijk} is the kth observation in the ith group of A and the jth group of B.
μ is an expected mean, estimated from the overall mean of all observations.

Table 10.8 Data layout for an $a \times b$ factorial design.

		Factor B_j ($j = 1, 2, \ldots, b$)				$X_{i\cdot\cdot}$	$\bar{X}_{i\cdot\cdot}$
		B_1	B_2	$\cdots$	B_b		
Factor A_i ($i = 1, 2, \ldots, a$)	A_1	X_{111}	X_{121}	$\cdots$	X_{1b1}	$X_{1\cdot\cdot}$	$\bar{X}_{1\cdot\cdot}$
		X_{112}	X_{122}	$\cdots$	X_{1b2}		
		$\vdots$	$\vdots$	$\cdots$	$\vdots$		
		X_{11n}	X_{12n}	$\cdots$	X_{1bn}		
	A_2	X_{211}	X_{221}	$\cdots$	X_{2b1}	$X_{2\cdot\cdot}$	$\bar{X}_{2\cdot\cdot}$
		X_{212}	X_{222}	$\cdots$	X_{2b2}		
		$\vdots$	$\vdots$	$\cdots$	$\vdots$		
		X_{21n}	X_{22n}	$\cdots$	X_{2bn}		
	$\vdots$	$\vdots$	$\vdots$	$\cdots$	$\vdots$	$\vdots$	$\vdots$
	A_a	X_{a11}	X_{a21}	$\cdots$	X_{ab1}	$X_{a\cdot\cdot}$	$\bar{X}_{a\cdot\cdot}$
		X_{a12}	X_{a22}	$\cdots$	X_{ab2}		
		$\vdots$	$\vdots$	$\cdots$	$\vdots$		
		X_{a1n}	X_{a2n}	$\cdots$	X_{abn}		
	$X_{\cdot j \cdot}$	$X_{\cdot 1 \cdot}$	$X_{\cdot 2 \cdot}$	$\cdots$	$X_{\cdot b \cdot}$	$X_{\cdots}$	—
	$\bar{X}_{\cdot j \cdot}$	$\bar{X}_{\cdot 1 \cdot}$	$\bar{X}_{\cdot 2 \cdot}$	$\cdots$	$\bar{X}_{\cdot b \cdot}$	—	$\bar{X}_{\cdots}$

where $X_{i\cdot\cdot} = \sum_{j=1}^{b}\sum_{k=1}^{n} X_{ijk}$, $X_{\cdot j \cdot} = \sum_{i=1}^{a}\sum_{k=1}^{n} X_{ijk}$, $X_{\cdots} = \sum_{i=1}^{a}\sum_{j=1}^{b}\sum_{k=1}^{n} X_{ijk}$, $\bar{X}_{i\cdot\cdot} = \sum_{j=1}^{b}\sum_{k=1}^{n} X_{ijk} \Big/ bn$,
$\bar{X}_{\cdot j \cdot} = \sum_{i=1}^{a}\sum_{k=1}^{n} X_{ijk} \Big/ an$, and $\bar{X}_{\cdots} = \sum_{i=1}^{a}\sum_{j=1}^{b}\sum_{k=1}^{n} X_{ijk} \Big/ abn$.

α_i is an expected mean representing the effect of the ith level of factor A, i.e., $\alpha_i = \mu_i - \mu$.

β_j is an expected mean representing the effect of the jth level of factor B, i.e., $\beta_j = \mu_j - \mu$.

$(\alpha\beta)_{ij}$ is an expected mean representing the interaction effect between factors A at the ith level and B at the jth level.

ε_{ijk} is an error term, which is assumed to be normally distributed with mean 0 and variance σ^2.

Model Assumptions

(1) The observations for any factor-level combination are approximately normally distributed.
(2) The variance is equal for all factor-level combination populations. The population variance is estimated from the within-cell mean square (i.e., the error mean square).
(3) The model should satisfy $\sum_i \alpha_i = 0$, $\sum_j \beta_j = 0$, and $\sum_i (\alpha\beta)_{ij} = \sum_j (\alpha\beta)_{ij} = 0$.

10.2.3 Procedure of ANOVA

1. Partitioning Sum of Squares of Deviations

The basic idea of ANOVA, partitioning the total variation, also applies to factorial design. The deviation between any individual observation and the overall mean can be represented as follows:

$$X_{ijk} - \bar{X}_{...} = (\bar{X}_{i..} - \bar{X}_{...}) + (\bar{X}_{.j.} - \bar{X}_{...}) + (\bar{X}_{ij.} - \bar{X}_{i..} - \bar{X}_{.j.} + \bar{X}_{...}) + (X_{ijk} - \bar{X}_{ij.}). \quad (10.16)$$

Square both sides of Formula 10.16 and sum the squared deviations for all observations, and the following relationship is obtained (because the sum of all cross-product terms on the right side of the formula is zero):

$$\begin{aligned} &\sum_i \sum_j \sum_k (X_{ijk} - \bar{X}_{...})^2 \\ &= bn \sum_i (\bar{X}_{i..} - \bar{X}_{...})^2 + an \sum_j (\bar{X}_{.j.} - \bar{X}_{...})^2 \\ &+ n \sum_i \sum_j (\bar{X}_{ij.} - \bar{X}_{i..} - \bar{X}_{.j.} + \bar{X}_{...})^2 + \sum_i \sum_j \sum_k (X_{ijk} - \bar{X}_{ij.})^2. \end{aligned} \quad (10.17)$$

The first term on the right-hand side represents the sum of squared deviation of the row mean from the overall mean and is called the *row effect*, that is, the main effect of factor A.

The second term on the right-hand side represents the sum of squared deviation of the column mean from the overall mean and is called the *column effect*, that is, the main effect of factor B.

The third term on the right-hand side represents the interaction effect of factors A and B.

The fourth term represents the sum of squared deviation of an individual observation from the group mean for that observation. The expression is an indication of within-cell variation and is the error term.

For each item in Formula 10.17, we have

$$SS_T = SS_A + SS_B + SS_{A\times B} + SS_E. \tag{10.18}$$

The various sums of squares used in two-factor factorial design and their equivalent computational formulas are as follows:

The total sum of squares is

$$SS_T = \sum_i \sum_j \sum_k \left(X_{ijk} - \bar{X}_{...}\right)^2. \tag{10.19}$$

The simplified formula is

$$SS_T = \sum_i \sum_j \sum_k X_{ijk}^2 - \frac{\left(\sum_i \sum_j \sum_k X_{ijk}\right)^2}{abn}, \tag{10.20}$$

where $\left(\sum_i \sum_j \sum_k X_{ijk}\right)^2 \Big/ abn$ is the correction term and is denoted by C.

The sum of squares factor A is

$$SS_A = bn \sum_i \left(\bar{X}_{i..} - \bar{X}_{...}\right)^2. \tag{10.21}$$

The simplified formula is

$$SS_A = \frac{1}{bn} \sum_i X_{i..}^2 - C. \tag{10.22}$$

The sum of squares factor B is

$$SS_B = an \sum_j \left(\bar{X}_{.j.} - \bar{X}_{...}\right)^2. \tag{10.23}$$

The simplified formula is

$$SS_B = \frac{1}{an} \sum_j X_{.j.}^2 - C. \tag{10.24}$$

The error sum of squares is

$$SS_E = \sum_i \sum_j \sum_k \left(X_{ijk} - \bar{X}_{ij.}\right)^2. \tag{10.25}$$

The simplified formula is

$$SS_E = \sum_i \sum_j \sum_k X_{ijk}^2 - \frac{1}{n} \sum_i \sum_j X_{ij.}^2, \tag{10.26}$$

where $X_{ij.} = \sum_{k=1}^{n} X_{ijk}$.

The sum of squares for the interaction between factors A and B is

$$SS_{A\times B} = n \sum_i \sum_j \left(\bar{X}_{ij.} - \bar{X}_{i..} - \bar{X}_{.j.} + \bar{X}_{...}\right)^2. \tag{10.27}$$

It can also be directly calculated using the following formula:

$$SS_{A\times B} = SS_T - SS_A - SS_B - SS_E. \tag{10.28}$$

2. Partitioning Degrees of Freedom
The degrees of freedom are partitioned the same way as the sums of squares (Table 10.9).

3. Formulation of Variances from Different Sources
The mean square MS_A,

$$MS_A = SS_A / (a-1), \tag{10.29}$$

refers to the variance between the sample mean at each level of factor A.
The mean square MS_B,

$$MS_B = SS_B / (b-1), \tag{10.30}$$

refers to the variance between the sample mean at each level of factor B.
The mean square $MS_{A\times B}$,

$$MS_{A\times B} = SS_{A\times B} / [(a-1)(b-1)], \tag{10.31}$$

refers to the variance of the effect of factor $B(A)$ at different levels of factor $A(B)$.
Error mean square MS_E,

$$MS_E = SS_E / [ab(n-1)], \tag{10.32}$$

refers to the effect of the random error after removing the effects of each treatment and interaction.

4. Hypothesis Testing for the Means

The first step: test for interaction between factors. The hypotheses are

$$H_{0A\times B}: (\alpha\beta)_{ij} = 0, \quad \text{for all } i, j$$
$$H_{1A\times B}: (\alpha\beta)_{ij} \neq 0, \quad \text{for some } i, j$$

The appropriate test statistic for this null hypothesis is

$$F_{A\times B} = \frac{MS_{A\times B}}{MS_E}$$

Table 10.9 Partitioning of degrees of freedom for an $a \times b$ factorial design.

Source of variation	**v**
Main effect A	$a-1$
Main effect B	$b-1$
Interaction $A\times B$	$(a-1)(b-1)$
Error	$ab(n-1)$
Total	$abn-1$

follows a F distribution with degrees of freedom $\nu_{A\times B}=(a-1)(b-1)$ and $\nu_E=ab(n-1)$.

If $F_{A\times B}>F_{(\nu_{A\times B},\nu_E),1-\alpha}$, then reject $H_{0A\times B}$; the interaction effect is significant.

In this case, we omit F_A and F_B tests, because the levels of factor A do not behave consistently across the levels of factor B, and vice versa.

The results are usually summarized in the form of Table 10.10.

If $F_{A\times B}\le F_{(\nu_{A\times B},\nu_E),1-\alpha}$, then do not reject $H_{0A\times B}$; this indicates that there is no interaction effect between factors A and B. The analysis should continue to the second step.

The second step: test the main effect of factor A or factor B. Test hypotheses are as follows.

$$H_{0A}:\ \alpha_1=\alpha_2=\cdots=\alpha_a=0,\ H_{1A}:\ \text{at least one } \alpha_i\ne 0$$
$$H_{0B}:\ \beta_1=\beta_2=\cdots=\beta_b=0,\ H_{1B}:\ \text{at least one } \beta_j\ne 0$$
$$(i=1,2,\ldots,a;\ j=1,2,\ldots,b)$$

To obtain the equivalent result using the ANOVA approach, the sum of squares for AB interaction and error are "pooled" and a new MS'_E is computed, where

$$\mathrm{MS}'_E=\frac{\mathrm{SS}_{A\times B}+\mathrm{SS}_E}{\nu_{A\times B}+\nu_E}=\frac{\mathrm{SS}_{A\times B}+\mathrm{SS}_E}{abn-a-b+1}. \tag{10.33}$$

Calculate the test statistic for the main effect of factor A

$$F_A=\frac{\mathrm{MS}_A}{\mathrm{MS}'_E}\sim F(\nu_A,\nu'_E),\ \nu_A=a-1,\ \nu'_E=abn-a-b+1. \tag{10.34}$$

If $F_A>F_{(\nu_A,\nu'_E),1-\alpha}$, then reject H_{0A}; the main effect of factor A is significant.

If $F_A\le F_{(\nu_A,\nu'_E),1-\alpha}$, then do not reject H_{0A}; the main effect of factor A cannot be considered significant.

To test the main effect of factor B, calculate the test statistic

$$F_B=\frac{\mathrm{MS}_B}{\mathrm{MS}'_E}\sim F(\nu_B,\nu'_E),\ \nu_B=b-1,\ \nu'_E=abn-a-b+1. \tag{10.35}$$

If $F_B>F_{(\nu_B,\nu'_E),1-\alpha}$, then reject H_{0B}, the main effect of factor B is significant.

Table 10.10 ANOVA table for an $a\times b$ factorial design.

Source of variation	SS	ν	MS	F	p value
Main effect A	SS_A	$a-1$	SS_A/ν_A		
Main effect B	SS_B	$b-1$	SS_B/ν_B		
Interaction $A\times B$	$\mathrm{SS}_{A\times B}$	$(a-1)(b-1)$	$\mathrm{SS}_{A\times B}/\nu_{A\times B}$	$\mathrm{MS}_{A\times B}/\mathrm{MS}_E$	*
Error	SS_E	$ab(n-1)$	SS_E/ν_E		
Total	SS_T	$abn-1$			

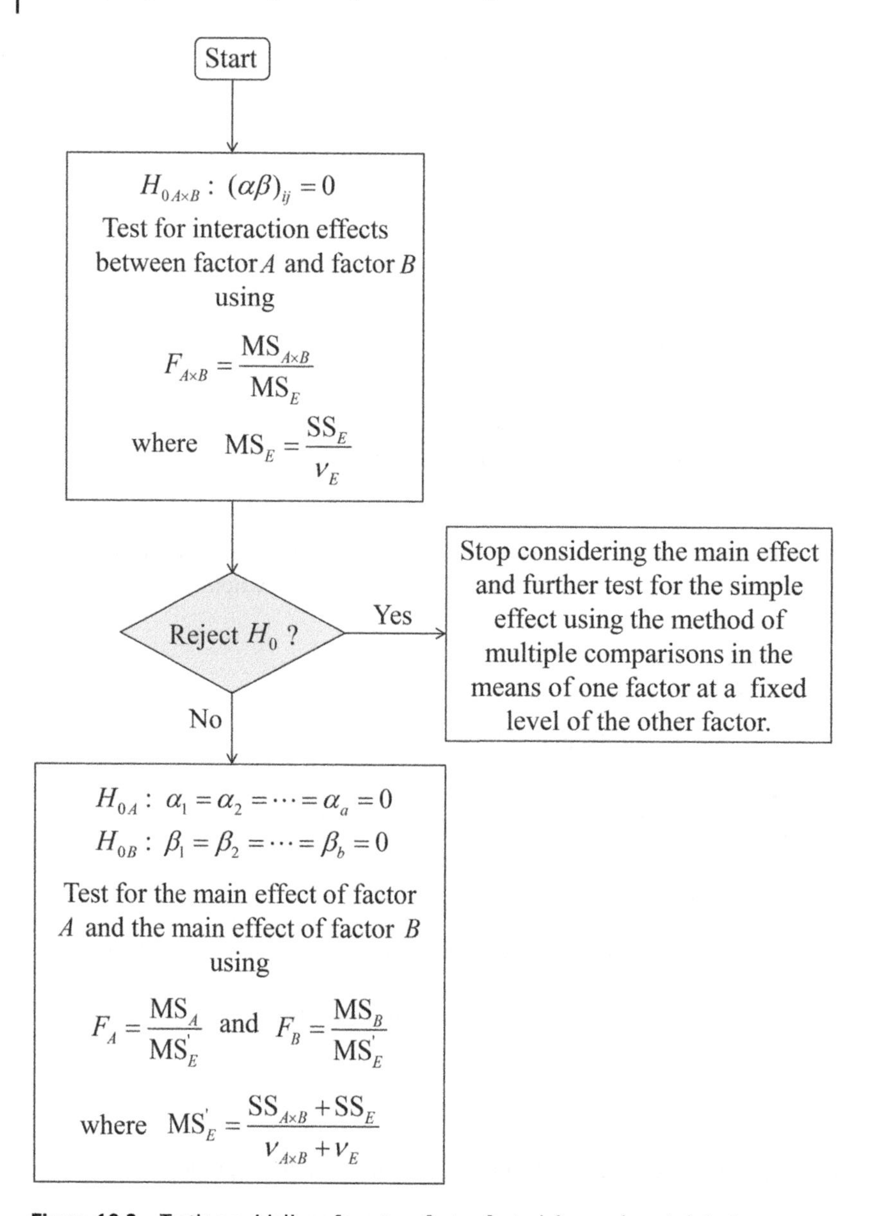

Figure 10.2 Testing guidelines for a two-factor factorial experimental design.

If $F_B \le F_{(\nu_B,\, \nu_E'),1-\alpha}$, then do not reject H_{0B}; the main effect of factor B cannot be considered significant.

Figure 10.2 presents the testing guidelines for a two-factor factorial experimental design.

Solution to Example 10.2

(1) State the hypotheses and select a significance level

$H_{0A\times B}$: there is no interaction effect between drug A and drug B

$H_{1A\times B}$: there is interaction effect between drug A and drug B

$$\alpha = 0.05$$

(2) Determine the test statistic and construct the ANOVA table

According to the data in Table 10.5, we have

$$C = \frac{\left(\sum_i \sum_j \sum_k x_{ijk}\right)^2}{abn} = \frac{21.93^2}{16} = 30.0578.$$

SS_T and ν_T are

$$SS_T = \sum_i \sum_j \sum_k x_{ijk}^2 - C = 30.7489 - 30.0578 = 0.6911,$$
$$\nu_T = abn - 1 = 16 - 1 = 15.$$

The SS_A, ν_A, and MS_A are

$$SS_A = \frac{1}{bn}\sum_i x_{i\cdot\cdot}^2 - C = \frac{1}{2\times 4}\times\left(11.90^2 + 10.03^2\right) - 30.0578 = 0.2186,$$
$$\nu_A = a - 1 = 2 - 1 = 1,$$
$$MS_A = \frac{SS_A}{\nu_A} = \frac{0.2186}{1} = 0.2186.$$

The SS_B, ν_B, and MS_B are

$$SS_B = \frac{1}{an}\sum_j x_{\cdot j\cdot}^2 - C = \frac{1}{2\times 4}\times\left(11.77^2 + 10.16^2\right) - 30.0578 = 0.1620,$$
$$\nu_B = b - 1 = 2 - 1 = 1,$$
$$MS_B = \frac{SS_B}{\nu_B} = \frac{0.1620}{1} = 0.1620.$$

The SS_E, ν_E, and MS_E are

$$SS_E = \sum_i \sum_j \sum_k x_{ijk}^2 - \frac{1}{n}\sum_i \sum_j x_{ij\cdot}^2 = 30.7489 - \frac{1}{4}\times\left(6.68^2 + 5.22^2 + 5.09^2 + 4.94^2\right)$$
$$= 0.2033,$$
$$\nu_E = ab(n-1) = 2\times 2\times(4-1) = 12,$$
$$MS_E = \frac{SS_E}{\nu_E} = \frac{0.2033}{12} = 0.0169.$$

$SS_{A\times B}$, $\nu_{A\times B}$, and $MS_{A\times B}$ are

$$SS_{A\times B} = SS_T - SS_A - SS_B - SS_E = 0.6911 - 0.2186 - 0.1620 - 0.2033$$
$$= 0.1072,$$
$$\nu_{A\times B} = (a-1)\times(b-1) = (2-1)\times(2-1) = 1,$$
$$MS_{A\times B} = \frac{SS_{A\times B}}{\nu_{A\times B}} = \frac{0.1072}{1} = 0.1072.$$

Table 10.11 ANOVA table for Example 10.2.

Source of variation	SS	ν	MS	F	p value
Main effect A	0.2186	1	0.2186		
Main effect B	0.1620	1	0.1620		
Interaction $A \times B$	0.1072	1	0.1072	6.34	0.0270
Error	0.2033	12	0.0169		
Total	0.6911	15			

The test statistic is

$$F_{A\times B} = \frac{\text{MS}_{A\times B}}{\text{MS}_E} = \frac{0.1072}{0.0169} = 6.34.$$

The results of the ANOVA are given in Table 10.11.

(3) Draw a conclusion

Under $H_{0A\times B}$, given $\alpha = 0.05$, $\nu_{A\times B} = 1$, and $\nu_E = 12$, the critical value of $F_{(1,12)}$ is $F_{(1,12),1-0.05} = 4.75$ (Appendix Table 6). Since $F_{A\times B} = 6.34 > F_{(1,12),1-0.05}$, $p < 0.05$. We reject $H_{0A\times B}$ and accept $H_{1A\times B}$ at the $\alpha = 0.05$ level. We have significant evidence to show that drugs A and B have an interaction effect on the hypoglycemic action in the rats.

As the interaction effect is significant in this example, the simple effect analysis should be performed. With multiple levels, drug B can be fixed at a certain level and the method of multiple comparisons (such as Tukey's test) can be used for multiple comparisons of the mean levels of drug A. Comparison of the mean levels of drug B is done the same way.

10.3 ANOVA for Repeated Measures Design

10.3.1 Characteristics of Repeated Measures Data

In practice, we are often interested in the change of a certain measurement index over time. For example, to know the growth and development of children, height, weight, and other indexes should be observed repeatedly. For diagnosis and treatment of diseases, some physiological, biochemical, or pathological parameters are measured at different times to understand the trend of change. For example, to detect lung cancer early, consecutive follow-up of patients with pulmonary nodules is required. These situations involve a new concept, *repeated measures*. This refers to multiple measurements of the same index in the same subject (such as human or animal) at different time points. The data obtained are called repeated measures data. Repeated measures data are more common in clinical trials than independent observation data. This section will introduce the

ANOVA method for one-sample repeated measures design data, which is the most commonly used in practice.

Example 10.3 To test the effect of an antiviral drug on serum levels of alanine aminotransferase (ALT, U/L) in patients with chronic hepatitis B, 10 patients with chronic hepatitis B were administered the drug at roughly the same time point. Their serum ALT levels were measured at 0 (baseline level), 10, 20, and 30 weeks after medication. The data are given in Table 10.12. Analyze the trend of changes in the ALT levels of patients with chronic hepatitis B taking the drug.

The data in Example 10.3 are from a single sample (10 patients) with only one factor (time). In this study, ALT levels were measured at four time points for each patient. In Figure 10.3, the patients' ALT levels generally showed a downward trend over time, but the characteristics of changes in different patients are not the same. In addition, the variation of ALT levels at baseline was large, and it became significantly smaller after 30 weeks of medication.

From the data structure perspective, the observations at different time points are correlated as they were obtained from the same patients.

The main purpose of the repeated measures design is to analyze the changing characteristics of a certain index of the subject over time. The main advantage of this design is that each subject can serve as their own control to remove the influence of between-subject variation, so the analysis can better focus on the effect of time; meanwhile, the between-subject variation can be partitioned from the error term to make its power of test higher, which is similar to the idea of block design.

Table 10.12 Serum ALT levels (U/L) of 10 patients with chronic hepatitis B at different time points.

Patient ID i	Time point j				$\sum_j x_{ij}$	$\bar{x}_{i\cdot}$
	0 weeks	10 weeks	20 weeks	30 weeks		
1	186	122	134	110	552	138.00
2	345	312	268	176	1101	275.25
3	98	84	52	61	295	73.75
4	288	98	91	85	562	140.50
5	176	86	130	99	491	122.75
6	210	188	143	120	661	165.25
7	271	322	86	65	744	186.00
8	415	332	265	186	1198	299.50
9	171	126	130	135	562	140.50
10	243	330	95	64	732	183.00
$\sum_i x_{ij}$	2403	2000	1394	1101	6898	—
$\bar{x}_{\cdot j}$	240.30	200.00	139.40	110.10	—	$\bar{x}_{\cdot\cdot} = 172.45$

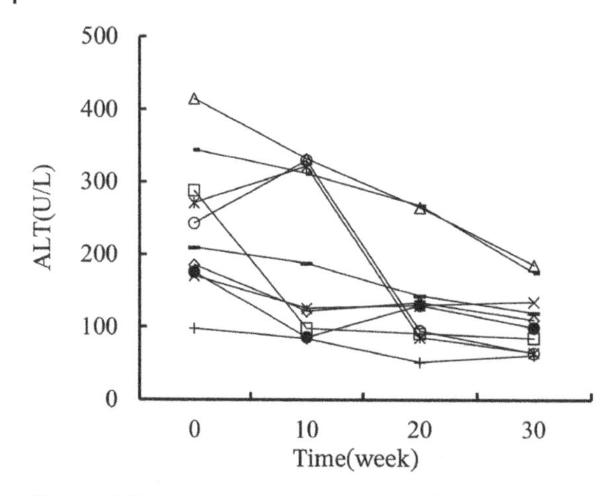

Figure 10.3 Trend of changes in serum ALT levels of patients with chronic hepatitis B at different time points.

10.3.2 Data Layout and Model Assumptions

Table 10.13 displays the data layout in which repeated measurements are obtained from a single sample.

In Table 10.13, $i = 1, 2, \ldots, n$; $j = 1, 2, \ldots, t$.

$\bar{X}_{i\cdot} = \sum_{j=1}^{t} X_{ij} / t$ denotes the mean of each subject over time, $\bar{X}_{\cdot j} = \sum_{i=1}^{n} X_{ij} / n$ denotes the means at each time point over subjects, and $\bar{X}_{\cdot\cdot} = \sum_{i=1}^{n}\sum_{j=1}^{t} X_{ij} / nt$ denotes the means of all subjects at all time points.

The ANOVA model in this situation is

$$X_{ij} = \mu + \beta_i + \alpha_j + \varepsilon_{ij}, \tag{10.36}$$

where:

X_{ij} is the observation of the ith subject at the jth time point.

μ is an expected mean, estimated from the overall mean of all observations.

β_i is the random effect of subject i, which is constant over all time points.

α_j is an expected mean of the jth time point.

ε_{ij} is the random error specific to subject i at time j, which is independent and follows a normal distribution $N(0, \sigma^2)$.

Model Assumptions

(1) *Normality*: the observations of the subject at each measurement time point are independent random samples, and the sampled population follows a normal distribution.

(2) *Homogeneity of variance*: the population variances at different measurement time points are equal.

(3) *Sphericity*: the covariance matrix of the observations at different measurement time points satisfies the sphericity (i.e., independent structure). See Section 10.3.4 for details.
(4) The model should satisfy $\sum_{j}\alpha_j = 0$, $\sum_{i}\beta_i = 0$.

10.3.3 Procedure of ANOVA

1. Partitioning Sum of Squares of Deviations
The process of partitioning variations for one sample repeated measures data still follows the basic idea of one-way ANOVA. The total variation of observations is partitioned into three parts: between-subject variation SS_B, between-time variation SS_W, and random error SS_E:

$$SS_T = SS_B + SS_W + SS_E. \tag{10.37}$$

The total sum of squares is

$$SS_T = \sum_{j}\sum_{i}\left(X_{ij} - \bar{X}_{..}\right)^2 = \sum_{j}\sum_{i}X_{ij}^2 - C, \tag{10.38}$$

where $C = \left(\sum_{j}\sum_{i}X_{ij}\right)^2 \Big/ nt$ is the correction term.

SS_T reflects the total variation of all observations.
The between-subject sum of squares is

$$SS_B = \sum_{i} t\left(\bar{X}_{i.} - \bar{X}_{..}\right)^2 = \frac{\sum_{i}\left(\sum_{j}X_{ij}\right)^2}{t} - C. \tag{10.39}$$

SS_B reflects the variation between subjects.
The between-time sum of squares is

$$SS_W = \sum_{j} n\left(\bar{X}_{.j} - \bar{X}_{..}\right)^2 = \frac{\sum_{j}\left(\sum_{i}X_{ij}\right)^2}{n} - C. \tag{10.40}$$

SS_W reflects the variation between repeated measurements at different time points within the subjects.
The error sum of squares is

$$SS_E = \sum_{j}\sum_{i}\left(X_{ij} - \bar{X}_{i.} - \bar{X}_{.j} + \bar{X}_{..}\right)^2 = SS_T - SS_B - SS_W. \tag{10.41}$$

SS_E reflects the random variation other than between subjects and between time points.

2. Partitioning Degrees of Freedom

Degrees of freedom can be partitioned in the same way. The number of degrees of freedom of SS_T is $\nu_T = nt - 1$; there are n subjects for SS_B, so $\nu_B = n - 1$; there are t time points for SS_W, so $\nu_W = t - 1$; and $\nu_E = (n-1)(t-1)$.

3. Formulation of Variance of Different Sources

The variances of different sources are as follows:

Between subject mean square:

$$MS_B = SS_B / \nu_B. \tag{10.42}$$

Between time mean square:

$$MS_W = SS_W / \nu_W. \tag{10.43}$$

Error mean square:

$$MS_E = SS_E / \nu_E. \tag{10.44}$$

4. Hypothesis Testing for the Means

Because the one sample repeated measures design mainly focuses on the changing characteristics of the index within the subject over time, we only conduct hypothesis testing on the variation between time points.

The hypotheses are

$H_0: \mu_1 = \mu_2 = \cdots = \mu_t$

$H_1: \mu_1, \mu_2, \ldots, \mu_t$ are not all the same, and

Determine a significance level α

Under H_0, the test statistic is

$$F = \frac{MS_W}{MS_E}, \tag{10.45}$$

Table 10.13 Data layout of one-sample repeated measures design.

Subject i	**Time point j**				$\sum_j X_{ij}$	$\bar{X}_{i\cdot}$
	1	**2**	...	t		
1	X_{11}	X_{12}	...	X_{1t}	$\sum_j X_{1j}$	$\bar{X}_{1\cdot}$
2	X_{21}	X_{22}	...	X_{2t}	$\sum_j X_{2j}$	$\bar{X}_{2\cdot}$
⋮	⋮	⋮	⋮	⋮	⋮	⋮
n	X_{n1}	X_{n2}	...	X_{nt}	$\sum_j X_{nj}$	$\bar{X}_{n\cdot}$
$\sum_i X_{ij}$	$\sum_i X_{i1}$	$\sum_i X_{i2}$	...	$\sum_i X_{it}$	—	—
$\bar{X}_{\cdot j}$	$\bar{X}_{\cdot 1}$	$\bar{X}_{\cdot 2}$	...	$\bar{X}_{\cdot t}$	—	$\bar{X}_{\cdot\cdot}$

Table 10.14 ANOVA table for one-sample repeated measures design.

Source of variation	SS	ν	MS	F	p value
Between-subject	SS_B	$n-1$	MS_B		
Between-time	SS_W	$t-1$	MS_W	$\frac{MS_W}{MS_E}$	*
Error	SS_E	$(n-1)(t-1)$	MS_E		
Total	SS_T	$nt-1$			

which follows an F distribution with degrees of freedom of $\nu_W = t-1$ and $\nu_E = (n-1)(t-1)$. The results are usually summarizd in the form of Table 10.14.

For a given α and degrees of freedom (ν_W, ν_E), the critical value $F_{(\nu_W,\nu_E),1-\alpha}$ can be obtained from the $F_{(\nu_W,\nu_E)}$ distribution (Appendix Table 6). If $F > F_{(\nu_W,\nu_E),1-\alpha}$, then reject H_0; otherwise, do not reject H_0.

Thus far, the calculation process of repeated measures ANOVA is similar to that for randomized block design (blocks here refers to subjects), but the conclusion is conditional. The conclusion can only be established when the sphericity assumption of the covariance matrix is satisfied, otherwise the correlation of the data will result in an inflated Type I error.

10.3.4 Sphericity Test of Covariance Matrix

The key of the ANOVA for repeated measures data lies in dealing with correlation among the repeated measurements from a subject, which is mainly reflected in the structure of the covariance matrix.

If the covariance matrix of the population of observations at t time points satisfies Formula 10.46, then the matrix is said to be of sphericity (i.e., independent structure).

$$\sum = \begin{bmatrix} \sigma^2 & 0 & \cdots & 0 \\ 0 & \sigma^2 & \cdots & 0 \\ \vdots & \vdots & \vdots & \vdots \\ 0 & 0 & \cdots & \sigma^2 \end{bmatrix} = \sigma^2 I_t, \tag{10.46}$$

where σ^2 is a constant, and I_t is a t-order identity matrix.

Observations satisfying the sphericity assumption have the following characteristics: (i) when $i=j$, $\sigma_{ii} = \sigma_{jj} = \sigma^2$ (both $i, j = 1, 2, \ldots, t$), that is, the population variances of the observations at each time point are equal; (ii) when $i \neq j$, $\sigma_{ij} = 0$, that is, the covariance between observations at different time points is 0.

The sphericity test of the covariance matrix is called the *Mauchly test*, which is realized by constructing a likelihood ratio statistic W (the calculating of W is beyond of this text). The closer the statistic W is to 1, the better the matrix satisfies sphericity. Under H_0, the test statistic is

$$\chi^2 = -\left[(n-1) - \frac{2(t-1)^2 + (t-1) + 2}{6(t-1)}\right] \ln W, \tag{10.47}$$

which approximately follows a χ^2 distribution with degrees of freedom $\nu = t(t-1)/2 - 1$.

For a given α and ν, the critical value $\chi^2_{\nu,1-\alpha}$ can be obtained from the χ^2_ν distribution (Appendix Table 5). If $\chi^2 > \chi^2_{\nu,1-\alpha}$ then reject H_0, we conclude that the covariance matrix does not satisfy sphericity; otherwise, do not reject H_0, and we do not have the evidence to show that sphericity is violated.

When the covariance matrix of the data does not satisfy sphericity conditions, to ensure the reliability of the results of ANOVA, the degrees of freedom of the numerator and denominator of the test statistic F corresponding to the measurement time points must be corrected. The commonly used correction coefficients are as follows. (i) *Greenhouse–Geisser correction coefficient* $\hat{\varepsilon}$, which is also called *G-G* $\hat{\varepsilon}$, $1/(t-1) \leq \hat{\varepsilon} \leq 1$. If the sample covariance matrix satisfies sphericity, then $\hat{\varepsilon} = 1$; a smaller $\hat{\varepsilon}$ indicates greater severity of the violation of sphericity. If $\hat{\varepsilon} \geq 0.7$, the statistical conclusions after correction with degrees of freedom using $\hat{\varepsilon}$ are conservative and the correction makes little sense. (ii) *Huynh–Feldt correction coefficient* $\tilde{\varepsilon}$, which is also called *H-F* $\tilde{\varepsilon}$ and is a correction of *G-G* $\hat{\varepsilon}$. $\tilde{\varepsilon}$ may be greater than 1, in which case we could simply take $\tilde{\varepsilon} = 1$.

For the F statistic, illustrated by *G-G* $\hat{\varepsilon}$, the corrected degrees of freedom are as follows:

Degrees of freedom for numerator:

$$\hat{\nu}_W = \nu_W \times \hat{\varepsilon}. \tag{10.48}$$

Degrees of freedom for denominator:

$$\hat{\nu}_E = \nu_E \times \hat{\varepsilon}. \tag{10.49}$$

Using the corrected degrees of freedom $\hat{\nu}_W$ and $\hat{\nu}_E$, we obtain the critical value $F_{(\hat{\nu}_W, \hat{\nu}_E), 1-\alpha}$ from the critical value of the F distribution (Appendix Table 6). As $\hat{\varepsilon}$ or $\tilde{\varepsilon}$ are both less than or equal to 1, the critical value after correction is greater than or equal to the critical value before correction.

Solution to Example 10.3

We proceed in two steps:

Step 1: Assuming that the covariance matrix of the data satisfies sphericity, the test procedure of ANOVA in this situation is identical to that for randomized block design.

(1) State the hypotheses and select a significance level

$H_0: \mu_1 = \mu_2 = \mu_3 = \mu_4$, that is, the population mean ALT levels of patients with chronic hepatitis B at different time points are the same

$H_1: \mu_1, \mu_2, \mu_3, \mu_4$ are not all the same

$$\alpha = 0.05$$

(2) Determine the test statistic and construct the ANOVA table

According to the data in Table 10.12, we have

$$\sum_j \sum_i x_{ij} = 6898,$$

$$\sum_j \sum_i x_{ij}^2 = 186^2 + 345^2 + \cdots + 64^2 = 1546538,$$

$$C = \left(\sum_j \sum_i x_{ij} \right)^2 \Big/ nt = 6898^2 / 40 = 1189560.10.$$

SS_T and ν_T are

$$SS_T = \sum_j \sum_i x_{ij}^2 - C = 1546538 - 1189560.10 = 356977.90,$$
$$\nu_T = nt - 1 = 40 - 1 = 39.$$

The SS_B, ν_B, and MS_B are

$$SS_B = \frac{\sum_i \left(\sum_j x_{ij} \right)^2}{t} - C = \frac{1}{4} \times \left(552^2 + 1101^2 + \cdots + 732^2 \right) - 1189560.10$$
$$= 169985.90,$$
$$\nu_B = n - 1 = 10 - 1 = 9,$$
$$MS_B = \frac{SS_B}{\nu_B} = \frac{169985.90}{9} = 18887.32.$$

The SS_W, ν_W, and MS_W are

$$SS_W = \frac{\sum_j \left(\sum_i x_{ij} \right)^2}{n} - C = \frac{1}{10} \times \left(2403^2 + 2000^2 + \cdots + 1101^2 \right) - 1189560.10$$
$$= 103424.50,$$
$$\nu_W = t - 1 = 4 - 1 = 3,$$
$$MS_W = \frac{SS_W}{\nu_W} = \frac{103424.50}{3} = 34474.83.$$

The SS_E, ν_E, and MS_E are

$$SS_E = SS_T - SS_B - SS_W = 356977.90 - 169985.90 - 103424.50$$
$$= 83567.50,$$
$$\nu_E = (n-1)(t-1) = (10-1)(4-1) = 27,$$
$$MS_E = \frac{SS_E}{\nu_E} = \frac{83567.50}{27} = 3095.09.$$

Calculate the test statistic F.

$$\text{Between-time } F_W = \frac{MS_W}{MS_E} = \frac{34474.83}{3095.09} = 11.14.$$

Construct the ANOVA table (Table 10.15).

Step 2: Mauchly test for sphericity

Table 10.16 gives the results of the Mauchly test, $p = 0.032 < 0.05$, which indicates that the data do not satisfy the sphericity condition. Therefore, it is necessary to correct the degrees of freedom of the numerator and denominator of the test statistic F corresponding to between-time in Table 10.15.

Table 10.15 ANOVA table for Example 10.3.

Source of variation	SS	ν	MS	F	p value
Between-subject	169985.90	9	18887.32		
Between-time	103424.50	3	34474.83	11.14	< 0.0001
Error	83567.50	27	3095.09		
Total	356977.90	39			

Table 10.16 Mauchly test for sphericity for Example 10.3

Between-time	Mauchly's W	Approx.χ^2	ν	p value	G-$G\hat{\varepsilon}$	H-$F\tilde{\varepsilon}$
	0.202	12.350	5	0.032	0.557	0.670

We can use either the correction coefficient G-$G\,\hat{\varepsilon}$ or H-$F\,\tilde{\varepsilon}$ to correct the degrees of freedom.

(1) G-$G\hat{\varepsilon}$ method
From the results in Table 10.16, we have G-$G\hat{\varepsilon} = 0.557$. Degrees of freedom for between time are $\nu_W = 3$, and associated corrected degrees of freedom are $\hat{\nu}_W = 3 \times 0.557 = 1.671 \approx 2$; degrees of freedom for the error term are $\nu_E = 27$, and associated corrected $\hat{\nu}_E = 27 \times 0.557 = 15.039 \approx 15$.

(2) H-$F\tilde{\varepsilon}$ method
H-$F\tilde{\varepsilon}$ method is used in the same way (therefore the details are omitted).

Table 10.17 gives the degrees of freedom before and after correction using the two methods and the corresponding critical values.

In Table 10.17, under H_0, using G-$G\hat{\varepsilon}$ method, the test statistic F_W follows the F distribution with degrees of freedom $\hat{\nu}_W = 2$ and $\hat{\nu}_E = 15$, the critical value is $F_{(2,15),1-0.05} = 3.68$ (Appendix Table 6). Similarly, using the H-$F\tilde{\varepsilon}$ method, the critical value is $F_{(2,18),1-0.05} = 3.55$. The corrected critical values obtained from the two correction methods are greater than the initial values, which indicates that the control of Type I error is improved. From the ANOVA table (Table 10.15), as $F_W > F_{(2,15),1-0.05}$ and $F_W > F_{(2,18),1-0.05}$, $p < 0.05$, we reject H_0 and accept H_1 at the $\alpha = 0.05$ level. We have significant evidence to show that the mean serum ALT levels of patients with chronic hepatitis B are not all the same at different time points.

10.3.5 Multiple Comparisons of Means

The statistical conclusion obtained in the above example is to reject the null hypothesis, that is, the mean ALT levels at different time points after taking the drug are not all the same. To analyze the specific differences, the means at different time points should be compared.

Table 10.17 Comparison of critical values before and after correction of degrees of freedom.

	Uncorrected	G - G $\hat{\varepsilon}$ method	*H* - *F* $\tilde{\varepsilon}$ method
ε	—	0.557	0.670
ν_W	3	2	2
ν_E	27	15	18
$F_{(\nu_W,\nu_E),1-0.05}$	2.96	3.68	3.55
p	< 0.0001	0.0016	0.0007

There are many methods to compare the means. We use one of the more commonly used methods, the *Bonferroni correction* (especially when $\hat{\varepsilon} < 0.7$) for multiple comparisons. The basic principle of the Bonferroni correction is to adjust the significance level, by $\alpha' = \alpha / g$, where g is the number of paired compared groups.

Example 10.4 Refer to Example 10.3. Assuming that the baseline level of ALT is determined as the reference in the design phase, we intend to evaluate the difference between the mean ALT level at each time point after taking the drug and the baseline level.

In this example, $t = 4$ and three paired comparisons $(g = 3)$ are required. Therefore, $\alpha' = \alpha / 3 = 0.017$; we take $\alpha' = 0.01$ as the significant level. According to Table 10.12, the differences between the ALT level of each patient $(i = 1, 2, \ldots, 10)$ at each time point $(j = 1, 2, 3)$ after taking the drug and the baseline level $(j = 0)$, denoted as d_{ij}, are given in Table 10.18.

Take 10 weeks $(j = 1)$ after taking the drug as an example.

(1) State the hypotheses and select a significance level

$$H_0: \mu_{\bar{d}_1} = 0$$

$$H_1: \mu_{\bar{d}_1} \neq 0$$

$$\alpha' = 0.01$$

(2) Determine the test statistics

$$s_{d_1} = \sqrt{\frac{\sum_i d_{i1}^2 - \left(\sum_i d_{i1}\right)^2 \Big/ n}{n-1}} = \sqrt{\frac{69149 - 403^2 / 10}{9}} = 76.67,$$

$$s_{\bar{d}_1} = \frac{s_{d_1}}{\sqrt{n}} = \frac{76.67}{\sqrt{10}} = 24.25,$$

$$t_1 = \frac{\bar{d}_1}{s_{\bar{d}_1}} = \frac{40.3}{24.25} = 1.66.$$

Table 10.18 Difference in serum ALT levels (U/L) in 10 patients before and after taking the drug.

Patient ID i	Difference at time point j with baseline		
	10 weeks	**20 weeks**	**30 weeks**
1	64	52	76
2	33	77	169
3	14	46	37
4	190	197	203
5	90	46	77
6	22	67	90
7	-51	185	206
8	83	150	229
9	45	41	36
10	-87	148	179
$\sum_i d_{ij}$	403	1009	1302
$\sum_i d_{ij}^2$	69149	136473	219158
$\bar{d}_j$	40.3	100.9	130.2

Table 10.19 Results of paired t-test for Example 10.4.

Comparison	n	$\bar{d}_j$	$s_{\bar{d}_j}$	t_j	p value
Baseline and 10 weeks	10	40.3	24.25	1.66	0.1313
Baseline and 20 weeks	10	100.9	19.63	5.14	0.0006
Baseline and 30 weeks	10	130.2	23.48	5.55	0.0004

The calculation of test statistics for comparing 20 and 30 weeks after treatment with the baseline is the same. Table 10.19 gives the calculation results; the specific process will not be repeated.

(3) Draw a conclusion

For the baseline and 10 weeks after taking the drug, under H_0, the test statistic t follows the t distribution with degrees of freedom $\nu = 10 - 1 = 9$; the critical value is $t_{9,1-0.01/2} = 3.250$ (Appendix Table 4). As $t = 1.66 < t_{9,1-0.01/2} = 3.250$, $p > 0.01$, we do not reject H_0 at the $\alpha' = 0.01$ level; the difference is not statistically significant. We do not have significant evidence to show a difference between the ALT levels of baseline and 10 weeks after taking the drug. For the baseline and 20 or 30 weeks after taking the drug, we have $p < 0.01$; then reject H_0 at the $\alpha' = 0.01$ level. We have significant evidence to show that compared with the baseline level, the mean ALT level of patients with chronic hepatitis B decreased at 20 and 30 weeks after they took the drug.

10.4 ANOVA for 2×2 Crossover Design

Crossover design is a special type of self-matching and self-control design commonly used in clinical trials. The effects of two or more treatments are observed on the same subject to control the variation between subjects, reduce experimental errors, and improve the power of the test.

In this section, we consider data obtained using a two-treatment and two-period (abbreviated 2×2) crossover design, taking a pharmaceutical trial as an example to introduce the ANOVA technique.

10.4.1 Concept of a 2×2 Crossover Design

Example 10.5 To evaluate the effect of sustained-release morphine on relieving refractory dyspnea, 14 patients with chronic obstructive pulmonary disease (COPD) who had not been treated with opioids were enrolled. They were randomly divided into groups A and B. Then, a crossover design trial was conducted. In the first period, patients in group A took 20-mg morphine sustained-release tablets (drug A) in the morning for four consecutive days, and group B took the placebo tablets (drug B). After a 4-day wash-out period, in the second period, the patients in group A took the placebo tablets (drug B) for four consecutive days, and the patients in group B took 20-mg morphine sustained-release tablets (drug A). The dyspnea scale scores collected at the end of each period are given in Table 10.20. Please analyze the data.

Table 10.20 shows an example of a typical crossover design. In this design, all eligible patients are randomly assigned to two groups (group A or B), and then the sequence

Table 10.20 Dyspnea scale score of 14 COPD patients.

	Patient ID	Period 1	Period 2	Total
Morphine	1	47.2	61.5	108.7
↓	2	20.6	28.4	49.0
Placebo	3	48.7	55.2	103.9
	4	14.9	23.4	38.3
	5	70.1	78.7	148.8
	6	57.8	60.1	117.9
	7	22.8	27.9	50.7
	Total	282.1	335.2	617.3
Placebo	8	78.3	59.5	137.8
↓	9	34.4	29.1	63.5
Morphine	10	28.1	12.2	40.3
	11	21.7	17.6	39.3
	12	72.8	53.3	126.1
	13	46.2	39.4	85.6
	14	78.3	71.1	149.4
	Total	359.8	282.2	642.0

Randomized	Time period		
	First period	Wash-out period	Second period
→ Group A	Drug A	- - ->	Drug B
→ Group B	Drug B	- - ->	Drug A

Figure 10.4 Illustration of 2×2 crossover design.

of medication is determined: patients in group A receive drug A (morphine) in the first period and drug B (placebo) in the second period. The sequence of medication for patients in group B is reversed, with patients receiving drug B in the first period and drug A in the second period. There is often a wash-out period between two administration periods. The process is shown in Figure 10.4.

The purpose of a 2×2 crossover design is to compare treatment effects. Different treatments are administered; then there is a "crossover" during the trial to balance the influence of the sequence of medication. In this way, the effect of time period factors is separated to avoid their influence on the research results.

Before introducing the method of ANOVA for crossover design, we first explain two terms in crossover design.

Carryover effect, also referred to as residual effect, means that the drug in the first period has a residual biological effect in the second period.

Wash-out period refers to an adequate period between two treatment periods during which no treatment given. This is to prevent the drug effect in the first period affecting the drug effect in the second period. It ensures that the initial conditions of the two periods are consistent. The wash-out period length depends on the drug's metabolic period and usually requires more than 6–8 half-lives of the drug.

10.4.2 Data Layout and Model Assumptions

The data layout of ANOVA for a 2×2 crossover design is given in Table 10.21.

In Table 10.21, the observations have three subscripts (i, g, j): i is the subject number $(i = 1, 2, \ldots, n,\ n = n_1 + n_2)$; g is the group of drug D_g $(g = 1, 2)$; j is the time period $P_j\,(j = 1, 2)$.

The model of ANOVA for 2×2 crossover design is

$$X_{igj} = \mu + \alpha_g + \beta_j + \delta_{ig} + \varepsilon_{igj}, \tag{10.50}$$

where

X_{igj} is the observation on subject i of group g in period j.

μ is an expected mean, estimated from the mean of all observations.

α_g is an expected mean representing the effect of the gth level of drug D.

β_j is an expected mean representing the effect of the jth period of period P.

δ_{ig} is the effect on the ith subject at the gth level of drug D (random effect between subjects).

ε_{igj} is the random error.

Model Assumptions

(1) The observations for any level of drug or any period are approximately normally distributed.

(2) The population variances are equal at each level of drug and in each period.

(3) No carryover effect of the drug and no interaction effect between drug and period, with constraints $\sum_g \alpha_g = 0, \sum_j \beta_j = 0$, and $\sum_g \sum_i \delta_{ig} = 0$.

(4) ε_{igj} follows a normal distribution $N\left(0, \sigma^2\right)$.

Table 10.21 Data layout of 2×2 crossover design.

	Subject ID i	Period 1 $(j = 1)$	Period 2 $(j = 2)$
Drug A	1	$X_{1,1,1}$	$X_{1,2,2}$
↓	2	$X_{2,1,1}$	$X_{2,2,2}$
Drug B	3	$X_{3,1,1}$	$X_{3,2,2}$
	⋮	⋮	⋮
	n_1	$X_{n_1,1,1}$	$X_{n_1,2,2}$
Drug B	$n_1 + 1$	$X_{n_1+1,2,1}$	$X_{n_1+1,1,2}$
↓	$n_1 + 2$	$X_{n_1+2,2,1}$	$X_{n_1+2,1,2}$
Drug A	$n_1 + 3$	$X_{n_1+3,2,1}$	$X_{n_1+3,1,2}$
	⋮	⋮	⋮
	$n_1 + n_2$	$X_{n_1+n_2,2,1}$	$X_{n_1+n_2,1,2}$

Table 10.22 ANOVA table for 2×2 crossover design.

Source of variation	SS	ν	MS	F	p value
Drug	$SS_D = \frac{1}{n}\sum_g \left(\sum_i X_{igj}\right)^2 - C$	1	MS_D	$F_D = \frac{MS_D}{MS_E}$	*
Period	$SS_P = \frac{1}{n}\sum_j \left(\sum_i X_{igj}\right)^2 - C$	1	MS_P	$F_P = \frac{MS_P}{MS_E}$	*
Between-subject	$SS_B = \frac{1}{2}\sum_i \left(\sum_g X_{igj}\right)^2 - C$	$n - 1$	MS_B	$F_B = \frac{MS_B}{MS_E}$	*
Error	$SS_E = SS_T - SS_D - SS_P - SS_B$	$n - 2$	MS_E		
Total	$SS_T = \sum_i \sum_j X_{igj}^2 - C$	$2n - 1$			

Note: $C = \left(\sum_i \sum_j X_{igj}\right)^2 \Big/ 2n$.

10.4.3 Procedure of ANOVA

In a 2×2 crossover design, the total sum of squares of deviations from the mean of all $2(n_1+n_2)$ observations is partitioned into four parts: between-subject variation, drug variation, period variation, and random error. We have

$$SS_T = SS_B + SS_D + SS_P + SS_E. \quad (10.51)$$

The illustration of partitioning of variation in a 2×2 crossover design is given in Table 10.22.

It should be noted that the variation between subjects is similar to the variation between blocks in block design and is considered potential noise. The focus of ANOVA is on the variation within subjects.

Solution to Example 10.5

(1) State the hypotheses and select a significance level

Drug effect:

H_{0D} : Morphine and placebo have the same effects

H_{1D} : Morphine and placebo have different effects

$\alpha = 0.05$

Period effect:

H_{0P} : The population means of dyspnea scale scores of the two periods are the same

H_{1P} : The population means of dyspnea scale scores of the two periods are different

$\alpha = 0.05$

Between-subject effect:

H_{0B} : The population means of dyspnea scale scores between subjects are the same

H_{1B} : The population means of dyspnea scale scores between subjects are not all same

$\alpha = 0.05$

(2) Determine the test statistic and construct the ANOVA table

First, calculate the correction term. We have

$$C = \left(\sum_i \sum_j x_{igj}\right)^2 \Big/ 2n = 1259.3^2 / 28 = 56637.02$$

The total sum of squares and the degrees of freedom are

$$SS_T = \sum_i \sum_j x_{igj}^2 - C = 69222.15 - 56637.02 = 12585.13,$$

$$\nu_T = 2n - 1 = 28 - 1 = 27.$$

The sum of squares, degrees of freedom, and mean square for drug are as follows:

$$SS_D = \frac{1}{n}\sum_g \left(\sum_i x_{igj}\right)^2 - C = \left(\frac{564.3^2}{14} + \frac{695.0^2}{14}\right) - 56637.02 = 610.09,$$

$$\nu_D = 2 - 1 = 1,$$

$$MS_D = \frac{SS_D}{\nu_D} = \frac{610.09}{1} = 610.09.$$

The sum of squares, degrees of freedom, and mean square for period are as follows:

$$\begin{aligned}
SS_P &= \frac{1}{n}\sum_j\left(\sum_i x_{igj}\right)^2 - C = \left(\frac{641.9^2}{14} + \frac{617.4^2}{14}\right) - 56637.02 = 21.44,\\
\nu_P &= 2-1=1,\\
MS_P &= \frac{SS_P}{\nu_P} = \frac{21.44}{1} = 21.44.
\end{aligned}$$

The sum of squares, degrees of freedom, and mean square for between-subject are as follows:

$$\begin{aligned}
SS_B &= \frac{1}{2}\sum_i\left(\sum_g x_{igj}\right)^2 - C = \left(\frac{108.7^2}{2} + \frac{49.0^2}{2} + \cdots + \frac{85.6^2}{2} + \frac{149.4^2}{2}\right) - 56637.02\\
&= 11777.85,\\
\nu_B &= n-1 = 14-1 = 13,\\
MS_B &= \frac{SS_B}{\nu_B} = \frac{11777.85}{13} = 905.99.
\end{aligned}$$

Error sum of squares and the degrees of freedom and mean square are as follows:

$$\begin{aligned}
SS_E &= SS_T - SS_D - SS_P - SS_B = 12585.13 - 610.09 - 21.44 - 11777.85 = 175.75,\\
\nu_E &= n-2 = 14-2 = 12,\\
MS_E &= \frac{SS_E}{\nu_E} = \frac{175.75}{12} = 14.65.
\end{aligned}$$

Calculate the test statistic F:

Between drugs $F_D = \frac{MS_D}{MS_E} = \frac{610.09}{14.65} = 41.64$;

Between periods $F_P = \frac{MS_P}{MS_E} = \frac{21.44}{14.65} = 1.46$;

Between subjects $F_B = \frac{MS_B}{MS_E} = \frac{905.99}{14.65} = 61.84$.

List the ANOVA table (Table 10.23).

Table 10.23 ANOVA table for Example 10.5.

Source of variation	SS	ν	MS	F	p value
Drug	610.09	1	610.09	41.64	< 0.0001
Period	21.44	1	21.44	1.46	0.2502
Between-subject	11777.85	13	905.99	61.84	< 0.0001
Error	175.75	12	14.65		
Total	12585.13	27			

(3) Draw a conclusion

For drug effect, under H_{0D}, the test statistic F_D follows the F distribution with degrees of freedom $\nu_D = 1$ and $\nu_E = 12$, the critical value is $F_{(1,12),1-0.05} = 4.75$ (Appendix Table 6). As $F_D = 41.64 > F_{(1,12),1-0.05}$, $p < 0.05$, we reject H_{0D} and accept H_{1D} at the $\alpha = 0.05$ level; the difference is statistically significant. We conclude that the population mean of dyspnea scale scores of patients with COPD taking sustained-release morphine and a placebo are different. Similarly, we conclude that the population means of dyspnea scale scores between subjects have significant differences. However, we do not have significant evidence to show that the population means of dyspnea scale scores between periods have differences.

The limitation of crossover design is its relatively long research period, so it is not suitable for diseases with a short course or that require a long intervention period. In addition, the withdrawal of subjects greatly affects the trial results, and the missing data can undermine the comparability of self-control and increase the difficulty of the statistical analysis.

10.5 Summary

This chapter introduced ANOVA for randomized block design, factorial design, repeated measures design, and 2×2 crossover design. Although the design and number of factors considered are different, the basic philosophy and assumptions of ANOVA (independence, normality, and homogeneity of variance) remain unchanged.

The randomized block design is an extension of the paired samples design by division into blocks, and the comparison of different levels of treatment factors is limited to the same block to effectively control the influence of block factors and improve the experiment's efficiency. When the difference between the block means is not significant, the results should be cautiously interpreted.

Factorial design is mainly used to examine the interaction effects between factors, and the role of each factor in this design is the same. In the analysis, we should first infer through hypothesis testing whether the interaction effect exists. If the interaction effect is significant, further analysis of the simple effect should be performed; if the interaction effect is not significant, the main effect should be analyzed after combining the interaction term with the random error term.

The ANOVA for repeated measures data considers data correlation in the partitioning of variation. In addition to the normality and homogeneity of variance, the data also need to satisfy the sphericity of the covariance matrix of different measurement time points. It is necessary to construct a test statistic W for this hypothesis testing. When the sphericity condition is violated, the degrees of freedom of the numerator and denominator of the test statistic F corresponding to measurement time points should be corrected separately. Two commonly used methods are G-$G\hat{\varepsilon}$ and H-$F\,\tilde{\varepsilon}$ methods.

ANOVA for cross-over design is a method commonly used in clinical trials. The effect of time period factors is separated to avoid their influence on the research results. It is not suitable for diseases with a short course or those requiring a long intervention period.

In the next two chapters, we will extend the learning of hypothesis testing from the parametric field to the nonparametric field (including χ^2 test and rank sum test). The basic principles of hypothesis testing are the same, but the inference method will apply to data of broader characteristics and types.

10.6 Exercises

1. Answer the questions using the ANOVA tables given as follows:
   Design 1

Source of variation	SS	ν	MS	p value
Between groups	640.85	2	320.43	0.0135
Within groups	827.41	15	55.16	
Total	1468.27	17		

Design 2

Source of variation	SS	ν	MS	p value
Treatment	16.116	3	5.372	< 0.0001
Block	1.100	6	0.183	0.0104
Error	0.828	18	0.046	
Total	18.044	27		

Design 3

Source of variation	SS	ν	MS	p value
Factor A	15.68	1	15.68	< 0.0001
Factor B	0.11	1	0.11	0.0007
Interaction $A \times B$	0.05	1	0.05	0.0133
Error	0.10	16	0.01	
Total	15.94	19	0.80	

Design 4

Source of variation	SS	ν	MS	p value
Between-time	96221.000	3	32073.667	< 0.0001
Between-subject	171171.400	9	19019.044	
Error	83836.000	27	4517.972	
Total	351228.400	39		

Design 5

Source of variation	SS	ν	MS	p value
Drug	8.61	1	8.61	< 0.0001
Period	0.08	1	0.08	0.4901
Between-subject	6.33	11	0.58	0.0238
Error	1.55	10		
Total	16.57	23		

(a) What design does each table correspond to, and what is the primary purpose of each design?

(b) Although these designs serve different research purposes, what are the similarities between these designs and what is the common fundamental principle underlining them?

(c) Give the assumptions for each model.

(d) For design 2, which is the factor of interest to study? What role does the block factor play in this design? How can we benefit from incorporating block factor in the design?

(e) For design 3, what does interaction effect imply? What is main effect? What is simple effect? Why do we need to test simple effect following a significant interaction?

(f) For design 4, what is the advantageous characteristic of repeatedly measuring subjects?

2. To explore the protective effect of ginsenoside Rg1 on cadmium-induced testicular damage in rats, the researchers chose 10 litters of male rats of the same species with three rats in each litter. They randomly assigned them to three different treatment groups. The control group rats were intraperitoneally injected with normal saline. The cadmium chloride group rats were similarly injected with cadmium chloride solution. The rats in the Rg1 plus cadmium chloride group were given Rg1 by gavage before an intraperitoneal injection of cadmium chloride solution. After 2 weeks, the metallothionein (MT) levels in the rats' testes were measured (μg/g). The results are given in Table 10.24.

Table 10.24 MT levels in testes of rats (μg/g) after three different treatments.

Litter ID.	Control	Cadmium chloride	Rg1 plus cadmium chloride
1	40.6	78.3	116.3
2	44.8	86.0	124.6
3	36.7	72.1	149.0
4	49.9	95.4	128.8
5	59.8	99.2	134.1
6	54.5	95.9	133.0
7	38.4	76.4	115.6
8	41.6	79.9	117.0
9	46.8	86.5	128.4
10	44.7	85.3	124.3

Please answer the following questions:

(a) State the H_0 and H_1.
(b) What assumptions should the data satisfy when ANOVA is performed?
(c) Use appropriate methods to analyze the data and interpret the results.
(d) If the one-way ANOVA is performed not taking into consideration the block effect, what is its influence?
(e) What should be done if the block is not statistically significant? Give your reasons.

3. Researchers wished to investigate the effects of exposure to a certain toxicant and leucocyte increasing drugs on the phagocytic index of mice. They selected 20 mice and randomly allocated them to four groups according to whether they were exposed to the toxicant or were given leucocyte-increasing drugs. The measurement results are given in Table 10.25.

Table 10.25 Data of the phagocytic index of mice.

No toxicant exposure (A_1)		**Toxicant exposure (A_2)**	
No drug administration (B_1)	**Drug administration (B_2)**	**No drug administration (B_1)**	**Drug administration (B_2)**
3.80	3.85	1.85	2.14
3.84	3.90	2.01	2.25
3.96	4.01	2.10	2.33
3.87	3.92	1.92	2.16
3.80	3.84	2.04	2.28

Please answer the following questions:

(a) Please state the H_0 and H_1.
(b) What assumptions should the data satisfy when ANOVA is performed?
(c) Use appropriate methods to analyze the data, construct an ANOVA table, and interpret the meanings represented.
(d) Can the main effect be directly interpreted in (c) and why? If the interaction effect is statistically significant, how should the results be interpreted, and what does simple effect imply at this point?
(e) If the interaction effect is not statistically significant, how should the main effect be analyzed and interpreted?

4. To evaluate the effect of a certain drug on the bone density of rats, 12 rats were selected and injected with the drug. The bone density (mg/cm^2) of the rats over time was recorded. The results are given in Table 10.26.

Table 10.26 Bone density (mg/cm^2) of 12 rats over time.

ID	0 days	3 days	7 days	ID	0 days	3 days	7 days
1	219.16	220.62	231.62	7	208.36	218.08	230.15
2	214.24	216.36	231.02	8	205.75	216.73	230.39
3	209.28	217.20	235.83	9	220.83	230.71	244.46
4	205.57	218.05	245.99	10	210.28	218.76	236.86
5	215.35	217.97	233.36	11	208.18	218.49	233.39
6	218.80	222.23	239.22	12	220.73	231.18	242.18

Please answer the following questions:

(a) What is the main purpose of this design?
(b) What do normality and homogeneity of variance imply in a design with such repeated measures? How do you interpret the sphericity assumption in this case? Test these assumptions.
(c) Use appropriate methods to analyze the data and interpret the results.
(d) If necessary, use appropriate methods to conduct multiple comparisons.

5. To study the effects of two therapeutic regimes (A and B) on 12 hypertensive patients, a researcher randomly assigned patients 1, 2, 5, 8, 9, and 10 to be treated with regime A first, followed by regime B. Patients 3, 4, 6, 7, 11, and 12 were treated with regime B first, followed by treatment A. There is a certain wash-out period between the two regimes. The decrease in systolic blood pressure (SBP, mmHg) after treatment was recorded. The results are given in Table 10.27.

Table 10.27 SBP Decreases (mmHg) in patients with therapeutic regimes A and B.

	Patient ID											
Period	1	2	3	4	5	6	7	8	9	10	11	12
I	A	A	B	B	A	B	B	A	A	A	B	B
	17.6	28.0	10.3	14.0	24.4	17.0	15.1	26.0	30.2	31.8	14.0	17.5
II	B	B	A	A	B	A	A	B	B	B	A	A
	13.0	12.6	20.0	27.0	13.4	23.0	26.0	13.0	18.9	28.0	19.4	21.2

Please answer the following questions:

(a) What are the treatment factors in this design? What are the factors that are not of interest to the study but should still be considered?
(b) Use appropriate methods to analyze the data.

11

χ^2 Test

CONTENTS

In Chapters 7 to 10, we learned hypothesis testing for continuous variables. We presented methods for testing hypotheses concerning one, two, and more than two population means. The valid application of these tests and procedures requires specific assumptions, for example, the data characteristic under investigation being approximately normally distributed or relying on large samples for the application of the central limit theorem. They are called *parametric* methods. In practice, however, if little is known about the distribution and the small sample size cannot meet the central limit theorem or the data are categorical, parametric methods are not appropriate. In such cases, an alternative method that does not depend on the population distribution form or where the inference is not related to parameters would be used. These are called *nonparametric* methods. In this chapter and the next, we will present some nonparametric tests that require fewer or less stringent assumptions than those in the methods discussed in Chapters 7 to 10.

The *Pearson's χ^2 (chi-square) test* is used to test unknown probability/proportion for multiple experiments that involve $k(k \geq 2)$ possible categories of outcomes. Based on

Applied Medical Statistics, First Edition. Jingmei Jiang.

Companion website: www.wiley.com\go\jiang\appliedmedicalstatistics

the χ^2 distribution (see Chapter 6), herein, the Pearson's χ^2 test is used to determine the relationship between two categorical variables, which makes inferences by comparing the distribution between observed and expected frequencies. We introduce the 2×2 contingency table method, and the $R\times C$ contingency table method, and goodness-of-fit tests are also discussed for normal and Poisson distributions.

11.1 Contingency Table

We are often interested in how categorical variables are distributed among two or more populations. We may also wish to identify whether there is a relationship between two categorical variables. Let us look at an example.

Example 11.1 To investigate the effectiveness of two treatment regimens for treating infantile pneumonia, 207 patients were randomly allocated to two groups. In the experimental group, 104 patients were treated with a traditional Chinese herbal medicine mixture combined with cefuroxime sodium. In the control group, 103 patients were treated with only cefuroxime sodium. The two groups are the same in other routine treatments. The results are summarized in Table 11.1. Is there any difference between the effectiveness of these treatment regimens?

Table 11.1 is a *contingency table*. There are two categorical variables: the row variable X denotes the treatment regimen, which includes two categories (experimental and control); the column variable Y denotes the effectiveness, which includes two categories (effective and ineffective). There are four possible combinations (cells) of outcomes. For example, among 104 patients in the experimental group, the treatment was effective in 97 and ineffective in 7. Of the 103 patients in the control group, the treatment was effective in 73 and ineffective in 30.

Definition 11.1 An $R\times C$ contingency table is defined as a table with R rows and C columns. It displays the relationship between two categorical variables, where the variable in the rows has R categories, and the variable in the columns has C categories.

When the $R\times C$ contingency table just has two rows and two columns, such as Table 11.1, it is called a 2×2 contingency table (or *four-fold table*). It is the simplest and most common contingency table.

Table 11.1 Contingency table for treatment regimens and effectiveness.

Treatment X	Outcome Y		Total
	Effective	Ineffective	
Experimental group	97	7	104
Control group	73	30	103
Total	170	37	207

11.1.1 General Form of Contingency Table

According to Definition 11.1, suppose there are R and C categories in categorical variables $X_i\left(i=1,2,\ldots,R\right)$ and $Y_j\left(j=1,2,\ldots,C\right)$ respectively, where X_iY_j denote all possible outcomes of experiments, usually expressed as the form cell. n_{ij} is the observed frequency of each cell $\left(i,j\right)$, which denotes the frequency of event X_iY_j that occurs in n experiments; then the data layout of the $R\times C$ contingency table is usually presented in the form of Table 11.2.

Furthermore, it is customary to total.

(1) The *row margin total*, or row margin, denoted as $n_{i\cdot}$, is the sum of observed frequencies of each row, $n_{i\cdot}=\sum_{j=1}^{C}n_{ij}$. In Example 11.1, $n_{1\cdot}=104$, $n_{2\cdot}=103$.

(2) The *column margin total*, or column margin, denoted as $n_{\cdot j}$, is the sum of observed frequencies of each column, $n_{\cdot j}=\sum_{i=1}^{R}n_{ij}$. In Example 11.1, $n_{\cdot 1}=170$, $n_{\cdot 2}=37$.

(3) *Grand total*, denoted as n, is the sum of observed frequencies of $R\times C$ cells, $n=\sum_{j=1}^{C}\sum_{i=1}^{R}n_{ij}$. In Example 11.1, $n=104+103=170+37=207$.

The row, column, and joint probabilities corresponding to the cell counts in Table 11.2 are given in Table 11.3.

Row margin probability, denoted as $\pi_{i\cdot}=\sum_{j=1}^{C}\pi_{ij}$, represents the corresponding row probability totals. For example, the marginal probability for the first row is $\pi_{1\cdot}=\pi_{11}+\pi_{12}+\cdots+\pi_{1C}$. Obviously, $\sum_{i=1}^{R}\pi_{i\cdot}=1$.

Column margin probability, denoted as $\pi_{\cdot j}=\sum_{i=1}^{R}\pi_{ij}$, represents the corresponding column probability totals. For example, the marginal probability for the first column is $\pi_{\cdot 1}=\pi_{11}+\pi_{21}+\cdots+\pi_{R1}$. Obviously, $\sum_{j=1}^{C}\pi_{\cdot j}=1$.

Table 11.2 General form of an $R\times C$ contingency table.

X	**Y**				**Total $n_{i\cdot}$**
	Y_1	Y_2	$\cdots$	Y_C	
X_1	n_{11}	n_{12}	$\cdots$	n_{1C}	$n_{1\cdot}$
X_2	n_{21}	n_{22}	$\cdots$	n_{2C}	$n_{2\cdot}$
$\vdots$	$\vdots$	$\vdots$	$\vdots$	$\vdots$	$\vdots$
X_R	n_{R1}	n_{R2}	$\cdots$	n_{RC}	$n_{R\cdot}$
Total $n_{\cdot j}$	$n_{\cdot 1}$	$n_{\cdot 2}$	$\cdots$	$n_{\cdot C}$	n

$i=1,2,\ldots,R;\ j=1,2,\ldots,C.$

Table 11.3 Probabilities for $R \times C$ contingency table.

X	Y				$\pi_{i\cdot}$
	Y_1	Y_2	...	Y_C	
X_1	π_{11}	π_{12}	...	π_{1C}	$\pi_{1\cdot}$
X_2	π_{21}	π_{22}	...	π_{2C}	$\pi_{2\cdot}$
⋮	⋮	⋮	⋮	⋮	⋮
X_R	π_{R1}	π_{R2}	...	π_{RC}	$\pi_{R\cdot}$
$\pi_{\cdot j}$	$\pi_{\cdot 1}$	$\pi_{\cdot 2}$	...	$\pi_{\cdot C}$	1

$i = 1,2,\ldots, R; j = 1,2,\ldots, C.$

Joint probability, denoted as π_{ij}, represents the corresponding cell (i, j) probability. Obviously, $\sum_{j=1}^{C}\sum_{i=1}^{R}\pi_{ij} = 1$.

11.1.2 Independence of Two Categorical Variables

We know from Chapter 3 that the independence of events A and B implies $P(A \cap B) = P(A) \times P(B)$. Similarly, in a contingency table, a necessary and sufficient condition for two categorical variables to be independent of each other is that the joint probabilities of each cell are equal to the product of the marginal probabilities of the corresponding rows and columns. Thus, under the assumption of independence, in Table 11.3, we have

$$\pi_{ij} = \pi_{i\cdot}\pi_{\cdot j} \left(i = 1, 2, \ldots, R; j = 1, 2, \ldots, C\right). \tag{11.1}$$

Generally, π_{ij} is unknown and estimated by sample statistic p_{ij}, and the estimation is

$$p_{ij} = \frac{n_{ij}}{n}. \tag{11.2}$$

Thus, the estimations for marginal probabilities $\pi_{\cdot i}$ and $\pi_{\cdot j}$ are

$$p_{i\cdot} = \frac{n_{i\cdot}}{n}, \tag{11.3}$$

$$p_{\cdot j} = \frac{n_{\cdot j}}{n}. \tag{11.4}$$

Under the assumption of independence, the joint probability is estimated by the margin probabilities as

$$p_{ij} = p_{i\cdot}p_{\cdot j} = \frac{n_{i\cdot}}{n} \times \frac{n_{\cdot j}}{n} = \frac{n_{i\cdot}n_{\cdot j}}{n^2}. \tag{11.5}$$

11.1.3 Significance Testing Using the Contingency Table

The most important role of the contingency table method is to test the independence between two categorical variables. For example, we need to test whether treatment regimens and effectiveness are independent in Example 11.1. We call it the test of independence of categorical data. The test of independence is equal to the test of difference of rates discussed in Chapter 8, but approached from a different standpoint. The contingency table method draws an inference about independence by examining the difference between observed and expected frequencies using categorical variables. For this purpose, we need to develop an expected contingency table under the independence assumption.

(1) Calculate an expected contingency table

Null hypothesis H_0 : the two categorical variables are independent of each other, that is, $H_0:\ \pi_{ij}=\pi_{i.}\pi_{.j}$, for all $(i,\ j)$.

If H_0 is true, we may compute the expected table for the data in Table 11.1.

The *expected frequency* in the $(i,\ j)$ cell T_{ij} can be calculated as

$$T_{ij}=np_{ij}=np_{i.}p_{.j}=n\left(\frac{n_{i.}}{n}\right)\left(\frac{n_{.j}}{n}\right)=\frac{n_{i.}n_{.j}}{n}, \tag{11.6}$$

that is, the expected frequency is the product of the ith row margin and the jth column margin, divided by the grand total.

The calculated expected frequency of each cell based on Formula 11.6 is given in brackets in Table 11.4.

(2) Constructing the χ^2 test statistic

Intuitively, if H_0 is true, there will be good consistency between the observed contingency table and the expected one, otherwise H_0 is unlikely to be true. Therefore, we should choose a test statistic based on the difference of the observed frequencies and their expected frequencies. The question is how can we measure the difference? It has been shown that the best way is to calculate $\left(n_{ij}-T_{ij}\right)^2/T_{ij}$ in each cell and then summarize over all the cells. This test statistic was proposed by K. Pearson in 1900 (also called *Pearson's* χ^2 *statistic*), and under a large sample size, it can be shown that the test statistic (proof omitted) possess a sampling distribution that is approximately a χ^2 distribution.

$$\chi^2=\sum_{j=1}^{C}\sum_{i=1}^{R}\frac{\left(n_{ij}-T_{ij}\right)^2}{T_{ij}}\ \dot{\sim}\ \chi^2(\nu), \tag{11.7}$$

where $\nu=R\times C-1-\left(R+C-2\right)=\left(R-1\right)\left(C-1\right)$.

The reasoning for ν is that given $\sum_{i=1}^{R}\pi_{i.}=\sum_{j=1}^{C}\pi_{.j}=1$, there are $R+C-2$ parameters among $R\times C$ cells.

(3) Draw a conclusion

For a given significance level α:

If $\chi^2>\chi^2_{\nu,1-\alpha}$, then reject H_0;

If $\chi^2\le\chi^2_{\nu,1-\alpha}$, then do not reject H_0.

The rejection and non-rejection regions of χ^2 test are shown in Figure 11.1.

Table 11.4 The observed and expected frequencies for $R \times C$ contingency table.

X	Y				Total $n_{i\cdot}$
	Y_1	Y_2	...	Y_C	
X_1	$n_{11}(T_{11})$	$n_{12}(T_{12})$	...	$n_{1C}(T_{1C})$	$n_{1\cdot}$
X_2	$n_{21}(T_{21})$	$n_{22}(T_{22})$	...	$n_{2C}(T_{2C})$	$n_{2\cdot}$
⋮	⋮	⋮	⋮	⋮	⋮
X_R	$n_{R1}(T_{R1})$	$n_{R2}(T_{R2})$	...	$n_{RC}(T_{RC})$	$n_{R\cdot}$
Total $n_{\cdot j}$	$n_{\cdot 1}$	$n_{\cdot 2}$	...	$n_{\cdot C}$	n

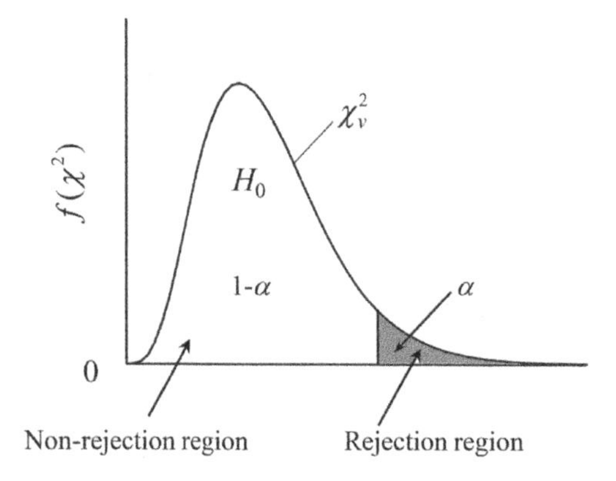

Figure 11.1 Illustration of rejection and non-rejection regions for the χ^2 test.

The assumptions of the Pearson's χ^2 test for a contingency table are as follows.

(1) The n observed counts are a random sample from the population of interest; we may then consider this from two different sampling methods. In one, a single random sample is drawn, and two categorical variables are observed, one with R categories and the other with C categories. In the other, independent random samples are drawn from R different populations, and a categorical variable with C categories as the outcome is observed.

(2) For the χ^2 approximation to be valid, each of the estimated expected frequencies is required to be no smaller than 5.

11.2 χ^2 Test for a 2×2 Contingency Table

11.2.1 Test of Independence

The χ^2 test of a four-fold table is different for a completely randomized design and paired samples design. For example, the data in Example 11.1 were collected using a completely randomized design, where the patients were randomly divided into two different treatment groups. This means that independent samples were used because the treatment and outcome of an individual patient would not impact that of another. Here we should pay attention to the difference of independence between individuals and independence between variables. The statements "the effective rate of the two treatment regimens is the same" and "treatment and outcomes are mutually independent" are equivalent, and either could be the null hypothesis for a significance test.

Solution to Example 11.1

Suppose the effective rate of the experimental treatment regime and control treatment regime is π_1 and π_2, respectively. The procedure is as follows:

(1) State the hypotheses and select a significance level

$H_0: \pi_1 = \pi_2$. The effective rate of the two treatment regimes is the same (the outcome is independent of the treatment)

$H_1: \pi_1 \neq \pi_2$. The effective rate of the two treatment regimes is not the same

$$\alpha = 0.05$$

(2) Determine the test statistic

Calculate the expected frequencies of each cell under H_0.

Based on Formula 11.6, the expected frequencies of the four cells are

$$T_{11} = \frac{n_{1.}n_{.1}}{n} = \frac{104 \times 170}{207} = 85.41$$

$$T_{12} = \frac{n_{1.}n_{.2}}{n} = \frac{104 \times 37}{207} = 18.59$$

$$T_{21} = \frac{n_{2.}n_{.1}}{n} = \frac{103 \times 170}{207} = 84.59$$

$$T_{22} = \frac{n_{2.}n_{.2}}{n} = \frac{103 \times 37}{207} = 18.41$$

The four-fold table is presented in Table 11.5 with observed frequencies followed by expected frequencies in brackets.

We can see from Table 11.5 that the sum of expected frequencies in each row (or each column) is equal to the corresponding row margin (or column margin). In practice, there may be minor rounding errors when the expected frequencies are kept to limited decimal places.

The test statistic is

$$\chi^2 = \sum_{j=1}^{2}\sum_{i=1}^{2}\frac{\left(n_{ij} - T_{ij}\right)^2}{T_{ij}}$$

$$= \frac{(97-85.41)^2}{85.41} + \frac{(7-18.59)^2}{18.59} + \frac{(73-84.59)^2}{84.59} + \frac{(30-18.41)^2}{18.41}$$

$$= 17.68,$$

$$\nu = (R-1)(C-1) = (2-1)(2-1) = 1.$$

Note that the absolute difference between observed and expected frequencies for each cell $\left|n_{ij} - T_{ij}\right| = 11.59$, is the same. This provides a convenient way to calculate the χ^2 statistic for a 2×2 contingency table.

Table 11.5 Observed and expected frequencies for Example 11.1.

Treatment X	Outcome Y		Total
	Effective	Ineffective	
Experimental group	97 (85.41)	7 (18.59)	104
Control group	73 (84.59)	30 (18.41)	103
Total	170	37	207

Formula 11.7 can be modified algebraically into a form that avoids the computation of expected frequencies. Consider the 2×2 contingency table. Let a, b, c, and d be n_{11}, n_{12}, n_{21}, and n_{22}, respectively; we have a shortcut for the calculation of the test statistic in a four-fold table:

$$\chi^2 = \frac{(ad-bc)^2 n}{(a+b)(c+d)(a+c)(b+d)}. \tag{11.8}$$

In this example, we have

$$\chi^2 = \frac{(ad-bc)^2 n}{(a+b)(c+d)(a+c)(b+d)} = \frac{(97\times30-73\times7)^2\times207}{170\times37\times104\times103} = 17.68$$

The results obtained using both Formulas 11.7 and 11.8 are the same.

(3) Draw a conclusion

Under H_0, the test statistic χ^2 approximately follows the χ^2 distribution with $\nu=(2-1)(2-1)=1$; given $\alpha=0.05$, the critical value is $\chi^2_{1,1-0.05}=3.84$ (Appendix Table 5). As $\chi^2=17.68>3.84$, $p<0.05$. We reject H_0 and accept H_1 at the $\alpha=0.05$ level, and the effective rates of the two treatment regimens are significantly different. We conclude that combination therapy is more effective than single therapy for infantile pneumonia.

Note that: (i) Because the distribution of the χ^2 test statistic under H_0 can only be approximated by the theoretical χ^2 distribution when the sample size is sufficiently large, the critical values in Appendix Table 5 are only approximate for the χ^2 statistic, and the sample size must be sufficiently large to ensure that the approximation is valid. A rule of thumb is that the above method is only appropriate when the binomial distribution approximates to a normal distribution, which requires the sample size to be large enough $(n\geq40)$ and the expected frequency of each cell to be at least 5 $(T\geq5)$. In practice, to prevent a small expected frequency T, fixed and balanced row or column margin totals are generally preferred in the study design. For example, in our Example 11.1, we may fix the row totals by randomly allocating the patients into the treatment groups (such as both groups allocating 100 patients). This would increase the likelihood that the estimated expected cell counts would be of adequate size. (ii) The χ^2 test is a two-sided test even though the rejection region, based on the χ^2 distribution, is one-sided. Thus, if we reject H_0, that means we accept H_1 regardless of whether $\pi_1<\pi_2$ or $\pi_1>\pi_2$. (iii). In addition, the sum of the expected frequencies across any row or column must equal the corresponding row or column margin, as is the case for 2×2 contingency tables. This fact provides a good check that the expected frequencies are computed correctly. The expected frequencies in Table 11.5 fulfill this criterion.

11.2.2 Yates' Corrected χ^2 Test for a 2×2 Contingency Table

Recall from Section 6.2.2 that the χ^2 distribution is continuous while the χ^2 values calculated from categories data are discrete, particularly for the small number of cells in the 2×2 contingency table. A continuity correction of the χ^2 statistic is therefore proposed to improve the approximation. This is called *Yates' correction*. It was proposed by F. Yates in 1934 using normal approximation theory based on the continuity correction of a binomial distribution. The test statistic is

$$\chi_C^2 = \sum_{j=1}^{2}\sum_{i=1}^{2}\frac{\left(\left|n_{ij} - T_{ij}\right| - 0.5\right)^2}{T_{ij}}. \tag{11.9}$$

We conduct continuity correction for each cell, and replace $\left(n_{ij} - T_{ij}\right)^2 / T_{ij}$ with $\left(\left|n_{ij} - T_{ij}\right| - 0.5\right)^2 / T_{ij}$. The statistic is called *Yates' corrected* χ^2.

Example 11.2 Calculate Yates' corrected χ^2 for Example 11.1.

Solution
Because $\left|n_{ij} - T_{ij}\right| = 11.59$, substituting this into Formula 11.9, we have

$$\chi_C^2 = (11.59 - 0.5)^2\left(\frac{1}{85.41} + \frac{1}{18.59} + \frac{1}{84.59} + \frac{1}{18.41}\right) = 16.19$$

The corresponding $p = 0.00006$.

Statisticians hold different opinions on whether continuity correction should be used. In general, the p value calculated by continuity correction is larger than no correction, which means it is not easy to derive a significant conclusion. The continuity correction method is more commonly used in research publications. When the results of correction and no correction are contradictory, Fisher's exact method is preferred (see Section 11.2.4).

Similarly, a simpler way for continuity correction of χ^2 statistics is

$$\chi_C^2 = \frac{\left(\left|ad - bc\right| - \frac{n}{2}\right)^2 n}{(a+b)(c+d)(a+c)(b+d)}. \tag{11.10}$$

Note that Formulas 11.10 and 11.9 also require a sample size $n \geq 40$ and all expected frequencies $T \geq 5$.

11.2.3 Paired Samples Design χ^2 Test

In biomedical studies, sometimes we need to examine the same batch sample using two different methods. Such data can be collected in the form of a paired samples

Table 11.6 Sputum culture results of two media.

Media *A*	Media *B*		Total
	+	−	
+	36	5	41
−	34	135	169
Total	70	140	210

design four-fold table, with the paired samples design χ^2 test (or *McNemar's test*) being used to conduct statistical inference.

Example 11.3 A batch of 210 sputum specimens was cultured in two media. The results are given in Table 11.6. Test the difference in the positive rates of the two media.

Of the 210 sputum specimens, the results of $171(36+135)$ specimens are the same (both positives or negatives), and they are therefore called consistent pairs; the results of the other $39(34+5)$ pairs were different, and they are called inconsistent pairs. From Table 11.6, the positive rate of media A is $41/210=19.5\%$, and that of media B is $70/210=33.3\%$. Because the two positive rates are not independent (both using 36 in the numerator), it it not suitable to calculate expected frequencies in the same way as in Pearson's χ^2 test method for the test of independence. As there are no differences in the two media in consistent pairs, we simply focus on the inconsistent pairs.

Let $n_{++}=a, n_{+-}=b, n_{-+}=c, n_{--}=d$. Table 11.7 presents the general form of a paired samples design four-fold table. In the inconsistent pairs, there are b pairs that are positive in media A and negative in media B, and there are c pairs that are positive in media B and negative in media A.

Analysis

The test hypotheses are

$$H_0: \pi_b=\pi_c=0.5$$

$$H_1: \pi_b \neq \pi_c$$

Usually let $\alpha=0.05$

When H_0 is true, cell count b and c follows binomial distribution, $E(b)=E(c)=(b+c)/2$, $Var(b)=Var(c)=(b+c)/4$ (according to the binomial distribution theorem). Under the assumption that a binomial distribution approximates to a normal distribution, a stricter condition of approximate validity is $np(1-p)=(b+c)/4\geq 5$, that is, $b+c\geq 20$, so the condition of the paired samples design test is $b+c\geq 20$.

The test statistic is

$$\chi^2=\frac{\left(b-\frac{b+c}{2}\right)^2}{\frac{b+c}{2}}+\frac{\left(c-\frac{b+c}{2}\right)^2}{\frac{b+c}{2}}=\frac{(b-c)^2}{b+c} \dot{\sim} \chi^2(\nu). \tag{11.11}$$

Table 11.7 Paired samples design four-fold table.

Media *A*	**Media *B***		**Total**
	+	−	
+	$a(++)$	$b(+-)$	$a+b$
−	$c(-+)$	$d(--)$	$c+d$
Total	$a+c$	$b+d$	n

The continuity correction formula is

$$\chi_C^2 = \frac{(|b-c|-1)^2}{b+c} \dot{\sim} \chi^2(\nu), \tag{11.12}$$

where degree of freedom $\nu = 1$.
For a given significance level α:
If $\chi^2 > \chi^2_{1,1-\alpha}$, then reject H_0;
If $\chi^2 \le \chi^2_{1,1-\alpha}$, then do not reject H_0.

Solution to Example 11.3

(1) State the hypotheses and select a significance level

H_0: The positive rates of the two media are the same
H_1: The positive rates of the two media are not the same

$\alpha = 0.05$

(2) Determine the test statistic

As $b+c = 5+34 = 39 > 20$, according to Formula 11.11, the test statistic is

$$\chi^2 = \frac{(b-c)^2}{b+c} = \frac{(5-34)^2}{5+34} = 21.56$$

To correct for continuity, use Formula 11.12,

$$\chi_C^2 = \frac{(|b-c|-1)^2}{b+c} = \frac{(|5-34|-1)^2}{5+34} = 20.10.$$

(3) Draw a conclusion

Under H_0, the test statistic χ^2 follows the χ_1^2 distribution with degrees of freedom $\nu = 1$, and the critical value is $\chi^2_{1,1-0.05} = 3.84$ (Appendix Table 5). As $\chi^2 > 3.84$ irrespective of whether continuity correction is used, $p < 0.05$, and we reject H_0 and accept H_1 at the $\alpha = 0.05$ level. There is evidence to show that the positive rates of the two media are not the same, and the positive rate of media B is higher.

If we test whether there is an association between the two categorical variables under the paired samples design, we can still use Formulas 11.7 or 11.8 to calculate the test statistics because the association includes consistent and inconsistent pairs.

11.2.4 Fisher's Exact Tests for Completely Randomized Design

The procedure for testing independence in a contingency table in Sections 11.2.1 to 11.2.3 is "approximate" because the χ^2 test statistic has an approximate χ^2 distribution. The larger the sample is, the better the test's approximation. For small samples (e.g., if $T < 5$ or the grand total $n < 40$); however, the p value from the χ^2 test may not be a good approximation for the actual (exact) p value of the test. In this case, we can employ a technique proposed by R.A. Fisher. For 2×2 contingency tables, Fisher developed a procedure for computing the exact p value for the test of independence. The theoretical foundation of *Fisher's exact test* is the *hypergeometric distribution*. We now provide the calculation steps in this test.

(1) Use the formula for the hypergeometric distribution to find the probability of the observed 2×2 contingency table:

Again we present the data layout of completely randomized design for a 2×2 contingency table, as in Table 11.8.

In Table 11.8, we denote the observed frequencies n_{ij} by the letters a, b, c, and d in the form of a four-fold table. When the row and column margins of the four-fold table are fixed, that is, the row margins of X_1 and X_2 are fixed at $a+b$ and $c+d$ respectively, the column margins of Y_1 and Y_2 are fixed at $a+c$ and $b+d$ respectively; then according to permutation and combination theory, it can be seen that the number of constituent methods of each row margin is

$$\frac{n!}{(a+b)!(c+d)!}$$

Similarly, the number of constituent methods of each column margin is

$$\frac{n!}{(a+c)!(b+d)!}$$

If X and Y are mutually independent, the number of constituent methods of row margin and column margin is

$$\frac{n!}{(a+b)!(c+d)!} \times \frac{n!}{(a+c)!(b+d)!}$$

Table 11.8 2×2 contingency table for completely randomized design.

X	Y		Total
	Y_1	Y_2	
X_1	a	b	$a+b$
X_2	c	d	$c+d$
Total	$a+c$	$b+d$	n

Furthermore, the number of possible combinations of (a, b, c, d) given fixed margins is

$$\frac{n!}{a!b!c!d!}$$

Therefore, the probability distribution of the four-fold table is

$$\frac{n!}{a!b!c!d!} \Big/ \left[\frac{n!}{(a+b)!(c+d)!} \times \frac{n!}{(a+c)!(b+d)!}\right] = \frac{(a+b)!(c+d)!(a+c)!(b+d)!}{a!b!c!d!n!}.$$

The formula for calculating the probability of the four-fold table is

$$p_i = \frac{(a+b)!(c+d)!(a+c)!(b+d)!}{a!b!c!d!n!}, \tag{11.13}$$

where i denotes the order of all possible four-fold tables that have the same margin totals as the observed table.

(2) Construct all possible 2×2 contingency tables that have the same margin totals as the observed table.
(3) Use Formula 11.13 to calculate the probability of all constructive four-fold tables in step (2).
(4) Sum the probabilities of all contingency tables that are at least as contradictory to the null hypothesis of independence as the observed table. (Note: include the probability of the observed table in the sum.) This sum represents Fisher's exact p value for a two-sided test.

Fisher's exact test theory described above may seem cumbersome at first glance. However, it may be easier to understand once we walk through the test procedure using the following example.

Example 11.4 Bilateral patella ligaments were examined by ultrasound in 14 female professional athletes and 19 healthy female volunteers; the results are given in Table 11.9. Compare the rate of synovitis in the athletes and healthy volunteers.

Table 11.9 Results of ultrasound examination of female professional athletes and healthy volunteers.

Group	Synovitis		Total
	Yes	No	
Professional athlete	7	7	14
Healthy volunteer	2	17	19
Total	9	24	33

Solution

In Table 11.9, the expected frequency of cell a is $T_{11} = \frac{14 \times 9}{33} = 3.82 < 5$ and $n < 40$, so Fisher's exact test should be used. Follow the following procedure:

(1) State the hypotheses and select a significance level

$H_0 : \pi_1 = \pi_2$ The rates of synovitis in these two groups are the same
$H_1 : \pi_1 \neq \pi_2$ The rates of synovitis in these two groups are not the same

$$\alpha = 0.05$$

(2) Construct all possible four-fold tables that have the same margin as the observed table

To find all the possible four-fold tables, we can just change one cell at a time; then the remaining cells are simultaneously determined as the row and column margins are fixed. In this example, we can simply start by entering 0 in cell a, which has the smallest margin $(a + c = 9)$, and stop by setting it as this smallest margin (9). Thus, we have $9 + 1 = 10$ possible tables, as shown in Figure 11.2.

(3) Calculate the exact probability of each possible table using Formula 11.13
The 8th table is the observed one, and its probability calculated from Formula 11.13 is

$$p_8 = \frac{14!19!9!24!}{7!7!2!17!33!} = 0.015217$$

The probabilities corresponding to other possible tables are calculated in the same way.

(4) Draw a conclusion

Notice that the sum of all p_i such that $p_i \leq p_8$ is the two-sided test p value in Fisher's exact test; the sum of all p_i such that $p_i \leq p_8$ and corresponding to a possible table to the left hand or right hand of the observed table is the one-sided test p value.

In this example, the two-sided probability is

$$\begin{aligned} p_{two-sided} &= p_1 + p_8 + p_9 + p_{10} \\ &= 0.002395 + 0.015217 + 0.001479 + 0.000052 \\ &= 0.0191. \end{aligned}$$

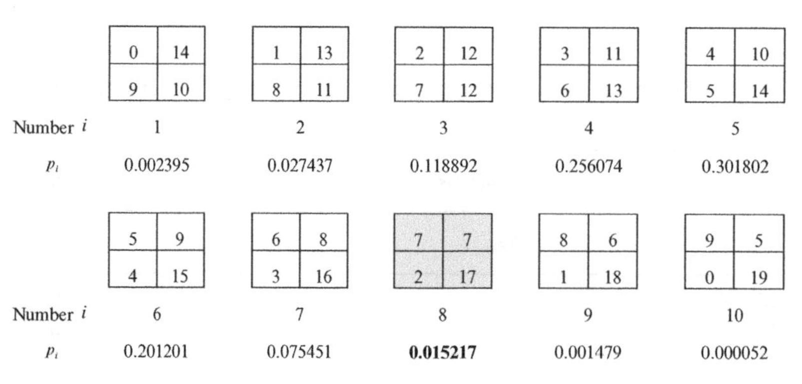

Figure 11.2 Possible four-fold tables when the row and column margins are fixed.

As $p < 0.05$, we reject H_0 and accept H_1 at $\alpha = 0.05$ level. There is evidence to show that the rates of synovitis of the two groups are not the same and the rate of synovitis in female athletes is higher.

If we conduct a one-sided inference for this example, $H_1 : \pi_1 > \pi_2$, that is, the synovitis incidence in female athletes is higher than in healthy female volunteers, then one-sided probability is

$$\begin{aligned} p_{one-sided} &= p_8 + p_9 + p_{10} \\ &= 0.015217 + 0.001479 + 0.000052 \\ &= 0.0167. \end{aligned}$$

The calculation of Fisher's exact p value is computationally complex, but is simplified with the current availability of statistical software. Therefore, we may conveniently select this approach even if the conditions for applying Pearson's χ^2 test are satisfied.

11.2.5 Exact McNemar's Test for Paired Samples Design

For a paired samples design four-fold table, when $b + c < 20$, it is not appropriate to use a normal distribution to approximate a binomial distribution. For such situations, the exact method is illustrated using the following example.

Example 11.5 To investigate the diagnostic results of two positron emission tomography tracers for lung cancer, the images of 20 patients using 3'-deoxy-3'-[^{18}F]fluorothymidine ([^{18}F]FLT) and 2-deoxy-2-[^{18}F]fluorodeoxyglucose ([^{18}F]FDG) tracers were obtained. The results are given in Table 11.10. Test for the difference of positive rates between these two tracers.

Solution In this example, $b + c = 8 < 20$; therefore, the conditions for the use of McNemar's test are not met. We could simply use binomial distribution to calculate the exact probability as follows:

(1) State the hypotheses and select a significance level

$H_0 : \pi_b = \pi_c = 0.5$; the positive rates of the two tracers are the same
$H_1 : \pi_b \neq \pi_c$; the positive rates of the two tracers are not the same

$$\alpha = 0.05$$

Table 11.10 Comparison of diagnostic results using [^{18}F]FLT and [^{18}F]FDG.

[^{18}F]FLT	[^{18}F]FDG		Total
	Negative	Positive	
Negative	3	7	10
Positive	1	9	10
Total	4	16	20

(2) Calculate the exact probability and draw a conclusion

When H_0 is true, the frequencies of either cell b or c follow a binomial distribution $B(b+c, 0.5)$. Let $k = \min(b, c)$, then the two-sided test p value is the sum of p_i such that $p_i \le p_k$.

In this example, $b+c=8$, $k=\min(7,1)=1$, and $\pi=0.5$, as binomial distribution $B(8, 0.5)$ is symmetric; therefore, the two-sided probability is

$$p_{two-sided} = 2\times(p_0 + p_1) = 2\times(0.00391 + 0.03125) = 0.0703$$

As $p > 0.05$, we do not reject H_0 at the $\alpha = 0.05$ level. There is no evidence to show that the positive rate of the two tracers is different.

11.3 χ^2 Test for $R\times C$ Contingency Tables

Generalizing our experience from the 2×2 contingency table, the expected table for an $R\times C$ contingency table under H_0 can be formed in the same way as a 2×2 table.

11.3.1 Comparison of Multiple Independent Proportions

Example 11.6 Suppose we are interested in knowing the effectiveness of three methods of preventing postpartum hemorrhage: oxytocin injection (A), misoprostol tablets (B), and oxytocin injection plus misoprostol tablets (C). We recruited 600 puerperal women and randomly assigned them to different treatment groups. The effectiveness of the preventive methods was defined as vaginal bleeding of less than 200 ml within 2 hours of delivery. The results are given in Table 11.11. Perform a significance test and draw conclusions.

Solution

(1) State the hypotheses and select a significance level

$H_0: \pi_A = \pi_B = \pi_C$; the effectiveness of different methods in preventing postpartum hemorrhage is the same

Table 11.11 Results of the three methods in preventing postpartum hemorrhage.

Method	Outcome		Total	Effective rate (%)
	Effective	Ineffective		
A	150	50	200	75.0
B	184	16	200	92.0
C	198	2	200	99.0
Total	532	68	600	88.7

$H_1 : \pi_A, \pi_B, \pi_C$ are not all the same; the effectiveness of different methods in preventing postpartum hemorrhage is not all the same

$$\alpha = 0.05$$

(2) Determine the test statistic

When H_0 is true, the expected frequency of each cell is

$$T_{11} = \frac{n_{1.}n_{.1}}{n} = \frac{200 \times 532}{600} = 177.33$$

$$T_{12} = \frac{n_{1.}n_{.2}}{n} = \frac{200 \times 68}{600} = 22.67$$

......

$$T_{32} = \frac{n_{3.}n_{.2}}{n} = \frac{200 \times 68}{600} = 22.67$$

The results are given in brackets in Table 11.12.
According to Formula 11.7, the test statistic χ^2 is

$$\begin{aligned}\chi^2 &= \sum_j \sum_i \frac{(n_{ij} - T_{ij})^2}{T_{ij}} \\ &= \frac{(150 - 177.33)^2}{177.33} + \frac{(184 - 177.33)^2}{177.33} + \cdots + \frac{(2 - 22.67)^2}{22.67} \\ &= 60.63.\end{aligned}$$

The degree of freedom $v = (3-1) \times (2-1) = 2$.

(3) Draw a conclusion

Refer to Appendix Table 5 and find that the critical value is $\chi^2_{2,1-0.05} = 5.99$. As $\chi^2 = 60.63 > 5.99$, $p < 0.05$; therefore, we reject H_0 at $\alpha = 0.05$. There is evidence to show that the effectiveness of different methods in preventing postpartum hemorrhage is not all the same.

Table 11.12 Observed and expected frequencies of the three methods.

Method	**Outcome**		**Total**
	Effective	**Ineffective**	
A	150 (177.33)	50 (22.67)	200
B	184 (177.33)	16 (22.67)	200
C	198 (177.33)	2 (22.67)	200
Total	532	68	600

As a shortcut, the χ^2 statistic of the $R \times C$ contingency table can be calculated as

$$\chi^2 = n\left(\sum_j \sum_i \frac{n_{ij}^2}{n_{i.}n_{.j}} - 1\right). \tag{11.14}$$

Although this avoids a calculation of expected frequencies, we should be careful with cells with a small expected frequency $(T < 5)$.

The continuity correction is not generally used for contingency tables other than 2×2, because statisticians have empirically found that the correction does not help with the approximation of the test statistic by the χ^2 distribution. χ^2 test should not be used for $R \times C$ tables if the expected frequencies of the cells are too small. Cochran studied the validity of the approximation in this case and recommended its use if: (i) no more than $1/5$ of the cells have expected frequencies less than 5; and (ii) no cell has an expected frequency less than 1.

When the conditions are not satisfied, consider the following approach to improve the accuracy of the results:

(1) The ideal way is to increase the expected frequency by increasing the sample size because that does not lead to any information loss in the present design.
(2) Refer to professional knowledge and combine the row (column) of this cell with its neighbors to increase the expected frequency. However, some information may be lost.
(3) Use Fisher's exact test.

11.3.2 Multiple Comparisons of Proportions

In Example 11.6, we concluded that the effectiveness of different methods in preventing postpartum hemorrhage is not the same. To know which pair of effective rates is different, we should continue with multiple comparisons. The analysis done here is analogous to the multiple comparisons in the analysis of variance. According to the purpose of comparison, $R \times C$ contingency tables are decomposed into multiple four-fold tables to test the difference of each pair of rates. The Bonferroni correction is the most commonly used for this purpose. To ensure that the total of Type I errors in multiple comparisons is no more than α, we need to correct the significance level by the times of comparisons to be made, and the adjusted significance level α' is

$$\alpha' = \frac{\alpha}{\text{number of comparison}}. \tag{11.15}$$

Example 11.7 Refer to the data in Example 11.6, and conduct pairwise comparisons using the Bonferroni correction.

Decomposing Table 11.11 into three four-fold tables, we obtain Tables 11.13(a), 11.13(b), and 11.13(c).

Table 11.13(a) Comparison of the prevention effectiveness of methods A and B.

Method	Outcome		Total
	Effective	Ineffective	
A	150	50	200
B	184	16	200
Total	334	66	400

Table 11.13(b) Comparison of the prevention effectiveness of methods A and C.

Method	Outcome		Total
	Effective	Ineffective	
A	150	50	200
C	198	2	200
Total	348	52	400

Table 11.13(c) Comparison of the prevention effectiveness of methods B and C.

Method	Outcome		Total
	Effective	Ineffective	
B	184	16	200
C	198	2	200
Total	382	18	400

Solution

Take the comparison of methods A and B for example:

(1) State the hypotheses and select a significance level

$H_0: \pi_A = \pi_B$, the effectiveness of methods A and B is the same
$H_1: \pi_A \neq \pi_B$, the effectiveness of methods A and B is not the same
The adjusted significance level is

$$\alpha' = \frac{0.05}{3 \times (3-1)/2} = 0.0167$$

Table 11.14 Results of multiple comparisons of prevention effectiveness of the three methods.

Comparison	χ^2	*p* value
A with *B*	20.98	<0.0001
A with *C*	50.93	<0.0001
B with *C*	11.40	0.0007

(2) Determine the test statistic

$$\chi^2_{AB} = \frac{(ad-bc)^2 n}{(a+b)(c+d)(a+c)(b+d)} = \frac{(150\times 16 - 50\times 184)^2 \times 400}{(150+50)\times(184+16)\times(150+184)\times(50+16)}$$

$$= 20.98,$$

$$\nu = (2-1)\times(2-1) = 1.$$

(3) Draw a conclusion

Calculate the corresponding probability $p = 0.0000046 < 0.0167$ using the value of χ^2_{AB}; reject H_0 and accept H_1 at the $\alpha' = 0.0167$ level. There is evidence to show that the effectiveness of methods A and B is different.

Similarly, according to Tables 11.13(b) and 11.13(c), the comparisons of A with C and B with C, are made; the results are given in Table 11.14.

From Table 11.14, we reject H_0 at the $\alpha' = 0.0167$ level. There is evidence to show that the effectiveness of the three methods is not the same.

Notice that it is appropriate to use the Bonferroni correction when there are only a few groups. If there were more groups, the conclusion would tend to be increasingly conservative the greater the number of comparisons.

The χ^2 test of an $R\times C$ contingency table introduced in this section is appropriate for the condition of bidirectionally unordered row and column variables. In case that one or both two variables are ordered, refer to the analysis methods described in Chapters 12 and 14.

11.4 χ^2 Goodness-of-Fit Test

In previous chapters on estimation and hypothesis testing, we assumed the data are from a specific underlying probability model and then proceeded either to estimate the parameters of the model or test hypotheses for different possible values of the parameters. This section presents a general method of testing for the goodness of fit of a probability model, that is, *Pearson's χ^2 goodness-of-fit test.*

The basic idea of Pearson's χ^2 goodness-of-fit test is that the assumption can be tested by first computing the expected frequencies in each group if the data came from an underlying specific distribution and then comparing these expected frequencies with the corresponding observed frequencies for inference. When H_0 is true, Pearson's χ^2 goodness-of -fit test statistic follows a χ^2 distribution approximately.

$$\chi^2 = \sum_{i=1}^{g} \frac{(n_i - T_i)^2}{T_i} \dot{\sim} \chi^2(v), \tag{11.16}$$

where $v = g - 1 - k$, g is the number of groups and k is the number of parameters estimated from the data used to compute the expected frequencies.

If $\chi^2 \leq \chi^2_{g-1-k,1-\alpha}$, $p \geq \alpha$, then do not reject H_0, and we conclude the fit is good.

11.4.1 Normal Distribution Goodness-of-Fit Test

Example 11.8 Refer to Example 2.1 in Chapter 2. We assume that the height measurements came from an underlying normal distribution. Besides the methods previously introduced in Chapters 5 and 9, how can the validity of this assumption be tested?

The procedure for the goodness-of-fit test is as follows:

(1) State the hypotheses and select a significance level α

H_0 : The height of girls X follows a normal distribution
H_1 : The height of girls X does not follow normal distribution

$\alpha = 0.05$

(2) Discretize continuous variables and calculate the number of observations

Divide interval $[a, b]$, the value range of X, into m mutually disjoint intervals: $I_1 = [a_1, a_2)$, $I_2 = [a_2, a_3)$,..., $I_{m-1} = [a_{m-1}, a_m)$, $I_m = [a_m, a_{m+1}]$, where $a_1 = a$, $a_{m+1} = b$, as shown in the first column in Table 11.15. Count n_i $(i = 1, 2, ..., m)$, the number of

Table 11.15 Frequency distribution of the heights (cm) of 153 healthy 10-year-old girls and calculation of goodness-of-fit test statistics.

Group i (1)	Observed frequency n_i (2)	$\Phi(z_i)$ (3)	$\Phi(z_{i+1})$ (4)	p_i (5) = (4) − (3)	Expected frequency T_i (6) = 153 × (5)
125.0–	2	0.0056	0.0180	0.0124	1.8972
128.0–	6	0.0180	0.0488	0.0308	4.7124
131.0–	9	0.0488	0.1118	0.0630	9.6390
134.0–	15	0.1118	0.2185	0.1067	16.3251
137.0–	26	0.2185	0.3680	0.1495	22.8735
140.0–	28	0.3680	0.5409	0.1729	26.4537
143.0–	20	0.5409	0.7063	0.1654	25.3062
146.0–	20	0.7063	0.8370	0.1307	19.9971
149.0–	12	0.8370	0.9225	0.0855	13.0815
152.0–	11	0.9225	0.9687	0.0462	7.0686
155.0–158.0	4	0.9687	0.9893	0.0206	3.1518
Total	$n = 153$	—	—	—	—

observations that fall into the ith interval $I_i (i=1,2,\ldots, m)$ (as shown in the second column of Table 11.15). This is the same as the procedure for constructing frequency distribution.

(3) Calculate the corresponding probability and expected frequency

When H_0 is true, calculate p_i the probability of falling into the ith interval I_i and $T_i = np_i$ the expected frequency of interval I_i.

In Table 11.15, suppose that the height follows a normal distribution; assume that the mean and standard deviation of this hypothetical normal distribution are given by the sample mean and standard deviation, respectively:

$\hat{\mu} = \bar{x} = 142.3$, $\hat{\sigma} = s = 6.82$. To be more specific, H_0 is $X \sim N(142.3, 6.82^2)$.

Therefore, the probability p_i of falling into the ith interval I_i is

$$p_i = \Phi\left[\left(a_{i+1} - \bar{x}\right)/s\right] - \Phi\left[\left(a_i - \bar{x}\right)/s\right] = \Phi\left(z_{i+1}\right) - \Phi\left(z_i\right)$$

and the corresponding expected frequency is $T_i = np_i$.

For instance, the probability of falling into the 1st $[125, 128)$ interval p_1 and the corresponding exacted frequency T_1 are

$$\begin{aligned} p_1 &= P\left(125 \le X < 128\right) = \Phi\left(\frac{128 - 142.3}{6.82}\right) - \Phi\left(\frac{125 - 142.3}{6.82}\right) \\ &= \Phi\left(-2.10\right) - \Phi\left(-2.54\right) = 0.0124, \\ T_1 &= np_1 = 153 \times 0.0124 = 1.8972. \end{aligned}$$

The calculation is completed in the same way; the results are shown in columns (5) and (6) of Table 11.15.

Note that the expected frequencies for the three intervals (125.0–, 128.0–, 155.0–158.0) are less than 5, which does not meet the conditions for Pearson's χ^2 goodness-of-fit test. Therefore, we need to modify the grouping by combination.

Combine 125.0– and 128.0– into one group, and $T = 6.61$, add the corresponding observed frequencies; then the number of groups changes from 11 into 10. There are $1/10$ cells whose expected frequency $T < 5$.

(4) Determine the test statistic

As in Example 11.8, $\chi^2 = \sum_{i=1}^{10} \frac{\left(n_i - T_i\right)^2}{T_i} = 0.2925 + 0.0424 + \cdots + 0.2283 = 4.58$

Degrees of freedom $\nu = 10 - 1 - 2 = 7$, because there are two parameters (μ and σ^2) that determine the normal distribution.

(5) Draw a conclusion

In the above example, under H_0, given that $\alpha = 0.05$ and $\nu = 7$, the critical value $\chi^2_{7,1-0.05} = 14.07$ can be obtained from the critical value of the χ^2_7 distribution (Appendix Table 5). As $\chi^2 = 4.58 < 14.07$, $p > 0.05$, and we do not reject H_0 at the $\alpha = 0.05$ level. There is no evidence to show that the height does not follow a normal distribution.

11.4.2 Poisson Distribution Goodness-of-Fit Test

Example 11.9 The daily numbers of lung cancer cases registered in Beijing in 2007 are given in Table 11.16. Test whether the daily numbers of lung cancer cases fit a Poisson distribution.

Solution

(1) State the hypotheses and select a significance level
H_0 : The daily numbers of lung cancer cases follow a Poisson distribution
H_1 : The daily numbers of lung cancer cases do not follow a Poisson distribution

$$\alpha = 0.05$$

If H_0 is true, that is, the daily numbers of lung cancer cases follow a Poisson distribution; the probability is $p(x) = e^{-\lambda}\dfrac{\lambda^x}{x!}$, where parameter λ is unknown, and the sample mean can be used as an estimate.

Table 11.16 Frequency distribution of the daily numbers of lung cancer cases and calculation of goodness-of-fit test statistics.

Daily number of cases x_i (1)	Observed frequency n_i (2)	$p(x_i)$ (3)	Expected frequency T_i (4) = 365 × (3)
3	1	0.0037	1.35
4	4	0.0102	3.72
5	9	0.0224	8.18
6	13	0.0411	15.00
7	22	0.0646	23.58
8	34	0.0888	32.41
9	41	0.1085	39.60
10	39	0.1194	43.58
11	48	0.1194	43.58
12	36	0.1094	39.93
13	37	0.0926	33.80
14	27	0.0728	26.57
15	16	0.0534	19.49
16	11	0.0367	13.40
17	8	0.0237	8.65
18	7	0.0145	5.29
19	6	0.0084	3.07
20	3	0.0046	1.68
21	3	0.0024	0.88
Total	$n = 365$		

In this example, $n = 365$; the estimate of λ, that is, the mean of daily numbers of lung cancer cases, is

$$\hat{\lambda} = \bar{x} = (1 \times 3 + 4 \times 4 + \cdots + 3 \times 21)/365 = 11$$

(2) Determine the test statistic

Using the estimate of λ, calculate the probability $p(x_i)$ of $x_i = 3, 4, 5, \ldots, 21$ using Formula 4.18.

$$p(3) = e^{-11}\frac{11^3}{3!} = 0.0037,$$
$$p(4) = e^{-11}\frac{11^4}{4!} = 0.0102,$$
$$\ldots\ldots$$
$$p(21) = e^{-11}\frac{11^{21}}{21!} = 0.0024.$$

The results are given in column (3) of Table 11.16, and the corresponding expected frequencies are given in column (4). Notice that the expected frequencies of the first two groups and the last three groups in column (4) are less than 5, and there are three cells with expected frequencies of about 1. Therefore, we combined the expected frequencies at each end, that is, $T_1 + T_2 = 5.07 > 5$ and $T_{17} + T_{18} + T_{19} = 5.63 > 5$. In this way, the number of groups decreases from 19 to 16.

Calculate test statistics based on columns (2) and (4) of the merged table:

$$\chi^2 = \sum_{i=1}^{16} \frac{(n_i - T_i)^2}{T_i} = 0.0010 + 0.0822 + \cdots + 7.2073$$
$$= 11.07.$$

The degrees of freedom $\nu = g - 1 - k = 16 - 1 - 1 = 14$.

(3) Draw a con3clusion

Under H_0, given that $\alpha = 0.05$ and $\nu = 14$, the critical value of $\chi^2_{14,1-0.05} = 23.68$ can be obtained from the critical-value table of χ^2_{14} distribution (Appendix Table 5). As $\chi^2 = 11.07 < 23.68$, $p > 0.05$, and we do not reject H_0 at the $\alpha = 0.05$ level. There is no evidence to show that the daily numbers of lung cancer cases do not follow a Poisson distribution with the parameter $\lambda = 11$.

11.5 Summary

In this chapter, we discussed the analysis methods for categorical data with a focus on Pearson's χ^2 test. Pearson's χ^2 test is used in many ways for hypothesis testing with one or more variables. Regardless of whether the population distribution is known, the principle is to decide the consistency (goodness of fit) between the observed frequency and the expected frequency calculated according to a certain hypothesis. Pearson's χ^2 test is applied so widely across several disciplines that it was selected as one of the 20 most important discoveries of the twentieth century.

The $R \times C$ contingency table is a cross-classification table of R rows and C columns. The simplest one is a 2×2 contingency table. Joint probability in a contingency table means the probability that an individual belongs in a cell according to its classification by variable attributes. The marginal probability is the probability obtained by summing the joint probabilities by row or column. An important role of the contingency table method is to test independence between two categorical variables, which is called the independence test or association test of categorical data. χ^2 test statistics are calculated as a measure of the distribution difference between the observed and expected frequency.

When considering the 2×2 contingency table, the approximation of test statistic χ^2 to the χ^2 distribution becomes poor when the sample size is small. Continuity correction could be used to improve this approximation. However, when the assumptions for the χ^2 test are not met, Fisher's exact test should be performed.

We also introduced McNemar's test for paired samples design data.

The χ^2 goodness-of-fit test is used to evaluate whether the data fit a theoretical population distribution. It has a wide range of practical applications.

11.6 Exercises

1. To compare the safety of two treatment methods for patients with diabetes, 161 patients were randomly divided into an experimental group and control group to observe the occurrence of adverse events such as hypoglycemia. The results are given in Table 11.17.

Please answer the following questions:

(a) What is the design of this study?

(b) Which methods can be used to test the difference in hypoglycemic incidence between the two groups? Please state H_0, H_1 and the necessary requirements for conducting the tests.

(c) Explain how the χ^2 distribution may be derived and the underlying rationale for testing the difference in the incidence of hypoglycemic events between the experimental and control groups.

(d) Explain the rationale behind the method of computing the expected frequencies in a test of independence.

(e) Compare the incidence of hypoglycemic events using the χ^2 test and interpret the results.

Table 11.17 Incidence of hypoglycemic events in the experimental and control groups.

Group	Hypoglycemic event	
	Yes	No
Experimental group	60	6
Control group	76	19
Total	136	25

2. Thirty-six patients with a COVID-19 were randomly assigned to treatment with drug A or drug B. The results are given in Table 11.18.
Please answer the following questions:
(a) Is it appropriate to conduct the χ^2 test in this study? Why?
(b) Which test could be employed to test the treatment effect between the two drugs? What distribution is the test based on?
(c) Please conduct the test and interpret the results.

Table 11.18 Treatment effect of the two drugs.

Drug	Cured	
	Yes	No
A	18	2
B	10	6
Total	28	8

3. In a toxicological study aiming to investigate whether there is any difference in toxicity between two doses of a new anticancer drug, 81 pairs of rats were matched according to litter, body weight, and age. Each pair of rats was randomly assigned to receive two injection doses. The results are given in Table 11.19.
Please answer the following questions:
(a) What is the design of this study?
(b) Is it appropriate to conduct a χ^2 test for an independent design to test the hypothesis? If the answer is no, why?
(c) Which method could be employed in this case? What distribution is the test based on, and what is the prerequisite for conducting the test? Please state H_0 and H_1.
(d) If the sample size is insufficient, which test could be used as an alternative? What distribution is the test based on?
(e) Test the hypothesis and interpret the result.

Table 11.19 Comparison of toxicity of two doses.

Dose A	Dose B		Total
	Dead	Alive	
Dead	6	33	39
Alive	24	18	42
Total	30	51	81

4. To investigate whether age is associated with the incidence of nosocomial angina among elderly patients with coronary heart disease after receiving noncardiac surgery, 1500 patients aged over 60 years who underwent noncardiac surgery were enrolled. The incidence of postoperative nosocomial angina in patients of different ages is summarized in Table 11.20.

Table 11.20 Incidence of postoperative nosocomial angina in noncardiac surgery patients of different age groups.

Age group	Nosocomial angina	
	Yes	No
60–	350	6
70–	462	13
80–	636	33

Please answer the following questions:

(a) What is the appropriate method in testing the difference of postoperative nosocomial angina in different age groups? Please state H_0 and H_1.

(b) Please test the hypothesis and interpret the result.

(c) What is the requirement for conducting a χ^2 test for this 3×2 contingency table? Is the requirement the same as for the 2×2 contingency table?

(d) Is it appropriate to conclude that the incidence of postoperative nosocomial angina increases with age?

5. In a pilot trial for a larger lung-cancer-screening program, the investigators enrolled patients who had a pulmonary nodule detected with low-dose computed tomography. The individual-level data of the first 12 patients are given in Table 11.21.

(a) Based on the collection information, state as many hypotheses as you can.

(b) Construct the 2×2 or $R \times C$ tables according to your hypotheses and perform the significance test.

(c) Suppose that you are provided with the full data (sample size = 240), will there be any changes in how you test the hypotheses? How many alternative ways are there to test the hypotheses? What are the conditions for applying the alternative test methods?

Table 11.21 Data of 12 pulmonary nodule patients.

ID	Sex	Smoking	Nodule solidity	Pathology diagnosis	Radiology diagnosis
1	Male	Yes	Solid	Cancer	Cancer
2	Male	No	Part solid	Cancer	No cancer
3	Male	No	Non solid	No cancer	No cancer
4	Male	Yes	Part solid	No cancer	No cancer
5	Male	Yes	Non solid	Cancer	No cancer
6	Male	No	Non solid	No cancer	No cancer
7	Female	Yes	Part solid	Cancer	Cancer
8	Female	No	Solid	Cancer	No cancer
9	Female	No	Non solid	No cancer	No cancer
10	Female	No	Part solid	No cancer	Cancer
11	Female	No	Part solid	Cancer	Cancer
12	Female	No	Part solid	No cancer	Cancer

12

Nonparametric Tests Based on Rank

CONTENTS

In this chapter, we continue our discussion about nonparametric methods focusing mainly on continuous variables. We assume that the data under study can be ordered without assuming any underlying distribution. The most popular nonparametric tests are based on a simple idea: sort the values from low to high and analyze only their ranks, ignoring the actual values. This approach is collectively termed rank-based nonparametric tests and ensures that the test is not considerably affected by outliers; these tests do not assume any particular distribution and are, therefore, also called distribution-free tests.

Rank-based nonparametric tests are versatile in application and simple in calculation. They enable simple hypothesis testing on data of various design types and have good approximate properties for large samples. In this chapter, we introduce rank-based tests for different designs. When distributions are not normal, these tests have greater statistical efficacy than their parametric counterparts.

12.1 Concept of Order Statistics

Order statistics, which are based on the ranks of observations, play a crucial role in many nonparametric hypothesis testing methods. They do not depend on the population distribution and are easy to use. We have partly introduced the basic idea of order statistics in Chapter 2, where we introduced percentiles.

Applied Medical Statistics, First Edition. Jingmei Jiang.

Companion website: www.wiley.com\go\jiang\appliedmedicalstatistics

Definition 12.1 Let $X_1, X_2, \ldots, X_n$ be a random sample drawn from a population X, and $X_i\,(i=1,2,\ldots,n)$ be *independent* and *identically distributed*. Sort the observed values of X_i from low to high,

$$X_{(1)} \leq X_{(2)} \leq \cdots \leq X_{(n)}; \tag{12.1}$$

then $\left(X_{(1)}, X_{(2)}, \ldots, X_{(n)}\right)$ are the order statistics of the sample $X_1, X_2, \ldots, X_n$, where $X_{(i)}\,(i=1,2,\ldots,n)$ is the ith order statistic. For example, $X_{(1)} = \min\limits_{1\leq i\leq n}\{X_i\}$ is the minimum order statistic (also called minimal sample value); $X_{(n)} = \max\limits_{1\leq i\leq n}\{X_i\}$ is the maximum order statistic (also called maximal sample value); and $X_{(n)} - X_{(1)}$ is the range.

Any $X_{(i)}$ is a function of a sample $X_1, X_2, \ldots, X_n$, so according to Definitions 4.1 and 12.1, order statistics are also random variables (but not mutually independent). In theory, it can be proved that the order statistics have good statistical properties (such as sufficiency). Order statistics can be used to study the properties of percentiles for large sample sizes.

Percentiles and the estimation of percentile functions of population distribution are the basic content of nonparametric estimation. In most nonparametric tests, the population median is what we are interested in as an important measure of location.

Assuming $F(x)$ as the population distribution function and using median M to represent the central position of the population, we have $F(M)=P(X \leq M)=0.5$.

The median divides the area of population distribution into two parts; the probability that any observation is to the right or left side of M is 0.5. For a random sample with n observations, the number of observations on the left side of M will follow a binomial distribution $B(n, 0.5)$, so the probability that k observations are exactly to the left side of M is

$$P(X_{(k)} < M \leq X_{(k+1)}) = C_n^k (0.5)^k (0.5)^{n-k} = C_n^k (0.5)^n$$

Let $X_{(r)} > M$ denote that the rth order statistic exceeds the median M; it is equivalent to having no more than $r-1$ observations in the sample to the left of M,

$$P\left(X_{(r)} > M\right) = \sum_{k=0}^{r-1} C_n^k (0.5)^n$$

The median is not sensitive to a difference in the shape of the population distribution but is sensitive to a difference in the central location. Owing to this property, the median plays an important role in rank-based nonparametric tests.

12.2 Wilcoxon's Signed-Rank Test for Paired Samples

Wilcoxon's signed-rank test was proposed by F. Wilcoxon in 1945. It is a signed rank test of paired samples that is analogous to the paired samples t-test. We illustrate the process of hypothesis testing using the following example.

Example 12.1 To investigate the antifatigue effect of a Chinese herbal compound, a researcher selected 20 pairs of mice matched for sex, age, and weight. The mice in each pair were randomly assigned to two dose groups of the compound. After being exhausted by a swimming exercise, the mice's hepatic glycogen level was measured (mg/100 g). The results are summarized in Table 12.1. Is there any difference in the hepatic glycogen levels between mice treated with different doses of the herbal compound?

Analysis

This example is a paired samples design with a small sample size. Calculate the difference d between the low- and high-dose groups (given in column (4) of Table 12.1). The result of the Shapiro–Wilk test of normality for d is $W = 0.828$, $p = 0.031$. At a significance level of $\alpha = 0.05$, we reject the assumption that the difference follows a normal distribution. The paired samples t-test is not preferred, and we use Wilcoxon's signed-rank test instead.

Similar to the paired samples t-test, Wilcoxon's signed-rank test converts the test of the difference between two populations into a test of one population. An exception is that Wilcoxon's signed-rank test is about the median of the population of differences. The underlying idea of the hypothesis is that if H_0 is true, i.e., the effect of the two treatment levels is the same, the population distribution of difference d should be symmetric, and its median M_d should be close to 0. In other words, the sum of the positive ranks (larger than the median 0, shown in column (6) Table 12.1), should be close to the sum of the negative ranks (smaller than the median 0). If the difference between the sum of positive and negative ranks is too large to be simply due to random error, we have the evidence to reject H_0, and the median of the distribution of the differences may not be 0.

Assumptions in Wilcoxon's Signed-Rank Test

Like the paired samples t-test, Wilcoxon's signed-rank test assumes that the pairs are randomly selected from (or at least representative of) a larger population and that each

Table 12.1 Hepatic glycogen levels (mg/100 g) of 20 pairs of mice in different dose groups.

Pair ID i (1)	Low dose (2)	High dose (3)	Difference d_i (4) = (3) − (2)	$\lvert d_i \rvert$ (5) = $\lvert(4)\rvert$	Rank (6)
1	958.5	958.5	0.0	0.0	—
2	838.4	866.5	28.1	28.1	5
3	641.2	788.9	147.7	147.7	8
4	812.9	815.2	2.3	2.3	1.5
5	739.0	783.2	44.2	44.2	6
6	899.4	910.9	11.5	11.5	3
7	758.5	760.8	2.3	2.3	1.5
8	695.0	870.8	175.8	175.8	9
9	749.7	862.3	112.6	112.6	7
10	815.5	799.9	−15.6	15.6	−4
				Positive rank sum $T_+ = 41$	
				Negative rank sum $T_- = 4$	

pair is selected independently from the others. Unlike the paired samples t-test, Wilcoxon's signed-rank test does not assume a normal distribution of the differences.

Solution

(1) State the hypotheses and select a significance level

$H_0 : M_d = 0$, i.e., the population median difference is equal to 0
$H_1 : M_d \neq 0$, i.e., the population median difference is not equal to 0

$\alpha = 0.05$

(2) Assign ranks and calculate the rank sum

Wilcoxon's test uses *rank sum* as the test statistic. To do that, we should rank the difference between each pair of observations according to sample data and then calculate the sums of the positive and negative ranks. It works via the following steps:

(i) Calculate the difference of observations, as given in column (4) of Table 12.1.

(ii) Rank the differences by their absolute value $|d_i|$. Ignore the value when the difference is 0 (e.g., the 1st pair) and rank the remaining values of difference from the lowest to the highest. We say there is a "*tie*" if the groups of differences have the same absolute value and assign tied values their average rank when the signs of the values are different. Otherwise, we can assign tied values either the average rank or the ordinal ranks (e.g., $d = 2.3$ for pairs 4 and 7, so either the average rank $(1+2)/2 = 1.5$ or ordinal ranks 1 and 2 will lead to the same rank sum). Then, mark the differences with the appropriate sign (+ or −), as given in column (6) of Table 12.1.

(iii) Add up the ranks of all the positive differences and all the negative differences. Let T_+ and T_- be the rank sums for positive and negative d, respectively, and they would total to $T_+ + T_- = n(n+1)/2$ (n is the number of nonzero differences that are ranked). In this example, $n = 9$, $T_+ = 41$, $T_- = 4$, and $T_+ + T_- = n(n+1)/2 = 45$.

Notice the difference in the meanings of rank and rank sum: rank is the sequence of all observations arranged in a certain order and reflects the grade to some extent, whereas rank sum is the sum of ranks in the same group (positive or negative) and reflects the distribution of the grade. Rank sum could be used as a test statistic because when H_0 is true, T_+ will be close to T_-; otherwise, a T_+ (or T_-) that is too large or too small is not supportive of H_0.

(3) Determine the test statistic T

After step (2), we can take the smaller rank sum as the test statistic $T = \min(T_+, T_-)$. In this example, $T = T_- = 4$.

(4) Draw a conclusion

There are two methods to draw a statistical inference depending on size n of the sample (number of untied pairs of observations).

(i) Critical-value method

When $5 \leq n < 30$, refer to Appendix Table 13 to identify the critical values T_0 at different significance level α and the number of pairs n. For the same α level, the larger n is, the larger is T_0; for the same n, the larger α is, the larger is T_0.

If $T < T_0$, then reject H_0;
If $T \geq T_0$, then do not reject H_0.

In this example, $n=9, T=4$, two-sided $\alpha=0.05$, and the corresponding critical value $T_0=6$. Because $T<T_0$, we reject H_0 and accept H_1 at the $\alpha=0.05$ level, and the difference has statistical significance, so it can be considered that the hepatic glycogen level of mice treated with different doses of the compound is different, and a higher dose of the Chinese herbal compound can lead to higher hepatic glycogen level.

Note that the critical values for the rank sum in Appendix Table 13 are accurate when no ties exist and only approximate otherwise. When ties exist, the normal approximation method for a large sample size would be more appropriate.

(ii) Normal approximation method

When $n>16$, according to the central limit theorem, the sampling distribution of statistic T approximates normal distribution under H_0,

$$T \dot{\sim} N\left(\frac{n(n+1)}{4}, \frac{n(n+1)(2n+1)}{24}\right). \tag{12.2}$$

In particular, T follows a normal distribution with mean $n(n+1)/4$ and variance $n(n+1)(2n+1)/24$. The test statistic would approximate the standard normal distribution after standardizing T.

A better approximation of the binomial by the normal distribution is obtained if we use a continuity-corrected version of the test statistic, as

$$Z=\frac{\left|T-\frac{n(n+1)}{4}\right|-0.5}{\sqrt{\frac{n(n+1)(2n+1)}{24}}}, \tag{12.3}$$

where n is the number of pairs for which the differences are not equal to 0 and 0.5 is a coefficient of continuity correction.

If $Z<z_{\alpha/2}$ or $Z>z_{1-\alpha/2}$, then reject H_0;

If $z_{\alpha/2} \leq Z \leq z_{1-\alpha/2}$, then do not reject H_0.

There could be several ties given a large sample size, and the following correction formula should be used, especially when the proportion of ties is greater than 25%:

$$Z_C=\frac{\left|T-\frac{n(n+1)}{4}\right|-0.5}{\sqrt{\frac{n(n+1)(2n+1)}{24}-\frac{\sum_{i=1}^{g}(t_i^3-t_i)}{48}}}, \tag{12.4}$$

where t_i is the number of observations with the same rank in the ith tie, and g is the number of ties.

Example 12.2 As the sample size in Example 12.1 is small, another experiment was performed using 32 pairs of mice under the same conditions to verify the conclusion. The results are given in Table 12.2. Perform a significance test.

Table 12.2 Hepatic glycogen levels (mg/100 g) of 32 pairs of mice in different dose groups.

Pair ID i	Low dose	High dose	Difference d_i	Rank	Pair ID i	Low dose	High dose	Difference d_i	Rank
(1)	(2)	(3)	(4)	(5)	(1)	(2)	(3)	(4)	(5)
1	946.3	1090.4	144.1	16	17	690.2	895.6	205.4	31
2	288.5	286.4	−2.1	−1	18	703.3	683.0	−20.3	−5
3	137.0	265.7	128.7	13	19	796.4	809.1	12.7	3
4	769.4	667.0	−102.4	−11	20	895.6	879.3	−16.3	−4
5	456.2	634.4	178.2	25	21	940.4	950.6	10.2	2
6	793.3	968.3	175.0	24	22	769.9	949.6	179.7	26
7	910.3	1048.9	138.6	15	23	741.3	904.5	163.2	21
8	745.4	937.9	192.5	28	24	682.4	513.4	−169.0	−22
9	645.9	804.8	158.9	20	25	784.2	976.8	192.6	29
10	796.3	726.9	−69.4	−8	26	846.6	677.2	−169.4	−23
11	632.6	737.9	105.3	12	27	847.1	976.8	129.7	14
12	805.2	889.9	84.7	10	28	764.0	1063.7	299.7	32
13	910.4	874.0	−36.4	−6	29	903.9	1090.5	186.6	27
14	764.2	909.5	145.3	17	30	705.2	625.6	−79.6	−9
15	865.4	1069.0	203.6	30	31	694.2	845.7	151.5	18
16	941.4	895.4	−46.0	−7	32	815.2	662.2	−153.0	−19
								Positive rank sum $T_+ = 413$	
								Negative rank sum $T_- = 115$	

Solution

Calculate the rank sum first (shown in last two rows in Table 12.2). Take the smaller rank sum T_{-} as the test statistic T; because the sample size is large $(n > 16)$, the sampling distribution of T approximates a normal distribution and there are no ties, we use Formula 12.3 rather than correction Formula 12.4:

$$z = \frac{\left|T - \frac{n(n+1)}{4}\right| - 0.5}{\sqrt{\frac{n(n+1)(2n+1)}{24}}} = \frac{149 - 0.5}{\sqrt{2860}} = 2.78.$$

As $z = 2.78 > z_{1-0.05/2} = 1.96$, $p < 0.05$. We reject H_0 and accept H_1 at the $\alpha = 0.05$ level to determine that the difference is statistically significant.

It can be seen that Wilcoxon's signed-rank test of paired samples data makes good use of the distribution symmetry of differences. This is reflective of the general principle of statistical analysis, of using as much information as possible. In addition, the inference conclusions are the same in Examples 12.1 and 12.2, even though the sample size and analysis methods are different. This strengthens our confidence in the conclusion and reflects the general principle of statistics to test and retest natural phenomena.

12.3 Wilcoxon's Rank-Sum Test for Two Independent Samples

A powerful nonparametric test, also developed by F. Wilcoxon, compares entire probability distributions and not just the medians. This test, called *Wilcoxon's rank-sum test*, tests whether the probability distributions associated with the two populations are identical.

Wilcoxon's rank-sum test is based on the rank sums for two samples. The basic idea of the test is as follows: assign ranks to the values of the two samples as if they were one sample; then take any of the rank sums of the individual samples as the test statistic. If the test statistic is too small or too large, then reject H_0 (that the two samples are not from the same population); otherwise, do not reject H_0.

Like Wilcoxon's signed rank test, the Wilcoxon's rank sum test can also be conducted using the Z test when the sample size is large ($n_1 \geq 10$ and $n_2 \geq 10$).

Wilcoxon's test can be applied to both continuous data and ordered categorical data. We will illustrate these applications with the two examples below.

Example 12.3 A cardiac surgeon plans to compare length of stay (LOS, days) between patients undergoing mitral valve replacement and mitral valvuloplasty. The data of 16 patients aged 45–70 are presented in Table 12.3. Perform a significance test.

Solution

This example has two independent samples and a small sample size. The result from the Shapiro–Wilk test of normality shows that at the significance level $\alpha = 0.05$, the LOS of patients with mitral valve replacement does not follow a normal distribution $(W = 0.712,\ p = 0.002)$; so we prefer to use Wilcoxon's rank-sum test.

The procedure for the test is as follows:

(1) State the test hypotheses and select a significance level

H_0: The population distributions of LOS are identical

H_1: The population distributions of LOS are not identical

$$\alpha = 0.05$$

Table 12.3 Length of stay (days) of patients undergoing mitral valve replacement and mitral valvuloplasty.

Mitral valve replacement		**Mitral valvuloplasty**	
Length of stay (1)	**Rank (2)**	**Length of stay (3)**	**Rank (4)**
38	8.5	32	3
29	1	42	11
35	5.5	44	12.5
33	4	81	16
38	8.5	35	5.5
41	10	46	15
31	2	37	7
		45	14
		44	12.5
$n_1 = 7$	$T_1 = 39.5$	$n_2 = 9$	$T_2 = 96.5$

(2) Assign ranks and calculate the rank sum

(i) Assign ranks. Assume H_0 is true. The two samples are drawn from one population, so the observations can be mixed and ranked from lowest to highest. Take either the average or ordinal rank for tied values in the same group; take the average rank for tied values in two groups. In Table 12.3, because the mitral valve replacement group has two "44" values, we can either take the ordinal rank (12, 13) or average rank $(12+13)/2=12.5$; both groups have the same value 35; we take the average rank $(5+6)/2=5.5$ because they are in two groups, as given in columns (2) and (4) of Table 12.3.

(ii) Calculate the rank sum separately. Let T_1 denote the rank sum of the replacement group and T_2 denote the rank sum of the valvuloplasty group. In this sample $T_1=39.5$ and $T_2=96.5$. See columns (2) and (4) of Table 12.3.

(3) Determine the test statistic T

Assuming that $n_1<n_2$ regarding the sample sizes of the two groups, we take the rank sum of the group with the smaller sample size n_1 as the test statistic T.

The sample size of the mitral valvuloplasty group is smaller in this example, and we take test statistic $T=T_1=39.5$.

(4) Draw a conclusion

(i) Critical-value method

When $n_1 \leq 10$, $n_2-n_1 \leq 10$, refer to Appendix Table 14. If T is not within the boundary determined by the critical values corresponding to n_1, n_2-n_1, p is less than the corresponding significance level α; if T is within the boundary, p is greater than significance level α.

In this example, $n_1=7$, $n_2-n_1=2$, and $\alpha=0.05$, and the boundary determined by the critical values is 40–79 (Appendix Table 14). As $T=39.5$ is beyond the critical-value boundary, $p<0.05$. We reject H_0 and accept H_1 at the $\alpha=0.05$ level. The difference is statistically significant, suggesting that the distributions of LOS of patients undergoing the two types of surgery are different. The mitral valve replacement patients generally have a longer LOS.

(ii) Normal approximation method

Like Wilcoxon's signed-rank test, the Wilcoxon's rank-sum test can also be conducted using the Z test when the sample size is large $(n_1 \geq 10 \text{ and } n_2 \geq 10)$.

Let $n = n_1 + n_2$, so the total average rank of the mixed sample is $(n+1)/2$. Under H_0, the expected value of T is equal to the average rank of the corresponding group: $E(T) = E(T_1) = n_1 \times \text{average rank of the mixed sample} = n_1(n+1)/2$ and variance $Var(T) = Var(T_1) = n_1 n_2 (n+1)/12$. The sampling distribution of the rank sum T approximately follows a normal distribution, that is,

$$T \dot{\sim} N\left(\frac{n_1(n+1)}{2}, \frac{n_1 n_2 (n+1)}{12}\right). \tag{12.5}$$

Wilcoxon's rank-sum test statistic is symmetric about $\mu = E(T) = n_1(n+1)/2$.

If there are no or a few ties, T after standardization is

$$Z = \frac{\left|T - \frac{n_1(n+1)}{2}\right| - 0.5}{\sqrt{\frac{n_1 n_2 (n+1)}{12}}}. \tag{12.6}$$

If there are several ties (>25%), the corrected formula is

$$Z_C = \frac{\left|T - \frac{n_1(n+1)}{2}\right| - 0.5}{\sqrt{\frac{n_1 n_2}{12}\left[(n+1) - \sum_{i=1}^{g} \frac{t_i(t_i^2 - 1)}{n(n-1)}\right]}}, \tag{12.7}$$

where t_i is the number of observations with the same rank in the ith tie and g is the number of ties. Formula 12.7 is widely used for ordered categorical data.

If $Z < z_{\alpha/2}$ or $Z > z_{1-\alpha/2}$, then reject H_0;

If $z_{\alpha/2} \leq Z \leq z_{1-\alpha/2}$, then do not reject H_0.

The step is the same when using Z_C as the test statistic.

Example 12.4 To investigate whether intraocular pressure (IOP) is the same in cataract patients after modified modern extracapsular extraction with different anesthesia methods, 128 older male cataract patients were enrolled in a study and randomly assigned into two groups. There were 61 and 67 patients in the surface anesthesia and retrobulbar anesthesia groups, respectively. The data of postoperative operative-side IOP in each group are given in Table 12.4. (grade I: ultralow; grade II: low; grade III: modest; grade IV: high.) Compare the IOP grade distribution between patients administered surface anesthesia and retrobulbar anesthesia.

Solution

IOP is ordinal categorical data in this example. Wilcoxon's rank-sum test with correction for several ties is preferred.

Table 12.4 Grade of patients' intraocular pressure between the two groups

Intraocular pressure grade	Anesthesia type					Rank sum	
	Surface anesthesia	Retrobulbar anesthesia	Total	Rank range	Average rank	Surface anesthesia	Retrobulbar anesthesia
(1)	(2)	(3)	(4)	(5)	(6)	(7) = (2) × (6)	(8) = (3) × (6)
I	5	18	23	1–23	12.0	60.0	216.0
II	38	34	72	24–95	59.5	2261.0	2023.0
III	17	12	29	96–124	110.0	1870.0	1320.0
IV	1	3	4	125–128	126.5	126.5	379.5
Total	$n_1 = 61$	$n_2 = 67$				$T_1 = 4317.5$	$T_2 = 3938.5$

(1) State the test hypothesis and select a significance level

H_0 : The population distributions of IOP with two anesthesia types are identical
H_1 : The population distributions of IOP with two anesthesia types differ in location

$\alpha = 0.05$

(2) Assign ranks and calculate the rank sum

(i) Assign ranks. The total number of patients corresponding to each IOP grade is shown in column (4) of Table 12.4. There are $5+18=23$ grade I patients assigned ranks 1–23, so they are assigned the average rank $(1+23)/2=12.0$. Assign ranks to other grades the same way. Columns (5) and (6) of Table 12.4 display the rank range and average rank of each grade.

(ii) Calculate the rank sum. Rank sum $=\sum$ (the average rank of each grade $\times$ the number of patients of each grade). As shown in the last row, columns (7) and (8) of Table 12.4.

(3) Determine the test statistic T

In this example, $n_1 = 61 < n_2 = 67$; therefore, $T = T_1 = 4317.5$.

(4) Draw a conclusion

The sample size $n_1 = 61 > 10$ is beyond the range of the T critical-value table. However, there are many ties, so an approximate calculation is made using the correction Formula 12.7,

$$z_c = \frac{\left|T - \frac{n_1(n+1)}{2}\right| - 0.5}{\sqrt{\frac{n_1 n_2}{12}\left[(n+1) - \sum_i \frac{t_i(t_i^2-1)}{n(n-1)}\right]}}$$

$$= \frac{\left|4317.5 - \frac{61\times(128+1)}{2}\right| - 0.5}{\sqrt{\frac{61\times 67}{12}\left[(128+1) - \frac{(23^3-23)+(72^3-72)+(29^3-29)+(4^3-4)}{128\times 127}\right]}}$$

$$= 2.03.$$

As $z_c = 2.03 > z_{1-0.05/2} = 1.96$, $p < 0.05$, we reject H_0 and accept H_1 at the $\alpha = 0.05$ level. The difference between the groups is statistically significant. The population distribution location of IOP between the two anesthesia groups different, and we conclude that the median grade of IOP is higher in the surface anesthesia group than in the retrobulbar anesthesia group.

12.4 Kruskal-Wallis Test for Multiple Independent Samples

The nonparametric test analogous to one-way ANOVA is called the Kruskal–Wallis test. The test is also called nonparametric ANOVA. The *Kruskal–Wallis test* was proposed by W.H. Kruskal and W.A. Wallis in 1952 as an extension of Wilcoxon's rank-sum test. It tests the null hypothesis that all k populations have the same probability distribution against the alternative hypothesis that the distributions differ in location. The advantage of the Kruskal–Wallis test over the F-test is that fewer assumptions about the nature of the sampled populations are needed, and Kruskal–Wallis test can be applied to data of non-normal or unknown distributions and ordered categorical data.

Assumptions of the Kruskal-Wallis Test

(1) The k samples are random and independent.
(2) There are at least five observations in each sample to allow for an approximation to the χ^2 distribution.
(3) The observations can be ranked.

12.4.1 Kruskal-Wallis Test

Let us use an example to illustrate the testing process.

Example 12.5 In a study on liver disease, a researcher collected the prealbumin (PA, μmol/L) of 35 patients with different degrees of jaundice. The data are given in Table 12.5. Is there any difference in the PA of patients with different degrees of jaundice?

Analysis

There are four groups, each with a small sample size, and the results from the Shapiro–Wilk normality test show that the data of the no jaundice group do not follow a normal distribution ($W = 0.663, p = 0.0003$); so the Kruskal–Wallis test is applied.

(1) State the test hypothesis and select a significance level

H_0 : The four population distributions of PA are identical
H_1 : At least two of the four distributions of PA differ in location

$\alpha = 0.05$

(2) Assign ranks and calculate the rank sum

(i) Assign ranks. Combine the four groups of data and assign rank from the lowest to the highest. The ranks of tied observations are averaged in the same manner as for Wilcoxon's rank-sum test.
See columns (2), (4), (6), and (8) of Table 12.5.
(ii) Calculate the rank sum. Calculate the rank sum of each group $T_j (j = 1,2,3,4)$ and then the average rank in each group, $\overline{T}_j = T_j / n_j$, where n_j is the sample size of each group (see Table 12.5).

Table 12.5 PA (μmol/L) of patients with different degrees of jaundice.

No jaundice		Mild jaundice		Moderate jaundice		Severe jaundice	
PA (1)	Rank (2)	PA (3)	Rank (4)	PA (5)	Rank (6)	PA (7)	Rank (8)
17.25	25	21.25	31	2.78	3	3.47	4
19.20	30	9.03	14	16.89	24	9.85	15
17.43	26	10.25	17	5.32	8	7.48	12.5
18.33	28	7.48	12.5	30.59	33	10.20	16
41.96	35	21.48	32	1.89	1	5.28	7
10.28	18	2.48	2	17.45	27	10.53	19
14.57	20	5.72	9	4.39	5	4.80	6
15.29	22	16.55	23	7.39	11	5.88	10
14.76	21	36.24	34				
18.69	29						
$n_1 = 10$	$T_1 = 254.0$	$n_2 = 9$	$T_2 = 174.5$	$n_3 = 8$	$T_3 = 112.0$	$n_4 = 8$	$T_4 = 89.5$
	$\overline{T}_1 = 25.4$		$\overline{T}_2 = 19.4$		$\overline{T}_2 = 14.0$		$\overline{T}_4 = 11.2$

(iii) The rank of the mixed sample is $1, 2, \ldots, n$, the rank sum is $T = 1 + 2 + \ldots + n = n(n+1)/2$, and the average rank is $\overline{T} = (n+1)/2$.

(3) Determine the test statistic H

If H_0 is true, and the sample sizes in each group equal 5 or more, then the test statistic H approximately follows a χ^2 distribution with degrees of freedom $\nu = k - 1$ (where k is the number of comparison groups).

$$H = \frac{\sum_{j=1}^{k} n_j \left[\overline{T}_j - (n+1)/2\right]^2}{\frac{1}{n-1} \frac{n(n^2-1)}{12}} \sim \chi(\nu). \tag{12.8}$$

In Formula 12.8, n_j denotes the number of observations in group j, T_j denotes the rank sum for group j, and n denotes the total sample size, i.e., $n = n_1 + n_2 + \cdots + n_k$.

According to Formula 12.8, it is obvious that if H_0 is true, the average rank of each group $\overline{T}_j$ should approach the total average rank $\overline{T} = (n+1)/2$; If the difference between $\overline{T}_j$ and $(n+1)/2$ is too large, then it is reasonable to reject H_0.

By replacing $\overline{T}_j$ with T_j/n_j in Formula 12.8, a simpler formula for H is obtained as

$$H = \frac{12}{n(n+1)} \sum_{j=1}^{k} \frac{T_j^2}{n_j} - 3(n+1). \tag{12.9}$$

When there are too many ties (>25%), the H statistic calculated from Formula 12.9 is biased toward lower values, especially for ordinal categorical data. We should then calculate the corrected statistic H_c using the following formula:

$$H_C = \frac{H}{1-\sum_{i=1}^{g}(t_i^3 - t_i)\Big/(n^3-n)}, \tag{12.10}$$

where t_i is the number of observations with the same rank in the ith tie and g is the number of ties.

Calculate the test statistic for this example. Because there is no tie here, correction is not required.

$$\begin{aligned} H &= \frac{12}{n(n+1)}\sum_{j=1}^{k}\frac{T_j^2}{n_j} - 3(n+1) \\ &= \frac{12}{35(35+1)}\times\left(\frac{254.0^2}{10}+\frac{174.5^2}{9}+\frac{112.0^2}{8}+\frac{89.5^2}{8}\right) - 3\times(35+1) \\ &= 10.14. \end{aligned}$$

(4) Draw a conclusion

(i) Critical-value method

When the number of groups $k=3$ and $n_j \le 5$, refer to the H critical-value table (Appendix Table 15).

(ii) χ^2 approximation method

When $k \ge 3$, or $n_j > 5$, under H_0, the test statistic H approximately follows a χ^2 distribution with degrees of freedom $\nu = k-1$. See Formula 12.8.

Referring to the χ^2 critical-value table (Appendix Table 5),

If $H > \chi^2_{k-1,1-a}$, then reject H_0;

If $H \le \chi^2_{k-1,1-a}$, then do not reject H_0.

In this example, $H = 10.14$. According to $\nu = k-1 = 4-1 = 3$, $\alpha = 0.05$, find critical value $\chi^2_{3,1-0.05} = 7.81$ in Appendix Table 5. As $H = 10.14 > \chi^2_{3,1-0.05}$, $p < 0.05$. We reject H_0 and accept H_1 at the $\alpha = 0.05$ level, so the difference is statistically significant. We conclude that at least two of the distributions of PA differ in location.

12.4.2 Multiple Comparisons

As with ANOVA, when H_0 is rejected, we need to further infer which two groups have different distributions. We recommend the extended t-test, among other alternatives, and the formula is as follows:

$$t = \frac{\overline{T}_i - \overline{T}_j}{\sqrt{\frac{n(n+1)(n-1-H)}{12(n-k)}\left(\frac{1}{n_i}+\frac{1}{n_j}\right)}}, \quad \nu = n-k, \tag{12.11}$$

where $\bar{T}_i - \bar{T}_j$ is the difference between the average rank sums of the two groups ($i \neq j$) we want to compare, n_i and n_j are the sample sizes of the ith and jth groups, respectively, $n = n_1 + n_2 + \ldots + n_k$, k is the number of groups, and H is the test statistic of the Kruskal–Wallis test.

Example 12.6 Refer to Example 12.5. We already know that at least two of the distributions of PA are significantly different. Perform pairwise comparisons with the extended t-test method.

Solution

(1) State test hypotheses and select a significance level

H_0: The population distributions of PA in the ith and jth groups are identical

H_1: The population distributions of PA in the ith and jth groups differ in central location

Because type I errors would increase if we compared these multiple samples by comparing two groups several times, we correct the significance level using the Bonferroni method:

$$\alpha' = \frac{\alpha}{\frac{k(k-1)}{2}} = \frac{0.05}{\frac{4 \times 3}{2}} \approx 0.008.$$

(2) Determine the test statistic t

According to Table 12.5, the average rank sum of each group is as follows: $\bar{T}_1 = 25.4$, $\bar{T}_2 = 19.4$, $\bar{T}_3 = 14.0$, and $\bar{T}_4 = 11.2$. Take the comparison of the "no jaundice" and "mild jaundice" groups as an example. The test statistic is calculated using Formula 12.11:

$$t_{12} = \frac{\bar{T}_1 - \bar{T}_2}{\sqrt{\frac{n(n+1)(n-1-H)}{12(n-k)}\left(\frac{1}{n_1} + \frac{1}{n_2}\right)}}$$
$$= \frac{25.4 - 19.4}{\sqrt{\frac{35 \times (35+1) \times (35-1-10.14)}{12 \times (35-4)} \times \left(\frac{1}{10} + \frac{1}{9}\right)}}$$
$$= 1.45,$$

$$\nu = n - k = 35 - 4 = 31.$$

Table 12.6 Pairwise comparison of four samples.

Group i,j	$\bar{T}_i - \bar{T}_j$	Difference standard error	t	p value
No vs. Mild	6.0	4.131	1.45	0.157
No vs. Moderate	11.4	4.264	2.67	0.012
No vs. Severe	14.2	4.264	3.33	0.002
Mild vs. Moderate	5.4	4.368	1.24	0.224
Mild vs. Severe	8.2	4.368	1.88	0.070
Moderate vs. Severe	2.8	4.495	0.62	0.540

Other comparison results are given in Table 12.6.

(3) Draw a conclusion

At the significance level $\alpha' = 0.008$, there is only one statistically significant difference of PA distribution between patients in the "no jaundice" and "severe jaundice" groups. It is concluded that the prealbumin of patients without jaundice is higher than that of patients with severe jaundice.

To examine a dose-response relationship between PA and degrees of jaundice, see Spearman rank correlation in Chapter 14.

12.5 Friedman's Test for Randomized Block Design

The Kruskal–Wallis test introduced in Section 12.4 is for independent samples. In this section, we will introduce the nonparametric *Friedman's test* corresponding to ANOVA for the randomized block design. This test, proposed by M. Friedman in 1937, is appropriate for comparing the relative locations of k or more population distributions when the normality or homogeneity of variance assumptions required for an analysis of variance are not satisfied.

Assumptions

(1) Each subject in each block is randomly assigned to one of k treatment groups.
(2) For the test statistic to approximate to a χ^2 distribution, either the number of blocks b or the number of treatments k should exceed 5.
(3) Tied observations are assigned ranks equal to the average of the ranks that would have been assigned to the observations had they not been tied.

Example 12.7 To investigate the influence of three anesthetics on sleep duration, a researcher first recorded the spontaneous activity levels of 21 mice. According to the results, the mice were divided into seven blocks, and each of the mice in a block was then randomly assigned to one of three treatment groups that received three anesthetics A, B, and C. The results of the sleep duration (min) of the mice are given in Table 12.7. Perform a significance test.

Solution

This example uses randomized block design. The Shapiro–Wilk normality test results show that the data of anesthetic C does not follow a normal distribution ($W = 0.708$, $p = 0.005$), so Friedman's test is applied.

(1) State the test hypotheses and select a significance level

H_0: The distributions of the mice's sleep duration between the three treatments are the same

H_1: At least two of the distribution medians of the mice's sleep duration among the three treatments differ

$$\alpha = 0.05$$

Similar to ANOVA for randomized block design, the key point is the effect among different treatments.

Table 12.7 Sleep duration (min) of mice treated with three anesthetics.

Block	*A*		*B*		*C*	
	Sleeping time	Rank	Sleeping time	Rank	Sleeping time	Rank
(1)	(2)	(3)	(4)	(5)	(6)	(7)
1	19.90	1	24.20	3	22.60	2
2	24.30	2	30.90	3	18.70	1
3	21.30	2	41.60	3	19.40	1
4	32.70	1	38.80	2	45.10	3
5	37.70	1	52.10	3	43.70	2
6	15.41	1	29.45	3	18.74	2
7	13.01	1	41.87	3	17.33	2
T_j		$T_1 = 9$		$T_2 = 20$		$T_3 = 13$

(2) Assign ranks and calculate the rank sum

The data layout of Table 12.7 is the same as that for ANOVA for randomized block design; i, j $(i = 1, 2, \ldots, b;\ j = 1, 2, \ldots, k)$ denote the row (block) and column (treatment), respectively.

For the block effect, ranking the values across blocks makes no sense because the activity levels of different blocks are different. Therefore, the sleep duration may be different, which would influence the estimation of the treatment effect of the three anesthetics. It is thus only appropriate to compare these treatments for mice in the same block. Therefore, we should rank the values within blocks. The specific procedure is as follows:

(i) Assign ranks. Assign rank for the observations within each block from the lowest to the highest. Calculate the average rank for tied values. See columns (3), (5), and (7) in Table 12.7.

(ii) Calculate the rank sum. Let R_{ij} denote the rank of the ith block and the jth treatment; the rank sum of each treatment $T_j = \sum_i R_{ij}$ $(j = 1, 2, \ldots, k)$. In this example, $T_1 = \sum_i R_{i1} = 1 + 2 + 2 + 1 + 1 + 1 + 1 = 9$; other rank sums can be found in Table 12.7.

(3) Determine the test statistic

The average rank of each treatment $\bar{T}_j = T_j / b$; under H_0, $\bar{T}_j$ has the following properties:

$$E(\bar{T}_j) = \frac{k+1}{2}$$

$$Var(\bar{T}_j) = \frac{k^2 - 1}{12b}$$

Friedman's test statistic,

$$M = \frac{12b}{k(k+1)} \sum_{j=1}^{k} \left(\bar{T}_j - \frac{k+1}{2} \right)^2, \tag{12.12}$$

where b is the number of blocks and k is the number of treatment groups. The farther $\bar{T}_j$ is from $E(T_j) = \frac{k+1}{2}$, the less likely it is to be supportive of H_0.

By replacing $\bar{T}_j$ with T_j, a simpler formula for Friedman's test statistic is

$$M = \frac{12}{bk(k+1)} \sum_{j=1}^{k} T_j^2 - 3b(k+1). \tag{12.13}$$

In this example, both the number of blocks and treatments are small: $b = 7$ and $k = 3$, therefore, we calculate the test statistic using Formula 12.13,

$$\begin{aligned} M &= \frac{12}{bk(k+1)} \sum_j T_j^2 - 3b(k+1) \\ &= \frac{12}{7 \times 3 \times (3+1)} \times \left(9^2 + 20^2 + 13^2\right) - 3 \times 7 \times (3+1) \\ &= 8.86. \end{aligned}$$

(4) Draw a conclusion

(i) Critical-value method

When $b \le 10$ and $k \le 6$, refer to the M critical-value table (Appendix Table 16). In this example, $b = 7$, $k = 3$; we find $M_{(7,3),1-0.05} = 7.143$. As $M = 8.86 > M_{(7,3),\,1-0.05}$, $p < 0.05$. We reject H_0 and accept H_1 at the $\alpha = 0.05$ level. We conclude that the distributions of the mice's sleep duration for all three anesthetics are not the same.

(ii) χ^2 approximation method

When b and k are large $b \ge 10$ and $k \ge 6$, under H_0, according to the center limited theory, M can be approximated by a χ^2 distribution with $\nu = k - 1$.

If $M > \chi^2_{k-1,0.05}$, then reject H_0;

If $M \le \chi^2_{k-1,0.05}$, then do not reject H_0.

When there are several ties, use the correction formula

$$M_C = \frac{M}{1 - \frac{\sum_{i=1}^{g} \left(t_i^3 - t_i\right)}{bk\left(k^2 - 1\right)}}. \tag{12.14}$$

Notice that when b is large or k is small, Friedman's test is not preferable because the ranks are within each block to eliminate the block effect. In such circumstances, we can refer to the modified rank sum analysis for randomized block design.

12.6 Further Considerations About Nonparametric Tests

The term "nonparametric" can only be applied to statistical tests, not to data.

The advantage of nonparametric tests is clear. They do not assume that data follow or approximately follow a normal distribution, and so nonparametric tests can be used when the validity of that assumption is dubious. When the assumption is not met, nonparametric tests have more power than parametric tests in detecting differences.

If the data are sampled from normal populations, nonparametric tests are less powerful than parametric tests when the sample size is small. This is easy to understand because nonparametric tests only consider the ranks and not the original data; they essentially give away some information. However, when the sample size is large, the nonparametric tests are almost as powerful as the parametric tests.

In practice, we need to avoid mistakes such as running both parametric and nonparametric tests and picking the result with the smaller p value, because p values can only be interpreted when the test is chosen as part of the experimental design. If you run two tests and report the results of the one that gives the lowest p value, you cannot interpret the actual meaning of the p value.

Furthermore, in this text, we classify the χ^2 test and Fisher's exact test in the nonparametric category, considering that under existing assumptions, these tests can only be tested based on empirical distribution. However, there is no distinction between parametric and nonparametric tests when analyzing dichotomous data. Many people would call these tests nonparametric, but some do not.

12.7 Summary

In this chapter, we introduced rank-based nonparametric test methods. Wilcoxon's signed-rank test and Wilcoxon's rank-sum test correspond to the paired samples t-test and two independent samples t-test, respectively; the Kruskal–Wallis test and Friedman's test are the methods corresponding to one-way ANOVA and two-way ANOVA without replication, respectively. Although these analysis methods are different in many aspects, the most important factor distinguishing the types of test is that parametric tests use the original observations, while nonparametric tests use the converted rank.

Because of loss of information during data conversion, if we use the nonparametric method when the sample(s) is/are from a normal distribution or the central limit theorem holds, the test's power would be reduced, especially when the sample size is small. Therefore, we should choose a parametric method when the conditions are met. If there is no information to examine the conditions, especially given samples with unknown distribution and small sample size, a nonparametric test would be appropriate as it will yield more robust conclusions.

12.8 Exercises

1. A oral health education program aimed at promoting oral hygiene was conducted, and 28 adult volunteers with mild periodontal disease were enrolled. The periodontal scores (between 0 and 6) were measured before the program and

Table 12.8 Change in periodontal scores before and after an oral health education program.

Score change	Number of cases
+3	4
+2	5
+1	6
0	5
−1	4
−2	2
−3	2

6 months after its completion. After 6 months, the periodontal scores of 15 patients had improved (increased scores), those of 8 patients deteriorated (decreased scores), and those of 5 patients remained the same, as given in Table 12.8.
Please answer the following questions:

(a) What is the design of this study?

(b) Is it appropriate to use the paired samples t-test for testing whether the oral health education program could improve the periodontal condition? Why?

(c) Which method could be used for testing the hypothesis? What is the underlying idea of this method. State H_0 and H_1.

(d) State the assumptions necessary for the validity of your analyses.

(e) Test the hypothesis using the appropriate method and interpret the results.

2. In an experiment aimed at assessing the effects of prolonged inhalation of cadmium oxide, 35 laboratory rats were randomly allocated to an experimental group and a control group. The 20 rats in the experimental group were continuously exposed cadmium oxide for 6 weeks and no intervention was given to the 15 rats in the control group. The variable of interest was the hemoglobin level (g/dL) following the experiment. The results are given in Table 12.9.
Please answer the following questions:

   (a) What is the design of this study? Is it appropriate to conduct a two independent samples t-test test here? If not, choose an appropriate method, and explain what is the advantage over the two independent samples t-test in this case?

   (b) What is the underlying idea of this method? How do you rank the subjects in the process of testing?

   (c) State H_0 and H_1, test the hypothesis using the appropriate method and interpret the results.

3. In a clinical trial for the treatment of angina pectoris, 172 patients were randomly divided into two groups and were given either sustained-release tablets or ordinary tablets. The results are given in Table 12.10. The aim is to investigate whether there is any difference between the two groups in terms of treatment effectiveness.

Table 12.9 Hemoglobin levels (g/dL) of 35 laboratory animals.

Experimental group	Control group
14.4	17.4
14.2	16.2
13.8	17.1
16.5	17.5
14.1	17.5
16.6	17.4
15.9	16.9
15.6	15.0
14.1	16.3
15.3	16.8
15.7	17.5
16.7	15.0
13.7	16.0
15.3	14.3
14.0	13.7
13.4	
16.2	
15.4	
15.2	
13.7	

Table 12.10 Effectiveness of two tablets for the treatment of angina pectoris.

Group	Significant effective	Effective	Ineffective	Aggravation
Sustained-release tablet	62	18	5	3
Normal tablet	35	31	14	4

Please answer the following questions:

(a) To test the hypothesis, is it appropriate to conduct a χ^2 test here? Explain the reason. What is your choice?

(b) State H_0 and H_1.

(c) Choose a method discussed in this chapter to test the difference.

(d) Because there are many ties in this case, how should you deal with the ties? What could happen if the ties are not taken into account in the calculation process?

4. To investigate the plasma renin activity in cirrhosis patients with different degrees of ascites, patients were randomly selected. Their plasma renin activity (g/ml) was measured. The results are given in Table 12.11.

Table 12.11 Plasma renin activity (g/ml) in cirrhosis patients with different degrees of ascites.

No ascites (control)	Mild ascites	Moderate ascites	Severe ascites
0.00	0.33	2.30	13.10
0.41	2.10	7.50	9.60
0.52	3.50	4.60	5.20
0.74	0.87	6.70	9.40
0.64	0.72	5.80	13.80
0.83	0.64	7.20	24.70
0.65	0.46	5.00	
0.45		8.90	

Table 12.12 ESM-1 levels (ng/ml) of mice with different types of multiple trauma.

Litter ID	*A*	*B*	*C*
1	0.03	0.08	0.16
2	0.06	0.07	0.19
3	2.26	2.98	3.21
4	0.03	0.03	0.74
5	0.02	0.10	0.24
6	0.03	0.08	0.16
7	3.17	3.58	3.75
8	0.05	0.09	0.28
9	0.02	0.06	0.29
10	0.04	0.06	0.18
11	6.53	7.18	8.09
12	0.05	0.09	0.17

Please answer the following questions:

(a) Is the data appropriate to conduct ANOVA here? If not, choose an appropriate method and state H_0 and H_1.

(b) Please test whether there is any difference in the plasma renin activity level between the four groups?

(c) What is the conclusion if the global test rejects H_0? Which method can be used if we need to further infer which two groups have different distributions? Conduct the test and interpret the results.

5. To investigate the changes in serum endothelial cell-specific molecule-1 (ESM-1) after multiple trauma, 12 litters of three mice were randomly allocated to three groups. Three types of multiple trauma (types A, B, and C) models were built for each group. Then 4 ml of venous blood was collected, serum was separated, and ESM-1 level (ng/ml) was measured in batches. The results are given in Table 12.12.

Please answer the following questions:

(a) What is the design of this study? Choose an appropriate test method after observing data.

(b) Provide H_0 and H_1 for the design.

(c) What is the underlying idea of this method? How do you rank the results in the process of testing?

(d) Use appropriate methods to analyze the data and interpret the results.

13

Simple Linear Regression

CONTENTS

In this chapter, we present analyses to determine the strength of the relationship between two variables. The magnitude of one of the variables (the dependent variable y) is assumed to be determined by a function of the magnitude of the another variable (the independent variable x), whereas the reverse is not true. In particular, we will look for straight-line (or linear) changes in y as x changes. The term "dependent" does not necessarily imply a cause-and-effect relationship between the two variables. Such a dependence relationship is called *simple linear regression*, or *linear regression* in short. The term "simple" is used because there is only one independent variable x. Starting from the basic concepts, we will systematically introduce the modeling principles of linear regression, statistical inference of parameters, and the application of regression model. Multiple linear regression, which considers two or more independent variables, will be introduced in Chapter 15. For convenience, in this chapter, we use lower case letters x and y to denote the dependent and independent variables, where y is still a random variable.

13.1 Concept of Simple Linear Regression

Let us consider the following example:

Example 13.1 To determine the relationship between weight and lung function in schoolboys, a doctor measured the weight (kg) and forced vital capacity (FVC, L) of 20 15-year-old schoolboys. The data are given in Table 13.1.

Applied Medical Statistics, First Edition. Jingmei Jiang.

Companion website: www.wiley.com\go\jiang\appliedmedicalstatistics

Table 13.1 Weight (kg) and FVC (L) of 20 15-year-old schoolboys.

ID i	Weight x_i	FVC y_i	ID i	Weight x_i	FVC y_i
1	61	5.36	11	61	5.08
2	57	4.51	12	49	4.17
3	67	4.17	13	70	4.60
4	67	5.14	14	43	2.37
5	50	4.27	15	63	3.86
6	56	4.60	16	56	4.03
7	65	5.40	17	64	4.59
8	49	3.89	18	46	2.65
9	59	3.81	19	47	3.26
10	56	4.25	20	39	2.88

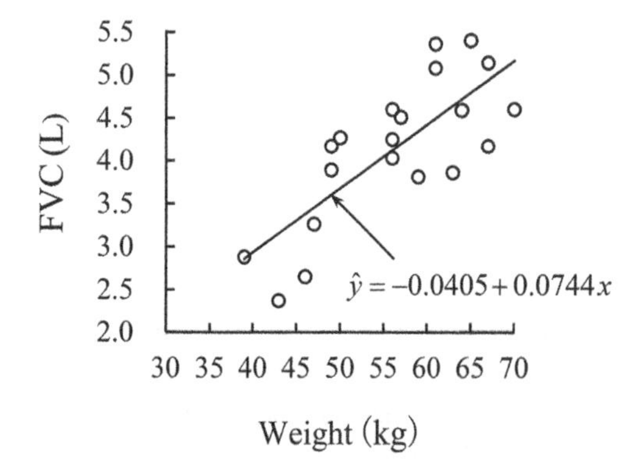

Figure 13.1 Scatterplot of the weight and FVC of 20 15-year-old schoolboys.

According to medical knowledge, weight and FVC have a functional dependence. However, how do we describe the relationship between these variables? It is convenient and informative to make a preliminary scatterplot of the data to determine whether there is any relationship between the two variables and, if so, what it might be. Figure 13.1 presents the plot of these data. It appears that x and y are approximately linearly related for this range of x values.

Figure 13.1 shows that FVC increases as weight increases. Although these points are scattered, most of them are scattered near a straight line, so it is natural to use a linear model to express this relationship between them.

We know that in mathematics, any linear equation can be written as

$$y = \alpha + \beta x,$$

where y is called the *dependent variable* or *response variable* and x is called the *independent variable* or *explanatory variable*. There are two parameters α and β in linear equations, where α represents the intercept of the line on the y-axis and β represents the slope of the line. If the parameters α and β are determined, then the line is uniquely determined. However, the data in Table 13.1 reveal that unlike in the equation $y=\alpha+\beta x$, the values of y and x do not have a one-to-one correspondence, that is, not all schoolboys with the same weight will have the same FVC. For instance, the weight of the third and fourth observations in Table 13.1 is the same (both 67 kg), but their FVCs are different (4.17 and 5.14 L). The way to solve this problem is to establish a probabilistic model of y and x, which can accommodate the random changes of the data near the line. The linear regression model is defined a follows:

Definition 13.1 For every given x, the expected value (population mean) of the random variable y can be drawn as a straight line, and the longitudinal distances of the points from the straight line are called residuals, denoted as ε. Thus, the simple linear regression model can be expressed by the following formula:

$$y_i=\alpha+\beta x_i+\varepsilon_i \left(i=1,2,\ldots,n\right), \tag{13.1}$$

where α and β are parameters; β, the slope of the regression line, is called *regression coefficient*. *Residuals* ε are random errors denoting the discrepancy between the actual y value and that predicted by the regression model, and residuals are independently identically distributed, $\varepsilon_i \sim N(0,\sigma^2)$.

For any given value of x, we are trying to predict y as a function of x, and we can inquire how the expected value of y changes with x. The probability distribution of y given x is referred to as a conditional distribution, indicating the regression of y on x. Assumptions of the simple linear regression model are as follows:

$$\begin{cases} y \mid x \sim N\left(\alpha+\beta x,\sigma^2\right) \\ E\left(y \mid x\right)=\alpha+\beta x \\ Var\left(y \mid x\right)=Var\left(\varepsilon\right)=\sigma^2 \end{cases}. \tag{13.2}$$

Formulas 13.1 and 13.2 can be expressed more concisely:

(1) For any given value of x, the corresponding value of y is normally distributed with an expected value $\alpha+\beta x$ and the same variance σ^2.
(2) For any two data points $\left(x_1,y_1\right),\left(x_2,y_2\right)$, the error terms ε_1, ε_2 are independent of each other.

Thus, we can see from Formula 13.2 that unlike the ordinary linear equation, the characteristic of the linear regression model is that its dependent variable y is a random variable, and the independent variable x is considered to be fixed. The effect of y is broken down into two sections: (i) a fixed part $\alpha+\beta x$, represented by expectation $E\left(y \mid x\right)$, is linearly associated with the change in x, and (ii) a random part, ε, results from the influence of other random factors.

In this way, one interpretation of the linear regression model in Example 13.1 is that for each schoolboy with a known weight x, the corresponding FVC y is a random variable and follows a normal distribution with mean $\alpha+\beta x$, that is, the average level of FVC y is a linear function of weight x; the variance is σ^2, which means that the dispersion of the FVC is a constant and does not change with x. If $\sigma^2=0$, then all the sample points fall on the regression line, and the larger the value of σ^2, the greater is the dispersion of the data points from the line.

13.2 Establishment of Regression Model

The main task of regression analysis is to study the linear dependence between two variables through a set of sample observations (x_i, y_i) $(i = 1, 2, \ldots, n)$. To select the best-fitting straight line of the dataset, it is necessary to try to determine the estimated values a and b of parameters α and β through the observed data so that the straight line can best reflect the relationship between x and y.

Definition 13.2 The predicted (or mean) value of y for a given value of x, as estimated from the fitted regression line, is given by

$$\hat{y}_i = a + bx_i, \tag{13.3}$$

thus, the point $(x, a + bx)$ is always on the regression line.

Similar to the straight line, a represents the intercept of the regression line on the y-axis, which is the estimate of $E(y)$ at $x = 0$; b is the estimate of the slope of the regression line, and its statistical meaning is that every time x changes by one unit, y changes by b units on average. Moreover, $b > 0$ means that the average level $\hat{y}$ increases linearly as x increases, $b < 0$ means that the average level $\hat{y}$ decreases linearly as x increases, and $b = 0$ means that the average level $\hat{y}$ is a constant and has no linear dependence on x.

13.2.1 Least Squares Estimation of a Regression Coefficient

Selecting the best-fitting straight line of the data set is equivalent to determining the "best" estimation of parameters α and β. Although numerous methods for estimating such parameters exist, the best known is the least squares estimation.

Definition 13.3 If the coordinates of the ith point are denoted by (x_i, y_i), the error of estimation will be a minimum if the sum of squares $\sum_{i=1}^{n}(y_i - \hat{y}_i)^2$ is minimum. This estimation method is called the *least squares estimation*.

Let $Q(\alpha, \beta)$ denote this sum. It is clear that this sum is a function of α and β only, i.e.,

$$Q(\alpha, \beta) = \sum_{i=1}^{n} \varepsilon_i^2 = \sum_{i=1}^{n} (y_i - \alpha - \beta x_i)^2. \tag{13.4}$$

It reaches a minimum

$$Q(a, b) = \min Q(\alpha, \beta). \tag{13.5}$$

According to the principle of extremum in calculus, a necessary condition for $Q(\alpha, \beta)$ to reach the minimum is that the first-order partial derivatives of Q with respect to α, β are equal to 0, i.e.,

$$\begin{cases} \dfrac{\partial Q}{\partial \alpha} = -2\sum_{i=1}^{n}(y_i - \alpha - \beta x_i) = 0 \\ \dfrac{\partial Q}{\partial \beta} = -2\sum_{i=1}^{n}(y_i - \alpha - \beta x_i)x_i = 0 \end{cases}. \tag{13.6}$$

After rearrangement of Formula 13.6, we have

$$\begin{cases} n\alpha + \beta\sum_{i=1}^{n} x_i = \sum_{i=1}^{n} y_i \\ \alpha\sum_{i=1}^{n} x_i + \beta\sum_{i=1}^{n} x_i^2 = \sum_{i=1}^{n} x_i y_i \end{cases} \tag{13.7}$$

The solutions of Formula 13.7 from the sample observation values are the estimated values of α and β.

It can be shown using calculus that a and b are given by the following formula:

$$a = \bar{y} - b\bar{x}, \tag{13.8}$$

$$b = \frac{\sum_{i=1}^{n}(x_i - \bar{x})(y_i - \bar{y})}{\sum_{i=1}^{n}(x_i - \bar{x})^2} = \frac{SS_{xy}}{SS_{xx}}, \tag{13.9}$$

where

$$SS_{xy} = \sum_i (x_i - \bar{x})(y_i - \bar{y}) = \sum_i x_i y_i - \frac{1}{n}\left(\sum_i x_i\right)\left(\sum_i y_i\right), \tag{13.10}$$

$$SS_{xx} = \sum_i (x_i - \bar{x})^2 = \sum_i x_i^2 - \frac{1}{n}\left(\sum_i x_i\right)^2. \tag{13.11}$$

Although the denominator in Formula 13.9 is always positive, the numerator may be positive, negative, or zero and the value of b can theoretically range from $-\infty$ to $+\infty$, including zero.

Thus, we obtain the regression line as specified by Formula 13.3. Because the straight line $\hat{y} = a + bx$ is estimated using least squares estimation, the line is also called the *least squares regression line*, where a and b are called the *least squares estimators* of α and β, respectively.

Solution to Example 13.1

For the data in Table 13.1, taking FVC as the dependent variable y and weight as the independent variable x, the steps for fitting a linear regression line are as follows:

(1) Draw a scatterplot (Figure 13.1). It seems that the two variables are linearly dependent, so a linear regression model can be fitted.

(2) Calculate the summary basic statistics $\sum_i x_i$, $\sum_i y_i$, $\sum_i x_i^2$, $\sum_i y_i^2$, $\sum_i x_i y_i$.

Here, $n = 20$, $\sum_i x_i = 1125$, $\sum_i y_i = 82.89$, $\sum_i x_i^2 = 64745$, $\sum_i y_i^2 = 357.2671$,

$\sum_i x_i y_i = 4771.48$,

$$\bar{x}=\frac{1}{n}\left(\sum_i x_i\right)=56.25,\ \bar{y}=\frac{1}{n}\left(\sum_i y_i\right)=4.1445,$$

$$SS_{xx}=\sum_i x_i^2-\frac{1}{n}\left(\sum_i x_i\right)^2=64745-\frac{1125^2}{20}=1463.7500,\text{ and}$$

$$SS_{xy}=\sum_i x_i y_i-\frac{1}{n}\left(\sum_i x_i\right)\left(\sum_i y_i\right)=4771.48-\frac{1125\times 82.89}{20}=108.9175.$$

(3) Calculate the regression coefficient b and intercept a according to Definition 13.3

$$b=\frac{SS_{xy}}{SS_{xx}}=\frac{108.9175}{1463.7500}=0.0744,$$

$$a=\bar{y}-b\bar{x}=4.1445-0.0744\times 56.25=-0.0405.$$

Here, b is positive, indicating that the FVC increases linearly as weight increases.

(4) Establish the regression model

$$\hat{y}=-0.0405+0.0744x,$$

It shows that for every 1-kg increase in weight, the FVC increases by 0.0744 L on average.

(5) Draw the regression line. We only need two points to determine a line. For instance, take $\hat{y}=3.6795$ at $x=50$ and $\hat{y}=4.4235$ at $x=60$; the straight line that connects these two points will be the regression line (Figure 13.1).

13.2.2 Basic Properties of the Regression Model

(1) The sum of squared residuals from observation point (x_i, y_i) to the regression line is the smallest, i.e., $Q(a, b)=\min Q(\alpha, \beta)=\min\sum_{i=1}^{n}\left(y_i-\hat{y}_i\right)^2=\min\sum_{i=1}^{n}\varepsilon_i^2$, and it can be proved that there is only one straight line that satisfies this condition.

(2) $\sum_{i=1}^{n}\left(y_i-\hat{y}_i\right)=0$, which means that the residuals can be positive or negative, but the sum must be 0. This is the characteristic of the regression model obtained using the least squares estimation.

(3) The regression line can thus be written as

$$\hat{y}_i=\bar{y}+b\left(x_i-\bar{x}\right),$$

so that it must pass through the geometric center of gravity $(\bar{x}, \bar{y})$ of the data.

In addition, we present the properties of least squares estimation, which is helpful for us in further understanding the regression line.

(1) The intercept a and the slope b of the regression line are minimum variance unbiased estimates of parameters α and β, respectively, and both the sampling distributions of a and b follow normal distributions.

$$a\sim N\left(\alpha,\left(\frac{1}{n}+\frac{\bar{x}^2}{SS_{xx}}\right)\sigma^2\right),\quad b\sim N\left(\beta,\frac{\sigma^2}{SS_{xx}}\right), \tag{13.12}$$

$$Cov(a,b) = -\frac{\overline{x}}{SS_{xx}}\sigma^2, \tag{13.13}$$

where $Cov(a,b)$ represents the covariance of a and b (see Chapter 14). It shows that coefficients a and b are correlated when $\overline{x} \neq 0$.

(2) For a given x_0, there is

$$\hat{y}_0 = a + bx_0 \sim N\left(\alpha + \beta x_0, \left(\frac{1}{n} + \frac{(x_0 - \overline{x})^2}{SS_{xx}}\right)\sigma^2\right). \tag{13.14}$$

Formula 13.14 shows that $\hat{y}_0 = a + bx_0$ is an unbiased estimate of $\alpha + \beta x_0$. It can also be seen from the formula that increasing the sample size is an effective way for improving the estimation precision of α and β.

13.2.3 Hypothesis Testing of Regression Model

The above-mentioned regression model $\hat{y} = a + bx$ only describes the linear dependence relationship between the variables y and x in the sample. The population regression model $E(y) = \alpha + \beta x$ needs to be tested to determine whether it truly reflects the statistical regularity between the two variables. Because the linear dependency of y on x is uniquely determined by the parameter β, for the simple linear regression model, the test of the regression model is equivalent to the test of the regression coefficient, that is, to test

$$H_0: \beta = 0, \ H_1: \beta \neq 0$$

It is obvious that y and x have no linear dependency relationship if $\beta = 0$. Accordingly, there are two alternatives: F-test, and t-test.

1. *F*-test

This test is also called the F-test. In the regression model, because x is a fixed variable, the variation of the dependent variable y can be decomposed to test whether there is a linear dependency of y on x. Take any point (x_i, y_i) as an example to illustrate the variation decomposition process for hypothesis testing (Figure 13.2).

Let $P(x_i, y_i)$ denote any point within the scope of x; the $(y_i - \overline{y})$ can be decomposed into two parts by the regression line: $(\hat{y}_i - \overline{y})$ and $(y_i - \hat{y}_i)$. Like one-way ANOVA, the decomposition of the sum of squares can be expressed using the following formula:

$$\sum_{i=1}^{n}(y_i - \overline{y})^2 = \sum_{i=1}^{n}(\hat{y}_i - \overline{y})^2 + \sum_{i=1}^{n}(y_i - \hat{y}_i)^2. \tag{13.15}$$

(1) The first term on the right side of Formula 13.15 is called *regression sum of squares*, denoted by SS_R; it represents the sum of squares of the deviance between the regression estimate $\hat{y}_i$ and the mean $\overline{y}$:

$$\begin{aligned} SS_R &= \sum_{i=1}^{n}(\hat{y}_i - \overline{y})^2 = \sum_{i=1}^{n}\left[a + bx_i - (a + b\overline{x})\right]^2 \\ &= SS_{xx}b^2 = SS_{xy}b. \end{aligned} \tag{13.16}$$

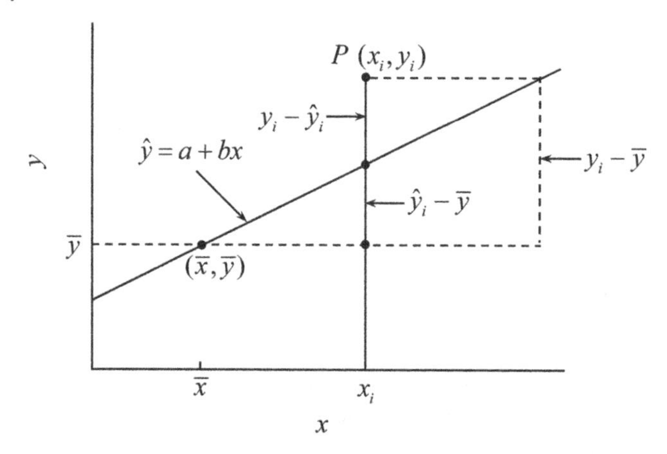

Figure 13.2 Variation decomposition of dependent variable y by regression line.

(2) The second term on the right side of Formula 13.15 is called the *residual sum of squares*, denoted by SS_E; it represents the sum of squares of the deviation of the observation value y_i from the regression estimate $\hat{y}_i$:

$$SS_E = \sum_{i=1}^{n} \left(y_i - \hat{y}_i\right)^2. \tag{13.17}$$

SS_E reflects the influence of factors that cannot be explained by the line regression. The smaller the value of SS_E, the better is the fit of the regression line.

Based on SS_E, we have

$$S_{yx}^2 = \frac{SS_E}{n-2} = \frac{\sum_{i=1}^{n} \left(y_i - \hat{y}_i\right)^2}{n-2}. \tag{13.18}$$

We call S_{yx}^2 the *residual mean square*, which is an unbiased estimator of σ^2 (i.e., the unbiased estimator of $Var(\varepsilon)$ in Formula 13.2).

The squared root of S_{yx}^2 is

$$S_{yx} = \sqrt{\frac{\sum_{i=1}^{n} \left(y_i - \hat{y}_i\right)^2}{n-2}}. \tag{13.19}$$

We call S_{yx} the *residual standard deviation*, which is an important index for the evaluation of the fit of the regression line.

In summary, Formula 13.15 indicates that the total sum of squares can be decomposed into regression and residual components, i.e.,

$$SS_{yy} = SS_R + SS_E. \tag{13.20}$$

Their corresponding degrees of freedom are as follows:

$$\nu_{yy} = \nu_R + \nu_E, \tag{13.21}$$

where $v_{yy} = n-1$, $v_R = 1$, $v_E = n-2$.

Under H_0, we have

$$\frac{SS_R}{\sigma^2} \sim \chi^2(\nu_R), \quad \frac{SS_E}{\sigma^2} \sim \chi^2(\nu_E)$$

where SS_R and SS_E are independent.

Test statistic

$$F = \frac{SS_R / \nu_R}{SS_E / \nu_E} \tag{13.22}$$

follows the F distribution with degrees of freedom $v_R = 1$ and $v_E = n-2$.

Formula 13.22 shows that if y and x do have a linear regression relationship, then the variation explained by the regression SS_R should be greater than the variation explained by other factors SS_E, which is exactly the basis of the F-test.

For a given α,

if $F > F_{(\nu_R,\nu_E),1-\alpha}$, then reject H_0;

if $F \leq F_{(\nu_R,\nu_E),1-\alpha}$, then do not reject H_0.

Example 13.2 Use the F-test to perform hypothesis testing for the regression line established in Example 13.1.

Solution

(1) State the hypotheses and select a significance level

$H_0 : \beta = 0$; there is no linear regression relationship between FVC and weight

$H_1 : \beta \neq 0$; there is a linear regression relationship between FVC and weight

$$\alpha = 0.05$$

(2) Determine the test statistic

$$SS_R = SS_{xx}b^2 = 1463.75 \times 0.0744^2 = 8.1024,$$

$$SS_E = SS_{yy} - SS_R = 13.7295 - 8.1024 = 5.6271,$$

$$F = \frac{SS_R / \nu_R}{SS_E / \nu_E} = \frac{8.1024/1}{5.6271/18} = 25.92.$$

The ANOVA results are given in Table 13.2.

Table 13.2 ANOVA table for Example 13.2.

Source of variation	SS	ν	MS	F	p value
Regression	8.1024	1	8.1024	25.92	<0.001
Residual	5.6271	18	0.3126		
Total	13.7295	19			

(3) Draw a conclusion

According to $\nu_R = 1$, $\nu_E = 18$, $\alpha = 0.05$, the critical value $F_{(1,18),\,1-0.05} = 4.41$ can be obtained from the $F_{(1,18)}$ distribution (Appendix Table 6). As $F = 25.92 > 4.41$, $p < 0.05$. We reject H_0 and accept H_1 at the $\alpha = 0.05$ level. We conclude that there is a linear regression relationship between FVC and weight in the 15-year-old schoolboys, and FVC increases linearly as weight increases.

2. *t*-test

The stability of the linear regression model depends on S_b, which is the estimated value of the standard error of the regression coefficient *b*. Because *b* is assumed to be from a normal population, the *t* statistic can be constructed from the sampling distribution of *b* for hypothesis testing.

Under $H_0: \beta = 0$, the test statistic follows a *t* distribution with degrees of freedom $\nu_E = n - 2$:

$$t = \frac{b - 0}{S_b} \sim t(\nu_E), \tag{13.23}$$

where $S_b = \dfrac{S_{yx}}{\sqrt{SS_{xx}}} = \sqrt{\dfrac{SS_E/(n-2)}{SS_{xx}}}$ is called the standard error of estimate.

The standard error of estimate is an overall indication of the precision with which the fitted regression function predicts the dependence of y on x.

For a given α and ν_E,

if $|t| > t_{\nu_E, 1-\alpha/2}$, then reject H_0;

if $|t| \le t_{\nu_E,\,1-\alpha/2}$, then do not reject H_0.

Example 13.3 Use the *t*-test to perform hypothesis testing for the regression model established in Example 13.1.

Solution

The hypotheses are the same as *F*-test.

Calculate s_b and the test statistic,

$$s_b = \frac{S_{yx}}{\sqrt{SS_{xx}}} = \sqrt{\frac{SS_E/(n-2)}{SS_{xx}}} = \sqrt{\frac{5.6271/(20-2)}{1463.75}} = 0.0146,$$

$$t = \frac{b-0}{s_b} = \frac{0.0744}{0.0146} = 5.10.$$

According to $\nu_E = 20 - 2 = 18$, $\alpha = 0.05$, the critical value $t_{18,\,1-0.05/2} = 2.101$ can be obtained from the t_{18} distribution (Appendix Table 4). As $t = 5.10 > 2.101$, $p < 0.05$, we reject H_0 and accept H_1 at the $\alpha = 0.05$ level. The conclusion is the same as that in Example 13.2.

For two-sided hypothesis testing of $H_0: \beta = 0$, either the F-test or t-test may be employed, with the same result; $F = t^2$, $F_{(1,n-2),1-\alpha} = t^2_{n-2,1-\alpha/2}$. The same concepts and procedures apply to one-sided hypothesis testing.

There may be several reasons for the linear regression model not being statistically significant: (i) The sample size is too small to reveal the intrinsic dependency between variables and can be expanded for further research if necessary; (ii) There is a relationship between x and y, but the influence is not linear (e.g., a curved relationship). In this case, a nonlinear regression method should be used; (iii) In addition to x, other important explanatory variables impact y and weaken the impact of x on y. In this case, a multiple linear regression method should be used to solve this problem (see Chapter 15).

The applicable range of the linear regression prediction generally corresponds to the range of the independent variable x. In medical practice, there may be different patterns between random variables in different ranges, and their correlation may also be different. Therefore, if there is no sufficient reason to prove that the linear regression relationship is still valid beyond the range of the independent variable, extension should be avoided.

13.3 Application of Regression Model

The purpose of establishing a regression line is to predict y from a known x, but it is not enough to present point estimates alone. The precision of the estimate should be considered, that is, interval estimation.

13.3.1 Confidence Interval Estimation of a Regression Coefficient

It can be seen from Formula 13.12 that the sampling distribution of b follows a normal distribution, and t is constructed according to the sampling distribution:

$$t = \frac{b-\beta}{S_b} \sim t(\nu_E), \tag{13.24}$$

where $\nu_E = n-2$, and

$$S_b = \frac{S_{yx}}{\sqrt{SS_{xx}}} = \sqrt{\frac{SS_E/(n-2)}{SS_{xx}}}.$$

Similar to the interval estimate in Chapter 6, the $(1-\alpha)\times 100\%$ CI of population regression coefficient β is

$$\left[b - t_{\nu_E,\,1-\alpha/2}S_b,\ b + t_{\nu_E,\,1-\alpha/2}S_b\right]. \tag{13.25}$$

Example 13.4 Estimate the two-sided 95% CI of β in Example 13.1.

Solution

Here, $n = 20$, $SS_E = 5.6271$, $SS_{xx} = 1463.75$, $b = 0.0744$, $s_b = 0.0146$.

According to $\nu_E = 18$, $\alpha = 0.05$, the critical value $t_{18,1\text{-}0.05/2} = 2.101$ can be obtained from the t_{18} distribution (Appendix Table 5). Then the two-sided 95% CI for β would be

$$\begin{aligned}
&[b - t_{18,1-0.05/2}s_b,\ b + t_{18,1-0.05/2}s_b] \\
&= [0.0744 - 2.101 \times 0.0146, 0.0744 + 2.101 \times 0.0146] \\
&= [0.0437, 0.1051].
\end{aligned}$$

13.3.2 Confidence Band Estimation of Regression Model

As shown in Definition 13.2, a regression model allows the estimation of the value of y (i.e., $\hat{y}$) existing in the population at a given value of x. However, $\hat{y}$ in $\hat{y}=a+bx$ is a statistic; it is only a point estimate of the population mean $\mu_{\hat{y}}$. Therefore, it is necessary to estimate the confidence intervals of the means, i.e., a confidence band of the population regression line.

Take any point on the regression line, for example, $\hat{y}_0=a+bx_0$ when $x=x_0$, and $\hat{y}_0$ follows a normal distribution (according to Formula 13.14):

$$\hat{y}_0=a+bx_0\sim N\left(\alpha+\beta x_0,\left(\frac{1}{n}+\frac{(x_0-\bar{x})^2}{\mathrm{SS}_{xx}}\right)\sigma^2\right).$$

The unknown σ can be estimated using $S_{yx}=\sqrt{\mathrm{SS}_E/(n-2)}$; then the random variable

$$t=\frac{\hat{y}_0-(\alpha+\beta x_0)}{S_{\hat{y}_0}}\sim t(\nu_E),\ \nu_E=n-2, \tag{13.26}$$

where

$$S_{\hat{y}_0}=S_{yx}\sqrt{\frac{1}{n}+\frac{(x_0-\bar{x})^2}{\mathrm{SS}_{xx}}}. \tag{13.27}$$

At any given $x=x_0$, the $(1-\alpha)\times 100\%$ CI of $\mu_{\hat{y}_0}$ for the corresponding $\hat{y}_0$ is

$$\left[\hat{y}_0-t_{\nu_E,1-\alpha/2}S_{\hat{y}_0},\hat{y}_0+t_{\nu_E,1-\alpha/2}S_{\hat{y}_0}\right]. \tag{13.28}$$

When x takes all possible values, the upper and lower limits of the $(1-\alpha)\times 100\%$ CI of the population mean $\mu_{\hat{y}_x}$ for the corresponding $\hat{y}_x$ are connected to form two arcs. The region between the arcs is the $(1-\alpha)\times 100\%$ *confidence band* of the regression line.

It can be seen from Formula 13.28 and Figure 13.3 that the confidence band is narrow in the middle and wide at both ends, and the SE determines its width. The

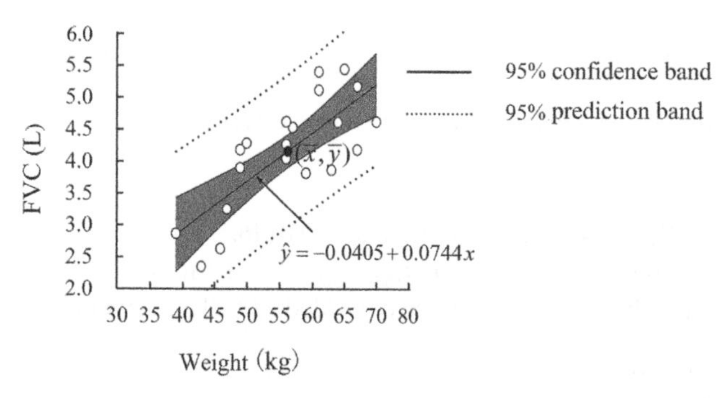

Figure 13.3 The 95% confidence band of the population regression line and the 95% prediction band of the response value.

specific influencing factors are as follows (assuming other conditions remain unchanged):

(1) The larger the S_{yx}, the wider the confidence interval and the lower is the precision of the estimated regression line.
(2) The larger the sample size n, the narrower the confidence interval and the higher is the precision of the estimated regression line.
(3) The larger the SS_{xx}, the more scattered the value of x, the narrower the confidence interval, and the higher is the precision of the estimated regression line.
(4) The position with the best estimated effect is $x_0 = \bar{x}$, and the estimation error here is the smallest.

Example 13.5 Calculate the 95% CI of the $\mu_{\hat{y}_0}$ for the FVC at $x_0 = 62$ for the regression model obtained in Example 13.1.

Solution
Here, $x_0 = 62, \hat{y}_0 = -0.0405 + 0.0744x_0 = 4.5723$,

$$
\begin{aligned}
s_{\hat{y}_0} &= s_{yx}\sqrt{\frac{1}{n} + \frac{(x_0 - \bar{x})^2}{SS_{xx}}} \\
&= \sqrt{\frac{5.6271}{18}} \times \sqrt{\frac{1}{20} + \frac{(62 - 56.25)^2}{1463.75}} \\
&= 0.5591 \times 0.2694 \\
&= 0.1506.
\end{aligned}
$$

According to $\nu_E = n - 2 = 18$, $\alpha = 0.05$, the critical value $t_{18,\,1\text{-}0.05/2} = 2.101$ can be obtained from the t_{18} distribution (Appendix Table 4). Substituting these values into Formula 13.28, we have

$$
\begin{aligned}
&[\hat{y}_0 - t_{18,1-0.05/2}s_{\hat{y}_0}, \hat{y}_0 + t_{18,1-0.05/2}s_{\hat{y}_0}] \\
&= [4.5723 - 2.101 \times 0.1506, 4.5723 + 2.101 \times 0.1506] \\
&= [4.2559,\ 4.8887].
\end{aligned}
$$

The 95% CI of FVC is [4.2559, 4.8887]L when the weight is 62 kg.

13.3.3 Prediction Band Estimation of Individual Response Values

Using the regression model, the $(1-\alpha) \times 100\%$ prediction interval of μ_{y_0} for individuals at a given x_0 can also be calculated.

According to Formula 13.2,

$$
y_0 \sim N\left(\alpha + \beta x_0,\ \sigma^2\right),
$$

Let variable $u = y_0 - \hat{y}_0$; then u follows a normal distribution,

$$
u \sim N\left(0, \left(1 + \frac{1}{n} + \frac{(x_0 - \bar{x})^2}{SS_{xx}}\right)\sigma^2\right). \tag{13.29}
$$

Here,

$$E(u) = E\left(y_0 - \hat{y}_0\right) = E(y_0) - E\left(\hat{y}_0\right) = \alpha + \beta x_0 - \alpha - \beta x_0 = 0,$$

$$\begin{aligned} Var(u) &= Var\left(y_0 - \hat{y}_0\right) = Var(y_0) + Var\left(\hat{y}_0\right) \\ &= \sigma^2 + \left[\frac{1}{n} + \frac{(x_0 - \bar{x})^2}{\mathrm{SS}_{xx}}\right]\sigma^2 = \left[1 + \frac{1}{n} + \frac{(x_0 - \bar{x})^2}{\mathrm{SS}_{xx}}\right]\sigma^2. \end{aligned}$$

The unknown σ can be estimated using $S_{yx} = \sqrt{\mathrm{SS}_E/(n-2)}$; then the random variable

$$t = \frac{u - E(u)}{\sqrt{Var(u)}} = \frac{\left(y_0 - \hat{y}_0\right) - 0}{S_{y_0}} \sim t(v_E), \tag{13.30}$$

where $v_E = n - 2$.

$$S_{y_0} = S_{yx}\sqrt{1 + \frac{1}{n} + \frac{(x_0 - \bar{x})^2}{\mathrm{SS}_{xx}}}. \tag{13.31}$$

The $(1-\alpha)\times 100\%$ prediction interval of y_0 is

$$\left[\hat{y}_0 - t_{v_E, 1-\alpha/2} S_{y_0},\ \hat{y}_0 + t_{v_E, 1-\alpha/2} S_{y_0}\right]. \tag{13.32}$$

When x takes all possible values, the upper and lower limits of the $(1-\alpha)\times 100\%$ prediction interval of y are also connected to form two arcs. The region between the arcs is called the $(1-\alpha)\times 100\%$ *prediction band* of y. For example, the region between the two dotted lines in Figure 13.3 is the 95% prediction band.

Example 13.6 Calculate the 95% prediction interval of y_0 at $x_0 = 62$ for the regression model obtained in Example 13.1.

Solution

According to Formula 13.31,

$$\begin{aligned} s_{y_0} &= s_{yx}\sqrt{1 + \frac{1}{n} + \frac{(x_0 - \bar{x})^2}{\mathrm{SS}_{xx}}} \\ &= \sqrt{\frac{5.6271}{18}} \times \sqrt{1 + \frac{1}{20} + \frac{(62 - 56.25)^2}{1463.75}} \\ &= 0.5591 \times 1.0357 \\ &= 0.5791. \end{aligned}$$

Substituting this into Formula 13.32, we have

$$\begin{aligned}&[\hat{y}_0 - t_{18,1-0.05/2}s_{y_0}, \hat{y}_0 + t_{18,1-0.05/2}s_{y_0}]\\&=[4.5723-2.101\times0.5791, 4.5723+2.101\times0.5791]\\&=[3.3556,\ 5.7890].\end{aligned}$$

This means that the 95% prediction interval of FVC is [3.3556, 5.7890] L when the weight is 62 kg.

Figure 13.3 shows the 95% confidence band of the population regression line $\mu_{\hat{y}}$ and the 95% prediction band of the response value y.

Comparing Formulas 13.32 and 13.28, we can see that for a given x, the 95% prediction band of the individual value μ_y is wider than the 95% confidence band of the population regression line $\mu_{\hat{y}}$. This has the same meaning as the estimation of the reference interval introduced in Chapter 5 and the estimation of the parameter confidence interval introduced in Chapter 6, except that the estimation in previous chapters is for a single variable.

13.4 Evaluation of Model Fitting

After fitting a regression line, how can we assess the goodness of fit of the regression line? Here we introduce two basic measures.

13.4.1 Coefficient of Determination

One way to assess the goodness of fit of the regression line is to measure the contribution of x in predicting y, i.e., to consider how much the errors in the prediction of y can be reduced using the information provided by x.

In Formula 13.20, we have the following equation:

$$SS_{yy} = SS_R + SS_E,$$

(1) If x has no contribution to the prediction of y or the contribution is very small, the regression sum of squares $SS_R \approx 0$; then the total sum of squares $SS_{yy} = \sum_i (y_i - \bar{y})^2$ and the residual sum of squares $SS_E = \sum_i (y_i - \hat{y}_i)^2$ are almost equal, that is, the deviation of the observed point from the regression line is approximately equal to its deviation from the mean $\bar{y}$.
(2) If a contribution of x to the prediction of y exists, then SS_R will be much larger than SS_E. If all points fall on the regression line, then $SS_E = 0$.

Therefore, a simple calculation method is to divide the regression sum of squares SS_R by the total sum of squares SS_{yy}. This ratio is called the *coefficient of determination*.

Definition 13.4 The coefficient of determination, denoted as R^2, is

$$R^2 = \frac{SS_R}{SS_{yy}}. \tag{13.33}$$

It represents the proportion of the deviance of y values from their predicted values $\hat{y}$ that can be attributed to a linear relationship between y and x. In simple linear correlation, it may also be computed as the square of the coefficient of correlation r (see Section 14.1).

The value range of R^2 is always between 0 and 1. Therefore, we may say that R^2 reflects the extent of fitness of the regression line or the explanatory ability of the regression model. The closer each observation point is to the regression line, the greater the value of SS_R / SS_{yy}, the closer the coefficient of determination to 1, and the better is the fit of the line.

For example, according to Definition 13.4, the coefficient of determination in Example 13.1 is

$$R^2 = 8.1024 / 13.7295 = 0.59,$$

which means that about 60% of the variation in FVC can be explained by the weight in this sample.

13.4.2 Residual Analysis

According to Formula 13.2, four conditions have to be satisfied for applying the simple linear regression model: linearity, independence, normality, and equality of variance. In general, we do not know for certain whether these conditions are satisfied. The question becomes, how far can we deviate from these conditions and still expect regression analysis to yield results that will have the reliability stated in this chapter? How can we detect departures (if they exist) from the conditions? Analysis of the residual ε can help provide answers to these questions.

We can obtain the standardized residual using the standardization procedure given as follows:

$$\varepsilon_i' = \frac{\varepsilon_i - 0}{S_\varepsilon} = \frac{y_i - \hat{y}_i}{S_\varepsilon}, \tag{13.34}$$

where S_ε is the standard deviation of the residual, estimated as S_{yx}, and $\varepsilon_i' \sim N(0,1)$.

Residual analysis can be used to analyze the rationality and stability of the model. It analyzes the reliability, periodicity, and the relationship between the data and model through the information provided by the residual data. It evaluates whether the actual data satisfy the regression model's assumptions. A residual plot can also be used to evaluate the model fitting and identify *outliers*.

Residual plot refers to a scatterplot with a certain residual as the ordinate and any other quantity as the abscissa in a Euclidean coordinate system. For example, in Figure 13.4, we take the standardized residual of the data in Example 13.1 as the ordinate and the independent variable weight as the abscissa.

Figure 13.4 shows that all standardized residuals ε_i' in this example are within $(-2, 2)$. They are approximately randomly scattered around 0 on the vertical axis, indicating that the error term ε meets the assumptions of $E(\varepsilon) = 0$. The scatterplots can also be used to check the assumption of a constant error variance. If the plot reveals a random pattern of points (no trends), then it is likely that the condition of constant error variance is reasonably satisfied, i.e., $Var(\varepsilon) = \sigma^2$ (just like Figure 13.4 of Example 13.1). However, if a strong pattern emerges on the residual plot, it indicates a violation of the condition.

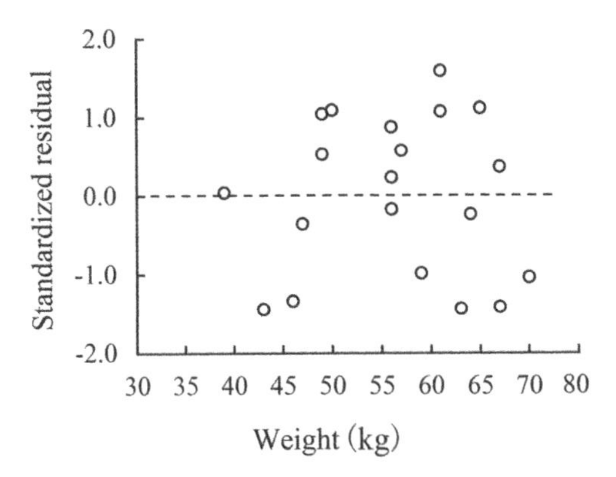

Figure 13.4 Standardized residual plot of the regression model in Example 13.1.

Finally, an outlier can be identified if $|\varepsilon_i'|$ of the residual point is larger than 2 or 3 (the choice depending on research objective and precision). The handling of outliers (by data curation or elimination) is necessary before performing regression analysis. However, be careful not to discard outliers routinely without careful evaluation because their omission may affect the conclusions. Always investigate the reasons for their presence and report them.

13.5 Summary

In this chapter, we learned the statistical inference of the dependence between two variables. A simple linear regression can be used for two continuous variables when we are interested in whether there is a linear dependency of a random dependent variable y on a fixed independent variable x.

Unlike the ordinary linear equation, the simple linear regression model $y_i = \alpha + \beta x_i + \varepsilon_i$ decomposes the random variable y into two parts: the fixed part of the linear change caused by x $\left(\text{i.e., } \alpha + \beta x\right)$ and the random part affected by other random factors (called residual ε). The regression model can be determined using the least squares estimation to find the optimal estimated values of parameters α and β.

The F-test of the simple linear regression model is equivalent to the t-test of the regression coefficient β.

Four conditions have to be satisfied before applying the simple linear regression model: linearity, independence, normality, and equal variance. Before modeling, we should first draw a scatterplot for primary judgment, then add the calculated regression line to the plot. Finally, we determine whether the regression model conditions are satisfied by simply and intuitively drawing a residual plot.

The $(1-\alpha)\times 100\%$ CI of β is estimated according to the t distribution and represents the estimated interval of the parameter. The confidence band $(1-\alpha)\times 100\%$ of the overall regression line is the area between the two arcs formed by connecting the upper and lower limits of the estimates of the overall mean $\mu_{\hat{y}}$ corresponding to all the values of the independent variables. Its middle is narrow and two ends are wide. This implies that the confidence level where the true regression line falls into the interval is $1-\alpha$; The $(1-\alpha)\times 100\%$ prediction interval of individual values refers to the prediction interval of the corresponding value of y at a given x_0. Notice that extension of the prediction should be avoided if there is insufficient reason to prove that the linear relationship is still valid.

Finally, it should be noted that the linear regression analysis must make sense, that is, regression analysis is not appropriate if the two phenomena are completely unrelated. It is necessary to determine whether a linear dependence between the two variables is expected according to professional knowledge, practical experience, and analysis purpose. Even if there is a linear regression relationship between the two variables, it is not necessarily a causal relationship. The context behind the data is important for deriving reasonable explanations and conclusions.

13.6 Exercises

1. To explore the relationship between weight and transverse cardiac diameter among children, the weight (kg) and transverse cardiac diameter (cm) data were obtained from 13 healthy 7-year-old boys. The data are given in Table 13.3.
Please answer the following questions:
(a) What are the dependent variable y and independent variables x in this study?
(b) Draw a scatterplot of x and y. Determine whether a linear regression line is appropriate for depicting the relationship between x and y.
(c) Provide H_0 and H_1 if the researcher would like to investigate the linear dependency between the weight and transverse cardiac diameter.
(d) What is the method for estimating the parameters in the regression equation? What is the basic rationale of this method?

Table 13.3 Weight (kg) and transverse cardiac diameter (cm) of 13 healthy 7-year-old boys.

ID	Weight	Transverse cardiac diameter
1	25.5	9.2
2	19.5	7.8
3	24.0	9.4
4	20.5	8.6
5	25.0	9.0
6	22.0	8.8
7	21.5	9.0
8	23.5	9.4
9	26.5	9.7
10	23.5	8.8
11	22.0	8.5
12	20.0	8.2
13	28.0	9.9

(e) Perform a regression analysis, construct the regression equation, and explain the meaning of slope of the regression equation.

(f) Based on the above result, draw a regression line on the scatterplot obtained in (b).

(g) Construct the 95% CI of regression coefficient β. How do you interpret its meaning in this case?

(h) Perform hypothesis testing of the regression equation using the t-test and F-test. How are these two test statistics related? Are the conclusions the same?

(i) What is the coefficient of determination? Calculate and interpret the coefficient of determination in this case.

(j) Draw a residual plot and use it to judge whether the assumptions for the linear regression analysis are satisfied.

(k) What are S_y, S_{yx}, and how do they differ? Interpret the difference with reference to the plot drawn in (f).

2. A high-sensitivity 32P marker analysis was used to determine a certain DNA adduct content (per 10^8 nucleotides) in the lung tissue of 12 patients with lung cancer. Their smoking amount (cigarettes/day) was also investigated. The data are given in Table 13.4.

(a) Draw a scatterplot and visually explore the relationship between smoking amount and DNA adduct content. Judge whether it is appropriate to fit a simple linear regression for these data.

(b) Perform a regression analysis and interpret the results you obtained.

(c) Check whether the underlying assumptions of linear regression was violated using a residual plot.

(d) Calculate and explain the meaning of coefficient of determination in this case.

Table 13.4 Smoking amount (cigarettes/day) and DNA adduct content (per 10^8 nucleotides) among lung cancer patients.

Smoking amount x	DNA adduct content y	Smoking amount x	DNA adduct content y
5	9.26	20	9.70
5	3.17	20	15.66
10	6.34	20	12.40
15	14.92	25	11.74
15	7.78	25	17.20
15	12.00	30	19.34

(e) Based on the regression equation you obtained in (b), predict the lung tissue DNA adduct content for patients who smoke 10 cigarettes per day. Calculate the 95% CI and 95% prediction interval and explain their implications and difference.

(f) Is it appropriate to predict the lung tissue DNA adduct content for patients smoking 40 cigarettes per day using the regression equation? Explain the reason.

(g) How do you identify outliers? What impact might they have? What will you do about them?

14

Simple Linear Correlation

CONTENTS

In Chapter 13, we discussed simple linear regression, which can be used to investigate the linear dependence relationship between dependent variable y and independent variable x. In practice, the regression method is not suitable when considering how two variables are mutually related. For example, it is not appropriate to construct a regression equation to predict the cholesterol level of a spouse using the level of the other; instead, studying the relationship between the levels of each spouse would make sense. Simple linear correlation is a simple method to address this issue. Simple linear correlation also considers the linear relationship between two variables, but neither is assumed to be functionally dependent on the other. The term "simple" refers to only two variables being considered simultaneously.

14.1 Concept of Simple Linear Correlation

14.1.1 Definition of Correlation Coefficient

Example 14.1 Consider Table 14.1 that shows the data on chest circumference x (cm) and weight y (kg) of 20 15-year-old schoolboys. Analyze whether there is a linear correlation between chest circumference and weight.

Applied Medical Statistics, First Edition. Jingmei Jiang.

Companion website: www.wiley.com\go\jiang\appliedmedicalstatistics

Table 14.1 Chest circumference (cm) and weight (kg) of 20 15-year-old schoolboys.

ID i	Chest circumference x_i	Weight y_i	ID i	Chest circumference x_i	Weight y_i
1	83	61	11	80	62
2	82	57	12	77	49
3	85	67	13	89	70
4	85	67	14	70	43
5	77	50	15	83	63
6	80	57	16	78	51
7	80	65	17	86	64
8	74	49	18	73	46
9	83	59	19	72	47
10	79	56	20	62	39

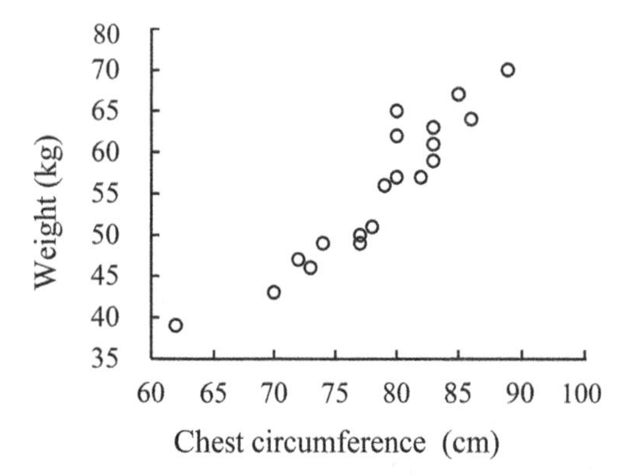

Figure 14.1 Scatterplot of the chest circumference and weight of 20 15-year-old schoolboys.

Every pair of measurements (x_i, y_i) $(i = 1, 2, \ldots, 20)$ in Table 14.1 can be located on a point in the Euclidean coordinate system, and all points are marked in this coordinate system to obtain a scatterplot (Figure 14.1).

Although the scatterplots in Figures 14.1 and 13.1 are similar, their assumptions about the data are different. Figure 14.1 indicates that the points correspond to a random sample of 20 schoolboys; consequently, both x and y are random variables. As shown in this scatterplot, there is a tendency for small values of chest circumference to correlate with small values of weight and large values of chest circumference to be correlated with large values of weight, that is, the trend of the scatter of chest circumference and weight is roughly a straight line. We say such a relationship between two random variables is a *simple linear correlation*, or *linear correlation* for short. The task of correlation analysis is to quantitatively describe and infer this assoication.

First, we discuss the related concept of covariance. *Covariance* is a measure used to quantify the relationship between two random variables.

Definition 14.1 The covariance between two random variables x and y is denoted by $Cov(x,y)$ and is defined as

$$Cov(x,y) = E\left[\left(x-\mu_x\right)\left(y-\mu_y\right)\right] \tag{14.1}$$

which can also be written as $E\left(xy\right)-\mu_x\mu_y$, where μ_x is the expected value of x, μ_y is the expected value of y, and $E\left(xy\right)=$ expected value of the product of x and y.

It can be shown that if the random variables x and y are mutually independent, then $Cov(x,y)$ is 0. If large values of x and y tend to occur among the same subjects (as well as small values of x and y), then the covariance is positive. If large values of x and small values of y (or conversely, small values of x and large values of y) tend to occur among the same subjects, then the covariance is negative.

One issue with covariance in quantifying the correlation between two random variables x and y is that the unit is that of x multiplied by that of y. Thus, it is difficult to interpret and compare the strength of correlation between pairs of variables from the magnitude of the covariance. To obtain a measure of correlation that is independent of the units of x and y, we consider the correlation coefficient.

Definition 14.2 The correlation coefficient between two random variables x and y is denoted by $Corr(x,y)$ or ρ and is defined as

$$\rho = Corr(x,y) = \frac{Cov(x,y)}{\sigma_x\sigma_y}, \tag{14.2}$$

where σ_x and σ_y are the standard deviations of x and y, respectively.

Unlike covariance $Cov(x,y)$, correlation coefficient $Corr(x,y)$ is independent of the units of x and y, and ranges between -1 and 1. Because the population correlation coefficient ρ is usually unknown, we need to use sample correlation coefficient r to estimate the population correlation coefficient ρ.

Definition 14.3 Let $\left(x_i, y_i\right)\left(i=1,2,\ldots,n\right)$ be a sample of size n randomly drawn from a bivariate normal population*; the sample *Pearson's product moment correlation coefficient* r, or *Pearson correlation coefficient* in short, is defined as

$$r = \frac{\sum_{i=1}^{n}(x_i-\bar{x})(y_i-\bar{y})}{\sqrt{\sum_{i=1}^{n}(x_i-\bar{x})^2\sum_{i=1}^{n}(y_i-\bar{y})^2}} = \frac{SS_{xy}}{\sqrt{SS_{xx}SS_{yy}}}, \tag{14.3}$$

where the computation of SS_{xy}, SS_{xx} is the same as in Formulas 13.10 and 13.11, and the computed SS_{yy} is similar to SS_{xx}.

*If the joint probability distribution of x and y is bivariate normal, then the marginal distributions of both x and y are also normal.

Pearson correlation coefficient r is a measure of the strength of the linear correlation between x and y in the sample. Because the sample covariance S_{xy}^2 is an unbiased estimator for the population covariance $Cov(x,y)$, and the sample variances S_x^2 and S_y^2 are also the unbiased estimators of population variances σ_x^2 and σ_y^2, it is reasonable that the correlation coefficient r is a good estimator of the population correlation coefficient ρ.

From the short-cut formula for the sum of squares and products, an alternative formula for the correlation coefficient, which is more convenient for computation, is

$$r = \frac{SS_{xy}}{\sqrt{SS_{xx}SS_{yy}}} = \frac{S_{xy}^2}{\sqrt{S_x^2 S_y^2}} = \frac{\sum_{i=1}^{n} x_i y_i - \left(\sum_{i=1}^{n} x_i\right)\left(\sum_{i=1}^{n} y_i\right) \Big/ n}{\sqrt{\left[\left[\sum_{i=1}^{n} x_i^2 - \left(\sum_{i=1}^{n} x_i\right)^2 \Big/ n\right]\left[\sum_{i=1}^{n} y_i^2 - \left(\sum_{i=1}^{n} y_i\right)^2 \Big/ n\right]\right]}}. \tag{14.4}$$

14.1.2 Interpretation of Correlation Coefficient

The correlation coefficient has two interpretations for the correlation between variables: (i) The sign is indicative of the direction of the correlation between two variables. If a linear correlation exists, we say it is a positive linear correlation $(r > 0)$ when random variables x and y increase or decrease in the same direction and a negative linear correlation $(r < 0)$ when variables x and y increase or decrease in the opposite direction. If the change in variable x is not related to the change in variable y, we say there is no linear correlation between two variables $(r = 0)$, i.e., zero correlation. (ii) The absolute value of the correlation coefficient $|r|$ indicates the strength of the linear relationship. $|r| = 1$ means perfect linear correlation; The closer $|r|$ is to 1, the stronger is the linear correlation. The closer $|r|$ is to 0, the weaker is the linear correlation. In general, r will not reach ± 1 in biological phenomena, and it is rare for r to be exactly 0.

The scatterplots of the correlation of various degrees and types are shown in Figure 14.2.

Notice that the Pearson correlation coefficient can only quantify the strength and direction of a linear relationship and is not suitable for nonlinear relationships. In other words, we need to be cautious in explaining $r = 0$. $r = 0$ only indicates that there is no linear correlation between the two variables. It does not exclude the existence of nonlinear correlation (see Figure 14.2(h)).

In addition, just as we explained in Chapter 13, the squared correlation coefficient is the fraction by which the sum of squares of the deviation of y from its mean is explained by (reduced by) the sum of squares because of the regression on x. The same applies to an interchange of x and y. For example, we have $r^2 = 1$ in Figures 14.2(b) and 14.2(d), $r^2 = 0$ in Figures 14.2(e)–14.2(h), and the sum of squares of either variable is unaffected by regression on the other, whereas in Figures 14.2(a) and 14.2(c), some reductions occur for either x or y because $0 < r^2 < 1$. For example, for fixed degrees of freedom, we say that the correlation association is weak when $|r| \le 0.5$, moderate when $0.5 < |r| < 0.8$, and strong when $|r| \ge 0.8$. The rationale is that even if $|r| = 0.5$ (then $r^2 = 0.25$) which means at most 25% of the observed variation of one variable can be explained by the other, the effect of the fitting regression line is low.

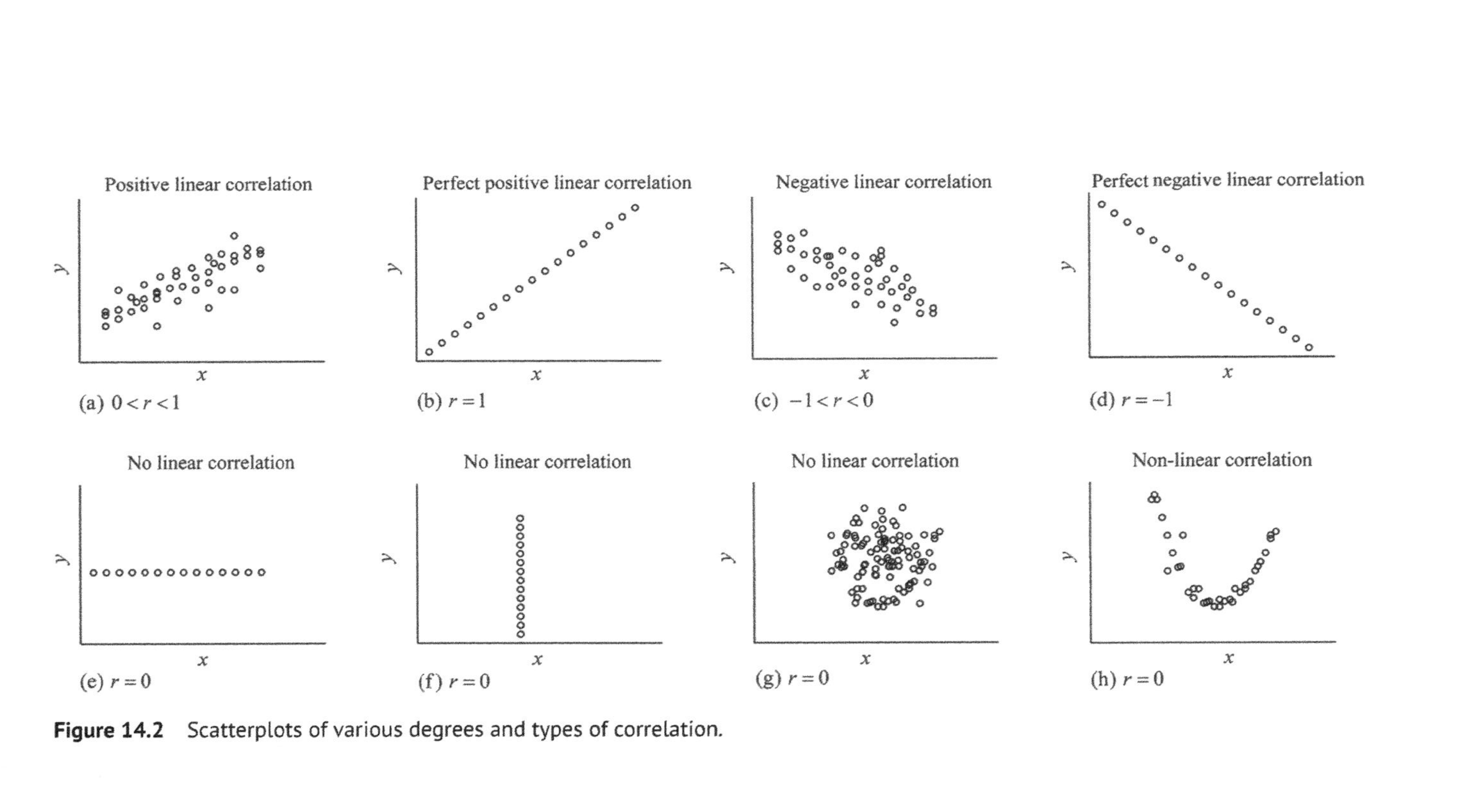

Figure 14.2 Scatterplots of various degrees and types of correlation.

Solution to Example 14.1

The analysis of the linear correlation between chest circumference and weight of the 20 15-year-old schoolboys is as follows:

(1) As shown by the scatterplot in Figure 14.1, there is likely to be a linear correlation between the two variables, and the trend is positive.

(2) Calculate the correlation coefficient r of the sample according to Definition 14.3. First, the basic summary statistics are obtained,

$$\sum_i x_i = 1578,\ \sum_i y_i = 1122,\ \sum_i x_i^2 = 125274,\ \sum_i y_i^2 = 64446,\ \sum_i x_i y_i = 89528.$$

Based on Formula 14.4, the correlation coefficient is

$$r = \frac{s_{xy}^2}{\sqrt{s_x^2 s_y^2}} = \frac{\sum_i x_i y_i - \left(\sum_i x_i\right)\left(\sum_i y_i\right)\Big/ n}{\sqrt{\left[\sum_i x_i^2 - \left(\sum_i x_i\right)^2 \Big/ n\right]\left[\sum_i y_i^2 - \left(\sum_i y_i\right)^2 \Big/ n\right]}}$$

$$= \frac{89528 - 1578 \times 1122 / 20}{\sqrt{\left(125274 - 1578^2/20\right) \times \left(64446 - 1122^2/20\right)}}$$

$$= 0.932.$$

Here, the correlation coefficient $|r| > 0.8$, which indicates a strong positive correlation is likely to be present between chest circumference and weight in schoolboys.

We must be careful not to jump to unwarranted conclusions. The high correlation does not imply causality. In real life, many other factors, such as height in this example, may contribute to the increase in weight.

14.2 Hypothesis Testing of Correlation Coefficient

Hypothesis testing of the sample correlation coefficient is needed to test whether it is of statistical significance, i.e., whether the population correlation coefficient ρ equals 0. We introduce two ways for making inferences on this.

1. *t*-test

(1) State the hypotheses and select a significance level

$H_0: \rho = 0$

$H_1: \rho \neq 0$

Usually let $\alpha = 0.05$

(2) Determine the test statistic

$$t = \frac{r - 0}{S_r} = \frac{r}{\sqrt{\dfrac{1 - r^2}{n - 2}}}, \qquad (14.5)$$

follows a t distribution with $\nu = n - 2$ degrees of freedom under H_0.

(3) Draw a conclusion

At a significance level α,
if $|t| > t_{\nu,1-\alpha/2}$ then reject H_0;
if $|t| \le t_{\nu,1-\alpha/2}$ then do not reject H_0.

Example 14.2 Perform a t-test for the correlation coefficient in Example 14.1.

Solution
(1) State the hypotheses and select a significance level

$H_0 : \rho = 0$, no linear correlation exists between chest circumference and weight
$H_1 : \rho \neq 0$, a linear correlation exists between chest circumference and weight

$\alpha = 0.05$

(2) Determine the test statistic

According to Formula 14.5,

$$t = \frac{r}{\sqrt{\frac{1-r^2}{n-2}}} = \frac{0.932}{\sqrt{\frac{1-0.932^2}{20-2}}} = 10.91,$$

$$\nu = n - 2 = 18$$

(3) Draw a conclusion

According to $\nu = 18$, $\alpha = 0.05$, find the critical value $t_{18,1-0.05/2} = 2.101$. As $t = 10.91 > 2.101 = t_{18,1-0.05/2}$, $p < 0.05$, we reject H_0 and accept H_1 at the $\alpha = 0.05$ level, and the correlation coefficient has statistical significance. We conclude that chest circumference and weight in 15-year-old schoolboys are correlated, and this relationship is strong.

2. Critical-Value Method
Statisticians have compiled a critical-value table of $|r|$ for hypothesis tests of correlation coefficients under different degrees of freedom ν (Appendix Table 11) so that a conclusion can be directly made after the calculation of r.

The underlying principles for this direct critical-value method are as follows:

The t-test of the correlation coefficient mentioned above is equivalent to the F-test of the regression coefficient given the same sample size, so we can obtain the relationship between r and F through formula transformation.

As the square of correlation coefficient r is the coefficient of determination in linear regression, we have

$$R^2 = \frac{SS_R}{SS_{yy}} = \frac{\frac{SS_R}{SS_E}}{\frac{SS_R}{SS_E}+1}, \tag{14.6}$$

while the test statistic F of the regression coefficient is

$$F = \frac{\frac{SS_R}{1}}{\frac{SS_E}{n-2}}. \tag{14.7}$$

Substituting F into Formula 14.6, the relationship between r and F is obtained as follows:

$$|r| = \sqrt{\frac{F}{F + (n-2)}}. \tag{14.8}$$

It can be proved that $|r|$ is strictly a monotone function of F, so that the quantile of $|r|$ can be obtained from the quantile of the F distribution. Thus, after obtaining the sample correlation coefficient, we can directly look up the critical-value $r_{\nu,1-\alpha/2}$ from Appendix Table 11 according to $\nu = n-2$ degrees of freedom and a given significance level α. We have

$$P\left(|r| > r_{\nu,1-\alpha/2}\right) = \alpha$$

If $|r| > r_{\nu,1-\alpha/2}$, then reject H_0; otherwise do not reject H_0.

Example 14.3 Perform a significance test for the correlation coefficient in Example 14.1 using the critical-value method.

Solution
According to $\nu = 18$, $\alpha = 0.05$, the critical value $r_{18,1-0.05/2} = 0.444$ is obtained from Appendix Table 11. As $|r| = 0.932 > 0.444$, $p < 0.05$. We reject H_0 and accept H_1 at the $\alpha = 0.05$ level, and the correlation coefficient has statistical significance. The conclusion is the same as in Example 14.2.

14.3 Confidence Interval Estimation for Correlation Coefficient

In Section 14.2, the t-test can be used for a significance test of the correlation coefficient. When H_0 is rejected, $\rho \neq 0$ is accepted at the $\alpha = 0.05$ level. Then we need to know the $(1-\alpha) \times 100\%$ CI of ρ. However, the sampling distribution of r is skewed when $\rho \neq 0$, and this cannot be corrected even in large samples. To establish a distribution that is more stable and approximates a normal distribution, we introduce the *Fisher's z transformation* for a transformed sample correlation coefficient so that it could be used to estimate the CI of ρ.

The Fisher's z transformation of sample correlation coefficient r is

$$z_r = \frac{1}{2} \ln \frac{1+r}{1-r}. \tag{14.9}$$

It can be proved that when the sample size increases, z_r approximately follows a normal distribution:

$$z_r \dot{\sim} N\left(\frac{1}{2} \ln \frac{1+\rho}{1-\rho}, \frac{1}{n-3}\right), \tag{14.10}$$

that is, the population mean of z_r is $\mu_{z_r} = \frac{1}{2}\ln\frac{1+\rho}{1-\rho}$, and variance is $\sigma_{z_r}^2 = \frac{1}{n-3}$.

In this way, we can estimate the $(1-\alpha)\times 100\%$ CI for ρ based on the principle of normal distribution using the following steps:

(1) Calculate the Fisher z transformation of r, $z_r = \frac{1}{2}\ln\frac{1+r}{1-r}$.

(2) According to formula 14.10, we have $\dfrac{z_r - \frac{1}{2}\ln\frac{1+\rho}{1-\rho}}{\sqrt{\frac{1}{n-3}}} \sim N(0,1)$

With simple algebraic manipulation, we obtain

$$[z_{r1}, z_{r2}] = \left[z_r - z_{1-\alpha/2}/\sqrt{n-3},\ z_r + z_{1-\alpha/2}/\sqrt{n-3}\right]. \tag{14.11}$$

(3) Invert the confidence limit of z_{r1} and z_{r2}; then the population correlation coefficient ρ is $[\rho_L, \rho_U]$, and the lower and upper limits of the CI are

$$\begin{cases} \rho_L = \dfrac{e^{2z_{r1}}-1}{e^{2z_{r1}}+1} \\ \rho_U = \dfrac{e^{2z_{r2}}-1}{e^{2z_{r2}}+1} \end{cases}. \tag{14.12}$$

Example 14.4 Referring to Example 14.1, calculate the 95% CI for ρ.

Solution

The correlation coefficient $r = 0.932$. Substitute the value into Formula 14.9,

$$z_r = \frac{1}{2}\ln\frac{1+r}{1-r} = \frac{1}{2}\ln\frac{1+0.932}{1-0.932} = 1.6734$$

$$s_{z_r} = \frac{1}{\sqrt{20-3}} = 0.2425$$

Based on Formula 14.11,
$z_{r1} = z_r - z_{1-\alpha/2}/\sqrt{n-3} = 1.6734 - 1.96\times 0.2425 = 1.1981$;
$z_{r2} = z_r + z_{1-\alpha/2}/\sqrt{n-3} = 1.6734 + 1.96\times 0.2425 = 2.1487$.
Substituting these values into Formula 14.12, we have

$$\rho_L = \frac{e^{2z_{r1}}-1}{e^{2z_{r1}}+1} = \frac{e^{2\times 1.1981}-1}{e^{2\times 1.1981}+1} = 0.833$$

$$\rho_U = \frac{e^{2z_{r2}}-1}{e^{2z_{r2}}+1} = \frac{e^{2\times 2.1487}-1}{e^{2\times 2.1487}+1} = 0.973$$

so, the 95% CI of ρ for chest circumference and weight in 20 15-year-old schoolboys is $[0.833, 0.973]$.

Note that the CI of ρ is asymmetric. The reason is that the Fisher z transformation is a nonlinear transformation of r except when $|r|$ is very small $(|r| \le 0.2)$.

14.4 Spearman's Rank Correlation

The statistical inference for the Pearson correlation mentioned in Section 14.1 is a parametric test as it requests that the two variables follow a bivariate normal distribution. When these conditions are not met, e.g., one or both of two variables are ordered or one or both are continuous but not normally distributed, we can use Spearman's rank correlation as a nonparametric alternative to analyze the association.

14.4.1 Concept of Spearman's Rank Correlation Coefficient

Spearman's rank correlation was proposed by C.E. Spearman in 1904. It uses Spearman's rank correlation coefficient to describe the degree and direction of the correlation. The basic idea of Spearman's rank correlation is that the ranks of x and y are obtained by first separately ordering their values from small to large and then computing the correlation between the two sets of ranks. The strength of correlation is denoted by the coefficient of rank correlation, named Spearman's rank correlation coefficient.

Definition 14.4 Let $(x_i, y_i)(i=1,2,\ldots, n)$ be a random sample obtained from a bivariable population. Let $\{x_i\}$ and $\{y_i\}$ be arranged in ascending order, and the ranks of x_i and y_i in their respective order be denoted by $R_i(x)$ and $R_i(y)$, respectively. Spearman's rank correlation coefficient of the sample is defined as

$$r_s = \frac{\sum_{i=1}^{n}\left(R_i(x)-\overline{R(x)}\right)\left(R_i(y)-\overline{R(y)}\right)}{\sqrt{\sum_{i=1}^{n}\left(R_i(x)-\overline{R(x)}\right)^2 \times \sum_{i=1}^{n}\left(R_i(y)-\overline{R(y)}\right)^2}}, \tag{14.13}$$

where $\overline{R(x)}=\frac{1}{n}\sum_{i=1}^{n}R_i(x)$, $\overline{R(y)}=\frac{1}{n}\sum_{i=1}^{n}R_i(y)$

The interpretation of *Spearman's rank correlation coefficient* r_s is similar to the Pearson correlation coefficient r, and r_s takes values from -1 to 1. The closer $|r_s|$ is to 1, the stronger the correlation between the ranks. The closer $|r_s|$ is to 0, the weaker is the correlation; $r_s=1$ indicates a perfect correlation of ranks, $r_s=-1$ indicates a perfect negative correlation of ranks, and $r_s=0$ indicates no linear correlation between ranks.

By comparing Formulas 14.13 and 14.3, we can see that the Spearman's rank correlation coefficient is based on the calculation of rank, and the variations of the original values of variables x and y are replaced by the variations of their corresponding ranks $R(x)$ and $R(y)$, and so are the covariances of x and y.

Example 14.5 For 10 infants with birth weights below 2000 g and born before 33 weeks of pregnancy, the mean values of serum thyroxine (μg/dL) in the first week after birth were measured. The data are given in Table 14.2. Analyze whether there is a correlation between thyroxine level and pregnancy period.

Table 14.2 Mean serum thyroxine (μg/dL) of 10 premature infants and pregnancy period (week) of the mothers.

Pregnancy period x	Rank $R_i(x)$	Mean serum thyroxine y	Rank $R_i(y)$
(1)	(2)	(3)	(4)
≤24	1	6.5	1
25	2	7.1	4
26	3	7.0	2
27	4	7.1	4
28	5	7.2	6
29	6	7.1	4
30	7	8.1	7
31	8	8.7	8
32	9	9.5	9
33	10	10.1	10

Solution

(1) Assign ranks

We arrange x and y separately in ascending order from small to large; the ranks are as shown in columns (2) and (4) of Table 14.2. Among the values, three values of y are the same (7.1 μg/dL); so the average rank is taken.

(2) Calculate Spearman's rank correlation coefficient r_s.

The basic calculations are first obtained:

$$\sum_i \left(R_i(x)-\overline{R(x)}\right)\left(R_i(y)-\overline{R(y)}\right)=(1-5.5)\times(1-5.5)+(2-5.5)\times(4-5.5)+\cdots+(10-5.5)\times(10-5.5)=76.5,$$

$$\sum_i \left(R_i(x)-\overline{R(x)}\right)^2=(1-5.5)^2+(2-5.5)^2+\cdots+(10-5.5)^2=82.5,$$

$$\sum_i \left(R_i(y)-\overline{R(y)}\right)^2=(1-5.5)^2+(4-5.5)^2+\cdots+(10-5.5)^2=80.5.$$

Substituting these values into Formula 14.13 (Definition 14.4), we have

$$r_s=\frac{\sum_i \left(R_i(x)-\overline{R(x)}\right)\left(R_i(y)-\overline{R(y)}\right)}{\sqrt{\sum_i \left(R_i(x)-\overline{R(x)}\right)^2\times\sum_i \left(R_i(y)-\overline{R(y)}\right)^2}}=\frac{76.5}{\sqrt{82.5\times 80.5}}=0.939$$

Here, the positive Spearman's rank correlation coefficient is indicative of a positive correlation between thyroid hormone level of premature infants and the pregnancy period of the mothers. The absolute value is 0.939, suggesting that the correlation between the two variables is strong.

14.4.2 Hypothesis Testing of Spearman's Rank Correlation Coefficient

Like the Pearson correlation coefficient, r_s is an estimation of the population correlation coefficient ρ_s and is subject to sampling error. Thus, hypothesis testing of $\rho_s = 0$ needs to be performed after calculating the sample r_s.

There are two methods of hypothesis testing depending on sample size:

(1) When $n \leq 50$, we can find the critical value of Spearman's rank correlation coefficient with the degrees of freedom $\nu = n-2$ from Appendix Table 12. Note that the critical value at the α level corresponds to a two-sided hypothesis.
(2) Hotelling and Pabst (1936) proved that Spearman's rank correlation coefficient enjoys a large sample property, that is, when $n \to \infty$, we have

$$Z = r_s\sqrt{n-1} \dot{\sim} N(0,1). \tag{14.14}$$

Therefore, we can adopt a normal approximate method to perform hypothesis testing when n exceeds the range of the critical-value table.

Example 14.6 Perform a significance test for the correlation coefficient in Example 14.5.

Solution
Here $n = 10$; we use the critical-value table method to perform hypothesis testing. According to $\nu = n-2 = 8$ and $\alpha = 0.05$, we find $r_{s(8,1-0.05/2)} = 0.738$ in Appendix Table 12. As $|r_s| = 0.939 > 0.738$, $p < 0.05$. We reject H_0 and accept H_1 at the $\alpha = 0.05$ level and conclude that the mean serum thyroxin level and pregnancy age in premature infants are strongly correlated.

An easy way to think about the difference between the two types of correlation is to recognize that the Pearson correlation quantifies the linear relationship between x and y, while the Spearman correlation coefficient quantifies the monotonic relationship between x and y.

14.5 Summary

Unlike the relationship in simple linear regression, where one variable is functionally dependent on another, linear correlation is preferred when studying a bidirectional linear relationship between two variables. The correlation coefficient is used to quantify the strength and direction of the linear correlation of two variables.

In linear correlation analyses, the observed values must be independent of each other. Pearson correlation coefficient is suitable for data following a bivariate normal distribution. It is not the best way to capture the information of deviation within and between variables and is thus not suitable for analysis of correlation. Spearman's correlation coefficient, based on the ranks of the data, is a good alternative in such cases.

Whether a correlation exists needs to be judged based on hypothesis testing. The test methods can be divided into *t*-test and critical-value method. Nevertheless, the decision on whether there is a real relationship between the two variables should be primarily based on background knowledge rather than simply depending on the statistical significance of the test of the correlation coefficient.

14.6 Exercises

1. Twelve 20-year-old men were randomly chosen from a university, and their height (cm) and length of forearm (cm) were measured and recorded. The data are given in Table 14.3.

Please answer the following questions:

(a) Inspect the relationship between height and forearm length by drawing a scatterplot. Make a preliminary visual judgment of whether a linear or nonlinear relationship exists between them.

(b) Test whether there is a relationship between height and length of forearm? Provide H_0 and H_1.

(c) What are the assumptions for conducting such procedures? Check whether such assumptions hold.

(d) Calculate the correlation coefficient between height and length of forearm, conduct the test procedure, and interpret the result.

(e) Provide a 95% CI for ρ.

(f) Is it appropriate to build a regression equation on this sample?

Table 14.3 Height (cm) and length of forearm (cm) of 12 20-year-old men.

ID	1	2	3	4	5	6	7	8	9	10	11	12
Height	170	173	160	168	173	188	178	183	179	169	175	174
Length of forearm	45	42	44	41	47	50	47	46	49	43	46	47

2. A study was conducted to investigate the association between platelet count and bleeding symptoms, 14 patients were inducted, and their platelet count ($\times 10^9$/L) as well as their bleeding symptoms were measured. The results are presented in Table 14.4.

Please answer the following questions:

(a) Consider the types of data collected in this study. Is it appropriate to assess the correlation between platelet count and bleeding symptoms by calculating the Pearson correlation coefficients? Why?

(b) Choose an appropriate method discussed in this chapter to assess the correlation between platelet count and bleeding symptoms. Then, conduct a statistical test for the correlation coefficient obtained and interpret the result.

Table 14.4 Patients' platelet count ($\times 10^9$/L) and bleeding symptoms.

Patient ID	Platelet count	Bleeding symptoms	Patient ID	Platelet count	Bleeding symptoms
1	120	++	8	1060	−
2	130	+++	9	1260	−
3	160	±	10	1230	−
4	310	±	11	1440	±
5	420	+	12	1600	−
6	540	+	13	1800	−
7	740	−	14	2000	−

3. In a survey of 447 women who had just given birth, the investigator recorded the lactation level of the women at different ages. You are provided with the summarized data, as given in Table 14.5, for help with the statistical issues below.

(a) The investigator wants to use a χ^2 test to see whether age is associated with lactation level. Is it appropriate? Why? If not, what is your suggestion?

(b) Suppose that the investigator is interested in whether there is a difference in the lactation levels of the three age groups or between different age groups. What is your analysis plan? What if the question is whether there is a difference in the lactation levels between women aged below and over 30 years?

(c) Suppose that the investigator presents you with the individual-level raw data regarding age and lactation amount (both as continuous data). Would there be any changes in the analysis plans for question (a)?

Table 14.5 Lactation level in women at different ages.

Age group (years)	Lactation level			
	None	Few	Barely sufficient	Adequate
<25	4	6	11	200
25–	6	18	113	80
30–	10	26	12	1

15

Multiple Linear Regression

CONTENTS

In our discussion of simple linear regression in Chapter 13, we were concerned with the linear relationship between the mean value of dependent variable y and an independent variable (or, predictive variable) x. In practice, most applications of regression analysis use more complex models. Often, there is more than one independent variable, and we would like to evaluate the relationship between each of the independent variables $x_1, x_2, \ldots, x_k$ and the dependent variable y after considering the remaining independent variables. This type of problem falls into the domain of multiple regression analysis. Different regression methods are available for different types of data. In this chapter, we discuss multiple linear regression, in which the outcome variable is continuous. In Chapter 16, we discuss logistic regression (categorical outcome), and in Chapter 17, we discuss Cox's proportional hazards regression for modeling time-to-event outcomes. All these regression methods are widely applied and effective in biostatistical research.

Applied Medical Statistics, First Edition. Jingmei Jiang.

Companion website: www.wiley.com\go\jiang\appliedmedicalstatistics

15.1 Multiple Linear Regression Model

15.1.1 Concept of the Multiple Linear Regression

Let us consider the following example:

Example 15.1 Recall Example 13.1, in which we explored the linear relationship between weight and forced vital capacity (FVC) of 20 schoolboys. We can use the linear regression model to predict the mean value of FVC given the value of weight. However, we know that FVC may be affected by several other factors, such as age, hip circumference, and height. Intuitively, we should be able to improve our predictive ability by including more independent variables in such a model. Therefore, we add age to the analysis to examine the combined effects of age (years) and weight (kg) on the lung function of the schoolboys, with FVC (L) as a measurement of lung function. The data of 60 schoolboys are given in Table 15.1. How do we describe and test the relationship between these variables?

As in simple linear regression, first, we want to know whether y has a linear relationship with each x. Therefore, before analyzing the data, we construct scatterplots of the relationships between the variables. This is accomplished by making separate plots of each pair of variables, (x_1, y), (x_2, y), and (x_1, x_2). A software package such as SPSS can display each combination simultaneously in a matrix format, as shown in Figure 15.1.

The scatterplots indicate that there are positive linear correlations between FVC and age and FVC and weight. Furthermore, we can see that there is a positive linear correlation between age and weight (we will discuss the correlation between independent variables in Section 15.4.1).

Suppose a relationship is postulated between FVC (y), age (x_1), and weight (x_2), which can be expressed as

$$y_i = \beta_0 + \beta_1 x_{i1} + \beta_2 x_{i2} + \varepsilon_i \ (i = 1, 2, \ldots, n). \tag{15.1}$$

We wish to make an inference about the linear function. For example, we may wish to estimate $E(y)$ given by

$$E(\text{FVC}) = \beta_0 + \beta_1 \text{age} + \beta_2 \text{weight},$$

where $E(\text{FVC})$ represents the mean FVC for the settings of the predictive variables, age and weight.

More generally, if we consider regressing one dependent variable on k independent variables, we may obtain the definition of the multiple linear regression model.

Definition 15.1 Assume that the expectation (mean) of y is a function of a set of independent variables $x_1, x_2, \ldots, x_k$, where the function is linear in a set of unknown parameters. Then for y, the expression

$$y_i = \beta_0 + \beta_1 x_{i1} + \beta_2 x_{i2} + \cdots + \beta_k x_{ik} + \varepsilon_i \ (i = 1, 2, \ldots, n) \tag{15.2}$$

is called a *multiple linear regression model*, where dependent variable y is decomposed into two components: ε is an error component, which is the random component of the

Table 15.1 Data for age (years), weight (kg), and FVC (L) in 60 schoolboys.

ID	Age	Weight	FVC	ID	Age	Weight	FVC
	x_1	x_2	y		x_1	x_2	y
1	11	37	2.21	31	16	70	4.60
2	11	29	2.64	32	17	79	5.29
3	11	49	2.64	33	14	67	4.20
4	10	37	2.09	34	11	33	2.75
5	13	38	2.89	35	17	56	4.15
6	12	36	2.11	36	14	51	3.93
7	15	48	3.24	37	13	34	2.80
8	15	47	3.29	38	12	32	2.57
9	13	46	3.04	39	10	33	2.69
10	11	37	2.33	40	16	56	4.25
11	17	58	3.79	41	12	33	2.49
12	15	38	2.85	42	14	46	3.24
13	11	35	2.35	43	12	33	2.51
14	13	35	2.43	44	11	33	1.96
15	12	31	1.91	45	11	43	2.80
16	14	65	4.41	46	15	77	5.10
17	17	67	5.36	47	10	49	3.24
18	14	54	3.55	48	14	51	2.99
19	17	52	3.99	49	12	33	2.50
20	12	35	2.73	50	16	59	3.81
21	16	67	5.14	51	16	46	2.65
22	12	45	3.23	52	14	68	4.54
23	12	55	2.94	53	18	62	4.30
24	12	46	3.89	54	15	50	3.40
25	14	57	4.11	55	17	61	3.74
26	12	40	2.33	56	15	60	4.43
27	16	47	3.26	57	10	41	2.26
28	15	49	3.89	58	15	76	5.67
29	15	45	3.47	59	15	51	3.84
30	14	41	2.59	60	10	29	1.86

model, $E(y) = \beta_0 + \beta_1 x_1 + \cdots + \beta_k x_k$ is the systematic component of the model, $\beta_1, \ldots, \beta_k$ are called the *partial-regression coefficients*, and β_0 is called the *intercept*.

The partial-regression coefficient $\beta_{j'}$ represents the amount by which y changes on average when $x_{j'}$ changes by one unit and all the other $x_j (j \neq j')$ remain constant. Here variables $x_1, x_2, \ldots, x_k$ can be continuous or categorical.

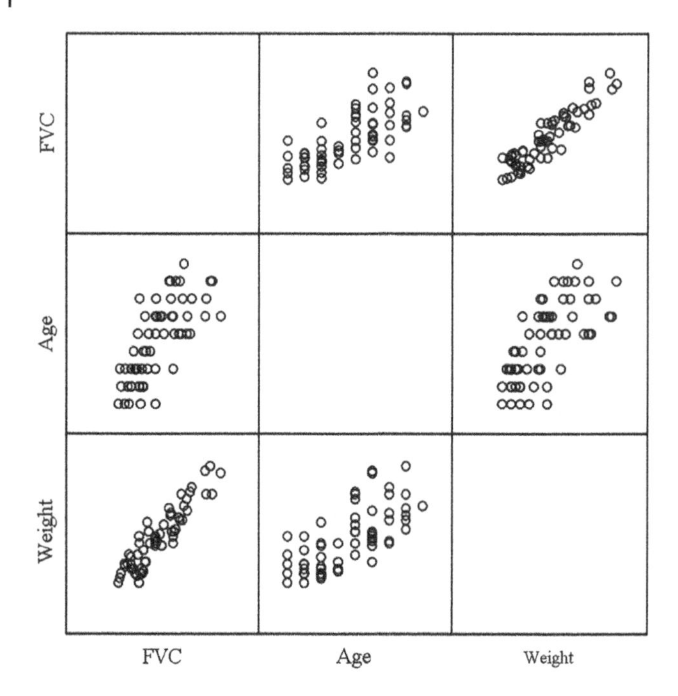

Figure 15.1 Scatterplots of the relationships between variables

Note: The symbols $x_1, x_2, \ldots, x_k$ may represent higher-order terms for numerical predictors, such as x^2.

Model Assumptions

(1) The mean of ε is 0, that is, $E(\varepsilon) = 0$, indicating that the mean of y is equivalent to the systematic component of the model, i.e., $E(y) = \beta_0 + \beta_1 x_1 + \cdots + \beta_k x_k$.
(2) For all settings of the independent variables $x_1, x_2, \ldots, x_k$, the variance of ε is constant.
(3) The error components ε are mutually independent and normally distributed.

These assumptions do not impact the calculation of regression statistics if they are violated, but they do underlie the performance of hypothesis testing and the expression of confidence intervals. Fortunately, regression analysis is robust to some deviation from these assumptions, especially when n is large.

In the multiple linear regression model (Definition 15.1), the partial-regression coefficient $\beta_j\left(j = 1, 2, \ldots, k\right)$ is unknown, the estimated b_j can be obtained by fitting the regression model with the sample data; then the multiple linear regression model can be estimated as

$$\hat{y}_i = b_0 + b_1 x_{i1} + b_2 x_{i2} + \cdots + b_k x_{ik} \left(i = 1, 2, \ldots, n\right), \tag{15.3}$$

where $\hat{y}$ is the predicted value of y and $b_0, b_1, b_2, \ldots, b_k$ are the estimates of $\beta_0, \beta_1, \beta_2, \ldots, \beta_k$, respectively.

Once a model has been chosen to relate $E(y)$ to a set of independent variables $x_1, x_2, \ldots, x_k$, the steps of a multiple linear regression analysis parallel those of a simple regression analysis. The only differences are that the mathematical theory and the computations are considerably more complex; the former is beyond the scope of this text. In the following sections, we will present the methods for estimating and hypothesis testing the model parameters. Because most multiple regression analyses are performed on a computer, we also present how to interpret the output produced by statistical software.

15.1.2 Least Squares Estimation of Regression Coefficient

As introduced in Section 13.2.1 for simple linear regression, the least squares estimation in multiple linear regression also requires the minimum residual sum of squares.

Let $Q(\beta)$ denote this sum, where $\beta=(\beta_0,\beta_1,\beta_2,\ldots,\beta_k)$; it is clear that this sum is a function of $\beta=(\beta_0,\beta_1,\beta_2,\ldots,\beta_k)$ only, that is,

$$\begin{aligned} Q(\beta_0, \beta_1, \beta_2,\ldots, \beta_k) &= \sum_{i=1}^{n} \varepsilon_i^2 = \sum_{i=1}^{n} \left(y_i - E(y_i)\right)^2 \\ &= \sum_{i=1}^{n} \left(y_i - \beta_0 - \beta_1 x_{i1} - \beta_2 x_{i2} - \cdots - \beta_k x_{ik}\right)^2. \end{aligned} \tag{15.4}$$

For this function to have the minimum value, the partial derivatives of $Q(\beta)$ in Formula 15.4 with respect to the parameters β_0 and $\beta_j (j=1,2,\ldots,k)$ must satisfy the following equations:

$$\begin{cases} \dfrac{\partial Q(\beta)}{\partial \beta_0} = -2\sum_{i=1}^{n}\left(y_i - \beta_0 - \sum_{j=1}^{k}\beta_j x_{ij}\right) = 0 \\ \dfrac{\partial Q(\beta)}{\partial \beta_j} = -2\sum_{i=1}^{n}\left(y_i - \beta_0 - \sum_{j=1}^{k}\beta_j x_{ij}\right)x_{ij} = 0\ (j=1,2,\ldots,k) \end{cases}. \tag{15.5}$$

Formula 15.5 produces the following equations:

$$\begin{cases} n\beta_0 + \sum_{i=1}^{n} x_{i1}\beta_1 + \sum_{i=1}^{n} x_{i2}\beta_2 + \cdots + \sum_{i=1}^{n} x_{ik}\beta_k = \sum_{i=1}^{n} y_i \\ \sum_{i=1}^{n} x_{i1}\beta_0 + \sum_{i=1}^{n} x_{i1}^2\beta_1 + \sum_{i=1}^{n} x_{i1}x_{i2}\beta_2 + \cdots + \sum_{i=1}^{n} x_{i1}x_{ik}\beta_k = \sum_{i=1}^{n} x_{i1}y_i \\ \sum_{i=1}^{n} x_{i2}\beta_0 + \sum_{i=1}^{n} x_{i1}x_{i2}\beta_1 + \sum_{i=1}^{n} x_{i2}^2\beta_2 + \cdots + \sum_{i=1}^{n} x_{i2}x_{ik}\beta_k = \sum_{i=1}^{n} x_{i2}y_i \\ \vdots \\ \sum_{i=1}^{n} x_{ik}\beta_0 + \sum_{i=1}^{n} x_{i1}x_{ik}\beta_1 + \sum_{i=1}^{n} x_{i2}x_{ik}\beta_2 + \cdots + \sum_{i=1}^{n} x_{ik}^2\beta_k = \sum_{i=1}^{n} x_{ik}y_i \end{cases}. \tag{15.6}$$

Formula 15.6, which are obtained using the least squares estimation, are commonly called *normal equations*. Normal equations are the multivariate extensions of Formula 13.7. In general, a unique solution exists. $b_0, b_1, b_2, \ldots, b_k$ are called the *least squares estimates* of the model parameters $\beta_0, \beta_1, \beta_2, \ldots, \beta_k$, denoted by

$$Q(b_0, b_1, b_2, \ldots, b_k) = \min_{\beta_0, \beta_1, \beta_2, \ldots, \beta_k} Q(\beta_0, \beta_1, \beta_2, \ldots, \beta_k). \tag{15.7}$$

Example 15.2 Estimate the parameters of the multiple linear regression model using the data in Table 15.1.

Solution

Use the SPSS software program to obtain the least squares estimates. The results are given in Table 15.2.

According to the parameter-estimate column (unstandardized coefficient), $b_0 = -0.464$, $b_1 = 0.072$, and $b_2 = 0.059$. Then, the estimated multiple linear regression model is

$$\hat{y} = -0.464 + 0.072x_1 + 0.059x_2. \tag{15.8}$$

Example 15.3 Calculate the predicted (mean) FVC of a 12-year-old schoolboy weighing 40 kg using Formula 15.8.

Solution

The mean FVC is estimated as

$$-0.464 + 0.072 \times 12 + 0.059 \times 40 = 2.76\text{L}$$

Example 15.4 Interpret the partial-regression coefficients in Formula 15.8.

Solution

The estimated partial-regression coefficient for age $b_1 = 0.072$ L/year represents the estimated average increase in FVC per 1-year increase in age for schoolboys of the same weight. The estimated partial-regression coefficient for weight $b_2 = 0.059$ L/kg represents the estimated average increase in FVC per 1 kg increase in weight for schoolboys of the same age. Therefore, b_1 is an estimate of the relationship between y

Table 15.2 Estimator for the partial-regression coefficient and standard error.

Model	Unstandardized coefficient		Standardized coefficient	t	p value
	Coefficient	Standard error			
Intercept	−0.464	0.2896		−1.60	0.115
Age	0.072	0.0293	0.168	2.46	0.017
Weight	0.059	0.0050	0.805	11.78	<0.001

and x_1 after removing the effects of x_2 on y (i.e., holding x_2 constant) and b_2 estimates the relationship between y and x_2 after removing the effects of x_1 (i.e., holding x_1 a constant).

Points of note: (i) Partial-regression coefficients differ from simple linear regression coefficients; the latter represent the average increase in y per unit increase in x without considering any other independent variables. If there are relationships among the independent variables in a multiple regression model, then the partial-regression coefficients may differ from the simple linear regression coefficients obtained from considering each independent variable separately. (ii) If independent variables are highly correlated (called multicollinearity, see Section 15.4.1) in the model, then the interpretation of partial-regression coefficient becomes questionable, as does the testing of hypotheses about the coefficients.

15.1.3 Properties of the Least Squares Estimators

Some properties of these estimators are as follows (proof omitted):

(1) $E(b_j) = \beta_j (j = 0, 1, \ldots, k)$ and b_j is also the minimum variance unbiased estimator of β_j.
(2) The sampling distribution of each b_j is normally distributed.
(3) The variance of error $S^2 = SS_E / [n - (k+1)]$ is an unbiased estimator of σ^2. The statistics S^2 and b_j are mutually independent $(j = 0, 1, \ldots, k)$.

15.1.4 Standardized Partial-Regression Coefficient

In practice, we are often interested in ranking the effect of independent variables according to their predictive relationship with the dependent variable y. It is difficult to rank the variables based on the magnitude of the partial-regression coefficients because the independent variables are often in different units; for example, in Example 15.1, the units are years (age) and kilograms (weight). Therefore, the effect of different measurement units should be eliminated before the effects of each variable on the regression model are compared.

Definition 15.2 The estimated *standardized partial-regression coefficient*, denoted by b_j', represents the estimated average increase in y (expressed in standard deviation units of y) per standard deviation increase in x, after adjusting for all other variables in the model.

$$b_j' = \frac{S_{x_j}}{S_y} b_j, \tag{15.9}$$

where S_{x_j} is the standard deviation of the independent variable x_j, S_y is the standard deviation of the dependent variable, and b_j is its partial-regression coefficient. Because b_j' is unit-free, the absolute value of b_j' can be directly compared to reflect the effect of the independent variables on the dependent variable y. The greater the absolute value of b_j', the greater is the effect of x_j on y.

Example 15.5 Refer to Example 15.1. Compute the standardized partial-regression coefficients for age and weight using the data in Tables 15.1 and 15.2.

Solution

From Table 15.1, we have the basic summary statistics $s_y = 0.955$, $s_{x_1} = 2.23$, and $s_{x_2} = 13.13$. Then the standardized partial-regression coefficients using Definition 15.2 are as follows:

For age, $b_1' = \frac{s_{x_1}}{s_y} b_1 = \frac{2.23}{0.955} \times 0.072 = 0.168$

For weight, $b_2' = \frac{s_{x_2}}{s_y} b_2 = \frac{13.13}{0.955} \times 0.059 = 0.811$

Notice that here the difference with the result from Table 15.2, $b_2' = 0.805$, is because of a calculating error.

Thus, the average increase in FVC is 0.168 standard deviation units of FVC per standard deviation increase in age, holding weight constant, and 0.811 standard deviation units of FVC per standard deviation increase in weight, holding age constant. Thus, weight appears to be the more important variable for FVC in this model.

15.2 Hypothesis Testing

The partial-regression coefficient $b_j\left(j = 1, 2, \ldots, k\right)$ calculated from the sample is an estimate of β_j. Even if the estimate of the partial-regression coefficient b is not 0, the partial-regression coefficient β may be equal to 0. Therefore, as in simple linear regression, it is necessary to test the regression model and each partial-regression coefficient after establishing the regression model.

15.2.1 *F*-Test for Overall Regression Model

The F-test, that is, analysis-of-variance testing, can be used to examine the hypothesis of the multiple linear regression model. The basic principle is similar to that in simple linear regression, that is, to decompose the total variation in the dependent variable y into two parts. One part reflects the effect of the regression model on the variation of y, while the other part reflects the effect of all factors other than the regression model on the variation of y. By comparing the two parts of the variation, the overall regression model is tested to identify whether it is statistically significant.

(1) State the hypotheses and select a significance level

$H_0 : \beta_1 = \beta_2 = \cdots = \beta_k = 0$
H_1 : at least one of the $\beta_j \neq 0$ $(j = 1,2,\ldots,k)$
Let α be the significance level

(2) Determine the test statistic

(i) The decomposition of the sum of squares

The total variation of the dependent variable y is reflected by the total sum of squares SS_{yy}, which can be decomposed into two parts: the regression sum of squares SS_R and the residual sum of squares SS_E, that is

$$SS_{yy} = \sum_{i=1}^{n}(y_i - \bar{y})^2 = \sum_{i=1}^{n}(\hat{y}_i - \bar{y})^2 + \sum_{i=1}^{n}(y_i - \hat{y}_i)^2 \\ = SS_R + SS_E, \tag{15.10}$$

where $\hat{y}_i = b_0 + \sum_{j=1}^{k} b_j x_{ij}$.

(ii) The decomposition of degrees of freedom

The total degrees of freedom of the dependent variable can also be decomposed into two parts, the regression degrees of freedom ν_R and the residual degrees of freedom ν_E

$$\nu_{yy} = n-1 \\ \nu_R = k \\ \nu_E = \nu_{yy} - \nu_R = n-k-1, \tag{15.11}$$

where n is the sample size, and k is the number of independent variables in the model.

(iii) Compute mean square and the test statistic

$$MS_R = \frac{SS_R}{\nu_R}, \quad MS_E = \frac{SS_E}{\nu_E}. \tag{15.12}$$

When H_0 is true, the test statistic

$$F = \frac{SS_R / k}{SS_E / (n-k-1)} \sim F(\nu_R, \nu_E). \tag{15.13}$$

(3) Draw a conclusion

For a given α and degrees of freedom $\nu_R = k$, $\nu_E = n-k-1$, we can obtain the critical value $F_{(k,n-k-1),1-\alpha}$ from the F distribution (Appendix Table 6).

If $F > F_{(k,n-k-1),1-\alpha}$, then reject H_0

If $F \le F_{(k,n-k-1),1-\alpha}$, then do not reject H_0

Example 15.6 Refer to Example 15.1. Test whether the multiple linear regression model is significant.

Solution

(1) State the hypotheses and select a significance level

$H_0: \beta_1 = \beta_2 = 0$, i.e., age and weight have no linear relationship with FVC

H_1: at least one of β_1 and β_2 is not zero, i.e., at least age or weight has a linear relationship with FVC

$\alpha = 0.05$

Table 15.3 ANOVA table for Example 15.1.

Source of variation	Sum of squares	ν	Mean square	F	p value
Regression	46.5623	2	23.2812	182.65	<0.001
Residual	7.2652	57	0.1275		
Total	53.8275	59			

(2) Determine the test statistic and drawn a conclusion

From Table 15.3, we have $SS_R = 46.5623$, $\nu_R = 2$ and $SS_E = 7.2652$, $\nu_E = 57$. Thus, the test statistic

$$F = \frac{SS_R / \nu_R}{SS_E / \nu_E} = \frac{46.5623/2}{7.2652/57} = 182.65.$$

According to the values in Table 15.3 and $\alpha = 0.05$, $p < 0.05$, we then reject H_0 and accept H_1 at the $\alpha = 0.05$ level. We conclude that there is an overall linear regression relationship between FVC and at least one of the variables, age and weight.

15.2.2 *t*-Test for Partial-Regression Coefficients

F-test tests the significance of the joint relationship of y with the predictor variables. It is usually interesting to study the sampling variation of each $b_j\left(j=1,2,\ldots,k\right)$ separately. This not only provides information about the precision of the partial-regression coefficients but also enables each of them to be tested for a significant departure from zero. We introduce the t-test as it is commonly used to test the partial-regression coefficient in common statistical analysis software.

(i) State the hypotheses and select a significance level
$H_0: \beta_j = 0 (j=1,2,\ldots,k)$, $\beta_{j'} \neq 0$ $(j' \neq j)$(let $X_{j'}$s remain constant)
$H_1: \beta_j \neq 0$, $\beta_{j'} \neq 0$ $(j' \neq j)$
Let α be the significance level
(ii) Determine the test statistic
When H_0 is true, the test statistic

$$t_j = \frac{b_j - 0}{S_{b_j}} \sim t\left(\nu\right), \tag{15.14}$$

where $\nu = \nu_E = n-k-1$, S_{b_j} is the standard error of b_j and k is the number of independent variables.
(iii) Draw a conclusion
For a given α and degrees of freedom $n-k-1$, we can obtain the critical value $t_{n-k-1,1-\alpha/2}$ from the t distribution (Appendix Table 4),
If $t_j < -t_{n-k-1,1-\alpha/2}$ or $t_j > t_{n-k-1,1-\alpha/2}$, then reject H_0;
If $-t_{n-k-1,1-\alpha/2} \leq t_j \leq t_{n-k-1,1-\alpha/2}$, then do not reject H_0.

We ordinarily obtain the results using statistical software.

In addition, because the sampling distribution of b approximates to a normal distribution, the partial-regression coefficient and its standard error can be estimated, and the $(1-\alpha)\times 100\%$ CI for β_j is

$$\left[b_j - t_{n-k-1,1-\alpha/2}S_{b_j}, b_j + t_{n-k-1,1-\alpha/2}S_{b_j}\right]. \quad (15.15)$$

Example 15.7 Refer to Example 15.1. Test for the independent contributions of age and weight in predicting FVC in schoolboys using the output in Table 15.2.

Solution

First, we test the null hypothesis that age is irrelevant in predicting FVC.
State the hypotheses and select a significance level

$H_0: \beta_1 = 0,\ \beta_2 \neq 0$, the partial-regression coefficient for age is zero and that for weight is constant

$H_1: \beta_1 \neq 0,\ \beta_2 \neq 0$, the partial-regression coefficient for age is not zero and that for weight is constant

$\alpha = 0.05$

All the results are shown in Table 15.2.

For age: we have $b_1 = 0.072$ and $s_{b_1} = 0.0293$

Thus, the test statistic is $t = \dfrac{b_1 - 0}{s_{b_1}} = \dfrac{0.072}{0.0293} = 2.457$, $p = 0.017 < 0.05$

Similarly, for weight: we have $b_2 = 0.059$ and $s_{b_2} = 0.0050$

Thus, the test statistic is $t = \dfrac{b_2 - 0}{s_{b_2}} = \dfrac{0.059}{0.0050} = 11.800$, $p < 0.001 < 0.05$

In summary, we reject H_0 and accept H_1 at the $\alpha = 0.05$ level; both partial-regression coefficients are significant; each predictor variable (age and weight) contributes separately to the effectiveness of the overall regression. It is likely that the overall multiple regression fitted to the sample data applies to all schoolboys in that region.

Example 15.8 Refer to Example 15.1. Estimate the 95% CI for the population partial-regression coefficient of age and weight.

Solution

Here, $b_1 = 0.072$, $s_{b_1} = 0.0293$, and $b_2 = 0.059$, $s_{b_2} = 0.0050$ (Table 15.2.)

According to $\nu_E = 57$, $\alpha = 0.05$, the critical value $t_{57,1\text{-}0.05/2} = 2.002$ can be obtained from the t_{57} distribution (calculated by Excel). Then the two-sided 95% CI for age coefficient β_1 is

$$\begin{aligned}&[b_1 - t_{57,1\text{-}0.05/2}s_{b_1},\ b_1 + t_{57,1\text{-}0.05/2}s_{b_1}]\\&=[0.072 - 2.002\times 0.0293, 0.072+2.002\times 0.0293]\\&=[0.013, 0.131]\ \text{L/year}.\end{aligned}$$

Similarly, the two-sided 95% CI for weight coefficient β_2 is $[0.049, 0.068]$ L/kg.

Points of note:

(1) A final fitted regression model should not include predictive variables that have neither statistical significance nor clinical significance.
(2) F-test is about the overall model, and the t-test is about the individual partial-regression coefficients. Unless in the context of simple linear regression, the F-test and t-test cannot replace each other as they have different ways of dealing with the variations and random errors.
(3) Unstandardized and standardized partial-regression coefficients have distinct roles in multiple regression analysis. Partial-regression coefficients in their original form (unstandardized) describe the dependence of the dependent variable on the independent variables and are used for modeling purposes, whereas standardized partial-regression coefficients are used for making meaningful comparisons of the contributions of the independent variables to the dependent variable.

15.3 Evaluation of Model Fitting

Several methods can be used to comprehensively assess the goodness of fit of multiple linear regression model. The commonly used indicators include the coefficient of determination and adjusted coefficient of determination.

15.3.1 Coefficient of Determination and Adjusted Coefficient of Determination

The basis of the coefficient of determination is similar to that of simple linear regression:

$$R^2 = \frac{SS_R}{SS_{yy}} = 1 - \frac{SS_E}{SS_{yy}}, \tag{15.16}$$

which explains what proportion of the variation in the observed values of the response variable y is explained by the entire set of independent variables $x_1, x_2, \ldots, x_k$. R^2 ranges between 0 and 1, and the higher value of R^2, the better the model fit. In general, no meaning can be attached to the direction of a multiple correlation with more than one predictor variable, and the correlation coefficient is always given a positive value.

Example 15.9 Refer to Example 15.1. Compute R^2.

Solution
For the illustrative example in Table 15.3, we have $SS_{yy} = 53.8275$, $SS_R = 46.5623$. Thus

$$R^2 = \frac{SS_R}{SS_{yy}} = \frac{46.5623}{53.8275} = 0.865$$

Therefore, we say that 86.5% of the total variation in y is explained by the fitted regression, that is, by the linear relationship with age and weight.

However, R^2 is not a satisfactory measure of fit. In the process of variable selection, R^2 increases as further variables are introduced into a regression and therefore cannot be used to compare regressions with different numbers of variables. The value of R^2

may be adjusted to take account of the chance contribution of each variable included by subtracting the value that would be expected if none of the variables was associated with y. The *adjusted coefficient of determination*, denoted by R^2_{adj}, is

$$R^2_{adj} = 1 - \frac{\text{MS}_E}{\text{MS}_{yy}} = 1 - \frac{n-1}{n-k-1}\left(1 - R^2\right), \tag{15.17}$$

where n is the sample size and k is the number of independent variables in the fitted model.

Thus, in the process of variable selection for the regression model, when an independent variable with no significant effect is included in the regression model, R^2 will become larger than if that variable was omitted and R^2_{adj} will be smaller. Therefore, the larger R^2_{adj} is, the better the fitting effect of the regression model.

The range of R^2_{adj} is between 0 and 1. The closer it is to 1, the better is the fit of the linear regression model. The model that has the largest R^2_{adj} is the optimal linear regression model.

Example 15.10 Refer to Example 15.1. Compute the R^2_{adj}.

Solution

For our illustrative example in Table 15.3, we have $\text{SS}_{yy} = 53.8275$, $\nu_{yy} = 59$, and $\text{SS}_E = 7.2652$, $\nu_E = 57$. Thus,

$$R^2_{adj} = 1 - \frac{\text{MS}_E}{\text{MS}_{yy}} = 1 - \frac{\text{SS}_E / \nu_E}{\text{SS}_{yy} / \nu_{yy}} = 1 - \frac{7.2652 / 57}{53.8275 / 59} = 0.860$$

Because the effects of both age and weight on FVC are significant, both evaluation indicators R^2 and R^2_{adj} are similar. Therefore, we say that this regression model is a good fit after considering the number of variables.

It should be noted that, both R^2 and R^2_{adj} are statistics, so they should follow an F-test of the overall model, and should not be used to determine the model fit alone.

15.3.2 Residual Analysis and Outliers

In Chapter 13, we introduced the use of residual analysis to check whether the assumptions about random errors in simple linear models are satisfied. In the multiple regression model, it is also an important way to evaluate the fit of the linear regression model.

If the hypothesis of the multiple linear regression model is true and the fitted model describes this set of data well, the scatter in the residual plot with the predicted value $\hat{y}$ as the x-axis should be randomly distributed with no trend around the x-axis, and the residual will not change with the change in the index of the x-axis. Otherwise, there may be other variables that affect the dependent variable besides the independent variables in the model, or the relationship between the dependent and the independent variables is not linear.

In practice, the standard error of each of the fitted residuals is different and depends on the distance of the corresponding sample point from the average of the sample points used in fitting the regression line. Thus, we generally use the standardized residual, which is the residual value divided by standard deviation s. If a residual is greater than 3s (in absolute value), or, equivalently, a standardized residual is greater than 2 or 3 (in absolute value), we consider it an outlier and seek background information that may explain its large value. We can see from Figure 15.2 that all values of standardized residuals lie within $\pm$ 3, indicating that there are no outliers in this sample.

Example 15.11 Refer to Example 15.1. Assess the goodness of fit of the multiple regression model by residual plot.

Solution

We plot the standardized residuals against the predicted FVC (Figure 15.2(a)) and each of the independent variables age and weight (Figures 15.2(b) and 15.2(c)).

The three scatterplots show a relatively random scatter of points above and below a horizontal line at 0, this means that the linearity and homogeneity of variances assumptions are assumed to be met.

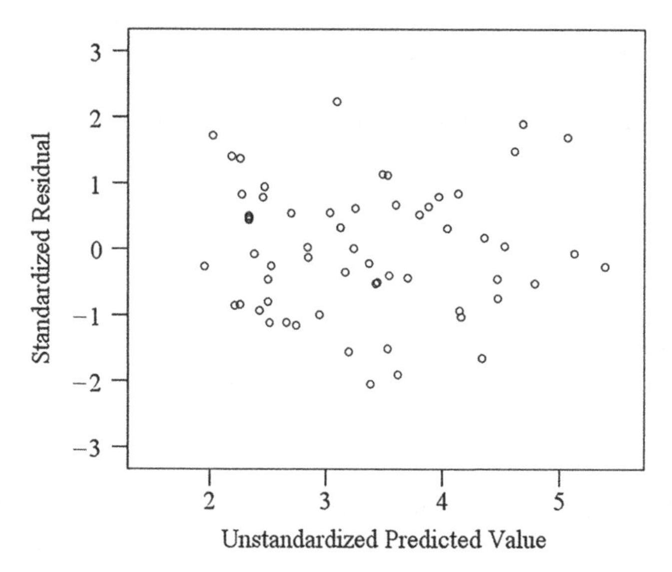

Figure 15.2(a) Plot of standardized residuals vs. predicted values of FVC for the multiple regression model in Example 15.1.

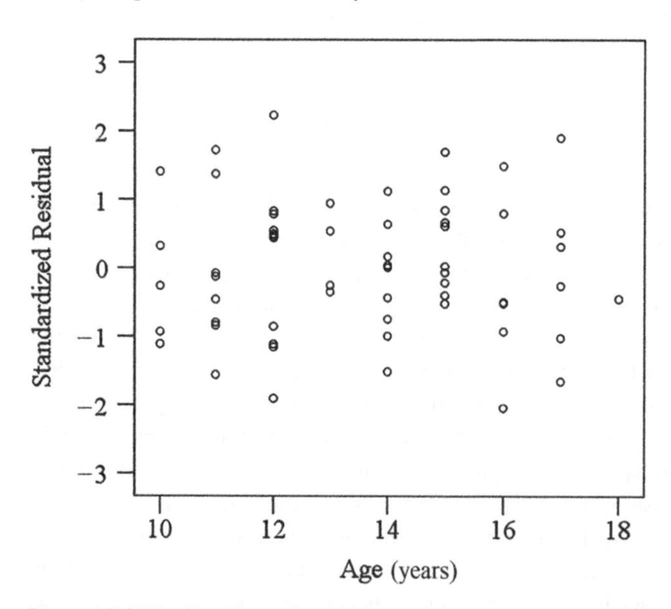

Figure 15.2(b) Plot of standardized residuals vs. age for the multiple regression model in Example 15.1.

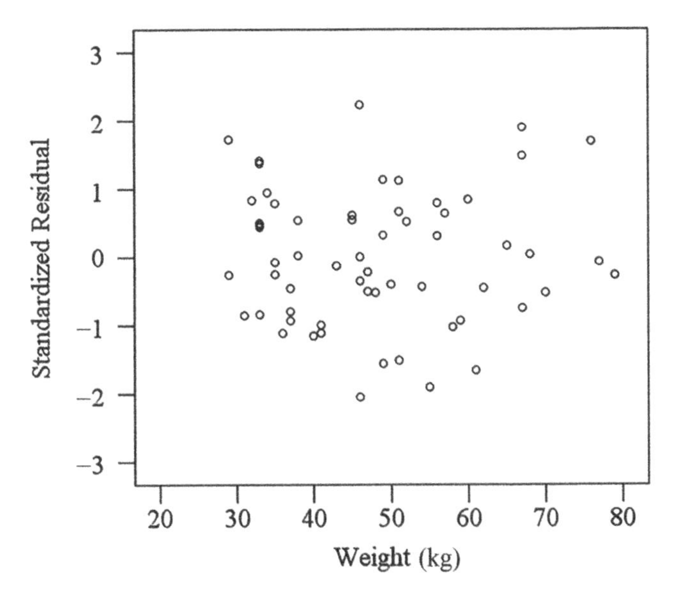

Figure 15.2(c) Plot of standardized residuals vs. weight for the multiple regression model in Example 15.1.

15.4 Other Aspects of Regression

15.4.1 Multicollinearity

Sometimes, two or more of the independent variables used in the model for $E(y)$ will contribute redundant information, that is, the independent variables will be correlated to each other. For example, in Figure 15.1, besides FVC and age and FVC and weight, age and weight also have a positive correlation. The Pearson correlation coefficient is 0.701 $(p<0.05)$. Thus, although both age and weight contribute information for the prediction of FVC, some of the information overlaps because age and weight are correlated. When the independent variables are corresponding, we say that *multicollinearity* exists. In practice, it is not uncommon to observe correlations among the independent variables. However, when serious multicollinearity is present, then the standard error of the partial-regression coefficient corresponding to x_j will be large (and confidence intervals of the β_j will be wide), significance testing will possess low power, and the interpretation of the effects of the x_j on y may be spurious or ambiguous.

Severe multicollinearity in the regression model can be detected by the following means:

(1) Significant correlations between pairs of independent variables in the model. If some correlation coefficients for pairs of x_j are very high (some researchers would say >0.80), such variables may be suspected to be collinear.

(2) Collinearity Statistics VIF and Tolerance

The *variance inflation factor* (*VIF*) refers to a relative measure of the increase in variance caused by the collinearity of the argument. For the jth $(j=1,2,\ldots,k)$ partial-regression coefficient,

$$\mathrm{VIF}_j=\frac{1}{1-R_j^2}, \tag{15.18}$$

where R_j^2 represents the unadjusted coefficient of determination for regressing the jth independent variable on the remaining ones.

Denote the reciprocal of VIF as *tolerance* (TOL):

$$\mathrm{TOL}_j=\frac{1}{\mathrm{VIF}_j}. \tag{15.19}$$

A $\mathrm{VIF}_j \geq 10$ (or equivalently, $\mathrm{TOL}_j \leq 0.1$) indicates severe multicollinearity.

(3) In cases where t-test for the individual parameters β_j yields non-significant results while the F-test for overall model adequacy is significant, multicollinearity should be considered.

(4) Opposite signs (from what is expected) in the estimated parameters indicate a potential of severe multicollinearity.

Example 15.12 Refer to Example 15.1. Suppose there is another variable, hip circumference, which may influence FVC. We investigate the effects of age (x_1), weight (x_2), and hip circumference (x_3) on FVC simultaneously. Check for collinearity.

Solution

The VIF of each variable is given in Table 15.4. The VIF of variable weight is 10.134 and that of variable hip circumference is 9.214, both close to 10. The Pearson correlation coefficient for weight and hip circumference $r=0.944$, $p<0.001$, which indicates

Table 15.4 Check of collinearity for Example 15.12.

Model	Unstandardized coefficient		Standardized coefficient	t	p value	Collinearity statistics	
	coefficient	Standard error				Tolerance	VIF
Intercept	0.669	0.9477		0.71	0.483		
Weight	0.071	0.0112	0.978	6.35	<0.001	0.099	10.134
Hip circumference	−0.021	0.0164	−0.185	−1.26	0.214	0.109	9.214
Age	0.072	0.0291	0.169	2.48	0.016	0.508	1.969

that the two variables are strongly correlated. The underlying reason may be that hip circumference and weight are both indicators of physique. In Figure 15.1, we can also see that age and weight have a positive correlation, and the Pearson correlation coefficient is 0.701, $p < 0.001$. We think the effect of multicollinearity is acceptable because it is within the VIF limit.

Several alternatives are available for solving multicollinearity problems, but the easiest way is to drop one or more of the correlated independent variables from the model. A screening procedure such as stepwise regression (see Section 15.4.2) is helpful in determining which variables can be dropped. In addition, the independent variables should be coded so that the first-, second-, and higher-order terms for a particular variable x are not highly correlated. In addition, strict care should be taken to ensure that the values of the x variables fall within the experimental region.

15.4.2 Selection of Independent Variables

Challenges facing the user of multiple regression analysis include concluding which of the independent variables have a significant effect on y in the population sampled. It is desirable to use a regression model with as many independent variables as required to provide a good determination of which of these variables produce a significant change in y in the population and to enable accurate predictions of y. However, the resulting regression model should comprise the minimum number of variables necessary for this purpose. This will minimize the time, energy, and expense in collecting further data or performing further calculations with the selected regression model to optimize statistical estimates. Therefore, to simplify the interpretations of the resultant regression model, a smaller number of variables will also tend to increase the precision of the predicted y.

Generally, there are three selection procedures (forward, backward, and stepwise) for selecting independent variables. Here we present the *stepwise regression* procedure (the other two procedures are similar in principle) for selecting independent variables using the dataset from Example 15.12.

Example 15.13 Refer to Example 15.12. Use the stepwise selection procedure to select independent variables.

Solution

Step 1. Consider all possible simple linear regressions (see Tables 15.5(a)–(c)). The predictor variable that explains the largest significant proportion of the variation in y, that is, the variable that has the largest correlation with the response is the first variable to enter the regression function. In this sample, variable weight is selected as it has the largest value of $|t|$.

Step 2. The next variable to enter is the one (out of those not yet included) that makes the largest significant contribution to the regression sum of squares. The significance

Table 15.5 (a) Simple linear regression analysis (age).

Model	Unstandardized coefficient		Standardized coefficient	t	p value
	Coefficient	Standard error			
Intercept	−0.939	0.5270		−1.78	0.080
Age	0.314	0.0383	0.732	8.19	<0.001

Table 15.5 (b) Simple linear regression analysis (weight).

Model	Unstandardized coefficient		Standardized coefficient	t	p value
	Coefficient	Standard error			
Intercept	0.102	0.1835		0.55	0.581
Weight	0.067	0.0040	0.922	18.18	<0.001

Table 15.5 (c) Simple linear regression analysis (hip circumference).

Model	Unstandardized coefficient		Standardized coefficient	t	p value
	Coefficient	Standard error			
Intercept	−4.274	0.6547		−7.22	<0.001
Hip circumference	0.095	0.0080	0.851	12.35	<0.001

of the contribution is determined by the partial F-test. The value of the F statistic (a "partial F," which is t^2) that must be exceeded before the contribution of a variable is deemed significant is often called the F to enter. In this step, we continue to establish the regressions possessing the weight selected and one of the other x, which yields the following statistics:

When adding age to the model (Table 15.6(a)), perform the partial F-test for age; $F = t^2 = 2.46^2 = 6.05,\ p < 0.05$.

When adding hip circumference (Table 15.6(b)), perform the partial F-test for hip circumference, $F = t^2 = \left(-1.18\right)^2 = 1.39,\ p > 0.05$.

Therefore, we exclude hip circumference from the model. The reason may be severe multicollinearity (discussed in Example 15.12). Hence, we include weight and age in the model.

Step 3. Once an additional variable has been included in the model, the individual contributions to the regression sum of squares of the other variables already in the-model are checked for significance using the partial F-test. As shown in Step 2,

Table 15.6 (a) Selection of more variables (weight and age).

Model	Unstandardized coefficient		Standardized coefficient	t	p value
	b	Standard error			
Intercept	−0.464	0.2896		−1.60	0.115
Weight	0.059	0.0050	0.805	11.78	<0.001
Age	0.072	0.0293	0.168	2.46	0.017

Table 15.6 (b) Selection of more variables (weight and hip circumference).

Model	Unstandardized coefficient			t	p value
	Coefficient	Standard error	Standardized coefficient		
Intercept	1.218	0.9624		1.27	0.211
Weight	0.080	0.0112	1.094	7.13	<0.001
Hip circumference	−0.020	0.0171	−0.181	−1.18	0.242

Table 15.6 (c) Selection of more variables (weight, hip circumference, and age).

Model	Unstandardized coefficient			t	p value
	Coefficient	Standard error	Standardized coefficient		
Intercept	0.669	0.9477		0.71	0.483
Weight	0.071	0.0112	0.978	6.35	<0.001
Hip circumference	−0.021	0.0164	−0.185	−1.26	0.214
Age	0.072	0.0291	0.169	2.48	0.016

perform a partial F-test for weight; $F = t^2 = (11.78)^2 = 138.77$, $p < 0.05$. Therefore, H_0 would be rejected, and we include weight.

Step 4. Steps 2 and 3 are repeated until all possible additions are nonsignificant and all possible deletions are significant. Thus, we continue to establish the regressions, with weight and age selected. Another variable, hip circumference, yields the following statistics (Table 15.6(c)):

Perform the partial F-test for hip circumference; $F = t^2 = (-1.26)^2 = 1.59$, $p > 0.05$. Therefore, H_0 would not be rejected for hip circumference, and the model established in step 3 represents the final model.

$$\hat{y} = -0.464 + 0.072x_1 + 0.059x_2$$

15.4.3 Sample Size

Multiple linear regression analysis requires a sufficient sample size. However, owing to uncertainty in the number of independent variables involved and corresponding parameters in the multiple linear regression model, there is currently no unanimously accepted accurate sample size estimation formula. Nevertheless, there is a consensus that the larger the number of independent variables, the greater is the sample size required. In general, the sample size should be more than 10 times the number of independent variables to ensure robustness and reliability of the regression parameters of the multiple linear regression model. When the sample size is too small, it is difficult to obtain good fitting accuracy and precision.

15.5 Summary

In this chapter, we used a least squares estimation to fit a multiple linear regression model to an experimental response. We assumed that the expected value of y is a function of a set of independent variables $x_1, x_2,\ldots, x_k$, where the function is linear in a set of unknown parameters $\beta_0,\beta_1,\beta_2,\ldots,\beta_k$. The methodology presented in this chapter is widely employed in medical biostatistics and all the sciences for exploring the relationship between a response and a set of independent variables. The estimation of $E(y)$ or prediction of y is usually the objective of many studies.

Inferential problems associated with the linear statistical model include estimation and tests of hypotheses related to the model parameters $\beta_0,\beta_1,\beta_2,\ldots,\beta_k$. Although the least squares estimation can be used to estimate model parameters in general situations, the formal inference-making techniques presented (based on the t and F distributions) are valid only under the assumptions that we have presented. Key assumptions include that the error terms in the model are of independence, normality, and homogeneity of variances.

The coefficient of determination, adjusted coefficient of determination, and residual analysis are often used to evaluate the fit of the regression model. In addition, some issues such as multicollinearity among independent variables, variable selection to optimize statistical estimates, and sample size have been addressed. These also play an important role in multiple linear regression analysis.

15.6 Exercises

1. The basal metabolic rate (Kcal/d) and several physical condition indicators of 70 children (aged 10-15 years) were investigated, as shown in Table 15.7. The research objective is to predict the basal metabolic rate using heart rate (beats per minute), blood pressure (mmHg), height (cm), and weight (kg).

(a) Identify the independent and dependent variables.

(b) What are the assumptions for the multivariable linear regression model?

(c) What is the method for estimating the parameters in the model? What is the principle of this method?

(d) Establish a multiple linear regression model for this data.

Table 15.7 Basal metabolic rate and physical condition indexes of 70 children.

ID	Height	Weight	Systolic pressure	Diastolic pressure	Heart rate	Metabolic rate	ID	Height	Weight	Systolic pressure	Diastolic pressure	Heart rate	Metabolic rate
1	144	32	118	71	66	776	36	149	38	99	66	93	943
2	136	30	106	76	67	843	37	150	46	94	63	94	927
3	140	28	96	59	73	701	38	136	37	111	95	95	864
4	158	49	94	58	73	988	39	139	30	104	63	96	850
5	146	35	111	67	74	836	40	142	31	113	78	96	963
6	132	28	111	78	75	575	41	139	32	111	71	96	968
7	137	28	117	73	76	622	42	144	38	109	74	97	901
8	146	51	121	67	77	773	43	139	29	89	64	98	971
9	157	42	122	83	78	932	44	142	46	106	80	98	910
10	142	29	117	52	79	682	45	142	35	113	70	98	956
11	128	26	117	52	80	734	46	151	39	103	68	99	893
12	151	43	120	56	81	1103	47	137	32	89	44	100	723
13	149	36	114	73	81	978	48	141	34	109	61	100	863
14	127	28	122	67	82	678	49	149	36	136	77	100	976
15	144	36	95	51	85	883	50	137	35	109	57	101	879
16	132	29	109	61	85	707	51	138	33	106	76	101	932
17	135	29	103	79	86	785	52	141	35	125	83	101	934
18	130	27	87	56	86	781	53	123	25	92	66	103	933
19	152	38	117	72	86	821	54	149	52	131	75	107	1129
20	138	32	97	60	87	827	55	129	24	82	54	109	1147

(Continued)

Table 15.7 (Continued)

ID	Height	Weight	Systolic pressure	Diastolic pressure	Heart rate	Metabolic rate	ID	Height	Weight	Systolic pressure	Diastolic pressure	Heart rate	Metabolic rate
21	145	35	97	64	87	836	56	144	29	110	75	110	933
22	146	35	95	56	87	978	57	146	38	121	86	110	992
23	152	43	106	53	87	861	58	155	48	130	113	113	1085
24	145	39	122	83	88	989	59	142	28	109	84	115	1082
25	138	31	89	67	89	938	60	151	43	122	75	115	1154
26	145	35	110	75	89	936	61	162	64	100	68	115	1311
27	138	33	118	79	89	742	62	152	35	89	60	117	927
28	148	35	109	68	90	920	63	143	36	106	82	118	947
29	132	29	107	68	91	766	64	150	39	108	75	118	978
30	143	33	123	56	91	814	65	142	30	104	57	120	1198
31	147	36	109	65	92	940	66	127	21	122	77	121	1164
32	149	39	109	68	92	955	67	136	27	115	78	122	1196
33	144	43	118	77	92	953	68	144	46	99	83	125	1050
34	136	30	100	56	93	843	69	153	43	124	66	128	1105
35	144	33	89	58	93	915	70	148	38	119	62	130	1138

(e) What is the difference between a simple linear regression coefficient and a partial-regression coefficient? How are they interpreted?

(f) How are the independent variables selected? How do you determine whether a certain variable is significant? Can you tell the difference between different variable selection methods?

(g) Which independent variable has the greatest impact? How do you determine this?

(h) Is the model a good fit? How can you measure and assess goodness-of-fit?

(i) Draw a plot to examine the assumptions for the model. Can you use the plot to assess goodness-of-fit?

(j) Are there any outliers in the data? How do you determine this and how are they handled?

(k) What is multicollinearity? How is multicollinearity identified and how can this issue be handled?

16

Logistic Regression

CONTENTS

The topic of this chapter is the analysis of categorical dependent (or response) variables. We describe logistic regression, which is a method that has become a more widely used analysis technique in public health and the biomedical sciences since the 1980s. As we discussed in Chapter 15, methods that fit regression models with two or more independent variables are called multiple regression methods. Multiple regression is, in fact, a family of methods. Because logistic regression is almost always used with two or more independent variables, it should be called *multiple logistic regression*. However, the word "multiple" is often omitted, but assumed.

Logistic regression represents another application of the linear model idea used in Chapter 13 and Chapter 15. Instead of predicting the mean of a dependent variable in multiple linear regression model, logistic regression models the probability of an event of interest for the dependent outcome based on one or more independent variables.

Applied Medical Statistics, First Edition. Jingmei Jiang.

Companion website: www.wiley.com\go\jiang\appliedmedicalstatistics

This is reflective of the basic idea of a family of logistic regression models that differ according to the type of study design and outcome. In this chapter, we introduce logistic regression models for a binary outcome under independent and paired designs, which lay the foundation for further study to extend logistic regression models.

16.1 Logistic Regression Model

In general, logistic regression model is also called unconditional logistic regression model. We introduce this topic using an example.

Example 16.1 In a large epidemiological survey on the prevalence and associated risk factors of adult female (age ≥ 18 years old) urinary incontinence (UI), the data of over 10,000 participants were collected, including age (years), delivery method, body mass index (BMI, kg/m^2), history of pelvic surgery, and UI. For a better illustration, 691 records of the participants were randomly extracted from the entire dataset of this survey (part of the data shown in Table 16.1), and 204 (29.5%) records referred to UI. The question of interest is whether a history of pelvic surgery increases the risk of UI.

Analysis

Logistic regression is often used in etiology study. In this example, there are four independent variables that could be associated with UI. We call the four independent variables risk factors, or exposure variable which refers to factors that are causally related to a change in the risk of a relevant health outcome. The aim of the example is to explore the association between the history of pelvic surgery and UI.

In this case, the dependent variable is UI, and we use 1 (yes) and 0 (no) to represent subjects "with" and "without" UI, respectively. For independent variables, age and

Table 16.1 Data extracted from an epidemiological survey on risk factors of UI.

ID	Age (years)	Delivery method	BMI (kg/m^2)	History of pelvic surgery	UI
1	33	Cesarean	< 24	Yes	No
2	47	No	≥ 24	No	No
3	96	No	< 24	No	Yes
4	61	Vaginal	≥ 24	No	Yes
5	57	Vaginal	≥ 24	Yes	Yes
6	29	Vaginal	< 24	No	Yes
7	37	Cesarean	< 24	No	No
8	26	No	< 24	No	No
9	40	Cesarean	≥ 24	Yes	No
10	51	Cesarean	≥ 24	No	No
…	…	…	…	…	…

Source: Zhu et al. (2009).

BMI are continuous variables. For ease of interpretation and illustration purposes, we reclass the BMI as a binary variable (overweight if BMI ≥ 24; otherwise not overweight. Hereafter, we use "overweight" instead of BMI). Delivery method is an unordered categorical variable with three levels categories.

Before proceeding with the logistic regression model, we introduce the concept of confounding. A confounding variable is associated with both the outcome and the exposure variable. Such a variable is usually adjusted when looking at an exposure–outcome relationship. For example, in this example, we want to know whether a history of pelvic surgery increases the risk of UI. Other risk factors need to be adjusted.

16.1.1 Linear Probability Model

Let y be a binary (dichotomous) variable, denoted by 1 (success) and 0 (failure) for a given trial. Let π denote the probability of success. Analogously to the linear regression model, we replace y directly with π; hence,

$$\pi\left(y=1 \mid x_1, x_2, \ldots, x_k\right)=\beta_0+\beta_1 x_1+\cdots+\beta_k x_k \tag{16.1}$$

is called the *linear probability model.*

Although this model is easy to interpret, it has a serious drawback: As π is a probability, $\beta_0+\sum_{j=1}^{k} \beta_j x_j$ has to be in $[0,1]$ for all possible values of x, which implies severe restrictions on β. Additionally, the typical assumptions of normality and homogeneity of variance of errors from the linear regression model are violated when the outcome is a binary variable, calling into question the validity of results from such an approach. Instead, when the outcome is binary, the logit transformation of π is often used as the dependent variable. We model the odds, or more specifically, we model the natural (base e) log of the odds, referred to as the logit of the distribution to avoid this limitation.

16.1.2 Probability, Odds, and Logit Transformation

1. Odds Versus Probability

Logistic regression models actually work with odds rather than probability. The key point is that odds and probability are two alternative ways to express precisely the same concept.

Definition 16.1 Let y be a binary variable. The *odds* of an event occurring equal the probability that that event will occur (success, denoted by $y=1$) divided by the probability that it will not occur (failure, denoted by $y=0$), defined as

$$Odds=\frac{\pi\left(y=1\right)}{\pi\left(y=0\right)}=\frac{\pi\left(y=1\right)}{1-\pi\left(y=1\right)}. \tag{16.2}$$

When the probability of success $\pi(y=1)$ is greater than the probability of failure $\pi(y=0)$, the odds are greater than 1; if the two outcomes are equally likely, the odds are approximately 1; and if the probability of success is less than the probability of failure, the odds are less than 1. Thus, all probabilities can be expressed as odds, and all odds can be expressed as probabilities.

2. Logit Transformation

Definition 16.2 Let $\pi(y=1)=\pi$ represent the probability of "success" or the outcome of interest. The logit transformation of π is often used as the dependent variable, which is defined as

$$\text{logit}(\pi)=\ln(Odds)=\ln\frac{\pi}{1-\pi}. \tag{16.3}$$

The logarithm of the odds is also referred to as the *log odds* or *logit*.

Unlike π, the logit transformation $\ln\frac{\pi}{1-\pi}$ can take any value on the entire real axis (i.e., from $-\infty$ to $+\infty$).

Thus far, we have discussed the following relationship: probabilities are transformed to odds, and odds are transformed to logits by taking the natural log. We use an example to intuitively illustrate the relationship between the three concepts.

Example 16.2 Given the probabilities in Table 16.2, compute the corresponding odds and logits, and describe the relationship between the probabilities and logits.

Solution

For example, based on Definitions 16.1 and 16.2, for probability 0.5, $Odds=\frac{0.50}{1-0.50}=1.00$, and logit $(0.5)=\ln(Odds)=\ln(1.00)=0$. Similar results are shown in Table 16.2.

The relationship between probabilities and logits is shown graphically in Figure 16.1.

Figure 16.1 indicates that the relationship is essentially linear for probabilities between 0.3 and 0.7 and nonlinear for lower and greater probabilities. A unit change in the logit results in greater differences in probabilities in the middle than at high and low levels.

Table 16.2 Comparison of probabilities, odds, and logits.

Probability (π_i)	0.01	0.10	0.20	0.30	0.40	0.50	0.60	0.70	0.80	0.90	0.99
odds	0.01	0.11	0.25	0.43	0.67	1.00	1.50	2.33	4.00	9.00	99.00
Logit: ln (odds)	−4.60	−2.20	−1.39	−0.85	−0.41	0.00	0.41	0.85	1.39	2.20	4.60

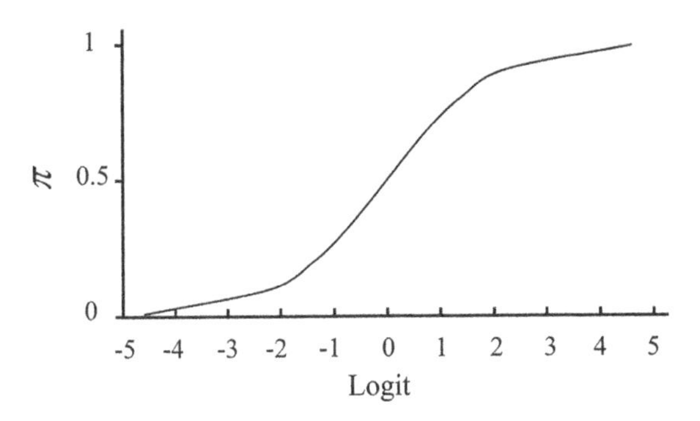

Figure 16.1 Relationship between probabilities and logits.

16.1.3 Definition of Logistic Regression

Definition 16.3 Let $x_1, x_2, \ldots, x_k$ be independent variables. For a binary dependent variable y, let $\pi(y = 1 | x_1, x_2, \ldots, x_k) = \pi(x)$ denote the "success" probability at value x. This probability is the parameter for the binomial distribution. The logistic regression model has a linear form for the logit of this probability:

$$\text{logit}[\pi(x)] = \ln\frac{\pi(x)}{1-\pi(x)} = \beta_0 + \beta_1 x_1 + \cdots + \beta_k x_k = \beta_0 + \sum_{j=1}^{k} \beta_j x_j. \tag{16.4}$$

The link function is the logit function $\ln\frac{\pi(x)}{1-\pi(x)}$ of $\pi(x)$, denoted by "logit$[\pi(x)]$," where $\pi(x)$ is restricted to the $0-1$ range. Logistic regression models are often called logit models. When the dependent variable is binary, we also call the model a binary logistic regression model.

Because $\ln\frac{\pi(x)}{1-\pi(x)}$ can take any value on the entire real axis, no restrictions on $\beta_0 + \sum_{j=1}^{k} \beta_j x_j$ and β have to be imposed.

The transformed model is linear in the parameters, which means that the effects of independent variables on the log of the odds are additive. Thus, the model is easy to work with and allows for the interpretation of variable effects that are exceptionally straightforward, and for model building strategies that mirror those of ordinary linear regression.

Solving for $\pi(x)$, we obtain the response function

$$\pi(x) = \frac{\exp\left(\beta_0 + \sum_{j=1}^{k} \beta_j x_j\right)}{1 + \exp\left(\beta_0 + \sum_{j=1}^{k} \beta_j x_j\right)}, \tag{16.5}$$

$$1-\pi(x)=\frac{1}{1+\exp\left(\beta_0+\sum_{j=1}^{k}\beta_j x_j\right)}, \tag{16.6}$$

where $\exp\left(\beta_0+\sum_{j=1}^{k}\beta_j x_j\right)=e^{\beta_0+\sum_{j=1}^{k}\beta_j x_j}$.

Note that compared with the multiple linear regression that ends with a random term ε (Formula 15.1), the "y" value in Formula 16.4 is the natural logarithm of odds, which can be transformed to a probability. Because it implicitly embodies uncertainty, there is no need to explicitly add a random term to the model.

For an intuitive impression of the logistic regression function distribution, we use the data from Example 16.1, and assume that the model has only an independent variable x to show its distribution.

Example 16.3 Referring to Example 16.1, using age alone as the independent variable (continuous) and UI as the dependent variable, describe the relationship between age and the probability that a woman of a given age will develop UI.

Solution

From the output of SPSS software for logistic regression, we obtained the estimators of the regression parameters $b_0=-2.360$ and $b_1=0.032$ (see Section 16.1.4 for the specific steps to estimate the parameter).

The estimated probability that a woman of a given age will develop UI is the simple analog of Formula 16.5; thus,

$$p_i=\frac{\exp(-2.360+0.032x_i)}{1+\exp(-2.360+0.032x_i)}$$

and the corresponding graph is shown in Figure 16.2.

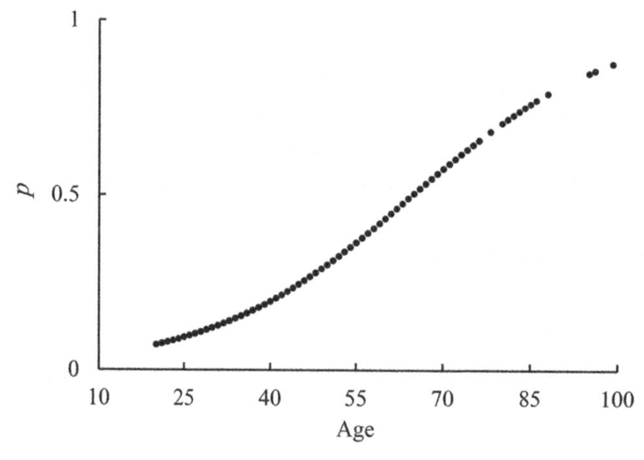

Figure 16.2 Graph of logistic regression for estimated probabilities of UI and predictive variable age.

Figure 16.2 shows the estimated probabilities of UI for the age range of the subjects enrolled in the study. Because the overall slope is positive, the probability of UI increases as the age of women increases.

Figure 16.2 shows an approximate S-shaped function with age. The logistic distribution function is also symmetric. In fact, the S-shaped curve in Figure 16.2 is the most important mathematical function in logistic regression. This is often the realistic shape for the relationship.

16.1.4 Inference for Logistic Regression

16.1.4.1 Estimation of Model Coefficient

Instead of least squares in multiple linear regression, logistic regression uses the *maximum likelihood (ML)* procedure to obtain the parameter estimates. The ML estimate requires a probability density function to be specified that is assumed to characterize the observed data. The ML estimate of a parameter is the parameter value for which the probability of the observed data takes its greatest value; that is, the *likelihood function* takes its maximum. The likelihood function is the probability of the observed data, which can be expressed as a function of the parameter.

In the case of binary logistic regression, the likelihood function, denoted by L, is constructed with reference to the binomial distribution probability mass function and multiplication rules of probability:

$$L=\prod_{i=1}^{n}\pi_i^{y_i}\left(1-\pi_i\right)^{1-y_i}$$
$$=\prod_{i=1}^{n}\left[\frac{e^{\beta_0+\sum_{j=1}^{k}\beta_j x_{ij}}}{1+e^{\beta_0+\sum_{j=1}^{k}\beta_j x_{ij}}}\right]^{y_i}\left[\frac{1}{1+e^{\beta_0+\sum_{j=1}^{k}\beta_j x_{ij}}}\right]^{1-y_i}, \tag{16.7}$$

where π_i is the probability of "success" for the ith subject, and y_i is 1 if the ith subject has "success" in an event, and 0 otherwise.

By taking the logarithm transformation of Formula 16.7, we obtain the log-likelihood function

$$\ln L=\sum_{i=1}^{n}y_i\ln\left[\frac{e^{\beta_0+\sum_{j=1}^{k}\beta_j x_{ij}}}{1+e^{\beta_0+\sum_{j=1}^{k}\beta_j x_{ij}}}\right]+\sum_{i=1}^{n}\left(1-y_i\right)\ln\left[\frac{1}{1+e^{\beta_0+\sum_{j=1}^{k}\beta_j x_{ij}}}\right]$$

Because of the monotony of the logarithm transformation, L reaches its maximum when $\ln L$ is at its maximum. Therefore, we could obtain the estimates of β_0 and β_j $(j=1,2,\ldots,k)$ by letting the first partial derivative of $\ln L$ be 0, that is, $\partial \ln L/\partial\beta_j=0$. A Newton–Raphson iterative method is generally used for solving the equation.

To make the function easy to understand and implement, we continue to use one independent variable (two levels) in the parameter estimation process.

Table 16.3 2×2 contingency table for a binary outcome and one binary predictive variable.

x	y		Total
	$y=1$	$y=0$	
$x=1$	n_{11}	n_{12}	$n_{11}+n_{12}$
$x=0$	n_{21}	n_{22}	$n_{21}+n_{22}$
Total	$n_{11}+n_{21}$	$n_{12}+n_{22}$	n

Table 16.4 Corresponding probability for Table 16.3 with logistic regression.

x	y	
	$y=1$	$y=0$
$x=1$	$\pi_1=\dfrac{e^{\beta_0+\beta_1}}{1+e^{\beta_0+\beta_1}}$	$1-\pi_1=\dfrac{1}{1+e^{\beta_0+\beta_1}}$
$x=0$	$\pi_0=\dfrac{e^{\beta_0}}{1+e^{\beta_0}}$	$1-\pi_0=\dfrac{1}{1+e^{\beta_0}}$

Table 16.3 is a 2×2 contingency table of counts $\{n_{ij}\}$ for which the two rows, as two levels of one binary independent variable, represent the exposure's status, that is, individuals who are exposed or not; and the two columns are the two levels of y, which represent the disease outcomes; that is, having or not having the disease according to the individuals' exposure status. The row totals, which are the numbers of trials for those binary variables, are naturally fixed.

The logistic predicted probabilities of data corresponding to Table 16.3 are shown in Table 16.4.

Then the likelihood function L of π according to Tables 16.3 and 16.4 is

$$\begin{aligned} L &= \pi_1^{n_{11}}\left(1-\pi_1\right)^{n_{12}}\pi_0^{n_{21}}\left(1-\pi_0\right)^{n_{22}} \\ &= \left(\frac{e^{\beta_0+\beta_1}}{1+e^{\beta_0+\beta_1}}\right)^{n_{11}}\left(\frac{1}{1+e^{\beta_0+\beta_1}}\right)^{n_{12}}\left(\frac{e^{\beta_0}}{1+e^{\beta_0}}\right)^{n_{21}}\left(\frac{1}{1+e^{\beta_0}}\right)^{n_{22}}, \end{aligned} \tag{16.8}$$

where $n_{11}+n_{12}+n_{21}+n_{22}=n$.

Additionally,

$$\ln L = n_{11}(\beta_0+\beta_1) - n_{11}\ln\left(1+e^{\beta_0+\beta_1}\right) + n_{21}\beta_0 - n_{21}\ln\left(1+e^{\beta_0}\right) - n_{12}\ln\left(1+e^{\beta_0+\beta_1}\right)$$
$$-n_{22}\ln\left(1+e^{\beta_0}\right).$$

We take the first partial derivatives of $\ln L$ with respect to β_0 and β_1. Let them be 0. Then, respectively,

$$\begin{cases} \dfrac{\partial \ln L}{\partial \beta_0} = n_{11}+n_{21} - \dfrac{(n_{11}+n_{12})e^{\beta_0+\beta_1}}{1+e^{\beta_0+\beta_1}} - \dfrac{(n_{21}+n_{22})e^{\beta_0}}{1+e^{\beta_0}} = 0 \\ \dfrac{\partial \ln L}{\partial \beta_1} = n_{11} - \dfrac{(n_{11}+n_{12})e^{\beta_0+\beta_1}}{1+e^{\beta_0+\beta_1}} = 0 \end{cases}. \tag{16.9}$$

Solving the equation, yields the ML estimates of β_0 and β_1:

$$\begin{cases} b_0 = \hat{\beta}_0 = \ln \dfrac{n_{21}}{n_{22}} \\ b_1 = \hat{\beta}_1 = \ln \dfrac{n_{11}n_{22}}{n_{12}n_{21}} \end{cases}. \tag{16.10}$$

Example 16.4 Referring to Example 16.1, estimate the intercept and regression coefficient of a logistic regression model for UI using the history of pelvic surgery alone as the independent variable.

Solution

In the case in which both the exposure and outcome variables are binary, a 2×2 contingency table can be built, as shown in Table 16.5.

From Table 16.5, n_{11}=74, n_{12}=122, n_{21}=130, $n_{22}=365$.

According to Formula 16.10, the ML estimates of β_0 and β_1 are

$$b_0 = \ln \frac{n_{21}}{n_{22}} = \ln \frac{130}{365} = -1.0324$$

$$b_1 = \ln \frac{n_{11}n_{22}}{n_{12}n_{21}} = \ln \frac{74\times365}{122\times130} = 0.5324$$

Therefore, according to Definition 16.3, the estimated logistic regression model is

$$\text{logit}(p) = -1.0324 + 0.5324x$$

The model indicates that the logit(p) increases by 0.5324, on average, for women with a history of pelvic surgery compared with women without a history of pelvic surgery. However, most of us do not think naturally on a logit (logarithm of the odds) scale, so we need to consider alternative interpretations (see Section 16.1.4.2).

The predictive probability of UI given an individual with a history of pelvic surgery is given by

$$p_i = \frac{\exp(-1.0324 + 0.5324x_i)}{1+\exp(-1.0324+0.5324x_i)}$$

We also provide the calculation results using SPSS software, shown in column 2 of Table 16.6.

Table 16.5 2×2 contingency table of the history of pelvic surgery and UI.

History of pelvic surgery	UI		Total
	Yes (1)	No (0)	
Yes (1)	74	122	196
No (0)	130	365	495
Total	204	487	691

Table 16.6 Results of the regression coefficient.

Model	Coefficient	Standard error	Wald statistic	p value	Odds ratio	95% confidence interval
Intercept	−1.0324	0.102	102.164	< 0.001	–	–
History of pelvic surgery	0.5324	0.179	8.819	0.003	1.703	[1.198, 2.420]
Likelihood ratio: $\chi^2 = 8.681$, $\nu = 1$, $p = 0.003$.						

When there are two or more independent variables in the model, the parameters can be estimated in the same manner, and the standard error can also be estimated using an iterative method through an estimation formula established by the first and second derivatives of the likelihood function. These procedures are more complex and can be completed using statistical analysis software.

Estimators based on the ML method are popular because they have good large-sample behavior. Most importantly, it is not possible to determine good estimators that are more precise, in terms of having small large-sample standard errors. Additionally, large-sample distributions of ML estimators are typically approximately normal.

16.1.4.2 Interpretation of Model Coefficient

How can the regression coefficients in Formula 16.10 be interpreted? The interpretation of the logistic regression coefficients uses the odds and the odds ratio (OR). We learned about the concept of odds in Section 16.1.2; hence, we discuss the OR next, which is another measure of association as a parameter in the most important type of model for categorical data.

1. Models with a Single Binary Independent Variable

We continue to use the case, in which both the independent and dependent variables are binary as an example to derive the OR.

Definition 16.4 Assume that the independent variable x, as an exposure variable, has two levels, that is, exposed (coded as 1) and not exposed (coded as 0); and the dependent variable y, as the outcome variable, has two levels, that is, disease occurs (coded as 1) and disease does not occur (coded as 0). According to Formula 16.2, the OR is defined as

$$OR = \frac{Odds_1}{Odds_0} = \frac{\pi_1 / (1-\pi_1)}{\pi_0 / (1-\pi_0)}, \tag{16.11}$$

According to Definition 16.4, the OR represents the odds in favor of disease for the exposed divided by the odds in favor of disease for the non-exposed.

The estimated OR equals the ratio of the sample odds in the two groups. According to Table 16.3,

$$\widehat{OR} = \frac{p_1 / (1-p_1)}{p_0 / (1-p_0)} = \frac{[n_{11} / (n_{11}+n_{12})] / [n_{12} / (n_{11}+n_{12})]}{[n_{21} / (n_{21}+n_{22})] / [n_{22} / (n_{21}+n_{22})]} = \frac{n_{11} / n_{12}}{n_{21} / n_{22}} = \frac{n_{11}n_{22}}{n_{12}n_{21}}. \tag{16.12}$$

From Formula 16.10, because $b_1 = \ln\frac{n_{11}n_{22}}{n_{12}n_{21}}$,

$$\widehat{OR} = e^{b_1}. \tag{16.13}$$

Example 16.5 Referring to Example 16.4, compute and interpret the estimated OR for the effect of the history of pelvic surgery on UI.

Solution

From Example 16.4, $b_1 = 0.5324$, and according to Formula 16.13,

$$\widehat{OR} = e^{b_1} = e^{0.5324} = 1.703$$

See the SPSS software outcome in Table 16.6 Odds Ratio column.

An $\widehat{OR}$ of 1.703 means that the risk of UI for a woman with a history of pelvic surgery is 1.703 times (or 70.3% increase) that of a woman without a history of pelvic surgery.

2. Models with Multiple Independent Variables

For more independent variables (including numerical and categorical), the explanation of the OR is the same. To demonstrate this, suppose we consider two individuals with different values of independent variables, as shown in Table 16.7, where the jth independent variable is a binary variable.

If we refer to variable x_j as exposure variables, then individuals A and B are the same for all other risk factors in the model, except the jth exposure variable, where individual A is exposed (coded as 1) and individual B is not exposed (coded as 0). According to Formula 16.4, the logits of the probability of success for individuals A and B, denoted by $\text{logit}(\pi_A)$ and $\text{logit}(\pi_B)$, are given by

$$\begin{cases} \text{logit}(\pi_A) = \beta_0 + \beta_1 x_1 + \cdots + \beta_{j-1}x_{j-1} + \beta_j \times 1 + \beta_{j+1}x_{j+1} + \cdots + \beta_k x_k, \\ \text{logit}(\pi_B) = \beta_0 + \beta_1 x_1 + \cdots + \beta_{j-1}x_{j-1} + \beta_j \times 0 + \beta_{j+1}x_{j+1} + \cdots + \beta_k x_k. \end{cases} \tag{16.14}$$

If we subtract $\text{logit}(\pi_B)$ from $\text{logit}(\pi_A)$ in Formula 16.14, we obtain

$$\text{logit}(\pi_A) - \text{logit}(\pi_B) = \beta_j$$

Table 16.7 Two hypothetical subjects with different values for a binary independent variable (x_j) and the same values for all other variables in a multiple logistic regression model.

	Independent Variable							
Individual	**1**	**2**	**...**	$j-1$	j	$j+1$	**...**	k
A	x_1	x_2	...	x_{j-1}	1	x_{j+1}	...	x_k
B	x_1	x_2	...	x_{j-1}	0	x_{j+1}	...	x_k

Because $\text{logit}(\pi_A) = \ln\frac{\pi_A}{1-\pi_A}$, $\text{logit}(\pi_B) = \ln\frac{\pi_B}{1-\pi_B}$,

$$\ln\left[\frac{\pi_A/(1-\pi_A)}{\pi_B/(1-\pi_B)}\right] = \beta_j. \tag{16.15}$$

If we take the antilog of each side of Formula 16.15, we obtain

$$\frac{\pi_A/(1-\pi_A)}{\pi_B/(1-\pi_B)} = e^{\beta_j}; \tag{16.16}$$

thus,

$$OR_j = \frac{Odds_A}{Odds_B} = e^{\beta_j}. \tag{16.17}$$

We can provide such an explanation of the meaning of the OR in logistic regression with multiple independent variables.

For OR relating the outcome to the jth exposure variable for two hypothetical individuals, subject A is exposed for the jth exposure variable and subject B is not exposed for the jth exposure variable, where the individuals are the same for all other risk factors considered in the model. Thus, this OR relating the outcome to the jth exposure variable, is adjusted for the levels of all other risk factors in the model. Formulas 16.11 and 16.17 have the same form and, essentially, the same interpretation, except that Formula 16.17 adjusts for other risk factors.

The values of OR are bounded below by 0, but have no upper bound; that is, they can range from 0 to infinity. An OR of 1.0 indicates that an exposure variable has no effect on the odds of the outcome. An OR larger than 1.0 indicates that the exposure variable has an increased effect on the odds of the outcome. An OR less than 1.0 indicates that the exposure variable has a decreased effect on the odds of the outcome.

16.1.4.3 Hypothesis Testing of Model Coefficient

How can the statistical significance of the partial regression coefficient estimates corresponding to the exposure (or any other risk factors) in Formula 16.10 be evaluated? The statistical significance of each of the independent variables after adjusting for all other independent variables in the model should be assessed. This task is typically achieved by performing one of the following tests.

1. Wald's Test

For the logistic regression model, $H_0: \beta_j = 0\,(j = 1,2,\ldots,k)$ states that the probability of success is independent of x_j. $H_1: \beta_j \neq 0$.

When H_0 is true, for large samples, the test statistic

$$Z = \frac{b_j - 0}{S_{b_j}} \tag{16.18}$$

has approximately a standard normal distribution $N(0,1)$.

If we square Z, we obtain the Wald's test statistic, which approximates the χ^2distribution with degrees of freedom $\nu = 1$.

$$\chi_W^2 = Z^2 = \left(\frac{b_j}{S_{b_j}}\right)^2 \dot{\sim} \chi^2(\nu),\ \nu = 1. \tag{16.19}$$

This type of statistic, which uses the standard error evaluated for the ML estimate, is called the Wald statistic. The Z or χ^2 test using this test statistic is called the Wald's test.

The Wald's test is typically used to examine whether a specific regression coefficient $\beta_j = 0$. When only one independent variable is considered, the significance test of the regression coefficient is equivalent to the likelihood ratio test.

2. Likelihood Ratio Test

Although the Wald's test is adequate for large samples, the *likelihood ratio test* is more powerful and more reliable for sample sizes often used in practice. Different from the Wald's test, the likelihood ratio test examines either the entire model or one specific regression coefficient.

For the likelihood ratio test, $H_0: \beta_1 = \beta_2 = \cdots = \beta_k = 0(j = 1,2,\ldots,k)$. In the simple case of only one independent variable β_j in the model, $H_0: \beta_j = 0$.

Recall that the likelihood function is the probability of the data, viewed as a function of the parameter once the data are observed. The likelihood ratio test determines the parameter values that maximize the likelihood function.

The test statistic is the deviance

$$\begin{aligned}\text{Deviance} &= -2\ \ln\left(\frac{\text{maximum likelihood when parameters satisfy } H_0(L_0)}{\text{maximum likelihood when parameters are unrestricted } (L_1)}\right)\\ &= -2\left(\ln(L_0) - \ln(L_1)\right).\end{aligned} \tag{16.20}$$

The test statistic value is nonnegative. When H_0 is false, the ratio of maximized likelihoods tends to be far below 1, for which the logarithm is negative; then, −2 times the log ratio tends to be a large positive number, more so as the sample size increases. It also has a large-sample χ^2 distribution with $\nu = 1$.

Example 16.6 Referring to Example 16.4, assess the significance of the effect of a history of pelvic surgery using the likelihood ratio test.

Solution

We begin with the model containing only the constant term and compare it with the model containing history of pelvic surgery. The −2 log-likelihood for the intercept-only model is 838.547, and the −2 log-likelihood for the model with the history of pelvic surgery variable is 829.866. According to Formula 16.20, the test statistic is $\chi^2 = 838.547 - 829.866 = 8.681$, as show in the last row in Table 16.6. Because $\chi^2 > \chi^2_{1,1\text{-}0.05} = 3.84$, $p < 0.05$, we reject H_0 at the 0.05 level, and conclude that β_1 is significantly different from 0.

16.1.4.4 Interval Estimation of Model Coefficient

1. Interval Estimation of β

Once the standard error of β_j is estimated by the ML method, with a sample of sufficient size, we can use a normal approximation method to show that the $(1-\alpha)\times 100\%$ CI of β_j, that is,

$$\left[b_j - z_{1-\alpha/2}S_{b_j},\ b_j + z_{1-\alpha/2}S_{b_j}\right], \tag{16.21}$$

where S_{b_j} is the estimated standard error of β_j and $z_{1-\alpha/2}$ is the critical-value of the standard normal distribution.

2. Interval Estimation of *OR*

Exponentiating the endpoints in Formula 16.21 yields an interval for e^{β_j}, thus, the $(1-\alpha)\times 100\%$ CI of OR_j is

$$exp\left[b_j \pm z_{1-\alpha/2}S_{b_j}\right]. \tag{16.22}$$

If the 95% CI of OR contains 1, we say that there is no significant difference of OR with 1, that is, there is no evidence to show that the outcome and exposure (or other risk factors) are associated.

Example 16.7 Referring to Examples 16.4 and 16.5, provide the 95% CI of the regression coefficients and OR.

Solution

In Example 16.4, from Table 16.6, $b_1 = 0.5324$, $s_{b_1} = 0.179$, and $z_{1-0.05/2} = 1.96$. According to Formula 16.21, the two-sided 95% CI for the history of pelvic surgery coefficient β_1 is

$$\begin{aligned}&[b_1 - z_{1-0.05}s_{b_1},\ b_1 + z_{1-0.05/2}s_{b_1}]\\&=[0.5324-1.96\times 0.179, 0.5324+1.96\times 0.179]\\&=[0.182, 0.883].\end{aligned}$$

According to Formula 16.22, the two-sided 95% CI of the OR regarding a history of pelvic surgery is

$$\begin{aligned}&\left[exp\left(b_1 - z_{1-0.05/2}s_{b_1}\right), exp\left(b_1 + z_{1-0.05/2}s_{b_1}\right)\right]\\&=\left[exp(0.182),\ exp(0.883)\right]\\&=[1.200, 2.418].\end{aligned}$$

Because of the rounding error in the manual calculation, there is a slight difference between the result in Table 16.6, which we can ignore. The interval of the OR does not contain 1, and the lower limit is greater than 1, which indicates that a history of pelvic surgery and UI are possibly associated.

Now that we have discussed the necessary "elements" of the logistic regression model, we return to the original example to establish the logistic regression model.

Table 16.8 Variables and corresponding values in the logistic regression model.

Variable	Value
Age (years)	Continuous
Delivery method	See Table 16.9
Overweight	1 = yes; 0 = no
History of pelvic surgery	1 = yes; 0 = no
UI	1 = yes; 0 = no

Table 16.9 Dummy variables for the delivery status variable.

Delivery method	Coding of dummy variables	
	Delivery method (1)	Delivery method (2)
No delivery	1	0
Cesarean delivery	0	1
Vaginal delivery	0	0

Example 16.8 Referring to Example 16.1, construct a logistic regression model for UI using a history of pelvic surgery, adjusting for the variables age, overweight, and delivery method. Calculate and interpret the OR and CI for each variable.

Solution

The four independent variables considered in the logistic regression model are presented in Table 16.8.

When considering a categorical variable with more than two categories in the model, we usually use dummy variables to distinguish the different categories of the variable. If the model contains an intercept term, then we can use $k-1$ dummy variables to distinguish the k categories. For example, because the delivery method in Table 16.8 contains three levels, we must create two dummy variables (delivery method (1) and delivery method (2)) to obtain a symbolic representation of this model. The dummy variables can be expressed as shown in Table 16.9.

We use the vaginal delivery status as the reference category and measure the effects of the other delivery methods from it. Thus, dummy variable delivery method (1) is 1 when the delivery method is no delivery and 0 otherwise; and delivery method (2) is 1 when the delivery method is cesarean delivery and 0 otherwise. Statistical software can create these dummy variables for the user conveniently. Therefore, the estimated logit can be expressed as

$$\text{logit}(\pi) = \beta_0 + \beta_1\text{Age} + \beta_2\text{Delivery method}(1) + \beta_3\text{Delivery method}(2) + \beta_4\text{Overweight} + \beta_5\text{History of pelvic surgery}.$$

Table 16.10 Logistic regression analysis of UI based on the variables age, delivery method, overweight, and history of pelvic surgery.

Model	Coefficient	Standard error	Wald statistic	*p* value	Odds ratio	95% confidence interval
Intercept	−2.002	0.319	39.298	< 0.001	0.135	–
Age	0.020	0.006	10.247	0.001	1.020	[1.008, 1.032]
Delivery method			24.084	< 0.001		
Delivery method (1)	−0.790	0.407	3.759	0.053	0.454	[0.204, 1.009]
Delivery method (2)	−1.895	0.410	21.393	< 0.001	0.150	[0.067, 0.335]
Overweight	0.447	0.184	5.933	0.015	1.564	[1.091, 2.242]
History of pelvic surgery	0.875	0.204	18.345	< 0.001	2.398	[1.607, 3.579]

Likelihood ratio: $\chi^2 = 85.095$, $\nu = 5$, $p < 0.001$.

We use SPSS software to analyze these data. First, perform univariate analysis for each independent variable. Each result shows that $p < 0.05$ for each independent variable. Then, perform multivariate analysis, and the results are shown in Table 16.10. The estimated values of the parameters of logit model as follows:

$$\text{logit}(p) = -2.002 + 0.020 \times \text{Age} - 0.790 \times \text{Delivery method}(1) - 1.895 \times \text{Delivery method}(2) + 0.447 \times \text{Overweight} + 0.875 \times \text{History of perlvic surgery.}$$

Similar to the significance test for logistic regression containing only one independent variable, Table 16.10 shows that, for the Wald's test, $p < 0.05$ for all the independent variables. Additionally, for the likelihood ratio test, $p < 0.05$ means that at least one variable in the model is statistically significant.

The results show that, when other factors are adjusted for, the OR regarding a history of pelvic surgery is 2.398, 95%CI: 1.607–3.579, that is, the odds in favor of UI for women with a history of pelvic surgery are 2.398 times the odds for women without a history of pelvic surgery (or we say women with a history of pelvic surgery are 2.398 times more likely to develop UI that those without a history of pelvic surgery). The OR regarding age is 1.020, 95%CI: 1.008–1.032, that is, the odds of UI increase by 2.0% with an increase of 1 year in age; and the OR regarding overweight is 1.564, 95%CI: 1.091–2.242, that is, the odds of UI in overweight women is 1.564 times the odds of those not overweight. For the dummy variables of the delivery method, compared with vaginal delivery, the ORs of no delivery and cesarean delivery are 0.454, 95% CI: 0.204–1.009, and 0.150, 95% CI: 0.067–0.335. The adjusted OR for no delivery is not statistically significant (the 95% confidence interval includes 1, corresponding to no effect). Clearly, the coefficient is far from statistically significant, so we would not want to place much confidence in this value. Because all dummy variables associated with the categorical variable are entered as a block, we still include this variable in the model. The adjusted OR for cesarean delivery indicates a lower risk of UI for cesarean delivery.

Note that a history of pelvic surgery is significantly associated with UI in Example 16.6 (without adjustment for other variables) and Example 16.8 (after adjustment); that is, the univariate and multivariate analysis results are mutually supportive. Additionally, the OR regarding a history of pelvic surgery in this example is 2.398, which is larger than 1.703 in Example 16.5. This may be caused by an adjustment for confounding factors.

We should now be familiar with the relationship between CIs and p values from Table 16.10. If the 95% CI of the OR does not contain 1 (the value 1 denotes no effect), then the p value must be less than 0.05. If the 95% CI of the odds ratio does contain 1, then the p value must be greater than 0.05.

16.1.5 Evaluation of Model Fitting

After a logistic regression model is fitted to the data, the goodness-of-fit of the model is needed. Similar to Pearson's χ^2 test, the goodness-of-fit test in logistic regression refers to testing whether the observed frequencies and expected frequencies predicted by the model are consistent. We can also use the residuals in logistic regression to examine the fit of the logistic model. Two common forms of residuals used in logistic regression are Pearson residuals and deviance residuals. These residual analyses are also useful for identifying outliers. Additionally, Hosmer–Lemeshow test is also discussed for large sample sizes.

1. Pearson Residual

For a logistic regression model, the *Pearson residual* that compares O_i to its fit is defined as

$$\text{Pearson residual} = e_i = \frac{O_i - n_i p_i}{\sqrt{n_i p_i (1 - p_i)}}, \tag{16.23}$$

where n_i is the number of observations with the ith pattern of independent variables (observed cross-classification of all levels of all the independent variables), $\sum_{i=1}^{I} n_i = n$ (where I is he number of patterns of independent variables), O_i is the number of observations with the outcome of interest among
n_i observations, and p_i is the predicted probability of the outcome of interest for the ith pattern of independent variables.

The form of Pearson residual is dividing the difference between an observed count and its fitted value by the estimated binomial standard deviation of the observed count. When n_i is large, e_i has an approximately standardized normal distribution,

$$e_i \mathrel{\dot\sim} N(0,1). \tag{16.24}$$

Based on Pearson residuals e_i, the Pearson's χ^2 test statistic is,

$$\chi_P^2 = \sum_{i=1}^{I} e_i^2 \mathrel{\dot\sim} \chi^2(\nu), \nu = I - (k+1), \tag{16.25}$$

where k is the number of independent variables.
If the test statistic $\chi_P^2 < \chi_{\nu,1-\alpha}^2$, then we conclude there is not enough evidence to show that the model has lack of fit.

We can also use the Pearson residuals to identify outlying values. A Pearson residual with absolute value larger than 2 or 3 are worth further checking.

2. Deviance Residual

The *deviance residual* is

$$d_i = \text{sgn}\left(O_i - n_i p_i\right)\left[2O_i \ln\left(\frac{O_i}{n_i p_i}\right) + 2\left(n_i - O_i\right)\ln\left(\frac{n_i - O_i}{n_i\left(1 - p_i\right)}\right)\right]^{1/2}, \tag{16.26}$$

where the symbol sgn is positive if the quantity in parentheses is positive and negative if the quantity is negative. The other symbols have the same definitions provided in Formula 16.23. When n_i is large, d_i has an approximately standardized normal distribution,

$$d_i \,\dot{\sim}\, N\left(0,1\right). \tag{16.27}$$

Similar to Pearson residual, deviance residual can also be used for diagnostics for casewise effects on the fit, as well as summary measures of fit.

Based on the deviance residuals d_i, the deviance χ^2 test statistic is

$$\chi_D^2 = \sum_{i=1}^{I} d_i^2 \,\dot{\sim}\, \chi^2\left(\nu\right),\ \nu = I - \left(k+1\right), \tag{16.28}$$

where I is the number of patterns of independent variables, and k is the number of independent variables.
If the test statistic $\chi_D^2 < \chi_{\nu,1-\alpha}^2$, then we conclude there is not enough evidence to show that the model has lack of fit.

The principles of the deviance residual test and Pearson residual test are similar: both use the χ^2 distribution to examine the difference between the observed and expected frequencies. The results are largely the same for a large sample size. For a small sample size, however, the approximation of the test statistics to the χ^2 distribution is not ideal in both tests, and when there are many independent variables (particularly when there are continuous variables), the degrees of freedom become too large for the results to be reliable. In such scenarios, the Hosmer–Lemeshow test is recommended.

3. Hosmer–Lemeshow Test

When there are many independent variables (particularly when there are continuous variables), the degrees of freedom become too large for the results to be reliable. In such scenarios, we recommend the *Hosmer–Lemeshow test* to assess the goodness-of-fit. However, this test relies on a large sample size (say $n \geq 400$). Specifically, the subjects are first divided into G groups according to their predicted probabilities, and then the Pearson's χ^2 test is performed with $G-2$ degrees of freedom. When there are many independent variables, we typically set $G = 10$ to control the level of degrees of freedom. Similar to statistic χ_P^2, the statistic for Hosmer–Lemeshow test is defined as

$$\chi_{HL}^2 = \sum_{g=1}^{G} \frac{\left(O_g - n_g p_g\right)^2}{n_g p_g \left(1 - p_g\right)} \dot{\sim} \chi^2(\nu),\ \nu = G - 2, \tag{16.29}$$

where n_g is the number of observations in the gth group, O_g is the number of observations with the outcome of interest among n_g observations, and p_g is the average predicted probability of the outcome of interest for the gth groups.
If the statistic $\chi_{HL}^2 < \chi_{\nu,1-\alpha}^2$, then we conclude there is not enough evidence to show that the model has lack of fit.

Example 16.9 Referring to Example 16.8, assess the goodness-of-fit of the model.

Solution
Table 16.11 shows the results of the goodness-of-fit tests for the model in Example 16.8 with three test methods (using SAS software for the deviance and Pearson residual tests). All demonstrate a good fit $(p > 0.05)$, which indicates that the logistic regression model obtained a good fit.

Figure 16.3 shows the residuals by subject. The y-axis in Figures 16.3(a) and 16.3(b) corresponds to standardized versions of Pearson residuals and deviance residuals. Because there appear to be some large residuals in Figures 16.3(a) and 16.3(b), it appears that some of the observations require further inspection.

Table 16.11 Goodness-of-fit test results for three testing methods for Example 16.8.

Test	χ^2	v	p value
Deviance	278.7764	261	0.2147
Pearson	244.7936	261	0.7565
Hosmer–Lemeshow	4.0978	8	0.8482

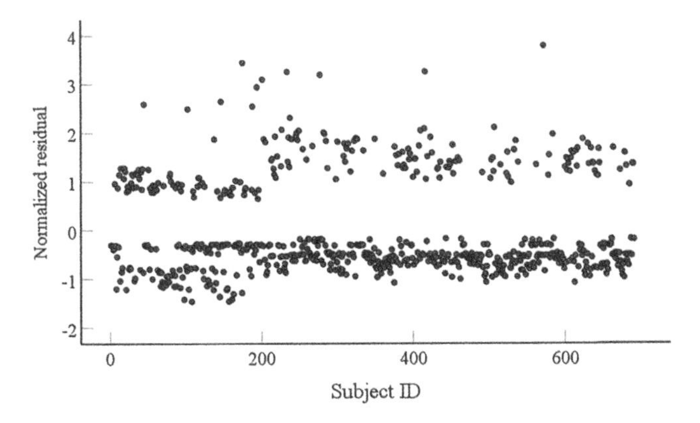

Figure 16.3a Pearson residual by subject for the data in Example 16.8.

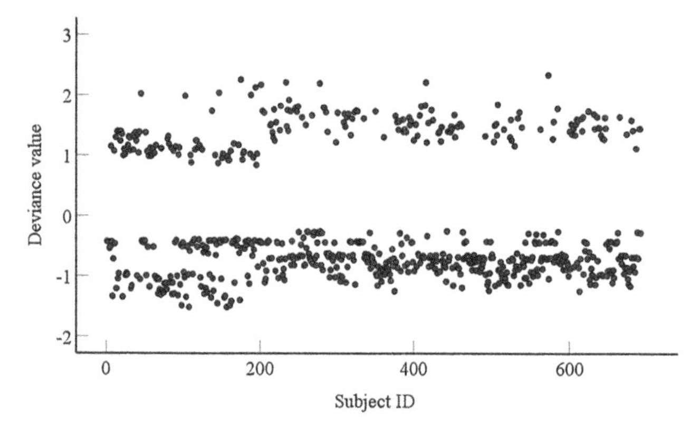

Figure 16.3b Deviance residual by subject for the data in Example 16.8.

Table 16.12 Goodness-of-fit test results for the three testing methods for Example 16.8.

Test	χ^2	v	p value
Deviance	250.1023	257	0.6093
Pearson	227.2097	257	0.9097
Hosmer–Lemeshow	9.8420	8	0.2763

Note: results obtained after deleting the outliers with Pearson residuals larger than 2

Outliers in logistic regression are typically identified by constructing appropriate diagrams and identifying points in them that appear to lie apart from the main body of the data. Note that a "point" in these circumstances relates to individuals with the same pattern of independent variables, not to a particular individual as in multiple regression. For example, outliers may be detected by plotting the logistic residual (e.g., the Pearson or deviance residual) against the subjects.

If we delete the outliers with standardized Pearson residuals larger than 2, the results of the goodness-of-fit tests change to the values shown in Table 16.12, in which the χ^2 of the deviance and Pearson residual tests becomes less than that in Table 16.11, and the p value becomes larger. This shows the effect of outliers on the goodness-of-fit.

16.2 Conditional Logistic Regression Model

Data from paired samples design can also be analyzed using a logistic regression approach. As we discussed in Chapter 8, matching is a way of balancing certain characteristics between two groups. If matching is used in the design phase of a study, a treatment is given to one member of a matched pair and a placebo is given to the other. In case-control studies (see Chapter 19), a case with a particular outcome is matched to a control without the outcome of interest and an examination of a possible relationship to an exposure is assessed retrospectively. Matching can be one-to-one or one-to-many controls. An approach to analyzing matched studies in multiple regression models is conditional logistic regression. *Conditional logistic regression* allows us to compare cases with controls in the same matched "set." In this scenario, the "outcome" is defined by the patient being a case (typically coded 1) or control (typically coded 0). We illustrate this method in the following example.

As seen in Example 16.1, an outcome may be affected by a number of risk factors, and when studying the association between an outcome with a specified factor (exposure), a confounding factor may have an impact on the reliability of casual inference. For the adjustment of one or a few confounding factors, the paired samples design is frequently used, and it is similar to what we have learned in Chapter 8 and later chapters. In a matched case-control study, each of the cases is paired with one or more controls that have identical, or at least similar, factors to the case, that is, 1:1 matching or 1:n matching. We introduce conditional logistic regression for the paired samples design case-control study data using 1:1 matching as an example.

Example 16.10 Referring to the multicenter study in Example 16.1, after identifying the outcome status, we selected 195 cases (subjects with UI) and paired each of the cases with one matched control who had the same delivery method and similar age (difference no greater than 5 years). Some of the data on the matched pairs are shown in Table 16.13. Perform multiple conditional logistic regression analysis.

Table 16.13 Data of matched pairs extracted from an epidemiological survey on risk factors of UI.

Pair ID	Age (years)	Delivery method	BMI (kg/m^2)	History of pelvic surgery	UI
1	68	Vaginal	< 24	No	No
1	69	Vaginal	≥ 24	Yes	Yes
2	37	Vaginal	< 24	No	No
2	42	Vaginal	< 24	No	Yes
3	44	Cesarean	< 24	Yes	No
3	49	Cesarean	≥ 24	Yes	Yes
4	63	Vaginal	< 24	Yes	No
4	60	Vaginal	≥ 24	Yes	Yes
5	21	No	< 24	No	No
5	21	No	< 24	No	Yes
6	51	Vaginal	< 24	No	No
6	48	Vaginal	< 24	No	Yes
7	80	No	≥ 24	No	No
7	81	No	≥ 24	No	Yes
8	33	Cesarean	< 24	Yes	No
8	31	Cesarean	< 24	No	Yes
9	72	No	< 24	Yes	No
9	74	No	≥ 24	No	Yes
10	68	Vaginal	< 24	No	No
10	69	Vaginal	< 24	Yes	Yes
...	...	...	...	...	...

16.2.1 Characteristics of Conditional Logistic Regression Model

Let y be a binary dependent variable, $y = 1$ for the case and $y = 0$ for the control, and $x_1, x_2, \ldots, x_k$ be independent variables. To fit a conditional logistic regression model, we take each matched pair as a stratum, and let $\pi(y = 1 | x_1, x_2, \ldots, x_k) = \pi(x)_i$ denote the probability of the case for the ith strata conditional on $x_1, x_2, \ldots, x_k$. Similar to unconditional logistic regression, the conditional logistic regression model is written as

$$\text{logit}(\pi(x)_i) = \beta_{i0} + \beta_1 x_1 + \cdots + \beta_k x_k.$$

If we take the exponential transformation, then

$$\pi(x)_i = \frac{\exp(\beta_{i0} + \beta_1 x_1 + \cdots + \beta_k x_k)}{1 + \exp(\beta_{i0} + \beta_1 x_1 + \cdots + \beta_k x_k)},$$

where $\beta_1, \beta_2, \ldots, \beta_k$ are the partial regression coefficients for the independent variables, which do not vary in different matched pairs.

In paired samples design, we are generally interested in estimating the effect of the independent variables $(\beta_1, \beta_2, \ldots, \beta_k)$ instead of the specific effect for each pair (β_{i0}); hence, we can omit the intercept β_{i0} from the conditional logistic equation. Thus, for the overall model,

$$\text{logit}(\pi(x)) = \beta_1 x_1 + \beta_2 x_2 + \cdots + \beta_k x_k. \tag{16.30}$$

16.2.2 Estimation of Regression Coefficient

1. Conditional Maximum Likelihood Estimation

To estimate the partial regression coefficients of conditional logistic regression, we use a *conditional likelihood function* instead of the likelihood function for ML estimation. Again, we walk through this procedure using a simple example in which there is only one binary independent variable x. To establish a conditional likelihood function, a four-fold contingency table for a matched pairs design case-control study is shown in Table 16.14.

We designate π_1 and π_0 as the probabilities of disease conditional on exposure and no exposure, respectively, according to the conditional logistic regression equation. Hence,

$$\pi_1 = \pi(D | E) = \frac{e^{\beta_0 + \beta}}{1 + e^{\beta_0 + \beta}}$$

$$\pi_0 = \pi(D | \bar{E}) = \frac{e^{\beta_0}}{1 + e^{\beta_0}}$$

Table 16.14 Four-fold table for a paired samples design case-control study.

Control $(\bar{D})$	Case (D)	
	Exposure (E)	**No exposure $(\bar{E})$**
Exposure (E)	n_{11}	n_{12}
No exposure $(\bar{E})$	n_{21}	n_{22}

For each matched pair (two individuals are denoted by A and B), where one is a case (diseased) and the other is a control (not diseased), we have the following possible conditions:

(1) Both A and B are exposed

The conditional probability that one is diseased and the other is not diseased is

$$
\begin{aligned}
&P(\text{only one is diseased}|\text{both are exposed})\\
&=P((\text{case } A \text{ control } B|\text{both are exposed})\cup(\text{control } A \text{ case } B|\text{both are exposed}))\\
&=P(\text{case } A \text{ control } B|\text{both are exposed})+P(\text{control } A \text{ case } B|\text{both are exposed})\\
&=\frac{1}{4}+\frac{1}{4}=\frac{1}{2}.
\end{aligned}
$$

(2) Both A and B are not exposed

The conditional probability that one is diseased and the other is not diseased is

$$
\begin{aligned}
&P(\text{only one is diseased}|\text{both are not exposed})\\
&=P((\text{case } A \text{ control } B|\text{both are not exposed})\cup(\text{control } A \text{ case } B|\text{both are not exposed}))\\
&=P(\text{case } A \text{ control } B|\text{both are not exposed})+P(\text{control } A \text{ case } B|\text{both are not exposed})\\
&=\frac{1}{4}+\frac{1}{4}=\frac{1}{2}.
\end{aligned}
$$

(3) Only one is exposed

The conditional probability that only the exposed is diseased is

$$
\begin{aligned}
&P(\text{the exposed is diseased}|\text{only one is exposed})\\
&=\frac{\pi_1(1-\pi_0)}{\pi_1(1-\pi_0)+\pi_0(1-\pi_1)}=\frac{\frac{e^{\beta_0+\beta}}{1+e^{\beta_0+\beta}}\times\frac{1}{1+e^{\beta_0}}}{\frac{e^{\beta_0+\beta}}{1+e^{\beta_0+\beta}}\times\frac{1}{1+e^{\beta_0}}+\frac{e^{\beta_0}}{1+e^{\beta_0}}\times\frac{1}{1+e^{\beta_0+\beta}}}=\frac{e^{\beta}}{1+e^{\beta}}.
\end{aligned}
$$

Table 16.15 Conditional probability distribution of the paired samples design case-control study.

Control	Case	
	Exposure (1)	**No exposure (0)**
Exposure (1)	$1/2$	$1/\left(1+e^{\beta}\right)$
No exposure (0)	$e^{\beta}/\left(1+e^{\beta}\right)$	$1/2$

The conditional probability that only the not exposed is diseased is

$$P(\text{the not exposed is diseased}|\text{only one is exposed})$$

$$=\frac{\pi_0\left(1-\pi_1\right)}{\pi_1\left(1-\pi_0\right)+\pi_0\left(1-\pi_1\right)}=\frac{\dfrac{e^{\beta_0}}{1+e^{\beta_0}}\times\dfrac{1}{1+e^{\beta_0+\beta}}}{\dfrac{e^{\beta_0+\beta}}{1+e^{\beta_0+\beta}}\times\dfrac{1}{1+e^{\beta_0}}+\dfrac{e^{\beta_0}}{1+e^{\beta_0}}\times\dfrac{1}{1+e^{\beta_0+\beta}}}=\frac{1}{1+e^{\beta}}.$$

Thus, the conditional probability distribution of the paired samples design case-control study is shown in Table 16.15.

The conditional likelihood function for Tables 16.14 and 16.15 is

$$L=\left(\frac{1}{2}\right)^{n_{11}}\left(\frac{1}{1+e^{\beta}}\right)^{n_{12}}\left(\frac{e^{\beta}}{1+e^{\beta}}\right)^{n_{21}}\left(\frac{1}{2}\right)^{n_{22}}.$$

If we take the logarithm transformation, then

$$\ln L=-\left(n_{11}+n_{22}\right)\ln 2+n_{21}\beta-\left(n_{12}+n_{21}\right)\ln\left(1+e^{\beta}\right).$$

Note that the likelihood function is free of the intercept β_0. Thus, we only need to take the first partial derivative of $\ln L$ with respect to β, and let it be 0 to estimate the regression coefficient β

$$\frac{\partial \ln L}{\partial \beta}=n_{21}-\left(n_{12}+n_{21}\right)\times\left(\frac{e^{\beta}}{1+e^{\beta}}\right)=0$$

The ML estimate for β is

$$b=\ln\frac{n_{21}}{n_{12}}, \tag{16.31}$$

and the ML estimate for OR in conditional logistic regression is

$$\widehat{OR}=\frac{n_{21}}{n_{12}}. \tag{16.32}$$

While advanced statistical packages may sometimes allow us to perform conditional logistic regression directly, it may be necessary to use the Cox's proportional hazards regression model in SPSS software.

Example 16.11 Referring to Example 16.10, estimate the regression coefficient and OR of a conditional logistic regression model for UI using a history of pelvic surgery alone as the explanatory variable.

Solution
When only a history of pelvic surgery is considered, n_{11}=17, n_{12}=16, n_{21}=49, n_{22} = 113; therefore

$$b = \ln\frac{n_{21}}{n_{12}} = \ln\frac{49}{16} = 1.119$$

$$\widehat{OR} = \frac{n_{21}}{n_{12}} = \frac{49}{16} = 3.063$$

The estimated OR 3.063 is larger than 1.703 estimated in Example 16.5, and we have a similar interpretation to the value 3.063.

16.2.3 Hypothesis Testing of Regression Coefficient

The hypothesis testing methods and goodness-of-fit tests for conditional logistic regression analysis are largely similar to those of unconditional logistic regression as introduced in Section 16.1.4.

Example 16.12 Referring to Example 16.10, estimate the regression coefficient and OR of a conditional logistic regression model for UI using the variables history of pelvic surgery and overweight.

Solution
The independent variables considered in the conditional logistic regression model are the same as those in Table 16.8, except that age and delivery method are not considered because they have been matched.

The partial regression coefficients can be estimated using SPSS software. Table16.16 shows the partial regression coefficient estimates, their standard errors, Wald's test results, and ORs.

Table 16.16 shows that the Wald's test $p < 0.05$ for two independent variables, that is, the two independent variables are statistically significant, which indicates that they are risk factors of UI. The odds of UI are 2.692 times greater among women with a history of pelvic surgery that those without. The impact of being overweight is interpreted in the same manner. Additionally, the likelihood ratio test $p < 0.05$ also means that the overall model is statistically significant.

Note that an appropriate paired samples design could help to improve the statistical power. As in this example, the sample size (195 + 195 = 390) is much smaller than that in Example 16.1 (208 + 487 = 691), and both estimates of the effects of a history of

Table 16.16 Estimate and significance test results for the regression coefficients.

Model	Coefficient	Standard error	Wald statistic	*p* value	Odds ratio	95% confidence intervel
Overweight	1.614	0.287	31.633	< 0.001	5.024	[2.862, 8.816]
History of Pelvic surgery	0.990	0.316	9.806	0.002	2.692	[1.449, 5.005]

Likelihood ratio: $\chi^2 = 59.699$, $\nu = 2$, $p < 0.001$.

pelvic surgery on UI are statistically significant. Additionally, the OR estimated in conditional logistic regression is 2.692, which is larger than the unconditional 2.398 in Example 16.8.

The major disadvantage to matching is that it can be costly, both in terms of the time and labor required to find appropriate matches and in terms of information loss caused by discarding the available controls that are not able to satisfy the matching criteria. In fact, if too much information is lost from matching, this may result in a loss of statistical power by matching.

When deciding whether to match or not on a given factor, the safest strategy is to match only on strong risk factors that are expected to cause serious confounding in the data. The factors considered for matching should be small, because over matching or improper matching could also lead to bias.

16.3 Additional Remarks

16.3.1 Sample Size

Overall, the sample size requirement is greater for logistic regression analysis than ordinary linear regression analysis because the dependent variable is categorical. Another requirement is that the sample size at each level of the categorical outcome has to be sufficient for logistic regression analysis. A rule of thumb is that the number of observations at each level should be more than 10 times (ideally more than 20 times) the number of independent variables to achieve good precision for the estimation. Additionally, there should not be too many unordered levels in the independent variables to avoid too many combinations of x and y, which may increase the chance of an insufficient sample size in each cell.

16.3.2 Types of Independent Variables

There are no strict restrictions for the types of independent variables in logistic regression analysis. Binary variables can be directly included in the logistic regression model, and its partial regression coefficient is the log-OR of two levels of events. For an unordered multiclass explanatory variable, each level of the variable makes no quantitative difference and there is no linear relationship between them, so it is necessary to set dummy variables for further analysis. A continuous explanatory variable can be directly included, and sometimes we can also transform it into a categorical variable. Although there may be some loss of information, this has been proved to be a useful approach to improve the linearity and interpretation of the results. An ordinal categorical variable can be set as a dummy variable, and the explanation of a partial regression coefficient is the same as that of an unordered categorical variable. If the degrees of each rank of the ordinal categorical variable are similar, they can also be assigned as a continuous value according to the rank order, and then included in the model as a continuous variable.

16.3.3 Selection of Independent Variables

Statistical modeling results on the same data may vary because of different study purposes and evaluation criteria, and, to a certain extent, selecting the "best" model is the art of the statistician.

Generally, variable selection methods in logistic regression are similar to those in multiple linear regression (so we omit this content in this chapter). When there are many candidate variables, the selection should be based on background knowledge and univariate analysis results, and the criterion for the latter could be relatively relaxed, for instance, using $\alpha = 0.1$ as the level of significance. Then the final model can be established using a forward method, backward method, or step-by-step method. In most cases, the results of regression models based on different variable selection methods are essentially the same. If the partial regression coefficients or the diagnostic model statistics of each model are greatly different, we should further deduce the reasons, and use interpretability, professional knowledge, and statistical significance to determine the most reasonable regression model.

16.3.4 Missing Data

Missing data are generally unavoidable. In the process of establishing a logistic regression model, only records with complete independent variables and response variables can be included in the model construction process; that is, a record will not be included in the equation if any variable in the record is missing. Therefore, if there are many variables in a study, and each factor has a certain number of missing records, the final regression model may contain fewer records than expected. Attention should be paid to this issue, and independent variables with a missing rate that is too high should be removed in the construction process of the logistic regression model. Clinical significance and statistical significance should also be considered to ensure the stability and accuracy of the model.

16.4 Summary

The goal of logistic regression in this chapter is to create an equation that can be used to estimate the probability of an event of interest for the dependent outcome based on one or more independent variables. The logistic regression model can be divided into different branches according to the type of research design, such as unconditional logistic regression for complete random design data and conditional logistic regression for paired samples design data.

The logistic regression model has no special requirements for the type of independent variables. Continuous, binary, unordered, and ordered variables can be included in the model as independent variables after proper handling.

The general interpretation of the partial regression coefficient is β_j, with all other variables held constant. For every unit of increase in the independent variable x_j, the log-OR of y as an event of interest over the reference event increases by β_j units on average.

The Wald's test and likelihood ratio test can be used for hypothesis testing of the partial regression coefficient in the logistic regression model. The Wald's test is mostly used to measure whether the contribution of a single independent variable to the model is significant. The likelihood ratio test is used to test all partial regression coefficients of the model as a whole; that is, to test the overall model fit.

16.5 Exercises

1. In a retrospective cohort study on the impact of low birth weight on the development of type 2 diabetes in middle and old age, 152 subjects with low birth weight (<2500 g) were selected using medical records from a hospital, and 738 subjects with normal birth weight (≥2500 g) were selected as the control. Data on age, sex (1 = Male, 2 = Female), birth weight, family history of type 2 diabetes (1 = Yes, 0 = No), serum lipid status (1 = Abnormal, 0 = Normal), and diagnosis of type 2 diabetes (1 = Yes, 0 = No) at investigation were collected and part of the data is shown in Table 16.17.

Table 16.17 Data in a study on the impact of low birth weight on the development of type 2 diabetes in middle and old age.

Id	Age (years)	Sex	Family history	Serum lipid	Birth weight (g)	Diabetes
1	82	Female	No	Normal	1784	No
2	72	Male	Yes	Normal	1865	Yes
3	74	Female	No	Normal	2000	Yes
4	71	Female	Yes	Normal	2320	Yes
5	62	Male	No	Normal	2390	No
6	73	Female	No	Normal	2334	Yes
7	76	Female	Yes	Abnormal	2435	No
8	70	Male	No	Normal	2340	No
...	...	...	...	...	...	...
890	52	Male	No	Normal	3300	No

Note: see the Appendix online for the complete data.

(a) In order to study the effect of low birth weight on type 2 diabetes, what model do you think is more suitable for analyzing this data? Please establish a suitable logistic regression equation.

(b) Write down the regression model structure and interpret the logit link function in your own words.

(c) How do you determine the partial regression coefficients? What is the difference with the least squares method?

(d) Perform significance tests of the partial regression coefficients and the overall fitted model. What are the differences between these tests? Can they replace each other?

(e) Is the regression model obtained by the stepwise regression method optimal? Why?

(f) From what perspectives could you assess the goodness-of-fit of the model?

(g) Given a 69-year-old man who has no family history of diabetes, abnormal serum lipid profiles, and was of normal birth weight, predict his probability of having type 2 diabetes.

(h) Suppose the data are collected using a paired samples design. What is the difference in the estimation method? Why is a paired samples design more efficient than the present design?

2. In a case-control study on the risk factors of type 2 diabetes, 1:1 paired samples design was applied. There were 91 pairs of case and control that were matched according to sex and similar age. Data on hypertension, obesity and family history of diabetes were collected and shown in Table 16.18 (Hypertension: 1 = Yes, 0 = No; Obesity: 1 = Yes, 0 = No; Family history of diabetes: 1 = Yes, 0 = No; Type 2 diabetes: 1 = Yes, 0 = No).

Table 16.18 Data from a case-control study on the risk factors of type 2 diabetes.

Pair ID	Hypertension	Obesity	Family history of diabetes	Type 2 diabetes
1	0	0	1	0
1	1	1	1	1
2	1	1	0	0
2	0	1	0	1
3	0	1	0	0
3	0	1	1	1
4	1	1	0	0
4	1	0	0	1
5	0	0	0	0
5	1	1	0	1
6	0	0	0	0
6	1	1	0	1

(Continued)

Table 16.18 (Continued)

Pair ID	Hypertension	Obesity	Family history of diabetes	Type 2 diabetes
7	1	1	0	0
7	0	1	0	1
8	0	0	0	0
8	1	1	0	1
9	0	0	0	0
9	1	1	0	1
10	0	1	0	0
10	1	1	0	1
…	…	…	…	…
91	0	0	0	0
91	0	0	1	1

Note: see the Appendix online for the complete data.

(a) What are the advantages of paired samples design and what we need to pay attention to when matching?

(b) Perform a multiple conditional logistic regression analysis.

(c) What method does conditional logistic regression use to estimate the model parameters, and how does the model equation differ from unconditional logistic regression?

(d) How would the results change if unconditional logistic regression is used? Why this is not suitable?

(e) If a family history of diabetes is considered as an exposure factor and obesity and hypertension are considered as potential confounders, how does the OR of family history of diabetes on the occurrence of diabetes change when adding all three factors to the model or deleting either or both of the potential confounders, and try to explain the changes.

17

Survival Analysis

Thus far, we have learned methods for the description and inference of numerical and categorical data, including some regression models that address the relationship between a numerical and categorical outcome and other explanatory variable(s). In this chapter, we will discuss survival data, which are a particular type of data that are of great interest in the biomedical field and typically collected in longitudinal studies, where we are not only interested in whether an event occurs (e.g., the onset of coronary heart disease or recurrence of a tumor), but also the length of time until the event occurs (i.e., time-to-event process). Survival data have two important characteristics: (i) the survival time is non-negative and typically positively skewed; and (ii) the full survival time is typically not observed for all individuals during the follow-up period. These features have hampered the application of traditional methods for the description, inference, and modeling of survival data, and have given rise to a family of statistical theories and methods collectively termed *survival analysis*, which has flourished in recent decades in biostatistics. In this chapter, we introduce basic methods for describing survival data, and compare different survival processes and a widely applied method – Cox's proportional hazards model – for identifying the risk (or prognostic) factors related to the survival outcome.

Applied Medical Statistics, First Edition. Jingmei Jiang.

Companion website: www.wiley.com\go\jiang\appliedmedicalstatistics

17.1 Overview

17.1.1 Concept of Survival Analysis

To set the framework for a discussion about the analysis of survival data, we first introduce several basic concepts.

1. Initial Event and Terminal Event

The *initial event* is a specific event that marks the starting point of the survival process of an individual, such as receiving surgery, diagnosis of a disease, or first medication. The *terminal event*, also known as the *failure event*, refers to the specific outcome of the individual that is of research interest, such as death or relapse. Clearly, the definitions of these events are crucial for survival analysis, so they should be clearly defined in the research design according to the research objectives, and strictly followed during the research process.

2. Survival Time

The time elapsed from the initial event to the terminal event is called the *survival time* (denoted by T), also called the *failure time*. Note that we call it the survival time because death is the prototypical event in the biomedical field; however, survival analysis does not necessarily relate to survival/death, but to the terminal event defined in specific research.

Example 17.1 To investigate the risk factors of a poor prognosis (relapse or death) in patients with primary esophageal cancer, a follow-up survey was conducted among postoperative patients discharged from hospital. The researcher observed and recorded the discharge date, terminal date for observation, and outcome status of each patient. Part of the data is shown in Table 17.1. Identify the initial and terminal events, and survival time.

Analysis
The initial event in this study is postoperative discharge, and the terminal event is the relapse of cancer or death. The survival time is the interval between the discharge date and date of relapse or death, that is, the terminal date of observation of patients.

Table 17.1 Follow-up records of five postoperative patients with esophageal cancer after discharge.

Patient ID	Sex	Age (years)	Discharge date	Terminal date	Outcome	Survival time (months)
1	Male	53	2015-07-08	2018-08-23	Loss to follow-up	37.5^{+}
2	Male	62	2015-07-01	2019-03-10	Death	44.3
3	Female	75	2015-07-16	2017-08-25	Death	25.3
4	Male	73	2015-08-18	2017-02-20	Relapse	18.1
5	Female	61	2015-10-10	2020-07-01	Survival	56.7^{+}

Note: Time values marked with a "+" sign represent right censored values (see below for definition of "right censored").

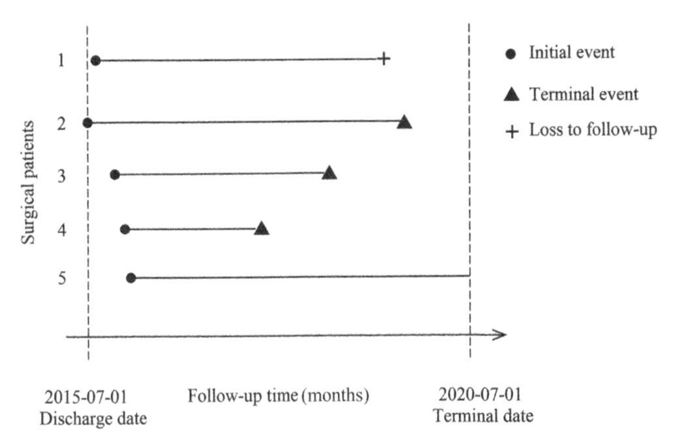

Figure 17.1 Schematic diagram of the follow-up data of five postoperative patients with esophageal cancer.

Schematic diagram of the follow-up data of five postoperative patients with esophageal cancer is shown in Figure 17.1.

Note that patients may leave the study for different reasons, and as shown in Figure 17.1, the information on the date of relapse or death was not available for all patients during the follow-up period. Generally, there are two categories of survival time data:

(1) Complete data: The exact survival time can be ascertained if the terminal event occurs before the end of the study. Such data are called *complete data*, which provide complete survival time information for the study. As in Example 17.1, patients ID 2 and 3 died before the end of the study, and patient ID 4 relapsed before the end of the study.
(2) Censored data: The exact survival time cannot be ascertained if the terminal event of the research object has not been observed, or has not been precisely determined in a time scale, for some reason, such as lost to follow-up (patient ID 1 in Table 17.1), no occurrence of the terminal event within the study period (patient ID 5), or withdrawal from the study. Such data are called *censored data*, or *incomplete data*, and only provide partial information on the survival time.

The condition in which the survival time is only partially known is termed *censoring*, and is a key analytic problem that most survival analyses must take into consideration. Censoring can be further classified into three categories:

(1) *Right censored* is typically identified by the superscripted symbol "+" in the observed survival time. For example, survival time for the first subject in Table 17.1 is 37.5^{+} (months), which indicates that actual survival time of the subject is longer than the observed time.
(2) *Left censored* indicates that actual survival time of the subject is shorter than the observed time.
(3) *Interval censored* means that the actual survival time of the subject is not known precisely, but instead, is only known to fall into a particular interval.

We focus only on right censored data in this chapter because they occur most frequently in the field of biomedical research.

17.1.2 Basic Functions of Survival Time

Survival time can be influenced by various random factors and is a random variable. Several functions are used to reflect the distribution characteristics of survival time in survival analysis. Here we introduce three most basic functions: density function, survival function, and hazard function, which play an important role in the description of, and inferences made from survival data.

1. Density Function

Definition 17.1 Let T be a non-negative continuous random variable that denotes the survival time. Its distribution form can be completely determined by the *density function*, which is defined as

$$\begin{aligned} f(t) &= \lim_{\Delta t \to 0} \frac{P(t \le T < t + \Delta t)}{\Delta t} \\ &= \lim_{\Delta t \to 0} \frac{P(\text{terminal event observed in } [t, t + \Delta t) \text{period})}{\Delta t}, \end{aligned} \tag{17.1}$$

where Δt refers to a very small period of time.

The density function to survival data is similar to its role to continuous variables introduced in Chapter 5. Note that the density function is not a probability but a rate, and reflects the instantaneous rate of the occurrence of the terminal event at any time t. The shape of the density function of survival time is typically right skewed.

The cumulative form of $f(t)$ over the time interval $[0, t]$ is known as the *distribution function* or *cumulative function* of T:

$$F(t) = P(T \le t) = \int_0^t f(x)dx. \tag{17.2}$$

2. Survival Function

Definition 17.2 *Survival function*, also known as the *cumulative survival probability* or *survival rate*, is defined as:

$$S(t) = P(T > t) = 1 - F(t) = \int_t^{\infty} f(x)dx. \tag{17.3}$$

$S(t)$ is the most intuitive description of the survival process, and it quantifies the probability that survival will be greater than time t.

According to Definition 17.2, $S(t)$ has two important properties: (i) it is monotone non-increasing; and (ii) $S(0) = 1$, and $S(\infty) = 0$. In practice, $S(t)$ is generally estimated by

$$\hat{S}(t) = \frac{\text{number of individuals whose survival time} > t}{\text{total number of follow-up individuals}}. \tag{17.4}$$

If we plot $S(t)$ against survival time t, then a *survival curve* can be obtained, such as that shown in Figure 17.2. Note that the survival curve is smooth in theory, but because non-parametric methods are often used to empirically estimate the survival rate, the curve may appear to be a staircase when the number of observations is small.

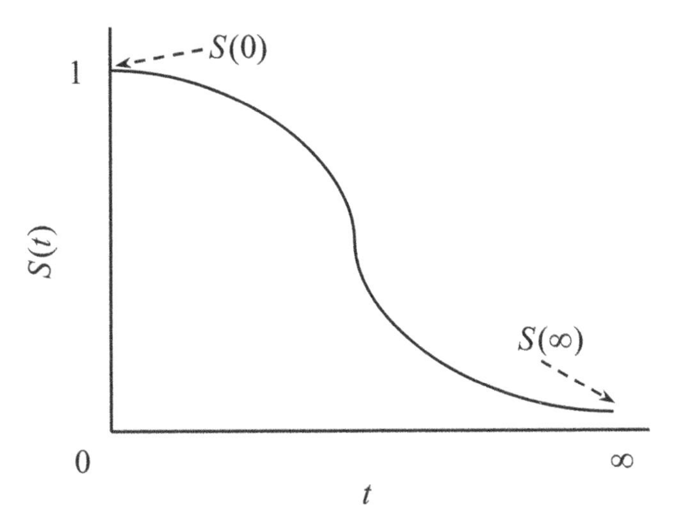

Figure 17.2 Illustration of survival curve.

3. Hazard Function

Definition 17.3 The *hazard function*, at time *t* is the instantaneous rate of failure at time *t*, and is defined as

$$h(t) = \lim_{\Delta t \to 0} \frac{P\left(t \leq T < t + \Delta t \mid T \geq t\right)}{\Delta t}. \tag{17.5}$$

Formula 17.5 expresses the hazard rate as the ratio of the conditional probability at *t* over an infinitesimal time change. Like *f(t)*, *h(t)* is not a probability but a rate. It is often referred to as *conditional hazard* or *instantaneous hazard*. In practice, it can be estimated by

$$\hat{h}(t) = \frac{\text{number of individuals with terminal events in}\,(t,\ t + \Delta t)}{\left(\text{number of surviving individuals at } t\right) \times \Delta t}. \tag{17.6}$$

According to Definition 17.3, $h(t)$ is in the range $\left[0,\ \infty\right)$ and can be a constant, an increasing or decreasing function, or even a complex shape. In practice, the laws of many natural phenomena can be described by $h(t)$, as shown in Figure 17.3.

In Figure 17.3, the hazard function represented by $h_1(t)$ is constant; this means the risk of death is independent of time, for example, the risk of death remains low for young adults. The hazard function represented by $h_2(t)$ increases with time, for example, the risk of death for elder people gradually increases with the person's age. The hazard function represented by $h_3(t)$ decreases as time increases, for example, the risk of death after a successful rescue from a car accident gradually decreases. The hazard function represented by $h_4(t)$ is U-shaped. The risk of the terminal event is high at the beginning, then gradually decreases, stabilizes at a lower level, and finally gradually increases, for example, the change in the risk of death for humans when viewed from a lifetime horizon. The hazard function represented by $h_5(t)$ is mountain-shaped. The risk of the terminal event at the beginning increases with time, and

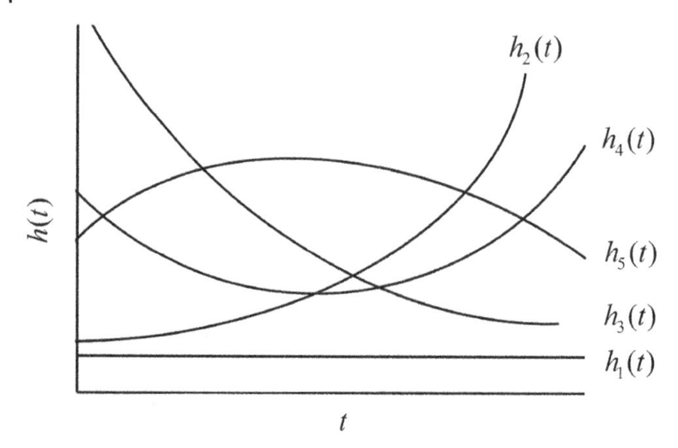

Figure 17.3 Illustration of common risk functions.

gradually decreases after reaching the peak. For example, tuberculosis patients have an increased risk of death at the beginning, and their risk gradually decreases after effective treatment. The identification of the shape of the hazard function helps us to fit the mathematical model so that is suitable for the survival data.

In fact, there is a close relationship among the functions $f(t)$, $S(t)$, and $h(t)$. Through the mathematical transformation of $h(t)$,

$$\begin{aligned} h(t) &= \lim_{\Delta t \to 0} \frac{P(t \le T < t + \Delta t \mid T \ge t)}{\Delta t} \\ &= \lim_{\Delta t \to 0} \frac{P(t \le T < t + \Delta t \ \& T \ge t)}{\Delta t \cdot P(T \ge t)} \\ &= \lim_{\Delta t \to 0} \frac{S(t) - S(t + \Delta t)}{\Delta t \cdot S(t)} \\ &= -\frac{\mathrm{d}(\ln S(t))}{\mathrm{d}t}. \end{aligned} \tag{17.7}$$

If both sides of Formula 17.7 are integrated,

$$S(\mathrm{t}) = e^{-\int_0^t h(u)du}. \tag{17.8}$$

Formula 17.8 can be used for the conversion between $S(t)$ and $h(t)$.

We can prove that when $\Delta t \to 0$,

$$\begin{aligned} h(t)\Delta t &= P(t \le T < t + \Delta t \mid T \ge t) = \frac{P(t \le T < t + \Delta t \ \& T \ge t)}{P(T \ge t)} \\ &= \frac{P(t \le T < t + \Delta t)}{P(T \ge t)} = \frac{f(t)\Delta t}{S(t)}. \end{aligned}$$

The relationship between the three functions $f(t)$, $h(t)$, and $S(t)$ can be expressed as

$$f(t) = h(t)S(t). \tag{17.9}$$

Through Formulas 17.8 and 17.9, we may obtain $f(t)$, $h(t)$, and $S(t)$ when any of them is known.

17.2 Description of the Survival Process

After obtaining the survival data, it is necessary to conduct descriptive analysis and consider whether parametric or non-parametric methods should be used. Although parametric methods assume that the survival time follows a certain distribution, such as the exponential distribution, Weibull distribution, or Gamma distribution, in practice, it is typically difficult to determine the distribution of the survival time. The non-parametric methods introduced in this section are more convenient and commonly applied in the description of survival data. We here introduce two commonly used methods: product limit method and life table method.

17.2.1 Product Limit Method

The *product limit method*, also called the *Kaplan–Meier (KM) method*, was introduced by E.L. Kaplan and P. Meier in 1958 to estimate the survival function for randomly censored data. The KM method is widely applied to ungrouped data, particularly in the case of small samples.

The basic principle of the KM method is to use the product of conditional probabilities to estimate the survival rate. Assume a sample of size n, where there are n potential survival times until all terminal events of interest (e.g., death) occur. We sort these survival times from smallest to largest:

$$t_1 \le t_2 \le t_3 \le \cdots \le t_n,$$

where $t_i\ (i = 1, 2, 3, \ldots, n)$ represents the time when the terminal event or right censoring occurred in individual i. If the survival time of the subject has no "tie" (some individuals may share the same survival times, which is referred to as the tied observation time), then total number of survival times is correspondingly equal to the number of observations. The survival times are expressed in order as

$$t_1 < t_2 < t_3 < \cdots < t_n.$$

In fact, because of the existence of a "tie," the total number of survival times is less than the number of observations n.

1. The Point Estimation of $S(t)$

Suppose n_i is the number of survivors exposed to a certain event risk at time t_i. Then $n_1 \ge n_2 \ge n_3 \ge \cdots \ge n_n$, where $n_n = 1$ represents the last survivor. Let d_i represent the number of people who have the terminal event at time t_i (if there is no tie at t_i, then $d_i = 1$). The formula for calculating the KM estimator of the survival rate at time t is

$$\hat{S}(t) = \prod_{t_i \le t} \frac{n_i - d_i}{n_i}. \tag{17.10}$$

Although not specifically noted, Formula 17.10 is inclusive of the censored scenario; that is, the occurrence of censoring does not affect the validity of the formula. For example, if we have $d_i = 0$ during t_{i-1} to t_i, then $n_i = n_{i-1} - 1$, and the conditional probability of survival from t_{i-1} to t_i is 1.

2. The Interval Estimate of $S(t)$

The sample survival rate calculated with the Formula 17.10 is the point estimate of the population survival rate, and $(1-\alpha)\times 100\%$ CI of the $S(t)$ is estimated using normal approximation as

$$\left[\hat{S}(t) - z_{1-\alpha/2}\sqrt{Var\left[\hat{S}(t)\right]},\ \hat{S}(t) + z_{1-\alpha/2}\sqrt{Var\left[\hat{S}(t)\right]}\right], \tag{17.11}$$

where the variance of $\hat{S}(t)$ is often estimated by the Greenwood method, and its approximate calculation formula is

$$Var\left[\hat{S}(t)\right] \approx \hat{S}(t)^2 \sum_{t_i \le t} \frac{d_i}{n_i\left(n_i - d_i\right)}. \tag{17.12}$$

It should be noted that the normal approximation may not be appropriate at either end of the survival curve, that is, when $\hat{S}(t)$ approaches 0 or 1 at this time. An alternative method is to calculate the survival rate and standard error after logarithmic transformation, and then calculate the confidence interval based on the principle of normal distribution for the transformed survival rate. Thus, the confidence interval can be obtained by inverting the corresponding confidence limit.

Example 17.2 Referring to Example 17.1, use the KM method to describe the survival process of the five esophageal cancer patients shown in Table 17.1.

Solution

The calculation procedure of the KM method is shown in Table 17.2.

(1) Sort the survival time of patients with terminal events and censored patients from smallest to largest (column (2) in Table 17.2).
(2) List the number of terminal events d_i at time t_i (column (3)). For instance, only patient ID 4 relapses at the 18.1th month, so $d_1 = 1$.
(3) List the number n_i of individuals still alive at time t_i, which is called the *risk set* (column (4)). For example, before the 44.3rd month, two patients had a terminal event and one patient was lost to follow-up, so the size of the risk set at the 44.3rd month was 2.
(4) Based on Formulas 17.10 and 17.12, the survival rate $\hat{S}(t_i)$ and variance $Var\left[\hat{S}(t_i)\right]$ at time t_i can be estimated (columns (5)–(7)).

The final calculated results are shown in Table 17.3.

We show the survival curve because it is more intuitive to observe the survival process (Figure 17.4). From Figure 17.4, we can see the KM estimator is a staircase function, and the time point when the terminal event occurs is the point of discontinuity. Each step (that is, when the survival curve drops to a lower value of $S(t)$) of the survival curve represents the occurrence of the terminal event: the three steps represent the death/relapse events of patients ID 4, 3, and 2. The time corresponding to the step is the

Table 17.2 Calculation process for estimating the survival rate using the KM method.

Serial number i	Time t_i	Number of terminal events d_i	Size of risk set n_i	Estimate of survival rate $\hat{S}(t_i)$	$\sum_i \frac{d_i}{n_i(n_i - d_i)}$	Estimate of variance $Var[\hat{S}(t_i)]$
(1)	(2)	(3)	(4)	(5)	(6)	(7)
1	18.1	1	5	$1-\frac{1}{5}=0.8$	$\frac{1}{5\times 4}=0.05$	$0.8^2\times 0.05=0.032$
2	25.3	1	4	$0.8\times\left(1-\frac{1}{4}\right)=0.6$	$0.05+\frac{1}{4\times 3}=0.13$	$0.6^2\times 0.13=0.047$
3	37.5^+	0	3	$0.6\times\left(1-\frac{0}{3}\right)=0.6$	$0.13+\frac{0}{3\times 3}=0.13$	$0.6^2\times 0.13=0.047$
4	44.3	1	2	$0.6\times\left(1-\frac{1}{2}\right)=0.3$	$0.13+\frac{1}{2\times 1}=0.63$	$0.3^2\times 0.63=0.057$
5	56.7^+	0	1	$0.3\times\left(1-\frac{0}{1}\right)=0.3$	$0.63+\frac{0}{1\times 1}=0.63$	$0.3^2\times 0.63=0.057$

Note: Time values marked with a "+" sign represent right censored values.

Table 17.3 Estimate of the survival rate and standard error using the KM method.

Time t	Survival rate $\hat{S}(t)$	Standard error $\sqrt{Var[\hat{S}(t)]}$
$0 \le t < 18.1$	1.0	0.000
$18.1 \le t < 25.3$	0.8	0.179
$25.3 \le t < 44.3$	0.6	0.217
$44.3 \le t < 56.7$	0.3	0.239

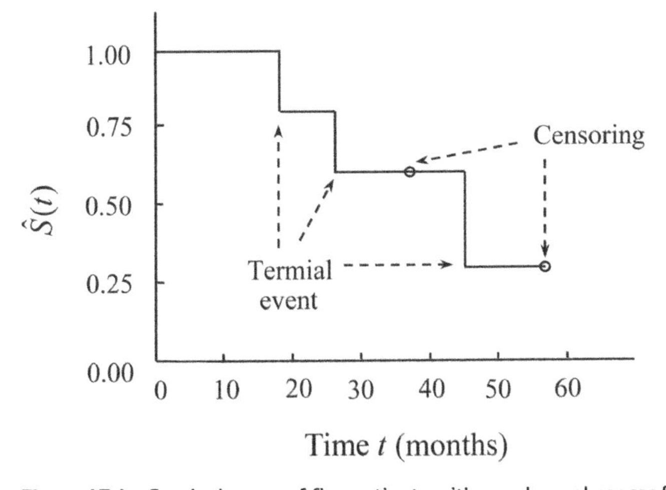

Figure 17.4 Survival curve of five patients with esophageal cancer from follow-up data.

point at which the terminal event occurs. The faster the step changes, the steeper the curve, which means the greater the number of terminal events. There is no step at the censored time points, but they are marked with a small circle (patients ID 1 and 5). As the largest survival time point in the data in this example is the censored data, the survival curve does not intersect the horizontal axis; otherwise, the survival curve finally declines to the x-axis at the maximum survival time. As the observation time increases, the number of observations decreases, so the survival rate shown at the tail of the curve is generally less precise.

The survival time is generally highly skewed, so, in practice, the median survival time is often used as a summary for the description of the average survival time. Because censored data always exist in the survival data, it is impossible to assess whether an individual lost to follow-up is dead or alive. Therefore, we cannot simply define the median survival time as the time when and only when 50% of the individuals survive. A more accurate definition of the median survival time should be the time t corresponding to the survival rate $S(t) = 0.5$.

17.2.2 Life Table Method

When the sample size is large, it is difficult to manually enumerate all the possible risk sets. For this condition, the observed value range of the survival time can be divided into several intervals that we want to display, and the *life table method* is used to describe the survival process.

Example 17.3 Table 17.4 shows the prognostic data of 352 inpatients with acute coronary syndrome. The follow-up period is six months. The time of the patient outcome (1 denotes recurrence; and 0 denotes free of recurrence, lost to follow-up, or other causes of death) is recorded. Estimate the survival process using the life table method.

Table 17.4 Prognostic follow-up data of 352 inpatients with acute coronary syndrome.

ID	Sex	Age (years)	Outcome	Survival time (days)
1	Female	74	1	53
2	Male	67	0	105^+
3	Female	77	0	137^+
4	Male	65	1	111
5	Female	69	0	140^+
6	Male	79	0	50^+
7	Male	71	0	105^+
8	Female	72	0	151^+
9	Male	73	0	88^+
10	Male	71	1	25
⋮	⋮	⋮	⋮	⋮

Note: Time values marked with a "+" sign represent right censored values.

Table 17.5 Life table calculation procedure for 352 inpatients for acute coronary syndrome.

Serial number i	Survival time (months) $[t_{i-1}, t_i]$	Number of terminal events d_i	Number of censored c_i	Number of initial observations n_i	Number of effective initial observations $n_i^* = n_i - c_i/2$	Survival probability $p_i = (n_i^* - d_i)/n_i^*$	Survival rate $\hat{S}(t_i)$
(1)	(2)	(3)	(4)	(5)	(6)	(7)	(8)
1	0–	11	0	352	352	0.968750	0.969
2	1–	7	41	341	320.5	0.978159	0.948
3	2–	10	48	293	269	0.962825	0.912
4	3–	8	54	235	208	0.961538	0.877
5	4–	6	80	173	133	0.954887	0.838
6	5–	2	85	87	45	0.955056	0.800

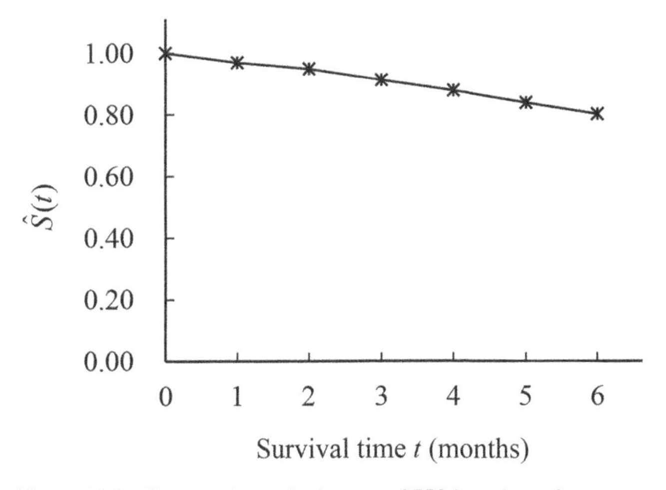

Figure 17.5 Prognostic survival curve of 352 inpatients for acute coronary syndrome.

The calculation procedure for the life table method is shown in Table 17.5.

(1) Divide the survival time of all subjects into small time intervals by "months" $[t_{i-1}, t_i)(i = 1,2,\ldots)$. Reorganize the time-to-event data into a frequency table, and calculate the frequency of terminal events d_i and censoring frequency c_i in each interval.
(2) Calculate the size of the risk set prior to each time interval, $n_i = n_{i-1} - d_{i-1} - c_{i-1}$.
(3) If censored observations exist, correct the size of the risk set. Assuming that censoring is uniformly distributed in the interval, subtract $c_i/2$ from the risk set, that is, the number of individuals at risk in each time interval is $n_i^* = n_i - c_i/2$.
(4) Calculate the survival probability of each time interval $p_i = (n_i^* - d_i)/n_i^*$.
(5) Estimate the survival rate at each time point as $\hat{S}(t_i) = p_1 \times p_2 \times \cdots \times p_i$. The survival curve for the data in Example 17.3 is plotted in Figure 17.5.

The life table method is essentially the same as the KM method; both calculate the survival rate through the product of a series of conditional probabilities. The difference between the two is that the life table method estimates the conditional probability between the intervals, whereas the KM method regards the observed time point as the "limit" of each interval, and estimates the conditional probability at the observation point. From this perspective, the KM method can be regarded as an extension of the life table method.

Because most survival analysis is performed after sorting the survival time, even a small rounding error may cause a difference to the sorted survival time and may affect the analysis result, particularly for small sample data.

17.3 Comparison of Survival Processes

In practice, we typically need to compare survival curves between two or more groups. Because of the influence of the sampling error, hypothesis testing is needed to determine whether the survival curves are statistically equivalent or different. Many test methods exist for this, and we introduce the log-rank test in detail because it is most commonly used.

17.3.1 Log-Rank Test

The log-rank test, introduced by Mantel in 1966, is a non-parametric method for comparing survival curves. It examines the distribution of the entire survival time rather than comparing the survival rate at specific time points.

In essence, the *log-rank test* is a χ^2 test. Consider the comparison of two survival processes, for instance, the null hypothesis of the log-rank test H_0: Survival curves of the two underlying populations are the same; and an alternative hypothesis H_1: Survival curves of the two populations are not the same. When H_0 is true, the observed and expected numbers of terminal events do not differ greatly. If the difference is too large, it is reasonable to believe that the difference is not only caused by the sampling error, that is, H_0 is not true, and the difference between the two survival curves is significant.

The log-rank test statistic is computed using the following steps:

(1) Under H_0, the survival curves of the two populations are the same, so the two sets of data can be merged and sorted by survival time from smallest to largest.

(2) Calculate the expected number $\left(e_{1j}, e_{2j}\right)$ of terminal events in each group at the time point when the jth terminal event occurred, denoted by

$$e_{1j} = \left(\frac{n_{1j}}{n_{1j}+n_{2j}}\right) \times \left(m_{1j}+m_{2j}\right),$$

$$e_{2j} = \left(\frac{n_{2j}}{n_{1j}+n_{2j}}\right) \times \left(m_{1j}+m_{2j}\right),$$

where m_{ij} denotes the number of terminal events in the ith$\left(i=1,\ 2\right)$ group at the jth time point, and n_{ij} denotes the number of initial observations in the ith$\left(i=1,\ 2\right)$ group at the jth time point.

(3) Sum the difference between the observed number of terminal events and the expected number of terminal events at all time points:

$$O_i - E_i = \sum_j \left(m_{ij} - e_{ij}\right) \quad \left(i = 1,\ 2\right)$$

Calculate its variance estimate

$$\widehat{Var}\left(O_i - E_i\right) = \sum_j \frac{n_{1j} n_{2j}\left(m_{1j} + m_{2j}\right)\left(n_{1j} + n_{2j} - m_{1j} - m_{2j}\right)}{\left(n_{1j} + n_{2j}\right)^2 \left(n_{1j} + n_{2j} - 1\right)} \quad \left(i = 1,\ 2\right). \tag{17.13}$$

(4) Calculate the test statistic of the log-rank test:

$$\chi^2 = \frac{\left(O_1 - E_1\right)^2}{\widehat{Var}\left(O_1 - E_1\right)} \text{ or } \chi^2 = \frac{\left(O_2 - E_2\right)^2}{\widehat{Var}\left(O_2 - E_2\right)}. \tag{17.14}$$

The statistic of the log-rank test can also be approximately estimated as

$$\chi^2 = \sum_{i=1}^{2} \frac{\left(O_i - E_i\right)^2}{E_i}, \tag{17.15}$$

which follows a χ^2 distribution with $\nu = 1$.

Formula 17.15 is an approximate estimation, for which the calculation is simpler but the result is more conservative compared with the precise method (generally used in statistical software).

Example 17.4 Twenty patients with a viral infectious disease were randomly assigned to treatment groups A and B. The outcome was viral suppression (<20 IU/ml) after treatment (1 = viral suppression, 0 = no viral suppression). The follow-up period was the 60th month and the survival data are shown in Table 17.6. The survival curves of the two groups of patients are shown in Figure 17.6. Perform a log-rank test on the prognosis of patients using different treatments.

Solution

(1) State the hypotheses and select a significance level

H_0 : Survival process of patients is the same using treatments A and B
H_1 : Survival process of patients differs using treatments A and B

$$\alpha = 0.05$$

(2) Determine the test statistic

According to the survival data of the two groups of patients in Example 17.4, the calculation process of the log-rank test is shown in Table 17.7.

Using the approximate estimation of the statistic of the log-rank test yields

$$\chi^2 = \frac{\left(9 - 5.96\right)^2}{5.96} + \frac{\left(7 - 10.04\right)^2}{10.04} = 2.47.$$

Table 17.6 Prognosis data of 20 patients with a viral infectious disease.

ID	Treatment group	Viral suppression	Survival time (months)
1	B	1	30
2	A	1	12
3	B	0	48^+
4	A	1	12
5	A	1	36
6	A	0	48^+
7	B	0	36^+
8	A	1	6
9	B	0	60^+
10	B	1	48
11	B	1	18
12	A	1	6
13	B	1	60
14	A	1	6
15	A	1	6
16	A	1	6
17	B	1	12
18	B	1	6
19	A	1	6
20	B	1	6

Note: Time values marked with a "+" sign represent right censored values.

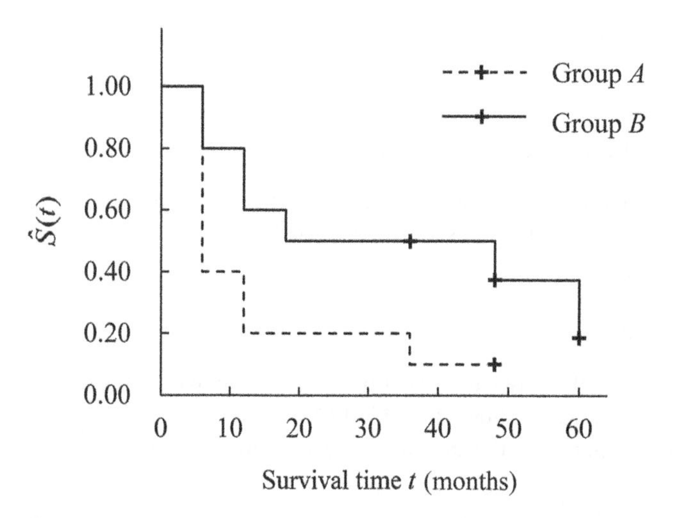

Figure 17.6 Survival curve of the treatment prognosis of 20 patients, with a viral infectious disease for two treatment groups.

Table 17.7 Calculation process of the log-rank test for 20 patients with viral infectious diseases.

Serial number j	t_j	Number of terminal events		Number of initial observations		Expected number		Observed number – Expected number	
		m_{1j}	m_{2j}	n_{1j}	n_{2j}	e_{1j}	e_{2j}	$m_{1j}-e_{1j}$	$m_{2j}-e_{2j}$
1	6	6	2	10	10	$(10/20)\times 8$	$(10/20)\times 8$	2.00	-2.00
2	12	2	1	4	8	$(4/12)\times 3$	$(8/12)\times 3$	1.00	-1.00
3	18	0	1	2	7	$(2/9)\times 1$	$(7/9)\times 1$	-0.22	0.22
4	30	0	1	2	6	$(2/8)\times 1$	$(6/8)\times 1$	-0.25	0.25
5	36	1	0	2	5	$(2/7)\times 1$	$(5/7)\times 1$	0.71	-0.71
6	48	0	1	1	4	$(1/5)\times 1$	$(4/5)\times 1$	-0.20	0.20
7	60	0	1	0	2	$(0/2)\times 1$	$(2/2)\times 1$	0.00	0.00
Total	-	9	7	-	-	5.96	10.04	3.04	-3.04

For given $\alpha = 0.05$ and $\nu = 1$, determine the critical value in Appendix Table 5. $\chi^2 < \chi^2_{1,1\text{-}0.05} = 3.84$, so $p > 0.05$. We do not reject H_0 at the $\alpha = 0.05$ level. We cannot consider that the survival curves of the two groups are different, that is, the prognoses of subjects under different treatments cannot be considered to be different.

The log-rank test can also be extended to testing the difference between three or more survival curves. The null hypothesis is H_0: Survival curves of multiple groups are the same. The calculation methods for the statistics are similar. The expected number and its total are calculated according to the number of initial observations of each group at different time points. The test statistic

$$\chi^2 = \sum_{i=1}^{k} \frac{\left(O_i - E_i\right)^2}{E_i} \tag{17.16}$$

approximately follows a χ^2 distribution with $\nu = k - 1$, where k denotes the number of comparison groups.

17.3.2 Other Methods for Comparing Survival Processes

In addition to the log-rank test, the Wilcoxon test (called the Breslow test in SPSS software), Tarone–Ware test, and Peto test can also be used. The difference lies in the weights assigned to the difference between the observed and expected number of terminal events at different time points. Consider the comparison of survival curves between the two groups as an example. The general form of the test statistics is

Table 17.8 Weights of several commonly used test statistics.

Test	Weight
Log-rank test	1
Wilcoxon test	n_j
Tarone–Ware test	$\sqrt{n_j}$
Peto test	$\hat{S}(t_j)$

$$\chi^2 = \frac{\left(\sum_j w(t_j)(m_{ij} - e_{ij})\right)^2}{\widehat{Var}\left(\sum_j w(t_j)(m_{ij} - e_{ij})\right)}, \tag{17.17}$$

where $w(t_j)$ denotes the weight and t_j denotes the time point. For the log-rank test, $w(t_j) = 1$; that is, the difference between the observed and expected number of terminal events at each time point is assigned the same weight. The power of the test is greatest when the hazard functions of two populations are proportional. For the Wilcoxon test, $w(t_j) = n_j$ and because the size of the risk set is larger in the early stage, this method assigns greater weights to the differences in the early stage. The weights of several commonly used test statistics are shown in Table 17.8.

17.4 Cox's Proportional Hazards Model

The above-mentioned methods apply to scenarios in which there is a single factor for analysis. Multivariate survival analysis methods are needed to comprehensively take into account the influence of multiple risk factors (or prognostic factors). The Cox's proportional hazards model, as a semi-parametric modeling approach for time-to-event data, was introduced by D.R. Cox in 1972. Compared with the parametric modeling approach, the Cox's proportional hazards model has no specific restrictions on the distribution of the survival time when analyzing the impact of risk factors on survival; thus, it has been widely used in medical research.

Example 17.5 To explore the prognostic factors of patients after breast cancer surgery, an oncologist in a hospital followed up with 74 patients after breast cancer surgery. The following observational data were included: age at diagnosis (x_1 years), type of first metastasis (x_2: 1 = multiple sites, 0 = a single site), survival status (1 = death, 0 = censored), and survival time (time, months). Part of the data is shown in Table 17.9.

We evaluate the impact of the type of first metastasis x_2 on the survival time of patients after surgery, controlling for age x_1. To facilitate the analysis, we set the age at diagnosis as a categorical variable:

$$x_1 = \begin{cases} 1, & \text{age at diagnosis} > 35 \text{ years old} \\ 0, & \text{age at diagnosis} \leq 35 \text{ years old} \end{cases}$$

Table 17.9 Follow-up data of 74 breast cancer patients in a certain hospital.

ID	Age at diagnosis (years)	Type of first metastasis (1 = multiple sites, 0 = single site)	Survival status (1 = death, 0 = censored)	Survival time (months)
1	34	1	1	120
2	28	1	1	35
3	31	1	0	28
4	51	1	1	63
5	36	0	1	95
6	33	0	0	130
7	31	1	1	100
8	44	0	0	128
⋮	⋮	⋮	⋮	⋮
74	46	0	1	120

In this example, there are two risk factors that could be associated with survival time. In order to explore the association between them, we can use Cox's proportional hazards model to address this question. Before proceeding, we should understand the following concepts.

17.4.1 Concept and Model Assumptions

1. Model Definition

Let $h(t \mid x_1, x_2, \ldots, x_k)$ be the hazard rate at time t for an individual with risk factors $x_1, x_2, \ldots, x_k$. The Cox's proportional hazards model is defined as

$$h(t \mid x_1, x_2, \ldots, x_k) = h_0(t) g(x_1, x_2, \ldots, x_k) = h_0(t) \exp\left(\sum_{j=1}^{k} \beta_j x_j\right), \tag{17.18}$$

where:

(1) $h_0(t)$ is *baseline hazard function* that represents how the risk changes over time, given that all risk factors are ignored or equal to 0.

(2) $g(x_1, x_2, \ldots, x_k) = \exp\left(\sum_{j=1}^{k} \beta_j x_j\right)$ is a function of a set of k independent variables (risk factors). It generally needs to satisfy $g(0) = 1$, and for any $x_1, x_2, \ldots, x_k$, $g(x_1, x_2, \ldots, x_k) > 0$. It represents the effect of variables $x_1, x_2, \ldots, x_k$ on the hazard.

(3) $\beta_j (j = 1, 2, \ldots, k)$ is the partial regression coefficient of x_j, that means the proportional change in hazard ratio (see Formula 17.20) with a 1-unit increase in x_j, with all other variables held constant (or, stated in another way, after adjustment for all the other variables in the model).

Cox's proportional hazards model is called a semi-parametric model because a parametric form is assumed only for the covariate effect. The baseline hazard rate $h_0(t)$ is treated nonparametrically.

2. Model Assumption

The key assumption for Cox's regression is the *proportional hazards (PH) assumption*. It assumes there is no interaction effect between independent variables and time. The reorganization of Formula 17.18 provides a formal way to interpret the PH assumption:

$$\frac{h(t)}{h_0(t)} = \exp\left(\sum_{j=1}^{k} \beta_j x_j\right). \tag{17.19}$$

It shows that the hazard function at any time point is proportional to the baseline hazard function, and the scale factor is $\exp\left(\sum_{j=1}^{k} \beta_j x_j\right)$, which is always a constant over time.

3. Hazard Ratio

Suppose there are two individuals with independent variables of $x_1, x_2, \ldots, x_k$ and $x_1^*, x_2^*, \ldots, x_k^*$, the ratio between hazard functions of two individuals is called the *Hazard ratio (HR)*, which can be expressed as

$$\begin{aligned} \text{HR} &= \frac{h\left(t \mid x_1, x_2, \ldots, x_k\right)}{h\left(t \mid x_1^*, x_2^*, \ldots, x_k^*\right)} \\ &= \frac{h_0(t)\exp\left(\sum_{j=1}^{k} \beta_j x_j\right)}{h_0(t)\exp\left(\sum_{j=1}^{k} \beta_j x_j^*\right)} \\ &= \exp\left(\sum_{j=1}^{k} \beta_j\left(x_j - x_j^*\right)\right). \end{aligned} \tag{17.20}$$

It should be noted that irrespective of how $h_0(t)$ varies over time, the ratio of one hazard to the other is $\exp\left(\sum_{j=1}^{k} \beta_j\left(x_j - x_j^*\right)\right)$, which is always a constant, and so the ratios of the two individuals remain proportional to each other.

When applied to etiology studies, the HR has a similar role to the *RR* (see Chapter 19), which means that the risk of a certain group of individuals' terminal events over that of another group is given by a multiplication factor. For example, in Example 17.5, according to Formula 17.20, we can calculate the HR of death in patients over 35 years old $\left(x_1 = x_1^* = 1\right)$ with first metastases at multiple sites $\left(x_2 = 1\right)$ over those with a first metastasis at a single site $\left(x_2^* = 0\right)$:

$$\text{HR} = \frac{h\left(t \mid x_1 = 1, x_2 = 1\right)}{h\left(t \mid x_1^* = 1, x_2^* = 0\right)} = \exp\left(\sum_{j=1}^{2} \beta_j\left(x_j - x_j^*\right)\right) = e^{\beta_1 \times (1-1) + \beta_2 \times (1-0)} = e^{\beta_2},$$

which means that the death risk of patients with breast cancer older than 35 years old with first metastases at multiple sites is e^{β_2} times that of patients with a first metastasis at a single site.

Note that the Cox's proportional hazard model does not require the estimation of the distribution of the baseline hazard function $h_0(t)$. In Formula 17.20, the baseline hazard function $h_0(t)$ that appears in the numerator and denominator can be offset; that is, the baseline hazard function does not need to be considered when calculating HR. Therefore, the establishment of the Cox's regression model does not need to assume the distribution of the survival time, which is also an important reason why the model is widely used in medical research.

17.4.2 Estimation of Model Coefficient

Parameter estimation in Cox's regression is performed by conditional death probability and uses the *partial likelihood function method.*

To construct the partial likelihood function, we take the following steps:

(1) Sort the survival times of n independent observed individuals in ascending order $t_1 \le t_2 \le \cdots \le t_i \le \cdots \le t_n$.
(2) Let R_i represent the risk set with survival time $T \ge t_i \ (i = 1,2,\ldots,n)$, which decreases in size as time increases. For each t_i, individuals in the risk set R_i are numbered $i, i+1, i+2, \ldots, n$, and every individual is at risk of the terminal event.
(3) Calculate the conditional probability of the terminal event for the individual numbered i as

$$q_i = \frac{h_0(t_i)\exp\left(\sum_{j=1}^{k} \beta_j x_{ij}\right)}{\sum_{m=i}^{n} h_0(t_i)\exp\left(\sum_{j=1}^{k} \beta_j x_{mj}\right)} = \frac{\exp\left(\sum_{j=1}^{k} \beta_j x_{ij}\right)}{\sum_{m \in R_i} \exp\left(\sum_{j=1}^{k} \beta_j x_{mj}\right)},$$

where $x_{i1}, x_{i2}, \ldots, x_{ik}$ represent independent variables for individuals numbered i. According to the probability multiplication principle, the probability of the terminal event for all individuals is the continuous product of the conditional probabilities over the survival process; therefore, the partial likelihood function can be expressed as

$$L_p(\beta) = \prod_{i=1}^{n} q_i = \prod_{i=1}^{n} \left[\frac{\exp\left(\sum_{j=1}^{k} \beta_j x_{ij}\right)}{\sum_{m \in R_i} \exp\left(\sum_{j=1}^{k} \beta_j x_{mj}\right)}\right]^{\delta_i}$$

where $L_p(\cdot)$ represents an incomplete likelihood function and δ_i is the censoring indicator such that $\delta_i = 1$ if t_i is an event time and $\delta_i = 0$ if t_i is an censored time. Thus, the equation above can be expressed as

$$L_p(\beta) = \prod_{i=1}^{d} q_i = \prod_{i=1}^{d} \left[\frac{\exp\left(\sum_{j=1}^{k} \beta_j x_{ij}\right)}{\sum_{m \in R_i} \exp\left(\sum_{j=1}^{k} \beta_j x_{mj}\right)}\right], \tag{17.21}$$

where d denotes the number of observations with complete data.

Clearly, although the partial likelihood function focuses on subjects who have the terminal event, survival time information prior to censorship is used for individuals who are censored.

(4) Once the partial likelihood function is constructed for a given model, we maximize the natural log of L as follows because it is easier for computation:

$$\ln L_p(\beta) = \sum_{i=1}^{d}\left[\left(\sum_{j=1}^{k}\beta_j x_{ij}\right) - \ln\sum_{m\in R_i}\exp\left(\sum_{j=1}^{k}\beta_j x_{mj}\right)\right]. \tag{17.22}$$

Then the estimation of the regression coefficients can be conducted by determining the first partial derivative of $\beta_j\,(j=1,2,\ldots,k)$ and setting $\partial \ln L_p(\beta)/\partial\beta_j = 0$ to obtain the following simultaneous equations:

$$\begin{cases} \dfrac{\partial \ln L_p(\beta)}{\partial\beta_1} = 0 \\ \dfrac{\partial \ln L_p(\beta)}{\partial\beta_2} = 0 \\ \vdots \\ \dfrac{\partial \ln L_p(\beta)}{\partial\beta_k} = 0 \end{cases}. \tag{17.23}$$

The solution $b_1, b_2, \ldots, b_k$ is the estimate of $\beta_1, \beta_2, \ldots, \beta_k$, which is typically obtained using the Newton–Raphson iterative method. The specific solution process is complicated; however, it may be obtained using statistical analysis software.

The above parameter estimation methods are for survival data when the survival time has no ties. If ties exist, the above partial likelihood function expression needs to be corrected.

Three correction methods exist. The first is the exact partial likelihood function method, which has a complicated calculation. The other two are the asymptotic expressions of the exact partial likelihood function proposed by N.E. Breslow (1974) and B. Efron (1977). Generally, the Efron parameter approach method is more accurate than the Breslow parameter approach method. However, the Breslow method can also obtain a satisfactory estimate when there are not too many ties.

Example 17.6 Fit a Cox's proportional hazards model to Example 17.5.

Solution

We applied the partial likelihood estimation method to estimate the regression coefficient using SPSS software.

The estimate of regression coefficient of the variable x_1 (age) $b_1 = 0.431$, with standard error $s_{b_1} = 0.346$; the estimate of regression coefficient of the variable x_2 (type of first metastasis) $b_2 = 0.637$, with standard error $s_{b_2} = 0.297$.

Then we obtain the Cox's proportional hazards model:

$$h(t) = h_0(t)\exp(0.431x_1 + 0.637x_2)$$

The results indicate that given the same first metastasis status, the hazard for the a patient aged 35 years old above is 1.539 ($e^{0.431} = 1.539$) times compared with a patient aged 35 years old or below. The interpretation of first metastasis is similar, that is, the risk of death for patients with multiple sites first metastasis is 1.891 ($e^{0.637}=1.891$) compared with patients with single site first metastasis .

17.4.3 Hypothesis Testing of Model Coefficient

After fitting a Cox's proportional hazards model, it is necessary to test whether the regression coefficients are statistically significant. Similar with logistic regression, we use Wald's test and the partial likelihood ratio test.

1. Wald's Test

Wald's test can be used to test whether independent variables in the model should be eliminated. When testing the coefficient of the jth regression variable in the model, the corresponding statistic is

$$Z=b_j/S_{b_j}$$

that is, the ratio of the estimate of the regression coefficient to the estimate of the standard error of the regression coefficient. For large samples, Z follows the standard normal distribution and Z^2 follows a χ^2 distribution with 1 degree of freedom. The test statistic of Wald's test is

$$\chi_W^2=\left(b_j/S_{b_j}\right)^2\sim\chi^2(1). \tag{17.24}$$

Using the Wald's test for the regression coefficient β_2 in Example 17.6,

$$\chi_W^2=\left(b_j/S_{b_j}\right)^2=\left(0.637/0.297\right)^2=4.60$$

For given $\alpha=0.05$, since $\chi_W^2=4.60>3.84$, $p<0.05$, we reject H_0 and accept H_1, and conclude that the variable for the type of first metastasis x_2 explains the survival time of patients after surgery.

2. Partial Likelihood Ratio Test

The *partial likelihood ratio test* is mainly used for the elimination of non-significant variables in the model, the introduction of new variables, and a comparison between models that contain different independent variables. When the Cox's regression model contains k independent variables and the jth independent variable is tested for whether it is statistically significant, the partial likelihood ratio test statistic χ_{LR}^2 is

$$\chi_{LR}^2=2\left[\ln L_p\left(\beta_k\right)-\ln L_p\left(\beta_{k-1}\right)\right], \tag{17.25}$$

where $\ln L_p\left(\beta_k\right)$ represents the log-partial likelihood function of the model containing all k independent variables, and $\ln L_p\left(\beta_{k-1}\right)$ represents the log-partial likelihood function of the model without the jth independent variable and containing the remaining $k-1$ independent variables. Under $H_0:\beta_j=0$, there is $\chi_{LR}^2\sim\chi^2(1)$.

Example 17.7 Referring to Example 17.6, perform a hypothesis test for the regression coefficient β_2 of variable x_2.

Solution

(1) State the hypotheses and select a significance level

$H_0: \beta_2 = 0, \beta_1 \neq 0$ (x_1 a constant)
$H_1: \beta_2 \neq 0, \beta_1 \neq 0$ (x_1 a constant)
$\alpha = 0.05$

(2) Determine the test statistic

Using SPSS software, we obtained the log-partial likelihood function value of the model containing two variables x_1 and x_2 as -167.224, and the log-partial likelihood function value of the model removing x_2 as -169.526. Then the test statistic is

$$\chi^2_{LR} = 2\left[\ln L_p(\beta_k) - \ln L_p(\beta_{k-1})\right] = 2\left[-167.224 - (-169.526)\right] = 4.60$$

(3) Draw a conclusion

For given $\alpha = 0.05$, since $\chi^2_{LR} = 4.60 > 3.84$, $p < 0.05$, we reject H_0 and accept H_1. The conclusion remains the same as that made from using the Wald's test.

17.4.4 Evaluation of Model Fitting

An objective approach to check the PH assumption is to use the goodness-of-fit test. We first introduce the statistics involved in the goodness-of-fit test method. For all individuals with a terminal event, the difference between the observed and expected value of each independent variable is called the *Schoenfeld residuals*, expressed as

$$\text{Schoenfeld residuals} = x_{ij} - \sum_{m \in R(t_i)} x_{mj} p_m$$

where x_{ij} is the observed value of the jth independent variable of the individual whose terminal event occurs at time point t_i, x_{mj} is the value of the jth independent variable of the individual m in the risk set at time point t_i, and p_m is the probability that individual m in the risk set will have a terminal event at time point t_i. $\sum_{m \in R(t_i)} x_{mj} p_m$ is the weighted average of the jth independent variable of all individuals in the risk set at time point t_i. Thus, the corresponding Schoenfeld residual can be calculated for each independent variable of all individuals with terminal events.

The idea of the goodness-of-fit test is that if a variable meets the PH assumption, then the Schoenfeld residual of the variable is not related to the survival time. The test procedure is as follows:

(1) Calculate the Schoenfeld residual of the variable to be tested.
(2) Rank the survival time of uncensored data, where the ranks are denoted by R.
(3) Perform a significance test of the correlation between the Schoenfeld residual and R. The null hypothesis is $H_0: \rho = 0$.

If H_0 is rejected, then the variable is not considered to meet the PH assumption.

17.5 Other Aspects of Cox's Proportional Hazard Model

17.5.1 Hazard Index

After fitting a Cox's regression model, the results can be used to quantify and compare the individual level of the hazard. It can be seen from the Formula 17.18 that the hazard of the terminal event of an individual is related to their risk factors and the regression coefficient corresponding to each factor. The index part of the Cox's regression model is called the *hazard index (HI)*:

$$\mathrm{HI} = \beta_1 x_1 + \beta_2 x_2 + \cdots + \beta_k x_k. \tag{17.26}$$

The HI is an indicator that reflects the prognosis of an individual. It represents the combined effect of various independent variables and can be used to predict the survival of an individual in the future. By substituting the values of the individual's risk factors into the model, the individual's HI can be obtained. The larger the HI, the higher the hazard of the terminal event or the worse the prognosis.

A hazard index of zero means the risk of the terminal event is at an average level; when the hazard index is less than zero the risk of the terminal event is below the average level; when the hazard index is greater than zero the risk of the terminal event is above the average level.

Example 17.8 Referring to Example 17.5, calculating the HI of patients ID 1 and ID 4.

Solution

From Example 17.6, $b_1 = 0.431$, $b_2 = 0.637$. Thus, for patient ID 1: $\mathrm{HI}_1 = 0.431 \times 0 + 0.637 \times 1 = 0.637$, for patient ID 4: $\mathrm{HI}_4 = 0.431 \times 1 + 0.637 \times 1 = 1.068$.

The HI for patients ID 1 and ID 4 are greater than 0, which means the risk of death after breast cancer surgery is higher than the average level. Additionally, the HI of the patient ID 4 is greater than ID 1, because of the difference in age.

17.5.2 Sample Size

The method for sample size estimation to compare survival curves between two groups under Cox's proportional hazards model is given as follows:

Suppose we wish to compare the survival curves between an experimental group (group E) and a control group (group C) in a clinical trial. n_1 and n_2 is the sample size of participants in group E and group C, respectively. The ratio of n_1 and n_2 is given by k and the maximum length of follow-up is t. We postulate a hazard ratio of *IRR* (incidence rate ratio) for group E compared with group C and wish to conduct a two-sided test with significance level α. The number of participants needed in each group to achieve a power of $1-\beta$ is

$$n_1 = \frac{mk}{k\pi_E + \pi_C}, \quad n_2 = \frac{m}{k\pi_E + \pi_C}, \tag{17.27}$$

where π_E and π_C are the probability of failure in group E and group C over the maximum time period of the study (t), respectively. m is the expected total number of events over both groups,

$$m = \frac{1}{k}\left(\frac{k \times IRR + 1}{IRR - 1}\right)^2 \left(z_{1-\alpha/2} + z_{1-\beta}\right)^2. \tag{17.28}$$

Example 17.9 A clinical research study is to be designed to compare a new form of chemotherapy with a standard treatment for patients with advanced primary liver cancer. According to the previous study, the death rate for patients receiving the standard treatment is 0.55 at the 3-year mark. Assume the accrual period is 24 months and the follow-up period is also 24 months, and the patients were recruited uniformly during the accrual period. If the two groups have same sample size, how many patients are required to enroll to ensure a power of 80% to find a decrease of 0.2 in the 3-year death rate with the new chemotherapy treatment using Cox's proportional hazards model at a 0.05 significance level.

Solution

The estimation process is divided into two stages.

(1) We estimate expected total number of events over both groups.

We have $p_E = 0.35$, $p_C = 0.55$, and $k = 1$. Thus $IRR = \frac{p_E}{p_C} = \frac{0.35}{0.55} = 0.636$.

With $z_{1-0.05/2} = 1.96$, $z_{0.8} = 0.84$, from Formula 17.28, we have

$$\begin{aligned} m &= \frac{1}{k}\left(\frac{k \times IRR + 1}{IRR - 1}\right)^2 \left(z_{1-0.05/2} + z_{0.8}\right)^2 \\ &= \left(\frac{0.636 + 1}{0.636 - 1}\right)^2 (1.96 + 0.84)^2 \\ &= 158.4. \end{aligned}$$

So, at least 158.4 events should be observed to find a decrease of 0.2 in the 3-year death rate for the new treatment.

(2) We estimate the number of patients needed in each group.

$$n_1 = n_2 = \frac{m}{p_E + p_C} = \frac{158.4}{0.35 + 0.55} = 176$$

Therefore, $176 \times 2 = 352$ patients should be recruited to achieve a power of 80%.

17.6 Summary

In this chapter, we introduced the basic features of survival data, survival time functions, non-parametric methods for estimating and comparing survival curves, and the semi-parametric method for modeling survival data.

Survival analysis is a type of statistical analysis method that comprehensively considers the terminal event and survival time.

When the occurrence of the terminal event changes greatly over time, the survival rate is an important statistic that best describes the process. In this chapter, we introduced the KM method for small samples and the life table method based on frequency table data. These two methods are essentially the same. Both methods are used to calculate the survival rate through the product of a series of conditional probabilities. The KM method can be regarded as an extension of the life table method.

The survival curve is the most intuitive description of the survival process. In this chapter, we focused on the log-rank test method based on the χ^2 test for a large sample, which is used to compare two or more populations regarding the survival curves.

The strategy of the Cox's proportional hazards model is similar to that of the multiple linear regression model and the logistic regression model; that is, single factor analysis is performed on each variable, and then multivariate analysis is performed on the related variables. It is worth noting that before fitting the model, it is necessary to check whether the data meet the PH assumption.

17.7 Exercises

1. A randomized trial was conducted to compare two treatment regimens for lung cancer and 137 patients with lung cancer were enrolled. Part of the data are shown in Table 17.10, including treatment regimens (treatment, 1 = standard therapy, 2 = test therapy), survival time (time, days), and survival status (status, 1 = event, 0 = censored). Answer the following questions.

(a) What are the characteristics of the survival data? How do you define the initial event, terminal event, and survival time in the data?

(b) What is the meaning of censored data? What caused censoring and what impact may censoring lead to?

(c) $S(t)$ is an important function for the description of the prognostic data. Interpret its meaning in your own words and explain its difference with other descriptive statistics introduced previously.

(d) What is the KM method? Use the KM method to estimate $S(t)$ for patients treated with the two treatment regimens and draw survival curves.

(e) Find the median survival time for patients treated with the two treatment regimens, respectively. What is the difference in median survival time? Can we use the t-test to compare the survival time?

(f) Is it appropriate to use the life table method to solve question (d)? Give your reason?

(g) Fit a Cox regression model to the data.

(h) What are the model assumptions regarding Cox's regression? How do you check the assumptions in this case?

(i) How do you interpret the regression coefficient?

(j) Suppose that other prognostic factors are collected such as tumor stage and type. How does this affect your analysis plan? How would you like to use the model results to compare survival of two patients given their specific prognostic factors?

Table 17.10 The data on two treatment regimens for 137 patients with lung cancer.

ID	Treatment	Time (days)	Status	ID	Treatment	Time (days)	Status	ID	Treatment	Time (days)	Status
1	1	72	1	47	1	92	1	93	2	13	1
2	1	411	1	48	1	35	1	94	2	87	1
3	1	228	1	49	1	117	1	95	2	2	1
4	1	126	1	50	1	132	1	96	2	20	1
5	1	118	1	51	1	12	1	97	2	7	1
6	1	10	1	52	1	162	1	98	2	24	1
7	1	82	1	53	1	3	1	99	2	99	1
8	1	110	1	54	1	95	1	100	2	8	1
9	1	314	1	55	1	177	1	101	2	99	1
10	1	100	0	56	1	162	1	102	2	61	1
11	1	42	1	57	1	216	1	103	2	25	1
12	1	8	1	58	1	553	1	104	2	95	1
13	1	144	1	59	1	278	1	105	2	80	1
14	1	25	0	60	1	12	1	106	2	51	1
15	1	11	1	61	1	260	1	107	2	29	1
16	1	30	1	62	1	200	1	108	2	24	1
17	1	384	1	63	1	156	1	109	2	18	1
18	1	4	1	64	1	182	0	110	2	83	0
19	1	54	1	65	1	143	1	111	2	31	1
20	1	13	1	66	1	105	1	112	2	51	1
21	1	123	0	67	1	103	1	113	2	90	1
22	1	97	0	68	1	250	1	114	2	52	1
23	1	153	1	69	1	100	1	115	2	73	1

24	1	59	1	70	2	999	1	116	2	8	1
25	1	117	1	71	2	112	1	117	2	36	1
26	1	16	1	72	2	87	0	118	2	48	1
27	1	151	1	73	2	231	0	119	2	7	1
28	1	22	1	74	2	242	1	120	2	140	1
29	1	56	1	75	2	991	1	121	2	186	1
30	1	21	1	76	2	111	1	122	2	84	1
31	1	18	1	77	2	1	1	123	2	19	1
32	1	139	1	78	2	587	1	124	2	45	1
33	1	20	1	79	2	389	1	125	2	80	1
34	1	31	1	80	2	33	1	126	2	52	1
35	1	52	1	81	2	25	1	127	2	164	1
36	1	287	1	82	2	357	1	128	2	19	1
37	1	18	1	83	2	467	1	129	2	53	1
38	1	51	1	84	2	201	1	130	2	15	1
39	1	122	1	85	2	1	1	131	2	43	1
40	1	27	1	86	2	30	1	132	2	340	1
41	1	54	1	87	2	44	1	133	2	133	1
42	1	7	1	88	2	283	1	134	2	111	1
43	1	63	1	89	2	15	1	135	2	231	1
44	1	392	1	90	2	25	1	136	2	378	1
45	1	10	1	91	2	103	0	137	2	49	1
46	1	8	1	92	2	21	1				

Source: D. Kalbfleisch and R.L. Prentice (1980), The Statistical Analysis of Failure Time Data. New York: Wiley.

2. In order to explore the factors affecting the prognosis of bone marrow transplantation, 137 leukemia patients undergoing bone marrow transplantation were followed up. Data collected are as follows (see Tables 17.11 and 17.12), please employ an appropriate method to analyze the data and answer the research question.

Table 17.11 Explanation and Assignment of Survival Data Variables of Leukemia Patients.

Variable	Explanation	Assignment
ID	No. of patient	–
x_1	Sex of patient	1 = Male, 0 = Female
x_2	Age of patient	Year
x_3	Age of bone marrow donor	Year
x_4	Platelet level has turned to normal	1 = Yes, 0 = No
x_5	Waiting time for surgery	Day
x_6	No. of hospital	1 = Hospital A, 2 = Hospital B, 3 = Hospital C, 4 = Hospital D
Time	Survival time	Day
Status	Terminal event	1 = Death, 0 = Alive

Table 17.12 Prognostic data of 137 leukemia patients undergoing bone marrow transplantation.

ID	x_1	x_2	x_3	x_4	x_5	x_6	Time	Status
1	1	13	24	1	90	1	1363	0
2	0	25	29	1	210	1	1030	0
3	0	25	31	1	180	1	860	0
4	1	21	15	1	120	1	414	1
5	0	25	19	1	60	1	2204	1
6	1	50	38	1	270	1	1063	1
7	1	35	36	1	90	1	481	1
8	1	37	34	1	120	1	105	1
9	1	26	24	1	90	1	641	1
10	1	50	48	1	120	1	390	1
11	1	45	43	0	90	1	288	1
12	1	28	30	1	90	1	522	1
13	0	43	43	0	90	1	79	1
14	1	14	19	1	60	1	1156	1

(Continued)

Table 17.12 (Continued)

ID	x_1	x_2	x_3	x_4	x_5	x_6	Time	Status
15	0	17	14	1	120	1	583	1
16	0	32	33	1	150	1	48	1
17	0	30	23	1	120	1	431	1
18	1	30	32	1	150	1	1074	1
19	0	33	28	1	120	1	393	1
20	1	18	23	1	750	1	2640	0
21	1	29	26	1	24	1	2430	0
22	1	35	31	1	120	1	2252	0
23	1	27	17	1	210	1	2140	0
24	0	36	39	1	240	1	2133	0
25	1	24	28	1	240	1	1238	0
26	0	22	21	0	210	1	491	1
27	1	22	23	1	300	1	162	1
28	0	8	2	0	105	1	1298	1
29	1	39	48	1	210	1	121	1
30	1	20	19	0	75	1	2	1
31	1	27	25	1	90	1	62	1
32	1	32	32	1	180	1	265	1
33	1	31	28	1	630	1	547	1
34	0	20	23	1	180	1	341	1
35	0	35	40	1	300	1	318	1
36	1	36	39	1	90	1	195	1
37	0	35	33	1	120	1	469	1
38	1	7	2	1	135	1	93	1
39	1	23	25	1	210	1	515	1
40	0	11	7	1	120	1	183	1
41	1	14	18	0	150	1	105	1
42	0	37	35	1	270	1	128	1
43	0	19	32	0	285	1	164	1
44	0	37	34	1	240	1	129	1
45	0	25	29	1	510	1	122	1
46	1	35	28	1	780	1	80	1
47	1	15	14	1	150	1	677	1
48	1	26	33	1	98	1	2081	0
49	1	21	37	1	1720	1	1602	0
50	1	26	35	1	127	1	1496	0
51	0	17	21	1	168	1	1462	0

(Continued)

Table 17.12 (Continued)

ID	x_1	x_2	x_3	x_4	x_5	x_6	Time	Status
52	1	32	36	1	93	1	1433	0
53	1	22	31	1	2187	1	1377	0
54	1	20	17	1	1006	1	1330	0
55	1	22	24	1	1319	1	996	0
56	0	18	21	1	208	1	226	0
57	1	18	14	1	110	1	418	1
58	1	15	20	1	824	1	417	1
59	0	18	5	1	146	1	276	1
60	1	20	33	1	85	1	156	1
61	1	27	27	1	187	1	781	1
62	0	40	37	1	129	1	172	1
63	1	22	20	1	128	1	487	1
64	1	28	32	1	84	1	716	1
65	0	26	32	1	329	1	194	1
66	0	39	31	1	147	1	371	1
67	1	15	20	1	943	1	526	1
68	1	20	26	1	2616	1	122	1
69	1	19	13	1	270	1	2569	0
70	1	31	34	1	60	1	2506	0
71	1	35	31	1	120	1	2409	0
72	1	16	16	1	60	1	2218	0
73	0	29	35	1	90	1	1857	0
74	1	19	18	1	210	1	1829	0
75	1	26	30	1	90	1	1562	0
76	1	27	34	1	240	1	1470	0
77	0	30	16	1	180	2	1258	0
78	1	34	54	0	240	2	10	1
79	0	33	41	0	180	2	53	1
80	0	30	35	0	150	2	80	1
81	0	23	25	0	150	2	35	1
82	1	27	21	1	690	2	1631	0
83	0	45	42	1	180	2	73	1
84	0	32	43	1	150	2	168	1
85	0	41	29	1	750	2	74	1
86	0	24	23	1	203	2	1182	0
87	0	27	22	0	191	2	1167	0
88	1	36	43	1	393	2	162	1
89	0	23	16	1	331	2	262	1

(Continued)

Table 17.12 (Continued)

ID	x_1	x_2	x_3	x_4	x_5	x_6	Time	Status
90	1	42	48	0	196	2	1	1
91	1	30	19	0	178	2	107	1
92	0	29	20	1	361	2	269	1
93	1	22	20	1	834	2	350	0
94	0	37	36	1	180	3	1850	0
95	0	34	32	1	270	3	1843	0
96	0	35	32	1	180	3	1535	0
97	0	33	28	1	150	3	1447	0
98	0	21	18	1	120	3	1384	0
99	1	28	30	1	120	3	222	1
100	1	33	22	1	210	3	1356	0
101	1	47	27	1	900	3	1136	0
102	0	40	39	1	210	3	845	0
103	1	43	50	1	240	3	392	1
104	1	44	37	1	360	3	63	1
105	1	48	56	0	330	3	97	1
106	0	31	25	1	240	3	153	1
107	1	52	48	1	180	3	363	1
108	1	24	40	1	174	3	1199	0
109	1	19	28	1	236	3	1111	0
110	1	17	28	1	151	3	530	0
111	0	17	20	1	937	3	1279	1
112	1	28	25	1	303	3	110	1
113	0	37	38	1	170	3	243	1
114	1	17	26	0	239	3	86	1
115	1	15	18	1	508	3	466	1
116	1	29	32	1	74	3	262	1
117	0	45	39	1	105	4	2246	0
118	0	33	30	1	225	4	1870	0
119	1	32	23	1	120	4	1799	0
120	0	23	28	1	90	4	1709	0
121	1	37	34	1	60	4	1674	0
122	1	15	19	1	90	4	1568	0
123	0	22	12	1	450	4	1527	0
124	1	46	31	1	75	4	1324	0
125	1	18	17	1	90	4	957	0
126	0	27	30	1	60	4	932	0
127	1	28	29	1	75	4	847	0

(Continued)

Table 17.12 (Continued)

ID	x_1	x_2	x_3	x_4	x_5	x_6	Time	Status
128	1	23	26	1	180	4	848	0
129	1	35	18	1	30	4	1499	0
130	0	29	21	1	105	4	704	1
131	1	23	16	1	90	4	653	1
132	0	35	41	1	105	4	2024	0
133	1	50	36	1	120	4	1345	0
134	0	27	36	0	180	4	16	1
135	0	33	39	1	180	4	248	1
136	0	39	43	1	150	4	732	1
137	0	17	14	1	210	4	105	1

Source: Klein, J.P. and Moeschberger, M.L. (2003). Survival Analysis: Techniques for Censored and Truncated Data, 2nd Edn. Springer Science & Business Media.

18

Evaluation of Diagnostic Tests

CONTENTS

In this chapter, we describe how statistical methods are used to evaluate the performance of diagnostic tests. A diagnostic test is aimed to identify patients with a disease or condition by assessing the signs, symptoms, or results of objective laboratory tests. In a broad sense, a good diagnostic test not only provides reliable information about the patient's physical condition, but also helps clinicians to make appropriate treatment plans. Because many diagnostic tests currently applied in clinical work cannot ensure perfect accuracy or are limited by invasiveness, high cost, or a long wait time, the evaluation of a growing number of new diagnostic tests can help inform clinicians' choices between candidate tests and ultimately improve the overall level of health care. Here we introduce several measures commonly used in the evaluation of diagnostic tests, as well as some basic methods for the analysis of diagnostic data.

18.1 Basic Characteristics of Diagnostic Tests

Accuracy is a crucial aspect for assessing a diagnostic test. Accuracy, which is also called validity, refers to a test's ability to correctly detect a condition when it is actually present (i.e., few missed diagnoses) and to correctly rule out the condition when it is

Applied Medical Statistics, First Edition. Jingmei Jiang.

Companion website: www.wiley.com\go\jiang\appliedmedicalstatistics

truly absent (i.e., few misdiagnoses). A diagnostic test has no value if its result is the same for different statuses of the disease, and a test would be perfect if its results divided different statuses of the disease with no overlap. In reality, both extremes are relatively rare in practice, and most diagnostic tests cannot completely rule out missed diagnoses and misdiagnoses simultaneously. Therefore, evaluating the validity of a diagnostic test requires a rigorous procedure involving the consideration of both aspects.

In the study design of a diagnostic test, there are two basic requirements: (i) sufficient amount of subjects with different disease statuses – typically, one group of subjects with the disease and one group of subjects without the disease; and (ii) a gold standard, which theoretically has an accuracy of 100% in classifying disease status. The basic logic of diagnosis test research is to compare the disease status of all study subjects as determined by the test being evaluated with these subjects' certified disease status as assessed with the gold standard as a reference. Because it is impractical to identify a reference test with 100% accuracy, the *gold standard* is usually the diagnostic test that is generally accepted by the medical community as the most valid (e.g., biopsy or pathology). Gold standard tests are more objective and accurate compared with other diagnostic tests, but they also have some disadvantages. For instance, coronary angiography as a gold standard for the diagnosis of coronary heart disease is very expensive, and histopathology as a gold standard for the diagnosis of gastric ulcer or cancer usually takes two or more days to complete. Thus, the evaluation of novel, convenient, or less expensive tests, kits, or instruments for diagnostic or screening purposes is of great clinical interest.

The layout of results in a typical diagnostic test is presented in Table 18.1. The rows of the four-fold table reflect the classification (D) of the study subjects according to the gold standard ($D=1$ for disease present; $D=0$ for disease absent), and the columns reflect their classification (T) according to the test being evaluated ($T=1$ for positive; $T=0$ for negative).

In Table 18.1, a is the number of "true-positive" cases (i.e., subjects with the disease who test positive), b is the number of "false-negative" cases or "missed diagnoses" (i.e., subjects with the disease who test negative), c is the number of "false-positive" cases or "misdiagnoses" (i.e., subjects without the disease who test positive), and d is the number of "true-negative" cases (i.e., subjects without the disease who test negative). Regarding the margins, $a+b$ is the total number of subjects with the disease, $c+d$ is the total number of subjects without the disease, $a+c$ is the total number of subjects testing positive, $b+d$ is the total number of subjects testing negative, and $n=a+b+c+d$ is the total number of subjects.

As can be seen in Table 18.1, a diagnostic test does not always give the "correct" answer; thus, it is important to be able to quantify how accurate a particular test is. There is no single statistical measure that can summarize accuracy because a test result may either fail to detect a case (false-negative) or falsely identify a case (false-positive). The following four measures are commonly used to summarize a test's performance:

(i) Sensitivity
(ii) Specificity
(iii) Positive predictive value
(iv) Negative predictive value

Of these four measures, sensitivity and specificity are measures of intrinsic accuracy – a test's inherent ability. These attributes are therefore considered fundamental to the tests themselves, and they do not change for different samples of patients with different disease prevalence rates. However, sensitivity and specificity do not directly help a clinician interpret the results of an individual test. Positive and negative predictive values are useful in clinical settings because these measures give the probability that an individual is truly positive given that they tested positive or truly negative given that they tested negative. We introduce these measures of diagnostic test characteristics in the following sub-sections.

18.1.1 Sensitivity and Specificity

Example 18.1 In a clinical study, 500 subjects for whom coronary heart disease was suspected underwent both coronary angiography and nuclide myocardial perfusion imaging. The former assessment was taken as the gold standard, and stenosis ($\geq 50\%$) in the left main coronary artery, left anterior descending branch, left circumflex branch, right main coronary artery, or the first-order branches of these was diagnosed as coronary heart disease. The study's purpose was to evaluate the diagnostic accuracy of nuclide myocardial perfusion imaging with hydrochloric higenamine injection as a cardiac stress test drug. The results are shown in Table 18.2.

Table 18.1 Four-fold table of a diagnostic test.

True disease status	Test results		Total
	Positive ($T = 1$)	Negative ($T = 0$)	
Present ($D = 1$)	a	b	$a + b$
Absent ($D = 0$)	c	d	$c + d$
Total	$a + c$	$b + d$	n

Table 18.2 Diagnostic test results for coronary heart disease.

Coronary angiography	Nuclide myocardial perfusion imaging with hydrochloric higenamine		Total
	Positive	Negative	
Present	156(a)	90(b)	246
Absent	23(c)	231(d)	254
Total	179	321	500

The combination of cells a, b, c, and d are presented as follows:

1. Sensitivity and the False-Negative Rate

Sensitivity (*Se*), also known as the true-positive rate, refers to the probability of testing positive given the presence of disease, $P(T=1 \mid D=1)$, and thus reflects a test's ability to correctly detect a disease. Sensitivity is estimated as

$$\widehat{\text{Se}} = \frac{a}{a+b} \times 100\%. \tag{18.1}$$

In Example 18.1, $\widehat{\text{Se}} = \frac{156}{246} \times 100\% = 63.41\%$.

The *false-negative rate* (*FNR*), also known as the *missed diagnosis rate*, refers to the probability of testing negative given the presence of disease, $P\left(T=0 \mid D=1\right)$. FNR is estimated as

$$\widehat{\text{FNR}} = 1 - \widehat{\text{Se}} = \frac{b}{a+b} \times 100\%. \tag{18.2}$$

In Example 18.1, $\widehat{\text{FNR}} = \frac{90}{246} \times 100\% = 36.59\%$.

2. Specificity and the False-Positive Rate

Specificity (*Sp*), also known as the true-negative rate, refers to the probability of testing negative given the absence of disease, $P(T=0 \mid D=0)$, and thus reflects a test's ability to correctly rule out a disease. Specificity is estimated as

$$\widehat{\text{Sp}} = \frac{d}{c+d} \times 100\%. \tag{18.3}$$

In Example 18.1, $\widehat{\text{Sp}} = \frac{231}{254} \times 100\% = 90.94\%$.

The *false-positive rate* (*FPR*), also known as the *misdiagnosis rate*, refers to the probability of testing positive given the absence of disease, $P(T=1 \mid D=0)$. FPR is estimated as

$$\widehat{\text{FPR}} = 1 - \widehat{\text{Sp}} = \frac{c}{c+d} \times 100\%. \tag{18.4}$$

In Example 18.1, $\widehat{\text{FPR}} = \frac{23}{254} \times 100\% = 9.06\%$.

3. Confidence Intervals of Sensitivity and Specificity

Because sensitivity and specificity are metrics that reflect diagnostic properties, their $(1-\alpha)\times 100\%$ CIs can be estimated. When the sample size is small or the sensitivity or specificity estimate is close to 0 or 1, the CI can be obtained using the exact probability method. Appendix Table 8 shows the exact 95% and 99% CIs for rates where $n \leq 50$.

When the sample size is sufficiently large, the standard errors of sensitivity and specificity can be calculated using the normal approximation method. The $(1-\alpha)\times 100\%$ CI of Se is calculated as

$$\left[\widehat{\text{Se}} - z_{1-\alpha/2}\sqrt{Var\left(\widehat{\text{Se}}\right)},\ \widehat{\text{Se}} + z_{1-\alpha/2}\sqrt{Var\left(\widehat{\text{Se}}\right)}\right], \tag{18.5}$$

where the standard error of $\widehat{\text{Se}}$ is $\sqrt{Var\left(\widehat{\text{Se}}\right)} = \sqrt{\dfrac{\widehat{\text{Se}}\left(1-\widehat{\text{Se}}\right)}{a+b}} = \sqrt{\dfrac{ab}{(a+b)^3}}$.

In Example 18.1, $\sqrt{Var\left(\widehat{\text{Se}}\right)} = \sqrt{\dfrac{ab}{(a+b)^3}} = \sqrt{\dfrac{156\times 90}{(156+90)^3}} = 0.0307$, and the 95% CI of Se is

$$\begin{aligned}&\left[\widehat{\text{Se}} - z_{1-\alpha/2}\sqrt{Var\left(\widehat{\text{Se}}\right)},\ \widehat{\text{Se}} + z_{1-\alpha/2}\sqrt{Var\left(\widehat{\text{Se}}\right)}\right]\\ &= \left[0.6341 - 1.96\times 0.0307, 0.6341 + 1.96\times 0.0307\right]\\ &= \left[57.39\%, 69.43\%\right].\end{aligned}$$

Similarly, the $(1-\alpha)\times 100\%$ CI of Sp is calculated as

$$\left[\widehat{\text{Sp}} - z_{1-\alpha/2}\sqrt{Var\left(\widehat{\text{Sp}}\right)},\ \widehat{\text{Sp}} + z_{1-\alpha/2}\sqrt{Var\left(\widehat{\text{Sp}}\right)}\right], \tag{18.6}$$

where the standard error of $\widehat{\text{Sp}}$ is $\sqrt{Var\left(\widehat{\text{Sp}}\right)} = \sqrt{\dfrac{\widehat{\text{Sp}}\left(1-\widehat{\text{Sp}}\right)}{c+d}} = \sqrt{\dfrac{cd}{(c+d)^3}}$.

In Example 18.1, $\sqrt{Var\left(\widehat{\text{Sp}}\right)} = \sqrt{\dfrac{cd}{(c+d)^3}} = \sqrt{\dfrac{23\times 231}{(23+231)^3}} = 0.0180$, and the 95% CI of Sp is

$$\begin{aligned}&\left[\widehat{\text{Sp}} - z_{1-\alpha/2}\sqrt{Var\left(\widehat{\text{Sp}}\right)},\ \widehat{\text{Sp}} + z_{1-\alpha/2}\sqrt{Var\left(\widehat{\text{Sp}}\right)}\right]\\ &= \left[0.9094 - 1.96\times 0.0180, 0.9094 + 1.96\times 0.0180\right]\\ &= \left[87.41\%, 94.47\%\right].\end{aligned}$$

18.1.2 Composite Measures of Sensitivity and Specificity

Frequently, it is difficult to decide which diagnostic test is better when comparing two or more tests because both sensitivity and specificity should be considered. As a solution to this problem, several composite measures of sensitivity and specificity can be used in practice. These measures include Youden's index and likelihood ratios.

1. Youden's Index

Youden's index, denoted by J, is the difference between the true-positive rate (sensitivity) and the false-positive rate. Youden's index is thus equivalent to the sum of sensitivity and specificity minus 1:

$$J = \text{sensitivity} - (1 - \text{specificity}) = \text{Se} + \text{Sp} - 1. \tag{18.7}$$

The value range of J is $[-1, 1]$. Higher values of J indicate higher *diagnostic validity*. $J = 1$ means perfect diagnostic performance because both sensitivity and specificity equal 1; $J \leq 0$ means no diagnostic value.

The $(1-\alpha)\times 100\%$ CI of J is

$$\left[\hat{J} - z_{1-\alpha/2}\sqrt{Var\left(\hat{J}\right)}, \hat{J} + z_{1-\alpha/2}\sqrt{Var\left(\hat{J}\right)}\right], \tag{18.8}$$

where the standard error of $\hat{J}$ is $\sqrt{Var\left(\hat{J}\right)} = \sqrt{\frac{\widehat{\mathrm{Se}}\left(1-\widehat{\mathrm{Se}}\right)}{a+b} + \frac{\widehat{\mathrm{Sp}}\left(1-\widehat{\mathrm{Sp}}\right)}{c+d}}$.

Example 18.2 A test kit was applied to test for allergy to chicken eggs among 714 patients in a multicenter study. The outcome is evaluated by the grades of specific IgE antibody levels. The results are displayed in Table 18.3.

The diagnostic validity evaluation result using different positive standards (called *cutoffs* or thresholds) is shown in Table 18.4. The estimated Youden's index $\left(\hat{J} = 0.714\right)$ is largest when using $+++$ as the cutoff ($\geq +++$ as the criteria for testing positive), and the $\widehat{\mathrm{Se}}$ and $\widehat{\mathrm{Sp}}$ are 86.0% and 85.4%, respectively.

In Table 18.4, it is clear that, when a higher cutoff is selected, sensitivity is lower and specificity is higher and that, when a lower cutoff is selected, sensitivity is higher, and specificity is lower. In clinical applications, however, the selection of thresholds depends on the purpose of the study. Usually, the cutoff can be selected on the basis of the largest J, which represents an optimal trade-off between sensitivity and specificity.

Table 18.3 Diagnostic test results for chicken egg allergy among 714 patients.

Gold standard	Specific IgE test result						Total
	−	±	+	++	+++	++++	
Allergic	2	8	17	24	88	226	365
Not allergic	156	72	34	36	33	18	349
Total	158	80	51	60	121	244	714

Table 18.4 Evaluation of diagnostic validity at different cutoffs.

Cutoff	$\widehat{\mathrm{Se}}$	$\widehat{\mathrm{Sp}}$	$\hat{J}$
−	1.000	0.000	0.000
±	0.995	0.447	0.442
+	0.973	0.653	0.626
++	0.926	0.751	0.677
+++	0.860	0.854	0.714
++++	0.619	0.948	0.567
>++++	0.000	1.000	0.000

For screening purposes, the cutoff can be selected to favor a higher sensitivity to reduce the false-negative rate (i.e., missed diagnoses); for confirmative diagnosis purposes, the cutoff can be selected to favor a higher specificity to reduce the false-positive rate (i.e., misdiagnoses).

2. Likelihood Ratios

As shown in Chapter 16, likelihood ratios are used to express a change in odds. They are also frequently applied in the realm of diagnosis as composite measures of sensitivity and test specificity.

The *positive likelihood ratio*, denoted by LR +, represents the probability of testing positive given the presence of disease over the probability of testing positive given the absence of disease; thus, the positive likelihood ratio is defined as the ratio of the true-positive rate and the false-positive rate:

$$\mathrm{LR}+=\frac{P\left(T=1\mid D=1\right)}{P\left(T=1\mid D=0\right)}=\frac{\mathrm{Se}}{1-\mathrm{Sp}}. \tag{18.9}$$

LR + can be estimated as

$$\widehat{\mathrm{LR}}+=\frac{\widehat{\mathrm{Se}}}{1-\widehat{\mathrm{Sp}}}=\frac{a\left(c+d\right)}{c\left(a+b\right)}. \tag{18.10}$$

The range of possible values of LR + is positive from 0 to infinity. Larger values of LR + indicate that the test is more informative. For instance, LR + equals 5 indicates that, using the test, there is a five-fold increase in the odds of having the disease in a subject with a positive test result, whereas LR + equals 1 means that the test is useless because the odds of a subject having the disease do not change after the test.

The sampling distribution of $\widehat{\mathrm{LR}}+$ is positively skewed, whereas the distribution of $\ln\left(\widehat{\mathrm{LR}}+\right)$ approximates normality, with a standard deviation

$$\sqrt{Var\left(\ln\left(\widehat{\mathrm{LR}}+\right)\right)}=\sqrt{\frac{1-\widehat{\mathrm{Se}}}{a}+\frac{\widehat{\mathrm{Sp}}}{c}}. \tag{18.11}$$

The $\left(1-\alpha\right)\times100\%$ CI of $\ln\left(\mathrm{LR}+\right)$ is

$$\ln\left(\frac{\widehat{\mathrm{Se}}}{1-\widehat{\mathrm{Sp}}}\right)\pm z_{1-\alpha/2}\sqrt{\frac{1-\widehat{\mathrm{Se}}}{a}+\frac{\widehat{\mathrm{Sp}}}{c}}, \tag{18.12}$$

and the $\left(1-\alpha\right)\times100\%$ CI of LR + is

$$\exp\left[\ln\left(\frac{\widehat{\mathrm{Se}}}{1-\widehat{\mathrm{Sp}}}\right)\pm z_{1-\alpha/2}\sqrt{\frac{1-\widehat{\mathrm{Se}}}{a}+\frac{\widehat{\mathrm{Sp}}}{c}}\right]. \tag{18.13}$$

The *negative likelihood ratio*, denoted by LR −, is the probability of testing negative given the presence of disease over the probability of testing negative given the absence of disease; thus, the negative likelihood ratio is defined as the ratio of the false-negative rate and the true-negative rate:

$$\text{LR}- = \frac{P(T=0 \mid D=1)}{P(T=0 \mid D=0)} = \frac{1-\text{Se}}{\text{Sp}}. \tag{18.14}$$

LR − can be estimated as

$$\widehat{\text{LR}}- = \frac{1-\widehat{\text{Se}}}{\widehat{\text{Sp}}} = \frac{b(c+d)}{d(a+b)}. \tag{18.15}$$

The range of possible values of LR − is positive from 0 to infinity. Smaller values of LR − indicate that the test is more informative. For instance, LR − valuing 0.1 indicates that, using the test, there is a 10-fold decrease in the odds of there being disease in a subject with a negative test result, whereas LR − valuing 1 is equivalent to LR + valuing 1 and means that the test is useless because the odds of disease being present do not change after the test. The $(1-\alpha)\times 100\%$ CI of LR − is:

$$\exp\left[\ln\left(\frac{1-\widehat{\text{Se}}}{\widehat{\text{Sp}}}\right) \pm z_{1-\alpha/2}\sqrt{\frac{\widehat{\text{Se}}}{b}+\frac{1-\widehat{\text{Sp}}}{d}}\right]. \tag{18.16}$$

The likelihood ratios for Example 18.2 are shown in Table 18.5.

As can be inferred from this table, when selecting a diagnostic cutoff, it is more convenient to use J instead of likelihood ratios. This is because the maximum value for J is 1, whereas likelihood ratios can be infinitely large, and the increasing (or decreasing) trends of LR + and LR − with different cutoffs are in the same direction.

18.1.3 Predictive Values

Positive predictive value, denoted by PPV, is the probability of disease given a positive test result. *Negative predictive value*, denoted by NPV, is the probability of no disease given a negative test result. From Table 18.1 and Bayes' rule, we can derive the defining formulas for these predictive values:

Table 18.5 Diagnostic accuracy measures at different diagnostic cutoffs.

Cutoff	$\widehat{\text{Se}}$	$\widehat{\text{Sp}}$	$\hat{J}$	$\widehat{\text{LR}}+$	$\widehat{\text{LR}}-$
−	1.000	0.000	0.000	1.000	−
±	0.995	0.447	0.442	1.799	0.011
+	0.973	0.653	0.626	2.804	0.041
++	0.926	0.751	0.677	3.719	0.099
+++	0.860	0.854	0.714	5.890	0.164
++++	0.619	0.948	0.567	11.904	0.402
>++++	0.000	1.000	0.000	−	1.000

$$\text{PPV} = P(D=1 \mid T=1) = \frac{P(D=1)P(T=1 \mid D=1)}{P(D=1)P(T=1 \mid D=1) + P(D=0)P(T=1 \mid D=0)}$$
$$= \frac{P \times \text{Se}}{P \times \text{Se} + (1-P) \times (1-\text{Sp})}, \tag{18.17}$$

$$\text{NPV} = P(D=0 \mid T=0) = \frac{P(D=0)P(T=0 \mid D=0)}{P(D=0)P(T=0 \mid D=0) + P(D=1)P(T=0 \mid D=1)}$$
$$= \frac{(1-P) \times \text{Sp}}{(1-P) \times \text{Sp} + P \times (1-\text{Se})}, \tag{18.18}$$

where $P = P(D=1)$ denotes the prevalence of the disease.

When the study sample is drawn randomly from the target population, the proportion with the disease $(a+b)/n$ can be taken as an empirical estimate of the disease prevalence; thus, the formulas for PPV and NPV can be simplified as

$$\widehat{\text{PPV}} = \frac{a}{a+c} \times 100\%, \tag{18.19}$$

$$\widehat{\text{NPV}} = \frac{d}{b+d} \times 100\%. \tag{18.20}$$

Why, then, would we bother to use sensitivity and specificity as measures of diagnostic validity instead of predictive values, which are more intuitive? We explain the answer to this question using the following example.

Example 18.3 Refer to Example 4.8. In this large epidemiological survey on pelvic disorders among women in China, Pelvic Organ Prolapse Quantification was used as the gold standard to evaluate the diagnostic value of a simplified pelvic dysfunction questionnaire. The results for 9000 women from North China and another 9000 women from South China are shown in Table 18.6.

Table 18.6 shows that the estimated sensitivities $(1456/1820 = 304/380 = 80\%)$ and specificities $(6821/7180 = 8189/8620 = 95\%)$ were equivalent for women in North

Table 18.6 Diagnostic results for pelvic disorders in North China and South China.

Location	Disease status determined by pelvic organ prolapse staging criterion	Result of simplified pelvic dysfunction questionnaire		
		Positive	**Negative**	**Total**
North China	Present	1456	364	1820
	Absent	359	6821	7180
	Total	1815	7185	9000
South China	Present	304	76	380
	Absent	431	8189	8620
	Total	735	8265	9000

and South China. However, the predictive values were very different; for instance, $\widehat{\text{PPV}}$ in North China $(1456/1815 = 80\%)$ was almost two times that in South China $(304/735 = 41\%)$. Why is this the case? Notice that the two groups of women have very different disease prevalence rates: $1820/9000 = 20.2\%$ in North China vs. $380/9000 = 4.2\%$ in South China. From this example, we can see that predictive values are not related only to the validity of the test (sensitivity and specificity); rather, these values are also sensitive to the disease prevalence in the locations where the study is carried out. Therefore, predictive values are not intrinsic measures of validity.

We now continue with another example.

Example 18.4 Suppose it is estimated that the sensitivity and specificity of serum alpha-fetoprotein (AFP) for detecting liver cancer is 90% and 95%, respectively.

(1) Knowing that the prevalence of liver cancer in a population undergoing routine physical examinations is 0.4%, what is the probability of liver cancer for a participant who has a positive AFP test result?

$$\widehat{\text{PPV}} = \frac{P \times \widehat{\text{Se}}}{P \times \widehat{\text{Se}} + (1-P) \times \left(1-\widehat{\text{Sp}}\right)} = \frac{0.004 \times 0.90}{0.004 \times 0.90 + (1-0.004) \times (1-0.95)} = 0.067$$

(2) Knowing that the prevalence of liver cancer among patients with hepatitis is 10%, what is the probability of liver cancer for a patient with hepatitis who has a positive AFP test result?

$$\widehat{\text{PPV}} = \frac{P \times \widehat{\text{Se}}}{P \times \widehat{\text{Se}} + (1-P) \times \left(1-\widehat{\text{Sp}}\right)} = \frac{0.10 \times 0.90}{0.10 \times 0.90 + (1-0.10) \times (1-0.95)} = 0.667$$

(3) Knowing that the prevalence of liver cancer among patients with cirrhosis is 40%, what is the probability of liver cancer for a patient with cirrhosis who has a positive AFP test result?

$$\widehat{\text{PPV}} = \frac{P \times \widehat{\text{Se}}}{P \times \widehat{\text{Se}} + (1-P) \times \left(1-\widehat{\text{Sp}}\right)} = \frac{0.40 \times 0.90}{0.40 \times 0.90 + (1-0.40) \times (1-0.95)} = 0.923.$$

Clearly, disease prevalence plays a very important role in the calculation of PPV and NPV.

It should be noted that study samples obtained from hospitals are not random samples of the population; therefore, we should calculate predictive values using Bayes' rule rather than the simplified direct calculation formula.

18.1.4 Sensitivity and Specificity Comparison of Two Diagnostic Tests

The two-sample inference methods for rates can be applied to the comparison of sensitivities and to the comparison of specificities because these measures are in essence proportional indicators. The study design is important for the choice of inference methods. For diagnostic studies with completely randomized designs, the Z-test, χ^2 test, or Fisher's exact test can be used, whereas McNemar's test can be used for diagnostic studies with paired samples designs.

1. Paired Samples Designs

Example 18.5 Referring to Example 18.1, the 500 subjects suspected to have coronary heart disease who underwent nuclide myocardial perfusion imaging used adenosine as the cardiac stress test drug, in addition to hydrochloric higenamine. Coronary angiography was used as the gold standard, and the results are shown in Table 18.7.

For nuclide myocardial perfusion imaging with hydrochloric higenamine, the sensitivity was $156/246 = 63.41\%$, and the specificity was $231/254 = 90.94\%$. For nuclide myocardial perfusion imaging with adenosine, the sensitivity was $146/246 = 59.35\%$, and the specificity was $234/254 = 92.13\%$. The sensitivities and specificities of the two cardiac stress test drugs are different, but are the differences statistically significant?

Notice that the same subjects were diagnosed using two test methods. This means the data were paired and thus not independent samples. The original data were therefore sorted into a four-fold table (Table 18.8) in the form of a paired samples design.

Solution

First, compare the sensitivities.

H_0 : The sensitivities of the two methods are the same

H_1 : The sensitivities of the two methods are not the same

$\alpha = 0.05$

$$\chi^2 = \frac{(b-c)^2}{b+c} = \frac{(16-26)^2}{16+26} = 2.38$$

Table 18.7 Diagnostic test results for coronary heart disease.

Coronary angiography	Hydrochloric higenamine		Adenosine		Total
	Positive	Negative	Positive	Negative	
Present	156	90	146	100	246
Absent	23	231	20	234	254
Total	179	321	166	334	500

Table 18.8 Paired samples design results for the comparison of sensitivity and specificity.

Adenosine	Disease			No disease		
	Hydrochloric higenamine			Hydrochloric higenamine		
	Positive	Negative	Total	Positive	Negative	Total
Positive	130	16	146	4	16	20
Negative	26	74	100	19	215	234
Total	156	90	246	23	231	254

According to the χ^2 distribution with $\nu = 1$ and $\alpha = 0.05$, we find that $\chi^2 < \chi^2_{1,1-0.05} = 3.84$, so $p > 0.05$. We do not reject H_0 at the $\alpha = 0.05$ level, and we conclude that the sensitivities of nuclide myocardial perfusion imaging with the two cardiac stress test drugs do not differ significantly.

Second, compare the specificities.

H_0 : The specificities of the two methods are the same

H_1 : The specificities of the two methods are not the same

$$\alpha = 0.05$$

$$\chi^2 = \frac{(b-c)^2}{b+c} = \frac{(19-16)^2}{19+16} = 0.26$$

According to the χ^2 distribution with $\nu = 1$ and $\alpha = 0.05$, we find that $\chi^2 < \chi^2_{1,1-0.05} = 3.84$, so $p > 0.05$. We do not reject H_0 at the $\alpha = 0.05$ level, and we conclude that the specificities of nuclide myocardial perfusion imaging with the two cardiac stress test drugs do not differ significantly.

2. Completely Randomized Designs

Example 18.6 In a clinical study, 135 of 186 subjects with lung cancer and 16 of 305 subjects without lung cancer had positive results for lung cancer with X-ray examination. In another study, 173 of 184 subjects with lung cancer and 13 of 298 subjects without lung cancer had positive results for lung cancer with enhanced computed tomography (CT). The results are displayed in Table 18.9. Does the diagnostic validity of X-ray vary from that of enhanced CT?

Solution

The diagnostic validity of X-ray examination and enhanced CT examination was evaluated in two independent clinical studies. The χ^2 test can be used to compare the sensitivity and specificity of the two examination methods.

First, compare the sensitivity among the subjects with lung cancer.

H_0 : The sensitivities of the two methods are the same

H_1 : The sensitivities of the two methods are not the same

$$\alpha = 0.05$$

$$\chi^2 = \frac{(ad-bc)^2 \times n}{(a+b)(c+d)(a+c)(b+d)} = \frac{(135\times 11 - 51\times 173)^2 \times 370}{186\times 184\times 308\times 62} = 30.48$$

Table 18.9 Results of X-ray examination and enhanced CT examination.

Examination	Lung cancer		No lung cancer	
	Positive	Negative	Positive	Negative
X-ray	135	51	16	289
Enhanced CT	173	11	13	285
Total	308	62	29	574

According to the χ^2 distribution with $\nu = 1$ and $\alpha = 0.05$, as $\chi^2 = 30.48 > 3.84$, $p < 0.05$. We reject H_0 and accept H_1 at the $\alpha = 0.05$ level. We conclude that the difference between the sensitivities of the two methods for diagnosing lung cancer is significant and that the sensitivity of enhanced CT $(173/184 = 94.02\%)$ is higher than that of X-ray $(135/186 = 72.58\%)$.

Second, compare the specificity among subjects without lung cancer.

H_0 : The specificities of the two methods are the same

H_1 : The specificities of the two methods are not the same

$$\alpha = 0.05$$

$$\chi^2 = \frac{(ad - bc)^2 \times n}{(a+b)(c+d)(a+c)(b+d)} = \frac{(16 \times 285 - 289 \times 13)^2 \times 603}{305 \times 298 \times 29 \times 574} = 0.26$$

According to the χ^2 distribution with $\nu = 1$ and $\alpha = 0.05$, as $\chi^2 = 0.26 < 3.84$, $p > 0.05$. We do not reject H_0 at the $\alpha = 0.05$ level. The evidence is insufficient to show that the specificities of enhanced CT $(285/298 = 95.64\%)$ and X-ray $(289/305 = 94.75\%)$ are different.

In summary, there is no statistically significant difference in the specificity of the two examination methods, whereas the sensitivity of enhanced CT examination is significantly higher than that of X-ray examination. Therefore, diagnostic validity is better for enhanced CT examination than for X-ray examination.

18.2 Agreement Between Diagnostic Tests

The calculation of sensitivity and specificity requires a definite gold standard to classify subjects into diseased and non-diseased statuses. In clinical practice, however, there is sometimes no widely accepted gold standard, and sensitivity and specificity thus cannot be precisely evaluated using the methods introduced in the previous section. In such a situation, measures of agreement are usually used to evaluate the value of diagnostic tests in an indirect way. By "agreement," we mean the consistency or similarity of results between two tests. In this section, we introduce the methods for evaluating agreement, first for categorical data and then for numerical data.

Table 18.10 X-ray results interpreted by two radiologists.

Interpretation by radiologist *B*	**Interpretation by radiologist *A***		**Total**
	Malignant	**Benign**	
Malignant	18(a)	25(b)	43
Benign	22(c)	33(d)	55
Total	40	58	98(n)

18.2.1 Agreement of Categorical Data

McNemar's test is sometimes misused to evaluate the agreement between two diagnostic tests and conclude that the tests are consistent if they have no significant difference in positive rates. In the following example, we illustrate why this approach is incorrect.

Example 18.7 Two radiologists independently interpreted X-ray results for 98 patients with lesions suspected to have thyroid tumor. Table 18.10 shows the summary of the results.

Using McNemar's test, $\chi^2 = \frac{(b-c)^2}{b+c} = \frac{(25-22)^2}{25+22} = 0.19$. Because $\chi^2 = 0.19 < 3.84$, $p > 0.05$, and the conclusion is that we do not reject the hypothesis that the interpretations of the two radiologists are consistent. However, in Table 18.10, we see that the two radiologists agreed on only 18 (18.37%) patients who both considered malignant and 33 (33.67%) patients who both considered benign; disagreements occurred for 47 (47.96%) patients. In other words, the two radiologists did not agree with each other on almost half of the patients. Obviously, McNemar's test failed in this evaluation of agreement between tests.

To address this issue, we introduce some commonly used measures of agreement between two tests.

(1) The *concordance rate*, also called the total concordance rate, total agreement rate, or observed agreement rate, refers to the proportion of subjects with the same test results. The formula to estimate its value is as follows:

$$\begin{aligned} \text{concordance rate} &= \frac{\text{number of subjects with the same test results}}{\text{total number of subjects}} \\ &= \frac{a+d}{n} \times 100\%. \end{aligned} \tag{18.21}$$

(2) The *positive concordance rate*, also called the positive agreement rate, refers to the proportion of subjects with positive results on the reference test (in this example, those who were classified as having malignant lesions by radiologist A) who had positive results on both tests (analogous to a sensitivity calculation). The formula to estimate its value is as follows:

$$\begin{aligned} \text{positive concordance rate} &= \frac{\text{number of subjects positive on both tests}}{\text{number of subjects positive on the reference test}} \\ &= \frac{a}{a+c} \times 100\%. \end{aligned} \tag{18.22}$$

(3) The *negative concordance rate*, also called the negative agreement rate, refers to the proportion of subjects with negative results on the reference test (in this example, those who were classified as having benign lesions by radiologist A) who had negative results on both tests (analogous to a specificity calculation). The formula to estimate its value is as follows:

$$\begin{aligned} \text{negative concordance rate} &= \frac{\text{number of subjects negative on both tests}}{\text{number of subjects negative on the reference test}} \\ &= \frac{d}{b+d} \times 100\%. \end{aligned} \tag{18.23}$$

(4) The *kappa coefficient*, denoted by κ, is an important measure of agreement for categorical data. It is defined as

$$\kappa = \frac{P_o - P_e}{1 - P_e}, \tag{18.24}$$

where P_o is the observed agreement between tests and is estimated as $\hat{P}_o = (a+d)/n$ and P_e is the expected probability, indicating chance agreement, and is estimated as $\hat{P}_e = \left[(a+b)(a+c)+(c+d)(b+d)\right]/n^2$. $P_o - P_e$ reflects the absolute agreement, and the kappa coefficient is a measure of the degree of absolute agreement that removes agreement by chance from the agreed and total test results.

The range of kappa is $[-1, 1]$. $\kappa = 1$ indicates perfect agreement, $\kappa = -1$ indicates complete disagreement, and $\kappa = 0$ means that the agreement is the same as would be expected by chance. Most of the time, the kappa coefficient falls between 0 and 1. Then, how much larger than 0 should κ be to indicate agreement in practice? The answer to this question depends on the clinical question being evaluated, although a rule of thumb is that $\kappa > 0.7$ indicates good agreement between two tests.

Example 18.8 A new specific allergen test kit was used among allergy patients. An approved ImmunoCAP test kit on the market was used as the reference test. The results for acaroid mite allergy among 1199 patients are shown in Table 18.11. Evaluate the agreement between these two tests.

Solution

Calculate the concordance rate.

$$\text{total concordance rate} = (a+d)/n = (512+526)/1199 \times 100\% = 86.57\%$$

$$\text{positive concordance rate} = a/(a+c) = 512/586 \times 100\% = 87.37\%$$

$$\text{negative concordance rate} = d/(b+d) = 526/613 \times 100\% = 85.81\%$$

Calculate the kappa coefficient.

$$\hat{P}_o = \text{total concordance rate} = 86.57\%$$

$$\hat{P}_e = \frac{(a+b)(a+c)+(c+d)(b+d)}{n^2} = 50.00\%,$$

$$\hat{\kappa} = \frac{\hat{P}_o - \hat{P}_e}{1 - \hat{P}_e} = \frac{86.57\% - 50.00\%}{1 - 50.00\%} = 0.7314$$

Table 18.11 Diagnosis results for allergy to acaroid mites using two test kits.

Specific allergen test kit.	**ImmunoCAP test kit as reference test**		**Total**
	Positive	**Negative**	
Positive	$512(a)$	$87(b)$	599
Negative	$74(c)$	$526(d)$	600
Total	586	613	$1199(n)$

Table 18.12 Results of multiclass categorical data for two diagnostic tests.

Test to be evaluated	Reference test				Total
	1	2	...	k	
1	a_{11}	a_{12}	...	a_{1k}	$n_{1\cdot}$
2	a_{21}	a_{22}	...	a_{2k}	$n_{2\cdot}$
⋮	⋮	⋮	⋮	⋮	⋮
k	a_{k1}	a_{k2}	...	a_{kk}	$n_{k\cdot}$
Total	$n_{\cdot 1}$	$n_{\cdot 2}$	...	$n_{\cdot k}$	n

The results show that the new specific allergen test kit has good agreement with the approved ImmunoCAP test kit for the detection of acaroid mite allergy.

For multiclass categorical data, the results can be summarized as shown in Table 18.12. Observed and chance agreement are estimated as follows:

$$\hat{P}_o = \frac{\sum_{i=1}^{k} a_{ii}}{n} = \frac{a_{11} + a_{22} + \cdots + a_{kk}}{n}, \tag{18.25}$$

$$\hat{P}_e = \frac{\sum_{i=1}^{k} n_{i\cdot} n_{\cdot i}}{n^2} = \frac{n_{1\cdot} n_{\cdot 1} + n_{2\cdot} n_{\cdot 2} + \cdots + n_{k\cdot} n_{\cdot k}}{n^2}. \tag{18.26}$$

Example 18.9 Two radiologists independently interpreted enhanced CT images for 311 patients suspected to have breast cancer. The results are shown in Table 18.13. Evaluate the two radiologists' agreement.

Solution

$$\hat{P}_o = \frac{a_{11} + a_{22} + a_{33}}{n} = \frac{58 + 12 + 196}{311} \times 100\% = 85.53\%$$

$$\hat{P}_e = \frac{n_{1\cdot} n_{\cdot 1} + n_{2\cdot} n_{\cdot 2} + n_{3\cdot} n_{\cdot 3}}{n^2} = \frac{77 \times 70 + 27 \times 34 + 207 \times 207}{311^2} \times 100\% = 50.82\%$$

Table 18.13 Interpretation of enhanced CT imaging for breast cancer by two radiologists.

Interpretation by radiologist *B*	Interpretation by radiologist *A*			Total
	Benign	Possibly malignant	Malignant	
Benign	58	14	5	77
Possibly malignant	9	12	6	27
Malignant	3	8	196	207
Total	70	34	207	311

$$\hat{\kappa} = \frac{\hat{P}_o - \hat{P}_e}{1 - \hat{P}_e} = \frac{85.53\% - 50.82\%}{1 - 50.82\%} = 0.7058$$

The results show that the two radiologists had good agreement in their interpretations of enhanced CT imaging for breast cancer.

Of note, $\hat{\kappa}$ is a sample estimate, and hypothesis testing is required for a final inference about the population. This can be done using statistical software.

18.2.2 Agreement of Numerical Data

Suppose that we are provided with a new kit for detecting leukocyte differentiation antigen CD8 or a new electronic sphygmomanometer. Can these new methods be used as alternatives to those that are currently used in clinical practice? In such cases, the results from both tests are numerical data. What is your study plan for the agreement evaluation?

Here are three possible solutions (note that some of them are flawed):

Option 1: Perform a paired samples *t*-test. If there is no statistically significant difference, the results of the two tests can be considered to have good agreement.

Option 2: Perform a correlation analysis. If the Pearson correlation coefficient or Spearman's rank correlation coefficient is large and statistically significant, the results of the two tests can be considered to have good agreement.

Option 3: Perform a linear regression analysis.

The first two options are both flawed. Regarding the first option, a paired samples *t*-test examines difference in means rather than individual-level differences between tests. In other words, nonsignificance in a paired samples *t*-test can only indicate that two tests have similar mean levels, and agreement between these tests is not guaranteed because the individual-level differences between the tests may be extremely large or small, as long as their sum approximates 0. Regarding the second option, correlation coefficients measure correlation rather than agreement, even if the result is close to 1. As an example of this, note that almost all the points in Figure 18.1 are arranged in a straight line. The Pearson correlation coefficient for these data is 0.999; however, the two tests do not agree because the results of one test are almost two times those of the other.

We are now close to the correct method of evaluating agreement for tests of numerical data, as in Option 3. The results of two tests that are in perfect agreement will exactly match along a diagonal line; thus, good agreement is indicated by a linear regression analysis in which the regression coefficient is not significantly different from 1 and the intercept is not significantly different from 0.

Example 18.10 The results of an agreement evaluation of a new electronic sphygmomanometer and a mercury sphygmomanometer are shown in Figure 18.2. A linear regression model was fitted: $\hat{y} = 0.485 + 0.992x$. The 95% CIs of the regression coefficient and the intercept were $[0.985, 1.000]$ and $[-0.134, 1.103]$, respectively. This means that the regression coefficient was not significantly different from 1 and that the intercept was not significantly different from 0. We can conclude that the results of the study indicated good agreement between the new electronic sphygmomanometer and the mercury sphygmomanometer.

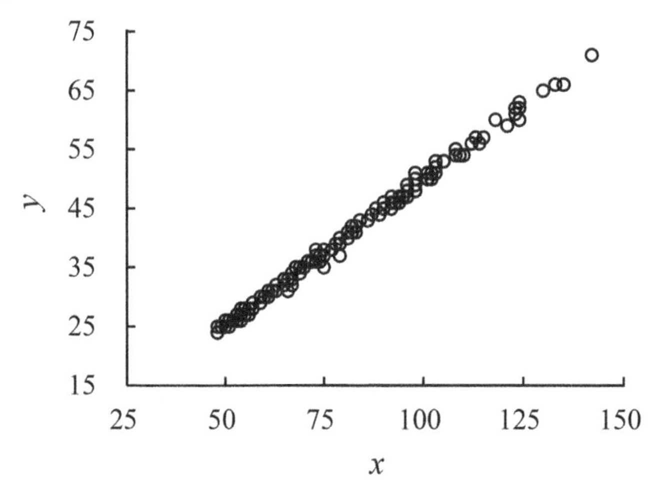

Figure 18.1 Scatterplot of the results of two tests (simulated).

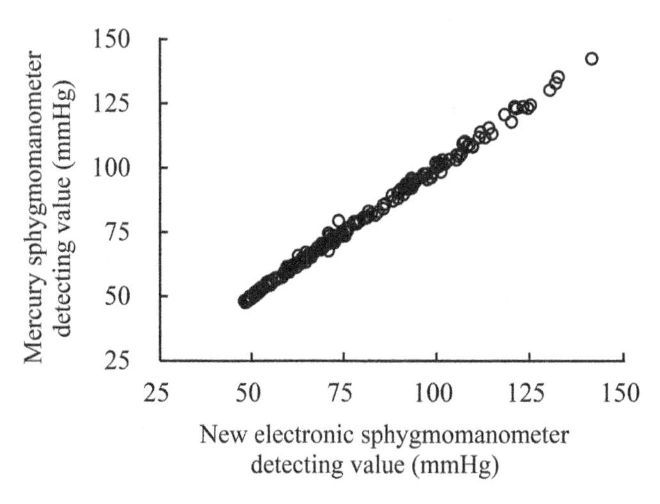

Figure 18.2 Scatterplots of blood pressure test results using the two sphygmomanometers.

For a quantitative measurement of the degree of agreement, one may refer to the literature on calculating the intraclass correlation coefficient (ICC). Although these measures are beyond the scope of this book, other methods of agreement evaluation for numerical data include the Bland–Altman plot, Deming regression, and Passing–Bablok regression. Under certain circumstances, we can also transform numerical data into categorical data for the evaluation of agreement between tests, provided that the results are clinically interpretable.

18.3 Receiver Operating Characteristic Curve Analysis

When a diagnostic test result extends from binary to an ordinal or continuous response, sensitivity and specificity may vary with different cutoffs. Problems then arise regarding how to comprehensively measure the validity of a test, how to select an

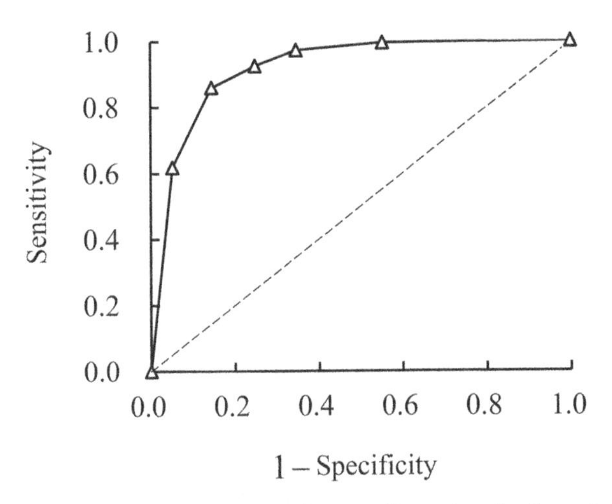

Figure 18.3 ROC curve for the egg allergy data for Example 18.2.

optimal cutoff, and how to compare different tests. *Receiver operating characteristic (ROC) curve* analysis provides a powerful framework for addressing these questions.

18.3.1 Concept of an ROC Curve

ROC curve analysis is a method that originated in the evaluation of the correctness of reception of radar signals in the 1940s. This method was introduced to the field of medical study by L.B. Lusted in 1960s. The ROC curve is a plot of sensitivity on the vertical axis against the false-positive rate $\left(1-\text{specificity}\right)$ on the horizontal axis, with both measures calculated at every possible cutoff of the test.

Figure 18.3 displays an empirical ROC curve for the test kit in Example 18.2. The dashed line running from the bottom left corner to the top right corner is called the diagnostic reference line or the chance line because, for a hypothetical "reference" test that is completely useless, we can expect sensitivity to equal 1 minus sensitivity at each given cutoff (i.e., subjects with and without the disease have equal "chances" of testing positive).

One advantage of ROC curve analysis is that it can help to identify an optimal cutoff. As a general rule, the cutoff corresponding to the point on the ROC curve that is closest to the upper left vertex of the coordinate system represents a reasonable trade-off between sensitivity and specificity, and it would be an optimal selection when we do not have a specific preference for optimizing sensitivity or specificity.

Example 18.11 Referring to Example 18.2, find an optimal cutoff for the test kit using ROC curve analysis (no specific preference for optimizing sensitivity or specificity is assumed).

Solution

When a cutoff of $+++$ is selected, $\widehat{\text{Se}}=0.860$, $\widehat{\text{Sp}}=0.854$, and $\left(1-\widehat{\text{Se}}\right)^2+\left(1-\widehat{\text{Sp}}\right)^2=0.041$, which is the smallest (the distance from the upper left vertex is the smallest) of the values corresponding to all possible cutoffs. Therefore, by using a criterion of $\geq +++$ for defining a positive test result, we may have a good trade-off between the minimization of missed diagnoses and misdiagnoses of egg allergy.

18.3.2 Area Under the ROC Curve

The *area under the ROC curve*, denoted as A, is the area defined by the contours of the ROC curve, the horizontal axis, and the vertical line $(1-\text{specificity}=1)$. It is also an important measure of the comprehensive diagnostic validity of a test, and it can be interpreted as the average sensitivity across all possible specificity values.

The range of A is 0–1, and, as A approaches 1, the diagnostic validity of the test becomes stronger. As A approaches 0.5, the diagnostic validity becomes weaker. An $A<0.5$ indicates that the way of defining a positive result is inconsistent with the clinical interpretation. In this case, the ROC curve analysis should be conducted after modifying the definition.

Parametric and nonparametric methods can be used for calculating A. Now we introduce a nonparametric method, the Hanley–McNeil method.

Let X and Y denote the test results of the groups with and without the disease, whereas n_1 and n_0 the corresponding sample sizes, respectively. Without loss of generalizability, we assume that A could be interpreted as the probability that a subject randomly selected from the diseased population has a higher test value compared with that of a subject randomly chosen from the non-diseased population:

$$A=P(X>Y)$$

This probability can be empirically estimated using a scoring method. To start, we pair every single value of X with a value of Y, and we then assign a score $S(X, Y)$ to each pair using the following rule:

$$S(X,Y)=\begin{cases}1, & X>Y\\ 1/2, & X=Y.\\ 0, & X<Y\end{cases} \tag{18.27}$$

A is then estimated as the sum of scores divided by the number of pairs:

$$\hat{A}=\frac{1}{n_1 n_0}\sum_1^{n_1}\sum_1^{n_0} S(X,Y). \tag{18.28}$$

The standard error of $\hat{A}$ can be estimated as

$$\sqrt{Var(\hat{A})}=\sqrt{\frac{\hat{A}\left(1-\hat{A}\right)+\left(n_1-1\right)\left(Q_1-\hat{A}^2\right)+\left(n_0-1\right)\left(Q_2-\hat{A}^2\right)}{n_1 n_0}}, \tag{18.29}$$

where Q_1, Q_2 are two statistics. Q_1 is the estimated probability that two subjects randomly selected from the diseased group have test values greater than the test value of one subject randomly selected from the non-diseased group; Q_2 is the estimated probability that one subject randomly selected from the diseased group has a test value greater than the test values of two subjects randomly selected from the non-diseased group.

The $(1-\alpha)\times 100\%$ CI for A is thus given by

$$\left[\hat{A}-z_{1-\alpha/2}\sqrt{Var\left(\hat{A}\right)},\ \hat{A}+z_{1-\alpha/2}\sqrt{Var\left(\hat{A}\right)}\right] \quad (18.30)$$

Hypothesis testing for an ROC curve can be done by comparing A with 0.5 using a Z-test.

(1) State the hypotheses and select a significance level.

$H_0: A=0.5$

$H_1: A\neq 0.5$

Usually let $\alpha=0.05$

(2) Determine the test statistic.

$$Z=\frac{\hat{A}-0.5}{\sqrt{Var\left(\hat{A}\right)}}. \quad (18.31)$$

(3) Draw a conclusion.

If $z>z_{1-\alpha/2}$, then reject H_0, and $A>0.5$ is considered statistically significant. We then conclude that the test has diagnostic value. Otherwise, do not reject H_0.

Example 18.12 Referring to Example 18.2 with the egg allergy data, calculate the area under curve and its 95% CI, and perform a significance test.

Solution

For the calculation of $\hat{A}$ and $\sqrt{Var\left(\hat{A}\right)}$, we can transform the data in Table 18.3 into the form displayed in Table 18.14. The first and second rows are the original data. In the third row, $\sum_{i=j+1}^{C} n_i^+$ (C is the number of grades among the subjects with egg allergy) represents the total numbers of subjects with egg allergy who have a diagnostic grade larger than j (e.g., the first number presented here is $8+17+24+88+226=363$). In the fourth row, $\sum_{i=1}^{j-1} n_i^-$ represents the total numbers of subjects without egg allergy who have a diagnostic grade smaller than j (e.g., the third number listed in this row is $156+72=228$). The fifth to seventh rows are calculated based on the first four rows (e.g., the first numbers in the fifth, sixth, and seventh rows are $156\times 363+2\times 156/2=56{,}784.0$, $2\times\left(0+0\times 156+156^2/3\right)=16{,}224.0$, and $156\times\left(363^2+363\times 2+2^2/3\right)=20{,}669{,}428.0$, respectively).

Calculate $\hat{A}$ and $\sqrt{Var\left(\hat{A}\right)}$ from Table 18.14.

$$\hat{A}=\frac{1}{n_1 n_0}\sum_1^{n_1}\sum_1^{n_0} S(X,Y)=\frac{T_1}{n_1 n_0}=\frac{117093.0}{349\times 365}=0.919$$

$$Q_1=\frac{T_3}{n_0 n_1^2}=\frac{40593295.3}{349\times 365^2}=0.873$$

Table 18.14 Calculation of the area under the receiver operating characteristic curve and its standard error.

Row	Calculation	Diagnostic grade (j)						Sum
		1	2	3	4	5	6	
(1)	Allergic	2	8	17	24	88	226	365
(2)	Not allergic	156	72	34	36	33	18	349
(3)	$\sum_{i=j+1}^{C} n_i^+$	363	355	338	314	226	0	
(4)	$\sum_{i=1}^{j-1} n_i^-$	0	156	228	262	298	331	
(5)	$(2)\times(3)+(1)\times(2)/2$	56,784.0	25,848.0	11,781.0	11,736.0	8910.0	2034.0	117,093.0(T_1)
(6)	$(1)\times\left[(4)^2+(4)\times(2)+(2)^2/3\right]$	16,224.0	298,368.0	1,022,063.7	1,884,192.0	8,712,088.0	26,131,702.0	38,064,636.7(T_2)
(7)	$(2)\times\left[(3)^2+(3)\times(1)+(1)^2/3\right]$	20,669,428.0	9,279,816.0	4,082,935.3	3,827,664.0	2,426,996.0	306,456.0	40,593,295.3(T_3)

$$Q_2 = \frac{T_2}{n_0^2 n_1} = \frac{38064636.7}{349^2 \times 365} = 0.856$$

$$\sqrt{Var(\widehat{A})} = \sqrt{\frac{0.919 \times (1-0.919) + (365-1)(0.873-0.919^2) + (349-1)(0.856-0.919^2)}{349 \times 365}}$$
$$= 0.011.$$

The 95% CI of A is

$$[0.919 - 1.96 \times 0.011, 0.919 + 1.96 \times 0.011]$$
$$= [0.897, 0.941].$$

Hypothesis testing for A:

$$H_0 : A = 0.5$$
$$H_1 : A \neq 0.5$$
$$\alpha = 0.05$$
$$z = \frac{\widehat{A} - 0.5}{\sqrt{Var(\widehat{A})}} = \frac{0.919 - 0.5}{0.011} = 38.09.$$

As $z > z_{1-0.05/2} = 1.96$, $p < 0.05$, we reject H_0 and accept H_1 at the $\alpha = 0.05$ level, the difference between A and 0.5 is statistically significant. Because $\widehat{A}$ is close to 1, we conclude that the test has a high diagnostic value for the detection of egg allergy.

18.3.3 Comparison of Areas Under ROC Curves

The ROC curve is not affected by the range of test results, and its shape remains the same under certain transformations of the test data. These properties and the ROC curve's visual presentation as a plot are particularly useful for making comparisons between different tests.

The Z-test can be used to compare the A values of two tests, and there are two methods for comparison, depending on the type of study design.

1. Completely Randomized Designs

When the sample size is sufficiently large, the test statistic for the comparison of two tests is

$$Z = \frac{\widehat{A}_1 - \widehat{A}_2}{\sqrt{Var(\widehat{A}_1) + Var(\widehat{A}_2)}}, \tag{18.32}$$

where $\widehat{A}_1$ and $\widehat{A}_2$ are the estimates of the area under the curve of two tests, and $Var(\widehat{A}_1)$ and $Var(\widehat{A}_2)$ are their squared standard errors.

Example 18.13 In a diagnostic test study, 1356 participants were randomly divided into two groups, and their egg allergy status was tested using two test kits, A and B, with one kit used for each group. ROC curves were plotted. For kit A, the group had 714 subjects, $\hat{A}_1 = 0.919$, and $Var(\hat{A}_1) = 0.011^2$; for kit B, the group had 642 subjects, $\hat{A}_2 = 0.847$, and $Var(\hat{A}_2) = 0.026^2$. Which test has a higher diagnostic validity?

Solution

(1) State the hypotheses and select a significance level

$H_0 : A_1 = A_2$

$H_1 : A_1 \neq A_2$

$\alpha = 0.05$

(2) Determine the test statistic

$$z = \frac{\hat{A}_1 - \hat{A}_2}{\sqrt{Var(\hat{A}_1) + Var(\hat{A}_2)}} = \frac{0.919 - 0.847}{\sqrt{0.011^2 + 0.026^2}} = 2.55$$

(3) Draw a conclusion

As $|z| > z_{1-\alpha/2} = 1.96$, $p < 0.05$, we reject H_0 and accept H_1 at the $\alpha = 0.05$ level, the difference between the two kits is statistically significant. We conclude that there is evidence to show that kit A has a higher diagnostic value for egg allergy compared with kit B.

2. Paired Samples Designs

When the sample size is sufficiently large, the test statistic for the comparison of two tests is:

$$Z = \frac{\hat{A}_1 - \hat{A}_2}{\sqrt{Var(\hat{A}_1) + Var(\hat{A}_2) - 2Cov(\hat{A}_1, \hat{A}_2)}}, \tag{18.33}$$

where $\hat{A}_1$ and $\hat{A}_2$ are the estimates of the area under the curve of the two tests, $Var(\hat{A}_1)$ and $Var(\hat{A}_1)$ are their squared standard errors, and $Cov(\hat{A}_1, \hat{A}_2)$ is the covariance of $\hat{A}_1$ and $\hat{A}_2$. The computation of $Cov(\hat{A}_1, \hat{A}_2)$ is relatively complex and can be done using statistical software.

Example 18.14 Two tests, A and B, were used for the detection of allergy to cat hair among 164 subjects who were in fact allergic to cat hair and 1026 subjects who were not allergic to cat hair. The results of each test have seven grades (0 to 6) and are shown in Table 18.15. Compare the diagnostic validity of the two tests.

Solution

Figure 18.4 displays the ROC curves for tests A and B.

Table 18.15 Results of two tests for allergy to cat hair.

			Test *B*							Total
			0	1	2	3	4	5	6	
Not allergic	Test *A*	0	900	11	19	3	0	0	0	933
		1	1	5	6	7	0	0	0	19
		2	2	6	15	8	0	0	0	31
		3	0	6	12	5	0	0	0	23
		4	0	0	9	1	2	0	0	12
		5	0	2	1	1	3	1	0	8
		6	0	0	0	0	0	0	0	0
		Total	903	30	62	25	5	1	0	1026
Allergic	Test *A*	0	26	7	24	9	0	0	0	66
		1	0	0	10	6	0	0	0	16
		2	0	1	8	15	1	0	0	25
		3	0	1	7	0	5	0	0	13
		4	0	0	4	4	4	2	0	14
		5	0	0	0	3	7	4	0	14
		6	0	0	0	0	2	6	8	16
		Total	26	9	53	37	19	12	8	164

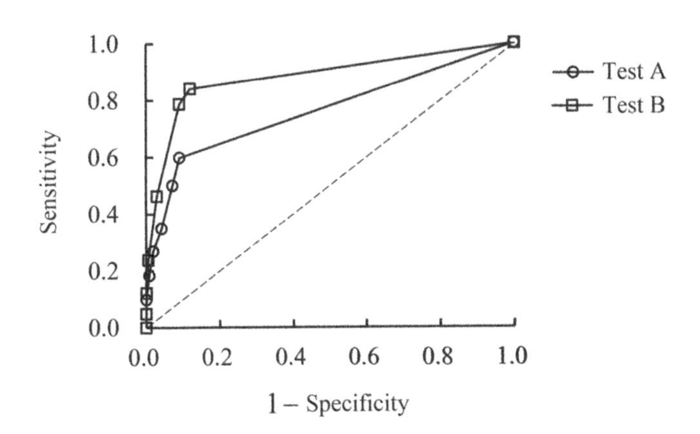

Figure 18.4 ROC curves for tests A and B.

(1) State the hypotheses and select a significance level

$H_0 : A_1 = A_2$

$H_1 : A_1 \neq A_2$

$\alpha = 0.05$

(2) Determine the test statistic

Calculated from the data in Table 18.15, we have:

$$\hat{A}_1 = 0.760,\ Var\left(\hat{A}_1\right) = 0.0201^2$$

$$\hat{A}_2 = 0.881,\ Var\left(\hat{A}_2\right) = 0.0157^2$$

$$Cov\left(\hat{A}_1, \hat{A}_2\right) = 0.0002$$

Substituting into Formula 18.33, the test statistic is:

$$z = \frac{\hat{A}_1 - \hat{A}_2}{\sqrt{Var\left(\hat{A}_1\right) + Var\left(\hat{A}_2\right) - 2Cov\left(\hat{A}_1, \hat{A}_2\right)}} = \frac{0.760 - 0.881}{\sqrt{0.0201^2 + 0.0157^2 - 2 \times 0.0002}} = -7.65.$$

(3) Draw a conclusion.

As $|z| > z_{1-\alpha/2} = 1.96$, $p < 0.05$, we reject H_0 and accept H_1 at the $\alpha = 0.05$ level. We conclude that test B has a higher diagnostic value for cat hair allergy compared with test A.

18.4 Summary

Sensitivity and specificity are the most basic and important properties of diagnostic validity. Sensitivity is the probability of testing positive given the presence of disease and thus reflects a test's ability to correctly detect a disease. Specificity is the probability of testing negative given the absence of disease and thus reflects a test's ability to correctly rule out a disease. These two indicators are independent of the prevalence of the disease and are thus intrinsic measures of a test's diagnostic validity.

Youden's index and likelihood ratios are composite measures of sensitivity and specificity. Youden's index is the difference between the true-positive rate and the false-positive rate (i.e., the sum of sensitivity and specificity minus 1). Higher values of Youden's index indicate better diagnostic validity. The positive likelihood ratio is the probability of testing positive given the presence of disease divided by the probability of testing positive given the absence of disease. The negative likelihood ratio is the probability of testing negative given the presence of disease divided by the probability of testing negative given the absence of disease.

Positive predictive value is the probability of disease given a positive test result, and negative predictive value is the probability of no disease given a negative test result. These two indicators are functions of the prevalence of the disease and thus are not measures of validity intrinsic to the test.

In Table 18.16, we summarize these measures in the form of conditional probabilities.

$D = 1$: diseased; $D = 0$: not diseased; $T = 1$: positive test result; $T = 0$: negative test result.

For the evaluation of agreement of categorical data, the concordance rate, and the kappa coefficient are commonly used. The concordance rate is the proportion of subjects with the same test results. The kappa coefficient is the ratio of the actual

Table 18.16 Measures of diagnostic value.

Measure	Notation	Expression
Sensitivity	Se	$P(T=1 \mid D=1)$
Specificity	Sp	$P(T=0 \mid D=0)$
Youden's index	J	$P(T=1 \mid D=1)-P(T=1 \mid D=0)$
Positive likelihood ratio	LR +	$P(T=1 \mid D=1)/P(T=1 \mid D=0)$
Negative likelihood ratio	LR −	$P(T=0 \mid D=1)/P(T=0 \mid D=0)$
Positive predictive value	PPV	$P(D=1 \mid T=1)$
Negative predictive value	NPV	$P(D=0 \mid T=0)$

agreement rate over the maximum possible value of this rate; kappa coefficient's range is $[-1, 1]$.

The ROC curve is a plot of sensitivity against the false-positive rate $(1-\text{specificity})$ calculated for every possible cutoff of the test, with the value range of $[0, 1]$. Advantages of the ROC curve include that it allows for selecting an optimal cutoff and that it provides a visual assessment and comparison of the diagnostic value of different tests.

18.5 Exercises

1. The results of two tests used to diagnose functional dyspepsia are displayed in Table 18.17.
   - **(a)** What is the study design?
   - **(b)** Estimate concordance rate, and its 95% CI.
   - **(c)** Estimate the Kappa coefficient. What is the difference between concordance rate and Kappa coefficient?
   - **(d)** Suppose that test B is the gold standard; construct a four-fold table.
   - **(e)** Using the table obtained in (d), calculate sensitivity (95% CI), specificity (95% CI), Youden's Index, likelihood ratios, and interpret the results.
   - **(f)** Using the table obtained in (d), can we predict the probability of functional dyspepsia given a positive result with test A? Why?

Table 18.17 Diagnostic results according to two tests for functional dyspepsia.

Test *A*	Test *B*	Frequency
Positive	Positive	129
Positive	Negative	12
Negative	Positive	16
Negative	Negative	369

2. Two tests are used to evaluate the level of serum potassium (mmol/L) of 10 samples, and the data are shown in Table 18.18. The Pearson correlation coefficient is $r = 0.925$ and $p < 0.001$.
   (a) Suppose we want to assess the agreement between the two tests, is the result of correlation analysis appropriate to conclude that this is a good agreement? Why?
   (b) Suppose we want to test the difference between the readings of two tests, what test method can be used? Can we use this result to evaluate agreement?
   (c) How do you determine agreement between the two tests? What is your conclusion.

Table 18.18 Level of serum potassium (mmol/L) determined by two tests.

Sample ID	1	2	3	4	5	6	7	8	9	10
Test *A*	3.74	4.09	4.54	5.76	5.05	4.88	4.36	4.55	4.98	5.16
Test *B*	3.68	4.10	4.24	5.18	4.87	4.19	4.14	4.44	4.78	5.06

3. A total of 72 subjects were tested for birch pollen allergy with a prick diagnostic kit, and 77 subjects were tested for *Fraxinus* pollen allergy, also with a prick diagnostic kit. The diagnostic test results are given as the diameter of wind mass (mm). After that, the two groups of subjects were divided into an allergic group and a control group according to the allergen sIgE test results (1 allergic, 2 nonallergic). The test results are shown in Table 18.19.
   (a) Does the prick diagnostic kit have diagnostic value for birch pollen allergy and for *Fraxinus* pollen allergy? Draw ROC curves and perform a significance test.
   (b) Determine an optimal cutoff for question (a) (assuming no specific preference between sensitivity and specificity) and calculate the 95% CI for sensitivity and specificity.
   (c) Is the diagnostic accuracy of the prick diagnostic kit the same for the two kinds of pollen? Make a comparison by using and not using the optimal cutoffs.

Table 18.19 Diagnostic test results (diameter of wind mass, mm) and allergy results (sIgE, 1 for allergic and 2 for nonallergic, as golden standard) to birch pollen and *Fraxinus* pollen.

Birch pollen				Fraxinus pollen			
Allergy (1)	Result (2)	Allergy (1)	Result (2)	Allergy (3)	Result (4)	Allergy (3)	Result (4)
1	6	2	1.5	2	2	1	4
1	27	1	2.5	1	3	1	6
2	1.5	1	9	2	2.5	2	1
2	1	1	8.5	1	3	1	3
1	13	2	3.5	1	7.5	1	5.5

(Continued)

Table 18.19 (Continued)

Birch pollen				Fraxinus pollen			
Allergy (1)	**Result (2)**	**Allergy (1)**	**Result (2)**	**Allergy (3)**	**Result (4)**	**Allergy (3)**	**Result (4)**
1	12	1	17	1	12	1	6
1	16	1	3.5	1	7	1	5
1	1.5	1	3.5	1	9	2	2
1	13.5	2	3	2	1	2	3.5
2	2	1	6	1	9	2	2.5
1	9.5	1	8	1	7.5	1	5
1	13.5	1	15	1	2.5	2	0.5
1	5.5	1	2.5	2	1	2	1.5
1	17	2	2	1	6.5	2	3
1	9	1	13.5	1	1.5	2	3.5
1	7.5	2	2.5	1	5	2	1
1	10.5	1	5.5	1	0.5	2	3
1	17.5	1	9	1	5	2	3
1	11.5	1	3.5	1	4.5	2	1.5
1	12	1	6	1	3.5	1	7
1	17.5	1	9.5	1	3	1	5
2	1	1	11	1	6.5	2	3.5
1	9	1	3.5	2	2	2	1
1	12.5	2	2.5	1	10	1	5.5
1	11	2	1.5	2	1	2	2
1	1	2	2.5	1	10	1	8
1	17	2	1	2	2	1	3
1	2.5	1	12	1	5.5	2	2
1	9.5	1	8	2	2	1	4
1	3.5	2	2.5	1	8	2	1
2	2	1	10	2	4	1	1.5
2	8.5	1	10	1	9.5	1	4.5
1	5	1	4.5	1	4.5	1	5.5
1	3.5	2	1.5	1	7.5	1	5.5
1	7	1	3.5	1	9	2	3
2	1.5	2	2.5	2	4	2	4.5
				2	2	2	1
				2	3.5	2	2
						2	1.5

19

Observational Study Design

CONTENTS

As we learned in Chapter 1 and subsequent chapters, the study design has profound impacts on not only the choice of the ensuing analytical methods but also the accuracy, reliability, rigor, and representativeness of the research results. Whereas poorly analyzed data can be reanalyzed at a later stage, defects in design cannot be corrected and may lead to failure of the entire study. As R.A. Fisher once said: "To call in the statistician after the experiment is done may be no more than asking him to perform a postmortem examination: he may be able to say what the experiment died of."

Study design, by definition, is the overall strategy and specific arrangement of the entire research process, to address the research questions in a logical way. *Statistical design* is one of the most important parts of the study design, and its main purpose is to reduce systematic and random errors. This involves specific tasks such as determination of the expected results of the study according to its objectives; specification of study participants and data to be collected; estimation of sample size; determination of random sampling and/or allocation approaches; planning statistical analyses; establishment and maintenance of databases; quality control approaches; etc. There are two categories of study design in biomedical research: observational and experimental. We focus on observational study designs in this chapter and introduce the latter in the following chapter.

Applied Medical Statistics, First Edition. Jingmei Jiang.

Companion website: www.wiley.com\go\jiang\appliedmedicalstatistics

Observational studies are used to describe or compare natural phenomena under given environmental condition(s). A feature that distinguishes observational studies from experimental studies is that the research participants are observed or measured in their "natural state," that is, researchers cannot actively exert intervention measures. There are three main types of observational study: cross-sectional studies, cohort studies, and case-control studies. In this chapter, the basic concepts are introduced first, followed by methods of determining samples sizes for each of these types of observational study.

19.1 Cross-Sectional Studies

19.1.1 Types of Cross-Sectional Studies

A *cross-sectional study*, also known as a prevalence survey, refers to research in which descriptive data at a specific time in a target population are collected, by means of a census, typical survey, or sample survey, so as to determine the distribution of a disease or explore the relationship between certain risk factors and diseases.

The specific types of cross-sectional study are as follows:

(1) *Census* is a cross-sectional study in which all members of the target population are enrolled in the investigation. This is generally used to understand the status of the target population at a specific time point, for example, the population census in China that is conducted every 10 years. Notice that statistical inference is not required in a census, as the result describes the target population itself.
(2) *Typical survey* is a cross-sectional study in which only typical cases are purposefully selected. This is normally used in the study of clinical cases of rare diseases.
(3) *Sample survey* refers to the process of selecting a portion of the target population and then estimating the overall characteristics using the obtained sample. We focus our interest on this type of cross-sectional study, as it is the most widely used in biomedical research.

19.1.2 Probability Sampling Methods

Sampling design is an important part of a cross-sectional study design. If each study participant could be selected according to a known probability, the representativeness of the sample can be ensured. We introduce some basic probability sampling methods that are commonly used in biomedical research.

1. Simple Random Sampling

Simple random sampling (*SRS*) refers to a simple way to obtain a random sample, where each individual in a target population has an equal probability of being selected. Although the same can be achieved using other random sampling methods, only simple random sampling ensures that every possible "combination of n units" is equally likely to be selected.

To conduct simple random sampling, first, all members of the target population, which composes the *sampling frame*, should be listed and each member assigned a unique number. Then, the researcher can choose random samples using random number tables by selecting an arbitrary starting point and reading down the column from the chosen arbitrary starting point, selecting any integers within the range of $1-N$. The selections are repeated and numbers greater than N are ignored; selection continues until n distinct units are obtained. To reduce labor during the selection process, a computer-based random number generator can be used instead of a random number table.

Example 19.1 Refer to Example 6.5. We are interested in estimating the hemoglobin level of mariners and plan to randomly select 10 out of 86 mariners employed in a shipping company. Draw a simple random sample.

Solution

Simple random sampling can be accomplished using the following procedures:

(1) Make a list of all mariners working in the shipping company.
(2) Assign a sequential number to each mariner, e.g., (1,2,...,86); this forms the sampling frame.
(3) Use Table of 2500 random digits in Appendix Table 1 to select the sample.

We start with 6th row, 3rd column, which reads: 87, **03**, **04**, **79**, 88, **08**, **13**, 13, **85**, **51**, **55**, **34**, **57**, 72, 69,.... Non-repeated numbers less than 87 are sequentially marked in bold, until we have 10 numbers. The 10 mariners corresponding to the numbers in bold are finally selected.

Advantages of simple random sampling include that it is easily operable and calculation of the corresponding statistics (mean, rate, and standard error) is straightforward. However, when the total number of members in the target population is large, it is not always possible to organize a sampling frame from which to sample randomly. This could limit the use of simple random sampling.

2. Systematic Sampling

Systematic sampling refers to a sampling technique in which the researcher selects study participants from the target population by randomly choosing a starting point, and subsequent participants are enrolled using a preset interval. The specific procedures for systematic random sampling are as follows:

(1) Establish a sampling frame.

Similar to simple random sampling, the researcher should define the target population and create a list to form a sampling frame. The individuals in the target population are numbered 1 to N and should not be in a periodic or cyclic order. Ideally, members can be listed in a random or random-like order to imitate the randomization effect of simple random sampling.

(2) Decide the sampling interval.

The sampling interval should be determined with consideration of the target sample size. To be more specific, we calculate the interval k by dividing the estimated population size N by the target sample size n, that is: $k = N / n$.

(3) Select the sample.

Select a random number i between 1 and k. After the first sampling unit is selected, select every kth unit after the ith unit of the population to include in the sample.

Example 19.2 Refer to Example 7.4. Assuming that we are interested in the birthweight of newborns girls in a hospital, and it is estimated that the annual number of newborn girls is approximately 1000. Considering restrictions of time and resources, we cannot access the information of all newborns girls in the hospital. In sample size estimation, we determined that at least 100 newborn girls should be selected. How can we obtain the sample using systematic sampling?

Solution

The specific procedures are as follows:

(1) The sampling frame can be defined as all newborns girls (excluding stillbirths, twins, and multiple births) with a birth ID number.
(2) As $N = 1000$ and $n = 100$, the sampling interval k can then be calculated as $k = N / n$, which is 10 in this case. Then, we can use the birth ID number and randomly choose a starting point from the remaining numbers (0–9), such as 4 in this case.
(3) After the starting point is determined, subsequent newborns can be chosen using a fixed interval, and the sampling procedure is repeated until 100 newborn girls are selected.

The advantages of systematic sampling are that it is very convenient and the cost is relatively low compared with simple random sampling. Additionally, the sampling units are spread more evenly across the target population so that no large proportions of the population are unrepresented. However, the downside of systematic random sampling is obvious: it is likely to be affected by certain hidden periodic traits, in other words, a systematic error could occur if the target population is ordered cyclically or periodically.

3. Stratified Sampling

Stratified sampling refers to a sampling technique in which the target population is first divided into mutually exclusive subgroups (called "strata"). Then, a certain number of individuals from each stratum is selected. The rationale underlying stratified sampling is to divide a target population with considerable variation into subgroups in which individuals within the same subgroup are more homogeneous.

The procedure for different strata is mutually independent across strata, and therefore it is possible to directly sum the variances of estimates for individual strata, to obtain the variance estimate for the whole population. Therefore, by partitioning the target population in such a way that the sampling units within a stratum are as similar as possible, even though one stratum might differ markedly from another stratum, a sample selected using stratified sampling would still be "representative" of the whole population if we guarantee inclusion of a sufficient number of units from each stratum of the target population.

The size of each stratum can be determined using the (1) equal allocation, (2) proportional allocation, or (3) optimal allocation method. In equal allocation, different strata have the same size, regardless of the actual size of the strata. In proportional allocation, the size of each stratum is proportional to the size of the stratum. For example, each stratum is sampled according to a proportion of 5% of the actual stratum size. In optimal allocation, both the size and variability of the strata are considered when determining the sample size in each stratum.

Example 19.3 The Surgical Safety Checklist (SSC) is a widely applied tool that was issued by the World Health Organization in 2008 to reinforce basic safety practices and foster better teamwork in the operating room. Although many studies have shown that the SSC has the potential to reduce operative complications, implementation of the SSC is not uniform and there remains resistance to the introduction of change. In the project on surgical safety discussed in Example 4.1, a sample survey was required to investigate the enthusiasm among operating theater staff toward the SSC.

Solution

The study participants were all surgery-related medical staff members (surgeons, anesthetists, and theater nurses), and these roles were used as the strata factor for designing a stratified sampling. Equal allocation was considered not appropriate as these roles have very different proportions, with surgeons being the absolute majority. Surgeons would be over-presented in the sample if proportional allocation is used. Therefore, an optimal allocation was used, and the distribution of roles in the final sample was about 50% surgeons, 20% anesthetists, and 30% theater nurses.

The advantage of stratified sampling is that appropriate stratification could improve the homogeneity within strata, which may lead to a reduction in sampling error and improvement in sample representativeness, as well as in precision of the study results. Moreover, stratified sampling can adopt different sampling methods for different strata and can be analyzed independently in each stratum, which is flexible and convenient in practice.

4. Cluster Sampling

Cluster sampling refers to a sampling technique in which we divide a target population into naturally existing clusters (such as districts, hospitals, or schools) and randomly select a sample from these clusters. Then, all the sampling units in the selected clusters would be incorporated into the sample. The basic sampling unit in cluster sampling is not a member of the target population but rather a group consisting of individuals. It should be noted that in cluster sampling, the between-cluster variance should be as small as possible, to obtain the most precise estimators of the population parameter. The ideal cluster should reflect the full diversity of the target population and every potential characteristic of the entire population.

Example 19.4 Nurse burnout can be caused by many different work-related issues such as emotional strain of losing patients and long shifts of 12 or more hours. Suppose that you are employed by the human resource department of a hospital with 24 clinical departments, how can you draw a sample to investigate mental well-being of nurses in the hospital.

Solution

As a hospital is a highly organized system, the cluster sampling method can be applied in this case. First, 8 departments are randomly selected from among 24 departments in the hospital. Then, the survey can be administered to all nursing staff in the selected department.

Clusters are usually naturally existing groups, and therefore cluster sampling is easy to implement and is more time- and cost-efficient than other probability sampling methods. This method is particularly appealing when the target population is spread across a wide geographical area. However, the sampling error in cluster sampling is generally greater than that in simple random sampling given the same sample size. The sampling error decreases with decreased heterogeneity among clusters. Sampling error can also be reduced by selecting a larger number of clusters.

5. Multistage Sampling

As suggested by its name, *multistage sampling* divides the entire sampling process into several stages (usually ≥ 2), with sampling units in each stage being sampled from the larger units chosen in the previous stage. This is particularly useful when an exhaustive list of all members of the target population is not available. For example, if we wish to investigate Chinese dietary characteristics, it is practically impossible to prepare a complete list of every individual in China.

Typical multistage sampling can be performed using the following procedures:

(1) In the first stage, a sampling frame is formed by numbering each group with a unique number, from which a small sample of relevant discrete groups is selected.
(2) On the basis of the relevant discrete groups selected in the previous stage, a sampling frame of relevant discrete subgroups is generated.
(3) Stage (2) is repeated, if necessary.
(4) Members of the sample group are chosen from the selected subgroups using the probability sampling methods introduced previously.

Example 19.5 Refer to Example 4.8. In the large epidemiological survey of pelvic disorders among about 18,000 adult Chinese women, a 3-stage sampling method was adopted in the survey.

Solution

The procedures are detailed as follows:

(1) In the first stage, all provincial administrative units in China are stratified into six administrative regions: Northeast, North, East, Northwest, Southwest, and Central China. One province (first-level sampling unit) is randomly selected from each administrative region.
(2) In the second stage, subregions in each province are stratified into rural and urban areas, and two to three counties and cities are selected from each rural and urban area (second-level sampling unit).
(3) In the third stage, a cluster including several villages or communities (third-level sampling unit) are selected from these counties and cities, and all eligible adult women aged 20 years and over in the selected villages and communities are included as the research participants.

The advantages of multistage sampling are: (i) it is highly cost- and time-effective because only the sampling frame of the sampling unit at each sampling stage is needed; it is sometimes the only option for data collection from a geographically dispersed population; and (ii) it is highly flexible because different sampling methods can be used in each sampling stage. However, estimation of sampling error is complicated with multistage sampling.

19.1.3 Sample Size for Surveys

Reliable conclusions can hardly be obtained with samples of limited size whereas a large sample beyond what is required will waste a lot of resources and sometimes even increase the systematic error. Therefore, determination of the minimum sample size that is required for answering the research question is an important component of the study design.

In sample surveys, the purpose is typically to infer the characteristics of a given population using information obtained in the sample. The question is how much error is allowed between the estimation and the population parameter. Therefore, the margin of error, which reflects the precision of estimation, should be considered.

1. Sample Size for Estimation of Population Mean

The sample size for estimation of population mean can be calculated according to the following formula:

$$n = \left(\frac{z_{1-\alpha/2}\sigma}{\delta}\right)^2, \tag{19.1}$$

where:

σ is standard deviation of the population.

δ is the margin of error, which, in this case, is the allowable difference in the population mean with its estimate (usually determined according to a previously available result).

$z_{1-\alpha/2}$ is the critical value of the standard normal distribution.

α is the significance level; generally $\alpha = 0.05$ (two-sided), with which $z_{1-0.05/2} = 1.96$.

Example 19.6 Refer to Example 2.1. For estimating the average height (cm) of 10-year-old girls in a certain region, we assume that the mean is 142 and the standard deviation is 6.8. With estimation errors not exceeding 0.5, 1.0, and 1.5, how many girls should be investigated with these three degrees of precision?

Solution

We have $\alpha = 0.05$, and $\delta_1 = 0.5$, $\delta_2 = 1.0$, $\delta_3 = 1.5$.

Substituting into Formula 19.1:

$$n_1 = \left(\frac{z_{1-\alpha/2}\sigma}{\delta_1}\right)^2 = \left(\frac{1.96 \times 6.8}{0.5}\right)^2 \approx 711,$$

$$n_2 = \left(\frac{z_{1-\alpha/2}\sigma}{\delta_2}\right)^2 = \left(\frac{1.96 \times 6.8}{1.0}\right)^2 \approx 178,$$

$$n_3 = \left(\frac{z_{1-\alpha/2}\sigma}{\delta_3}\right)^2 = \left(\frac{1.96 \times 6.8}{1.5}\right)^2 \approx 79.$$

Therefore, at least 711, 178, and 79 girls are required when the margin of error is 0.5, 1.0, and 1.5, respectively. It can be seen that a larger sample size is needed to improve the precision of the estimation.

2. Sample Size for Estimation of Population Rate

The sample size for estimation of the population rate π can be calculated according to the following formula:

$$n = \frac{z_{1-\alpha/2}^2 \pi(1-\pi)}{\delta^2}, \tag{19.2}$$

where:

π is the expected prevalence, which can be based on estimates from previous research.

δ is the margin of error, which, in this case, is the allowable difference in the population rate with its estimate.

$z_{1-\alpha/2}$ and α are the same as discussed above.

Example 19.7 Refer to Example 4.8. Suppose that a gynecologist is interested in estimating the prevalence of urinary incontinence in her city, which is not included in a large survey. The gynecologist refers to data in neighboring cities, and the expected prevalence is 20%. If the margin of error is to be controlled at 2%, how many people need to be investigated at minimum?

Solution

We have $\alpha = 0.05$, $\delta = 0.02$, and $\pi = 0.2$.

Substituting into Formula 19.2, we obtain

$$n = \frac{z_{1-\alpha/2}^2 \pi(1-\pi)}{\delta^2} = \frac{1.96^2 \times 0.2 \times (1-0.2)}{0.02^2} \approx 1537.$$

Thus, at least 1537 eligible participants are needed. If we further consider a nonresponse rate of approximately 20%, a total of $1537 \times 120\% = 1845$ participants would be needed for the investigation.

19.1.4 Cross-Sectional Studies for Clues of Etiology

In addition to estimation of population parameters, cross-sectional studies are sometimes used to explore the possible etiology of a disease. We illustrate this in the Example 19.8.

Example 19.8 Refer to Example 19.5. This large epidemiological survey was conducted not only to estimate outcomes (e.g., urinary incontinence) but also to collect and analyze risk factors (or called exposure factors) that may have a potential impact on the outcomes. The findings were used to provide an evidence base for government policy making.

Figure 19.1 illustrates the analysis framework of cross-sectional study design to investigate etiology for a specific exposure and outcome. Here the term "exposure" denotes that a participant has certain characteristics (low birthweight, certain genetic

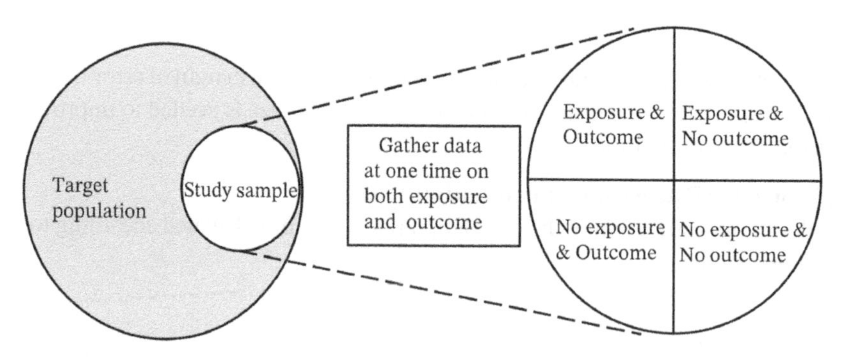

Figure 19.1 Analysis framework of cross-sectional study design.

defects, or chromosome abnormalities, and so on), is in a certain state (such as having depression), possesses a certain behavior or habit (e.g., smoking, alcoholism, engaging in homosexual sex), or has been exposed to certain substances (e.g., radiation, passive smoking). The term "outcome" refers to the health consequence (such as disease occurrence or death) that the researcher is interested in examining.

There are several advantages of a cross-sectional design, as follows: (i) a cross-sectional study can be conducted relatively fast and inexpensively; (ii) by determining the spatial and temporal distribution of a disease, the findings of cross-sectional studies may be useful for public health planning, monitoring, and evaluation; and (iii) the prevalence of outcomes or exposures obtained in cross-sectional studies could be useful for designing subsequent studies, for example, cohort studies and case-control studies, which are introduced in Sections 19.2 and 19.3.

19.2 Cohort Studies

A *cohort study*, also known as incidence study, refers to a type of observational study in which the study participants are divided into groups with different exposure levels (typically, an exposed and an unexposed group), and followed up over time so that the incidence rates of outcome(s) between groups can be compared, to determine whether there is any association between the exposure and outcome and the magnitude of the association. The overall design of a typical cohort study is illustrated in Figure 19.2.

19.2.1 Measures of Association in Cohort Studies

The most commonly used measure of association between exposure and outcome in a cohort study is *relative risk* (RR), also called the *risk ratio*, which is defined as follows:

$$RR = \frac{incidence\ in\ \text{exposure}\ group}{incidence\ in\ no\ \text{exposure}\ group}, \tag{19.3}$$

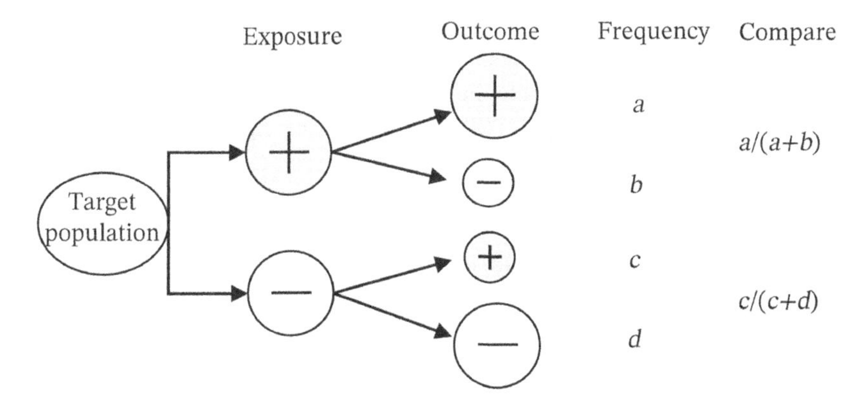

Figure 19.2 Illustration of cohort study design.

where RR is the ratio of the incidence rate (risk) in exposed participants to that of unexposed participants. Note that incidence is itself a rate and the unit is "per person-time." When there is no loss to follow-up, person-time can be omitted in the calculation of incidence rate. We can refer to the numbers shown in Figure 19.2 and use the Formula 19.4 to estimate RR:

$$\widehat{RR} = \frac{a/(a+b)}{c/(c+d)}. \tag{19.4}$$

A value RR = 1 indicates that there is no association between the exposure and the disease. An RR value less than 1 indicates a protective effect of the exposure, whereas an RR greater than 1 suggests that exposed people are more likely to develop the disease than their non-exposed counterparts.

Example 19.9 Consider a hypothetical cohort study investigating the association between smoking and cardiovascular disease (CVD) among men. A total of 10,792 men aged between 50 and 70 years are enrolled. All participants were free of CVD at baseline, and a self-administered questionnaire was used to obtain information on cigarette smoking. After 3 years of follow-up, a total of 106 new cases of CVD were identified, as shown in Table 19.1. To simplify the calculation, we assume no loss to follow-up. Calculate and interpret the RR.

Solution

From the data in Table 19.1, the association between smoking and CVD can be evaluated by estimating the RR using Formula 19.4:

$$\widehat{RR} = \frac{a/(a+b)}{c/(c+d)} = \frac{56/(56+4162)}{50/(50+6630)} = \frac{1.33\%}{0.75\%} = 1.77.$$

The result indicates that smoking is positively associated with CVD, and the risk of CVD is estimated to be 1.77 times more among smokers over that of non-smokers.

19.2.2 Sample Size for Cohort Studies

When drawing conclusions from a cohort study, RR should be tested against 1 to obtain valid conclusions. Let π_E and π_N denote the incidence rate in the exposed and non-exposed groups, respectively. Then $H_0: RR = \pi_E / \pi_N = 1$, or equivalently, $\pi_E = \pi_N$.

Table 19.1 Data obtained from a cohort study on smoking and CVD.

Exposure	CVD	No CVD	Total
Smoker	56	4162	4218
Non-smoker	50	6630	6680
Total	106	10,792	10,898

Thus, the formula for sample size calculation for the comparison of rates can be used for sample size determination in a cohort study (for the exposed group), as follows:

$$n = \frac{\left[z_{1-\alpha/2}\sqrt{(1+1/m)\bar{\pi}(1-\bar{\pi})} + z_{1-\beta}\sqrt{\pi_N(1-\pi_N)/m + \pi_E(1-\pi_E)}\right]^2}{(\pi_N - \pi_E)^2}, \quad (19.5)$$

where $\bar{\pi} = (\pi_E + m\pi_N)/(m+1)$, and m is a predefined ratio of unexposed participants over exposed participants, usually $m = 1$. When we have an estimate of π_E or π_N from previous research, we can use an anticipated RR to estimate the other using $\pi_E = \pi_N \times RR$.

$z_{1-\beta}$ and $z_{1-\alpha/2}$ are critical values corresponding to the desired power β and significance level α.

Notice that RR is a kind of effect size that we mentioned in Chapter 7.

Example 19.10 Refer to Example 19.9. Suppose the incidence rate of CVD is 450/100,000 person-years among men aged 50–70 years who do not smoke. If we anticipate an $RR = 2$ of smoking over no smoking for CVD and a preferred ratio of 1:1 between the exposed and unexposed groups, how many study participants should be enrolled to achieve 80% power to reject the $H_0 : RR = 1$ at a significance level of 0.05 (two-sided)?

Solution

Since $\alpha = 0.05$, $\beta = 0.2$, $\pi_N = 0.0045$, $\pi_E = RR \times \pi_N = 2 \times 0.0045 = 0.009$, and $m = 1$, we obtain $\bar{\pi} = (\pi_E + m\pi_N)/(m+1) = 0.00675$.

Substituting into Formula 19.5, we obtain

$$\begin{aligned} n &= \frac{\left[z_{1-\alpha/2}\sqrt{(1+1/m)\bar{\pi}(1-\bar{\pi})} + z_{1-\beta}\sqrt{\pi_N(1-\pi_N)/m + \pi_E(1-\pi_E)}\right]^2}{(\pi_N - \pi_E)^2} \\ &= \frac{\begin{bmatrix} 1.96 \times \sqrt{2 \times 0.00675 \times (1 - 0.00675)} \\ +0.84 \times \sqrt{0.0045 \times (1 - 0.0045) + 0.009 \times (1 - 0.009)} \end{bmatrix}^2}{(0.0045 - 0.009)^2} \\ &\approx 5191. \end{aligned}$$

Thus, at least 5191 eligible participants are needed in both the exposed and unexposed groups. Considering possible non-response, the actual number of individuals needed in each group is $5191 \times 120\% = 6230$ participants.

Notice that in a cohort study, the information about the exposure is determined prior to the observation of disease; thus, this study design is superior for determining etiology than a cross-sectional study. However, as suggested in this example, the sample size required in a cohort study is very large, especially for rare diseases with low incidence, in which only a few new cases may be observed despite a long-term follow-up, as this is usually insufficient to confirm a statistical association. In such situations, a case-control study is an efficient alternative.

19.3 Case-Control Studies

A *case-control study* is a type of observational study in which two existing groups of participants that differ in the outcome of interest are identified and compared based on some supposed exposure history. In case-control studies, the researcher first enrolls cases (participants with the outcome of interest) and controls (participants without the outcome) and then tries to trace back the exposure to a number of risk factors using face-to-face interviews, abstraction from existing records, and other methods. Therefore, case-control studies have a backward direction on the timeline and are always retrospective (Figure 19.3).

19.3.1 Measures of Association in Case-Control Studies

By comparing the history of exposure(s) between the case group and the control group, the association between exposure and outcome can be inferred. However, as there is no "follow-up" period, it is impossible to calculate the incidence rate, so RR cannot be calculated. Alternatively, we use the *odds ratio* (*OR*), which is calculated as follows, with reference to Figure 19.3.

$$OR = \frac{\text{odds of exposure in cases}}{\text{odds of exposure in controls}}, \tag{19.6}$$

that is, as the measure of association between exposure and outcome, the OR reflects the odds of having the exposure among diseased individuals in comparison with the odds of having the exposure among non-diseased individuals.
OR is estimated by

$$\widehat{OR} = \frac{[a/(a+b)]/[b/(a+b)]}{[c/(c+d)]/[d/(c+d)]} = \frac{a/b}{c/d} = \frac{ad}{bc} \tag{19.7}$$

OR approximates the RR for rare diseases (usually with an incidence less than 0.05). Thus, it can be interpreted in the same way as the RR under such conditions.

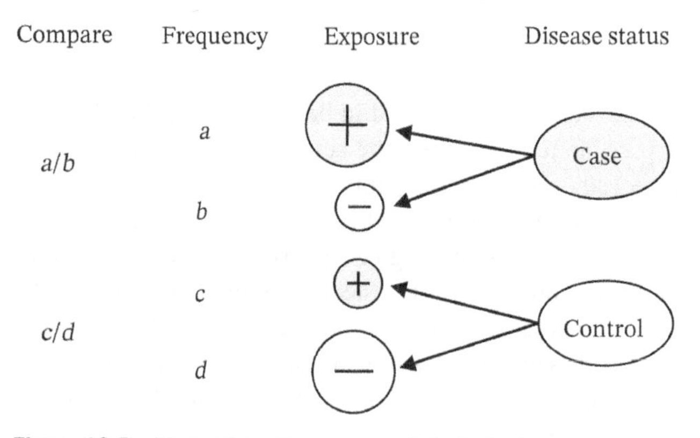

Figure 19.3 Illustration of case-control study design.

Example 19.11 To explore the association between smoking and pancreatic cancer, a case-control study was conducted. A total of 910 patients were included who were diagnosed with pancreatic cancer at a hospital. Another 910 participants who were healthy partners and genetically unrelated family members (spouses and in-laws) of patients in the same hospital, and who had cancers other than pancreatic, lung, or head and neck cancer (smoking-related cancers), were included as controls. The smoking status of participants was determined, as shown in Table 19.2. Calculate and interpret the OR.

Solution

The OR is estimated using Formula 19.7 as

$$\widehat{OR} = \frac{490/420}{370/540} = 1.70$$

The result indicates that smoking is positively associated with pancreatic cancer, and the risk of pancreatic cancer is estimated to be 1.70 times among smokers over that of non-smokers. Similarly, conclusions in case-control studies should be made by conducting a hypothesis testing.

19.3.2 Sample Size for Case-Control Studies

Let π_D and π_C denote the exposure rate in the case and control groups, respectively. The null hypothesis of $OR = 1$ can be written as: $H_0: OR = (\pi_D/(1-\pi_D))/(\pi_C/(1-\pi_C)) = 1$, or equivalently, $\pi_D = \pi_C$. Thus, the formula for sample size calculation in a case-control study (for the control group) is:

$$n = \frac{\left[z_{1-\alpha/2}\sqrt{(1+m)\bar{\pi}(1-\bar{\pi})} + z_{1-\beta}\sqrt{\pi_D(1-\pi_D) + m\pi_C(1-\pi_C)}\right]^2}{(\pi_D - \pi_C)^2}, \tag{19.8}$$

where $\bar{\pi} = (\pi_D + m\pi_C)/(1+m)$ and m is a predefined ratio of control participants over case participants.

With an estimate of π_D or π_C from previous research, we can use an anticipated OR to estimate the other using $\pi_D = \pi_C OR/(1 + \pi_C(OR-1))$.

$z_{1-\beta}$ and $z_{1-\alpha/2}$ are defined as above.

Notice that OR is also a kind of effect size.

Table 19.2 Data obtained from a case-control study on smoking and pancreatic cancer.

Exposure	Case	Control
Smoker	490	370
Non-smoker	420	540
Total	910	910

Example 19.12 Refer to Example 19.11. Assuming that the exposure rate in the control group is 41%, and the researcher decides to include the same number of individuals in both groups. How many participants should be enrolled to achieve 80% power to reject the null hypothesis of OR = 1 in favor of the alternative OR = 2, if the test is to be performed at a significance level of 0.05 (two-sided)?

Solution
Since $\alpha = 0.05$, $\beta = 0.2$, $\pi_C = 0.41$, $m = 1$, and $OR = 2$:

$$\pi_D = \frac{\pi_C OR}{1 + \pi_C (OR - 1)} = \frac{2 \times 0.41}{1 + 0.41 \times (2 - 1)} = 0.58$$

$$\bar{\pi} = \frac{\pi_D + m\pi_C}{1 + m} = 0.495$$

Substituting into Formula 19.8, we obtain

$$n = \frac{\left[z_{1-\alpha/2}\sqrt{(1+m)\bar{\pi}(1-\bar{\pi})} + z_{1-\beta}\sqrt{\pi_D(1-\pi_D) + m\pi_C(1-\pi_C)}\right]^2}{(\pi_D - \pi_C)^2}$$
$$= \frac{\left[1.96 \times \sqrt{2 \times 0.495 \times (1 - 0.495)} + 0.84 \times \sqrt{0.58 \times (1 - 0.58) + 0.41 \times (1 - 0.41)}\right]^2}{(0.58 - 0.41)^2}$$
$$\approx 135.$$

At least 135 eligible participants are needed for both the case and control groups.

In general, the sample size requirement in a case-control study is far smaller than that in a cohort study; thus case-control studies can be implemented in an inexpensive, quick, and labor-saving way. This type of design is well suited to studying the risk factors of rare diseases with a long latent period, especially for early exploratory research when there is little knowledge of the exact etiology of the disease investigated.

Notice that the sample size determination for observational studies only deals with random error, and multiple biases may exist in observational studies. For instance, in case-control studies, inappropriate selection of controls (a type of selection bias) would profoundly affect the validity of the results, and recall bias (a type of information bias) may exist because case-control studies are conducted retrospectively. These issues are beyond the scope of this text and readers should refer to relevant epidemiology literature.

19.4 Summary

In this chapter, we focused on observational study designs, in which research participants are observed or measured in their "natural state."

Three common types of observational study are cross-sectional studies, cohort studies, and case-control studies.

A cross-sectional study is generally used to estimate population characteristics within a sample. We were introduced to several probability sampling methods including simple random sampling, systematic sampling, stratified sampling, and cluster sampling. These sampling methods can be combined for use in multistage sampling.

A cohort study is conducted by dividing the research participants into exposed groups and comparing the incidence rates of an outcome between the groups during follow-up. Associations between the exposure and outcome in a cohort study are measured using RR, which is the ratio of the likelihood of an outcome in the exposed group to that in the unexposed group.

A case-control study is conducted by identifying case and control groups, determined according to the existence of an outcome of interest, and comparing their exposure histories in a retrospective investigation. The OR, as an alternative measure of association between the exposure and outcome, is used in case-control studies and can approximate relative risk when the outcome is rare.

Methods of sample size determination for these types of observational study were also discussed. In general, we need to specify a measure of precision for the estimation or an effect size for hypothesis testing, in addition to other necessary components for calculation of the minimum sample size required for statistical inference.

19.5 Exercises

1. Blood supply is critical in health care and knowledge of the characteristics and occupational satisfaction among employees in the blood supply system is important for making improvements. Specific jobs in the blood supply system vary, from blood collection, laboratory testing, and quality control to component preparation and delivery. Suppose that you need to design a survey among employees in the blood supply system. You decide to carry out a pilot study at a local blood center, with the aim to carry out a subsequent national survey.
   (a) How would you perform sampling in the pilot study at the local blood center and in the national survey? Is there any difference in the choice of sampling method for these two surveys with different scales? What are the advantages and disadvantages of your chosen method(s) over other possible alternatives?
   (b) What parameters do you need so as to calculate the sample size necessary to obtain sufficient data on age, sex, and job satisfaction among employees? Can we use estimates of the parameters obtained in the pilot study? Are there any alternative methods?
   (c) What errors may exist in the survey? How can they affect your results? How do you plan to control them?

2. Although tobacco smoking has been shown to increase the risk of multiple cancers, the association between smoking and melanoma remains controversial. You intend to undertake research on this subject; consider the following:
   (a) What types of study design can you use? What are the advantages and disadvantages of the different types of study designs in this case?
   (b) Select a study design and explain the method of sample size estimation in detail.

3. Suppose you are in a planning stage of research to estimate the incidence of children allergy and explore the potential risk factors, a questionnaire survey will be administered to the parents of children aged 0–3 years, please answer the following question.
   (a) Please design a sampling plan to get a representative sample from the city you are living to answer the research questions.
   (b) If we assume that the "estimated" incidence of allergy is 21.3%, how can we estimate the sample size to be investigated, and what other information is needed?
   (c) To investigate the potential risk factors of allergy among children, what else should be considered in sample size estimation?

20

Experimental Study Design

CONTENTS

In this chapter, we will discuss experimental study design. By "experimental," we mean that, rather than passively observing the study subjects, the researcher can actively impose one or more interventions on the research subjects to investigate the effects of the intervention(s). The research subjects in experimental studies can be randomly allocated to different treatment groups, and ideally, the conditions other than the treatment of interest between groups are controlled to examine a causal effect of the treatment.

Applied to different biomedical research fields, we can divide experimental studies into the following broad categories: (i) *Laboratory experiments*, which are the main research approach in basic medicine, in which the research subjects are usually experimental animals, cells, or other biomaterials; (ii) *Clinical trials*, referring to the application of an experimental study in a clinical setting, usually for investigating the safety, effectiveness, and efficacy of a treatment by recruiting patients with a certain disease; and (iii) *Community intervention trials*, which are used for the evaluation of intervention measures in public (e.g., lung cancer screening, toilet renovation projects). Some of these interventions may be difficult to implement at the individual level, and operate at the population level instead.

Applied Medical Statistics, First Edition. Jingmei Jiang.

Companion website: www.wiley.com\go\jiang\appliedmedicalstatistics

In this chapter, we provide an introduction to experimental study design, including its basic concepts and design methods, mostly using clinical trials for illustrative purposes, while the basic principles for other experimental studies are similar. We have introduced analysis methods for various types of experimental designs in Chapters 8 to 10, and herein we continue our discussion about their design aspects and sample size calculation methods.

20.1 Overview

20.1.1 Basic Components of an Experimental Study

There are three indispensable elements in experimental studies: research subjects, treatment factors, and experimental effects. In this section, we will introduce these key components.

1. Research Subjects
A *research subject* is the basic unit of experimental objects to which a treatment can be assigned, and may vary among different types of experimental study. As discussed earlier, in laboratory experiments, examples of research subjects include animals, cells, plasma samples, serum samples, and tissue samples; in clinical trials other than phase I clinical trials, patients suffering from a certain kind of disease are enrolled, and treated as research subjects. In community intervention trials, the research subject can be a community member, or the community as a whole.

In defining the research subjects, inclusion and exclusion criteria have an important impact on the target population that the research findings can be generalized to, and should be clearly specified according to the scientific question that the research is intended to answer. The *inclusion criteria* refer to characteristics (e.g., age, stage of disease) required for entering the study; the *exclusion criteria* refer to the conditions that make the subjects, although satisfying the inclusion criteria, not suitable for inclusion, possibly because they are likely to exhibit unfavorable effects, provide unreliable data, or drop out of the research. The example below provides a thorough description of the inclusion and exclusion criteria in a randomized clinical trial with regard to clinical transfusion decision.

Example 20.1 A randomized trial was conducted to determine whether a higher or lower threshold for blood transfusion would have an impact on functional recovery among patients with cardiacvascular disease who undergo surgery for hip fracture. The inclusion criteria are: (i) age of 50 years and older; (ii) undergoing primary surgical repair of a hip fracture; (iii) clinical evidence of or risk factors for cardiovascular disease; and (iv) a hemoglobin level of less than 10 g/dL within 3 days after surgery. The exclusion criteria are: (i) unable to walk without human assistance before hip fracture; (ii) declined blood transfusions; (iii) multiple trauma (defined as having had or planning to undergo surgery for non-hip-related traumatic injury); (iv) pathologic hip fracture associated with cancer; (v) history of clinically recognized acute myocardial infarction within 30 days before randomization; (vi) previous participation in the trial with a contralateral hip fracture; (vii) symptoms associated with anemia (e.g., ischemic chest pain); and (viii) actively bleeding at the time of potential randomization (Carson et al. 2011).

2. Treatment Factors

Treatment factor, also known as *experimental factors*, refers to the factors that the research subjects are exposed to, enabling their direct or indirect effects to be observed. A treatment factor could be an active intervention measure imposed by experimenters, such as hypolipidemic drugs delivered to patients in a clinical study to investigate their treatment efficacy, or different treatment regimes in a comparative study comparing the efficacy of treatment schemes among tumor patients.

The treatment factor, or a combination of treatment factors, is typicallly what a researcher is interested in. Although many other factors may also affect the research outcome, it is generally necessary to focus on only one or a few factors in one experiment, and the treatment should be defined clearly and remained as unchanged as possible throughout over the whole process. Factors that may affect the research outcome are called non-treatment factors, and the statistical design is largely focused on controlling their effects before, during, and after data is collected (for the discussion of the latter, see Chapters 15 to 17).

Example 20.2 Refer to Example 20.1. The treatment factor defined in the trial was liberal vs. restrictive transfusion. Patients in the liberal-strategy group received 1 unit of packed red cells and additional blood as needed to maintain a hemoglobin level of 10 g/dL or more. Patients in the restrictive-strategy group were permitted to receive transfusions if symptoms or signs of anemia developed or at the discretion of their physicians if the hemoglobin level fell below 8 g/dL. Blood was administered 1 unit at a time, and the presence of symptoms or signs was reassessed.

3. Experimental Effect

The *experimental effect* refers to the response caused by treatment factors. For assessing the effect, it is necessary to select appropriate indicators for measurement, which are called *outcome measures* or *effect measures*. This selection is highly important in designing an experiment.

Outcome measures can be classified into *subjective outcomes* and *objective outcomes*. An outcome is considered subjective if the evaluation of the results depends on personal judgment (e.g., degree of pain); whereas objective measures are usually obtained using measurement instruments and equipment (e.g., blood pressure). Because subjective outcomes are vulnerable to the influence of the psychological state of patients and observers, objective outcomes should be used as the primary endpoint. However, if an accurate and reliable objective measure is not available, an alternative option is quantifying or grading an existing subjective outcome.

The sensitivity and specificity of the outcome measure should also be prioritized when choosing and assessing the appropriate outcome measures. Sensitivity refers to the ability of the outcome measure to accurately measure an experimental effect when a treatment effect exists. In contrast, specificity refers to the likelihood that the treatment appears to be effective in the absence of a treatment effect. It should be noted that the choice of outcome measure is a highly context-dependent task, and these attributes themselves are specific to the population and settings of the measures used.

Example 20.3 In a study of arthritis, the degree of pain is an important experimental effect but an objective outcome measurement is lacking. For improving the quality of a possible measure, a visual analogue score (VAS) can be used. The score is determined by measuring the distance (mm) on the 10-cm line between the "no pain" anchor and the patient's mark, providing a range of scores from 0–10, with 0 indicating no pain, and 10 indicating the most severe pain. A higher score indicates greater pain intensity. Therefore, the amount of pain that a patient feels ranges across a continuum from none to an extreme amount of pain in a visual form.

20.1.2 Principles of Experimental Study Design

To avoid or reduce influence of systematic and random errors on the results of the study, several basic principles should be adhered to in the design stage to guarantee a valid research conclusion. The following subsections briefly describe these principles.

1. Setting Control Conditions

The purpose of setting control conditions is to provide a benchmark for evaluating the efficacy or effectiveness of treatments, providing relevant information about what would have happened to research subjects if they had not received (or received another) treatment. Many non-treatment factors can affect research results, such as subjects' age, subjects' psychological state, the subjective feelings of researchers, and external environmental factors such as climate, weather, and season.

Example 20.4 In a clinical study, 65 people with influenza were treated with a new flu antiviral drug, and 92.3% of patients recovered after 10 days. Consider whether a conclusion can be drawn regarding whether the drug is effective in treating influenza.

Solution

Without a control group, such a conclusion is apparently misleading, because influenza is a self-limiting illness and the symptoms last from a few days to several weeks for most patients even when no treatment is delivered. Therefore, a cure rate of 92.3% may fail to reflect the true efficacy of the drug. Therefore, it is reasonable to set up a concurrent parallel control group in the research and make sure the control group and experimental group are always treated in the same time and space during the whole research process.

Here we introduce several common concurrent controls:

(1) Placebo Concurrent Control

A *placebo concurrent control* group means that a group of research subjects are treated exactly the same as the patients who received treatment, except that no active treatment is given to these subjects. In medical research, it is not uncommon that treatments require manipulating the experimental units or subjects where the manipulation alone can produce a response that could be easily be mistaken for a "real" treatment effect. In such cases, it can be helpful to establish a placebo control group to overcome the influence of psychological factors of researchers, subjects, and analysts involved in evaluating efficacy and safety. The word "placebo" is Latin for "I will please," which originally referred to something a doctor would give a patient when asked for a remedy and none was available. Broadly speaking, a placebo is anything that seems to be a "real" intervention measure, which could be a pill, a shot, or some other type of "fake" treatment. The common characteristics shared by all placebos is they are designed to have no therapeutic value and do not contain any active substance affecting the health condition.

A placebo concurrent control is usually accompanied with a blinding protocol and attention should be paid to ensure that the use of a placebo control should never expose patients to unnecessary risks. Generally speaking, the application of a placebo concurrent control could be justified in the following scenarios: (i) there is no proven effective treatment for the condition under study; (ii) the disease is self-limiting or stable for a long time, and a delay in treatment would not lead to deterioration of the disease or bring any irreversible health consequence to the subjects; and (iii) there are compelling methodological reasons for using a placebo, and withholding treatment does not pose a risk of serious harm to participants.

(2) Active Treatment Concurrent Control

Active treatment concurrent control refers to a control group in which subjects allocated to the control group received an active intervention. This method is usually adopted when the research purpose is to compare the effectiveness of an experimental treatment with a known effective treatment to show that the experimental treatment is superior, as good as, or not substantially worse than a known effective treatment. For example, in a study of hypoglycemia, a researcher wants to investigate the hypoglycemic effects of oral insulin enteric-coated pills among moderate type 2 diabetic patients, and the subcutaneous medium-effect insulin injection is chosen as an active control. Active treatment concurrent controls can also be used when the placebo control group is not appropriate because of ethical constraints. In general, if many options are available, the treatment with the best efficacy and safety should be selected as a control.

(3) Historical Control

Historical control refers to the practice of using outcomes of patients in past studies and administrative databases to estimate potential responses to the treatment under investigation in an ongoing study. It is reasonable to use only historical control data to fully or partially replace a concurrent control due to either ethical concerns in recruiting patients for control arms in life-threatening diseases with no credible control arm or the disease of interest is too rare to set a parallel concurrent control. However, because a historical control is identified retrospectively, it is inherently vulnerable to the influence of selection bias or systematic difference among the groups in comparisons that could affect the final outcome. These biases might stem from a wide range of factors, such as the natural history of the disease, improvement of diagnostic techniques, or drug resistance.

(4) Self Control

Self control refers to a control method in which the same group of subjects is used for both the experimental and control groups, such that patients serve as their own controls. There are two kinds of self control: self concurrent control and pre-/post-treatment self control. In self concurrent control, different kinds of treatments are performed on the same subject at the same time, and most diagnostic tests adopt this kind of self-parallel control. For example, in a rapid diagnosis test of tuberculosis, one arm of a subject is randomly selected for a skin test with the test reagent, and the other arm is used as the control and treated with another diagnostic reagent. The accuracy of the two reagents for the diagnosis of tuberculosis can then be compared. Because the non-experimental factors are roughly balanced for self control, the systematic error of this control can be greatly reduced. In a pre-/post-treatment control, the outcome measure is assessed both before and after treatment for every research subject, making it a self-control design in nature. However, studies using self control without any other control can be vulnerable to the influence of subjective feelings, leading subjects to change their behavior or to report improved health status because they receive special attention by being in a study and not because of the study intervention itself.

2. Randomization

Generally speaking, *randomization* refers to the practice of randomly sampling research subjects from a population to ensure the *representative* of samples, or randomly allocating research subjects into different treatment groups to ensure the *comparability* between the treatment groups in terms of uncontrollable non-treatment factors, both known and unknown.

The randomization principle mainly includes random sampling (introduced in Chapter 19) and random assignment. Because of practical issues, random sampling is generally not feasible in clinical trials. Instead, to achieve the goal of minimizing the heterogeneity between groups for treatment effect evaluation, *random assignment* is required, in which every subject possesses an equal or defined opportunity to be allocated to each group. The combination of control and randomization is the most effective method for distinguishing the effects that can be attributed to the treatment factor from those caused by other factors.

Random allocation can be achieved using various methods, including a random number table, a random permutation table, and a random function. The specific operation method will be described in detail in the section on design methods.

3. Replication

Generally speaking, the principle of *replication* has two meanings: replication of studies and replication of research subjects. The replication of studies means multiple experiments are conducted under the same experimental conditions to improve the reliability and accuracy of the experimental results. In contrast, replication of research subjects means a sufficient number of research subjects should be involved to ensure the reliability of the estimates and reduce the influence of sampling errors.

20.1.3 Blinding Procedures in Clinical Trials

Blinding in clinical trials refers to the practice by which information that may influence participants (patients and/or investigators) in the trial is masked during the study, until after the research is complete. Blinding is used to avoid the influence of subjective factors and psychological factors of researchers, subjects, observers, and statisticians on the research results, controlling the bias that arises in conducting the clinical trial, and interpreting the results. If subjects know the group allocation information, regardless of whether a placebo control group, active control group, or experimental group is used, psychological effects might arise, potentially hindering or interfering with the research.

Example 20.5 Suppose you are a research doctor in a clinical trial. Without blinding, you know which of your patients is receiving an experimental drug or a standard treatment. You might pay more attention to patients in the experimental group and deliver excessive care to them. In addition, if your colleagues working in the computed tomography room know about the allocation of subjects, their behavior could affect the accuracy of their evaluation of the efficacy and diagnostic results. Similarly, you can imagine how you might feel or behave if you were a patient and you knew you were in the experimental group.

Generally speaking, blinding methods can be divided into the following categories.

1. ***Double-Blind***
In double-blind trials, neither the researchers nor participants know who is receiving a particular treatment during the research. This blinding procedure can greatly reduce the subjective psychological influence from both researchers and subjects. The blindness of random allocation is usually set up and preserved by a third-party agency. During the whole trial, blindness must be maintained. If the allocation of any patients is unmasked, it is regarded as a failed case that violates the protocol.

2. ***Single-Blind***
In single-blind trials, only researchers know the group assignment. A single-blind design is appropriate when double-blind is not applicable. For example, in a clinical study investigating the treatment of moderate and severe acute bacterial infection with Biapenem injection, the application of double-blindness could be hindered due to the difference in type of medication between the experimental group drugs and the control group drugs. Thus, single blindness is adopted, keeping the subjects unaware of their group assignment.

3. ***Open-Label***
In an open-label design, both the researchers and research subjects know which treatment is being administered. It is appropriate to adopt such a design under conditions in which it is impossible to blind the researchers delivering the medical care as well as the research subjects themselves. For example, it is impossible to blind the clinician and the patients in a study aiming to compare the effectiveness of surgery and chemotherapy among patients with nasopharyngeal carcinoma. However, a third-party evaluation of the outcomes generated in an open-label design is highly recommended to reduce bias. *Third-party evaluation* means the efficacy or diagnostic results assessor (medical imaging readers, endpoint committees, etc.) is blinded to the assignment. For example, in a clinical trial of norbrucine hydrochloric higenamine injection as a cardiac stress test drug in the diagnosis of coronary heart disease by nuclide myocardial perfusion imaging, a placebo control group was adopted. However, the efficacy of the test drug was so obvious that clinicians could recognize the drug type, resulting in bias in the results. To control the bias generated in the process of a clinical trial and interpretation of results, a third-party evaluation team was designated to analyze the imaging data blindly to ensure an objective and accurate evaluation of the diagnosis results.

20.2 Completely Randomized Design

20.2.1 Concept of Completely Randomized Design

Once the study objectives have been clearly defined, an appropriate randomized experimental design for the intended research can be chosen. In this section, we introduce the most common experimental design: completely randomized design.

A completely randomized design is a type of design in which each subject is randomly allocated to receive a single treatment. Therefore, this approach is also known as single-factor design. The simplest form of completely randomized design is the parallel design. Each treatment group usually (but not necessarily) contains approximately the same number of patients, and the design efficiency is highest when the sample size of each group is equal. A completely randomized design could also involve multiple groups and the sample size of each treatment group may be unequal.

Example 20.6 Referring to the study described in Example 9.1, how should the 15 mice be randomly allocated into 3 groups of 5 subjected to low-, medium-, or high-intensity exercise using the design we have described above?

Solution
Here we used a random number table to help perform random allocation. The process of random allocation was as follows:

(1) The mice are assigned a number, such as 1,2,...,15, according to their weight, from lowest to highest;
(2) A starting point is chosen from the table of 2500 random digits in Appendix Table 1, and 15 two-digit random numbers are selected sequentially. For example, starting from row (3), columns (7) and (8) are taken as the first random number "02," then the 15 two-digit random numbers are recorded from top to bottom, and replicated random numbers are deleted;
(3) Sorting the recorded random numbers from smallest to largest;
(4) Subjects with a rank order of 1–5 are allocated to group *A* (low-intensity exercise), those with a rank order of 6–10 are allocated to group *B* (medium-intensity exercise), and those with a rank order of 11–15 are allocated to group *C* (high-intensity exercise). The allocation results are shown in Table 20.1.

Completely randomized design is flexible and convenient to operate. The number of treatment groups and the sample size of each group are not limited. Moreover, in the process of the experiment, the dropping out of one subject would not influence the retrieval of information from other subjects, and therefore, the loss of experimental efficiency will be lower than in other design methods, making it the most popular design method in biomedical research. In addition, the statistical analysis method for completely randomized designs is also relatively simple. However, there are also clear disadvantages of completely randomized designs. First, this type of design can only analyze a single treatment factor. In addition, it can only rely on the random allocation of the subjects to balance the distribution of all non-treatment factors among groups. Therefore, the precision of this experimental design is low, and sometimes the balance between groups will be poor due to a relatively small sample size.

Table 20.1 Allocation by completely randomized design of 15 mice.

ID	1	2	3	4	5	6	7	8
Random number	2	71	26	64	54	70	30	33
Rank	1	13	4	11	10	12	6	7
Group	*A*	*C*	*A*	*C*	*B*	*C*	*B*	*B*

ID	9	10	11	12	13	14	15
Random number	95	41	42	27	84	17	24
Rank	15	8	9	5	14	2	3
Group	*C*	*B*	*B*	*A*	*C*	*A*	*A*

20.2.2 Sample Size for Completely Randomized Design

In Chapter 8, we discussed the sample size estimation for two population means using completely randomized design. In this section, we will introduce the sample size for comparison of means in a multiple group design using one-way ANOVA.

One-way ANOVA is the multi-group extension of the independent samples t-test, and, therefore, the goal of sample size estimation in one-way ANOVA is ensuring sufficient power for rejecting the null hypothesis for a global test when at least one pair of group means are significantly different from each other. Suppose we are planning to compare k population means, and the expected effect size is δ. Thus, for a balanced design with equal sample size across the treatment group, the required sample size in each group to detect a meaningful minimal difference of δ could be calculated as:

$$n = \frac{\left(q_{k,k(n_0-1),1-\alpha}\right)^2 \mathrm{MS}_E F_{k(n_0-1),\nu_{E'},1-\beta}}{\delta^2}, \tag{20.1}$$

where:

n_0 denotes a starting point value of sample size within each treatment group.

α is the significance level, and $1-\beta$ is the desired power.

$q_{k,k(n_0-1),1-\alpha}$ is the critical value of the q_k distribution (see multiple comparison in Chapter 9).

MS_E is the within mean square in ANOVA analysis which could be provided by a pilot study.

$\nu_{E'}$ is the degrees of freedom of the error in the pilot study.

$F_{k(n_0-1),\nu_{E'},1-\beta}$ is the β upper quantile of the F-distribution with $k(n_0-1)$ and $\nu_{E'}$ degrees of freedom.

It should be noted that, to use Formula 20.1 in estimating the required sample size, we need to set an initial value of n_0 (usually being a fairly large value), and, based on this, the values of $F_{k(n_0-1),\nu_{E'},1-\beta}$ and $q_{k,k(n_0-1),1-\alpha}$ can be obtained from Appendix Table 6 and Appendix Table 9, respectively.

The value of n calculated using Formula 20.1 can be further used to determine the values of $F_{k(n_0-1),\nu_{E'},1-\beta}$ and $q_{k,k(n_0-1),1-\alpha}$. Thus, the detectable difference when we involve n subjects in each group can be calculated using the following formula:

$$\delta' = \frac{q_{k,k(n-1),1-\alpha}\sqrt{\mathrm{MS}_E}\sqrt{F_{k(n-1),\nu_{E'},1-\beta}}}{\sqrt{n}}. \tag{20.2}$$

If δ' is slightly smaller than the predefined δ, n can be accepted as the final sample size for each group. If not, n should be slightly changed, and the previous procedure should be repeated using Formula 20.2 until δ' is close to δ.

Example 20.7 Refer to Example 9.1. Suppose in the planning stage the researcher wants to determine the required sample size and a difference of 11 seconds in cumulative paw-licking time is considered to be a meaningful difference. In addition, suppose that, based on the pilot research, the mean square error for the error term is 25, with 12 degrees of freedom. Assuming a significance level of 0.05 and a desired power of 0.9, how many mice would be required to detect a meaningful difference of 11 seconds in terms of mean paw-licking duration among mice with different exercise intensities?

Solution

First, we begin by choosing a fairly large value for n_0. To facilitate finding the critical value in Appendix Table 9, we could set $n_0 = 41$, which leads to $3\times(41-1)=120$. Therefore, as $MS_E = 25$, $\nu_E{}' = 12$, and $k=3$, we could easily find the critical value $q_{3,3\times(41-1),1-0.05} = 3.36$. Using the interpolation method in Appendix Table 6 leads to $F_{3\times(41-1),12,0.9} = 1.93$. Then, using Formula 20.1, we can calculate the sample size in each formula, as follows:

$$n = \frac{\left(q_{k,k(n_0-1),1-\alpha}\right)^2 MS_E F_{k(n_0-1),\nu_{E'},1-\beta}}{\delta^2} = \frac{3.36^2 \times 25 \times 1.93}{11^2} = 4.50.$$

We could let $n = 5$, with which we obtain $q_{3,3\times(5-1),1-0.05} = 3.77$, $F_{3\times(5-1),12,0.9} = 2.14$. Using Formula 20.2, we can calculate δ' as follows:

$$\delta' = \frac{q_{k,k(n-1),1-\alpha}\sqrt{MS_E}\sqrt{F_{k(n-1),\nu_{E'},1-\beta}}}{\sqrt{n}} = \frac{3.77\times\sqrt{25}\times\sqrt{2.14}}{\sqrt{5}} = 12.33$$

which is higher than 11. Therefore, we increase the sample size for each group to 6, which leads to $q_{3,3\times(6-1),1-0.05} = 3.67$, $F_{3\times(6-1),12,0.9} = 2.10$

$$\delta' = \frac{q_{k,k(n-1),1-\alpha}\sqrt{MS_E}\sqrt{F_{k(n-1),\nu_{E'},1-\beta}}}{\sqrt{n}} = \frac{3.67\times\sqrt{25}\times\sqrt{2.10}}{\sqrt{6}} = 10.86,$$

which is very close to 11. Thus, the required sample size for each group is 6 and the total sample size should be $6\times 3 = 18$ mice.

20.3 Randomized Block Design

20.3.1 Concepts of Randomized Block Design

In the completely randomized design, it is assumed that all experimental units are uniform, which is not always the case in practice. To ensure the balance and comparability of non-treatment factors among treatment groups, a randomized block design is commonly used.

Randomized block design, also known as compatibility group design, assumes that a population of experimental units can be divided into a number of relatively homogeneous subpopulations or blocks. The treatments are then randomly assigned to experimental units such that each treatment occurs equally often (usually once) in each block – i.e., each block contains all treatments. Blocks usually represent levels of naturally occurring differences or sources of variation that are unrelated to the treatments. For example, in animal experiments, animals with the same litter, sex, and similar weight are often grouped into the same block. In clinical studies, patients with the same sex, age, and severity of illness are grouped into the same block, which can improve the balance among the treatment groups. Each block can have two or more subjects. When there are only two subjects in each block, the design is sometimes referred to as a paired design, and can be treated as a special case of randomized block design.

Example 20.8 Refer to Example 10.1, in which the investigator adopted a randomized block design to investigate the effect of different feeds on the weight gain of rats. There are six litters of rats and three rats are randomly selected from each litter. Three different feeds are then randomly allocated to the three rats in each litter. The randomization procedure is then conducted.

Solution

The specific randomization procedures could be conducted as follows:

(1) Number the six litters of mice 1–6 (i.e., blocks (1–6));

(2) Select a certain number of rows in the table of random permutation (Appendix Table 2), with each row corresponding to a block. Then, numbers within each row are taken as random numbers. In the current study, we could select rows (1–6), which correspond to blocks (1–6), respectively. Then, we could select numbers "1," "2," and "3" within each row, which correspond to allocation to group *A*, *B*, and *C*. Take block (1) (row (1)) as an example: the first random number is 1 (column (8)), the second random number is 3 (column (10)), and the last random number is 2 (column (12)).

(3) Assign these random numbers sequentially to the rats within each block. The first rat selected is assigned the first random number, the second rat selected is assigned the second random number, and the third rat selected is assigned the third random number. In Table 20.2, For block (1) (row (1)), the rat first selected is assigned a random number of "1" and assigned to group *A*. The second rat selected is assigned a random number of "3" and assigned to group *C*. The third rat selected is assigned a random number of "2" and assigned to group *B*. The rest of the blocks can be performed in the same manner.

In a randomized block design, subjects are divided into blocks according to certain factors. Thus, the influence of many non-treatment factors on the experimental result could be reduced by increasing the balance among the groups and reducing the experimental error. Moreover, this process increases the block information and reduces the

Table 20.2 Allocation by randomized block design in Example 10.1.

ID	1	2	3	4	5	6	7	8	9
Block	1	1	1	2	2	2	3	3	3
Random number	1	3	2	2	1	3	1	2	3
Group	*A*	*C*	*B*	*B*	*A*	*C*	*A*	*B*	*C*

ID	10	11	12	13	14	15	16	17	18
Block	4	4	4	5	5	5	6	6	6
Random number	1	3	2	1	2	3	2	1	3
Group	*A*	*C*	*B*	*A*	*B*	*C*	*B*	*A*	*C*

individual differences among the subjects, thus reducing the sample size required and improving the statistical efficiency. The disadvantage of randomized block designs is that it is sometimes difficult to match subjects into blocks, thus losing information from some subjects. In addition, the impact is relatively substantial when subjects drop out in the blocks.

In clinical research in which many non-treatment factors influence the research results, it is often difficult to conduct pairings or match subjects one by one because it is often time- and energy-consuming to logistically identify and recruit research subjects with a number of matching factors being considered simultaneously. Moreover, poor compliance of the research subjects might also limit the application of matching. Thus, subjects are sometimes only matched according to the entry time to ensure that the time of enrollment of the subjects in each treatment group is relatively close. For example, in a clinical study, 100 patients with allergic purpura at a particular hospital were randomly assigned into an experimental group and a control group. According to the time at which they entered into the study, the first four patients were assigned to the first block. Likewise, all patients were assigned to 25 different blocks. Four subjects in each block were then randomly allocated into two treatment groups; that is, two of the four subjects in each block entered the experimental group and the other two entered the control group. Therefore, potential treatment imbalances that may occur periodically with complete randomization could be overcome.

20.3.2 Sample Size for Randomized Block Design

The sample size calculation for randomized block design is similar to that in one-way ANOVA, except that the degrees of freedom for the error are given by $(b-1)\times(k-1)$ in a randomized block design, where b is the number of blocks and k is the number of treatment groups, as described above.

Example 20.9 Refer to Example 10.1. Suppose that a study is in the planning stage, and it is necessary to determine how many litters of rats should be involved. Based on pilot research, it is known that the mean square of error term is 38, with 10 degrees of freedom. Suppose a weight gain of 12 g is considered to be meaningful. Assuming a significance level $\alpha = 0.05$ and a desired power of 0.9, how many litters are required to detect a difference of a size of 12 g in terms of mean weight gain between rats fed with feed A, B, and C?

Solution

Similar to Example 20.7, we need to set an initial value of n_0. Here, to facilitate finding the critical value, we could set the number of litter to $n_0 = 61$. Therefore, the degrees of freedom for the error term can be calculated as $(3-1)\times(61-1)=120$. Then, as $MS_E = 38$, $\nu_E{}' = 10$, and $k=3$, and we can find the $q_{3,(3-1)(61-1),1-0.05} = 3.36$ in Appendix Table 9. Then, by applying the interpolation method, we can obtain $F_{(3-1)\times(61-1),10,0.9} = 2.08$ using the critical value provided by Appendix Table 6.

Then, using Formula 20.1, we can calculate the sample size as follows:

$$n = \frac{\left(q_{k,k(n_0-1),1-\alpha}\right)^2 MS_E F_{k(n_0-1),\nu_{E'},1-\beta}}{\delta^2} = \frac{3.36^2 \times 38 \times 2.08}{12^2} = 6.2.$$

Therefore, we could let $n = 7$, then $q_{3,(3\text{-}1)\times(7-1),1-0.05} = 3.77$ and $F_{(3-1)\times(7-1),10,0.9} = 2.28$. Using Formula 20.2, we could calculate the δ' as follows:

$$\delta' = \frac{q_{k,k(n-1),1-\alpha}\sqrt{\text{MS}_E}\sqrt{F_{k(n-1),\nu_{E'},1-\beta}}}{\sqrt{n}} = \frac{3.77\times\sqrt{38}\times\sqrt{2.28}}{\sqrt{7}} = 13.26$$

13.26 is greater than the predefined value of 12, implying that we could fail to detect a significant difference of 12 g if we incorporate 7 litters of rats in this research. Therefore, we could increase n by 1, which leads to $q_{3,(3\text{-}1)\times(8-1),1-0.05} = 3.70$ and $F_{(3-1)\times(8-1),10,0.9} = 2.26$. Then, these values can be substituted into Formula 20.2, giving:

$$\delta' = \frac{3.70\times\sqrt{38}\times\sqrt{2.26}}{\sqrt{8}} = 12.12.$$

which is very close to the predefined $\delta = 12$. Therefore, we need at least eight litters, giving a total sample size of $8\times 3 = 24$ mice.

20.4 Factorial Design

In biomedical research, it is not uncommon for investigators to want to evaluate more than one factor simultaneously in one study. In such cases, a factorial design can be adopted to assess two or more interventions simultaneously. The main advantage of this design is its efficiency in terms of sample size, because more than one intervention can be assessed with the same participants. Moreover, a factorial design has an advantage in detecting potential interaction effects between interventions. Suppose there are two factors, A and B, both of which have two levels. Let A_1 and A_2 denote the two levels of factor A, and let B_1 and B_2 denote the two levels of factor B. Then, the four groups $(A_1B_1, A_1B_2, A_2B_1,\text{ and } A_2B_2)$ will be formed according to the combination of the levels of A and B, as illustrated below. The research subjects can then be randomly allocated into the four groups.

Example 20.10 Refer to the research described in Example 10.2, in which a factorial design was adopted to investigate the hypoglycemic effect of two drugs with different dose levels on 16 streptozotocin-induced diabetic male rats. How should the randomization procedures with a random number generator in SPSS be conducted?

Solution

As there are 4 combinations $(A_1B_1, A_1B_2, A_2B_1,\text{ and } A_2B_2)$, 4 groups can be formed, and the 16 rats can be randomly allocated into these groups. In this example, a random number generator in SPSS was used to generate 16 random numbers, and each rat was assigned a random number (Table 20.3). Then, similar to the process described in Example 20.1, the random numbers from smallest to largest and those with a rank order of 1–4 are allocated to group A_1B_1, those with a rank order of 5–8 are allocated to group A_1B_2, those with a rank order of 9–12 are allocated to group A_2B_1, and those with a rank order of 13–16 are allocated to group A_2B_2.

Table 20.3 Allocation by factorial design in Example 20.2.

ID	1	2	3	4	5	6	7	8
Random number	0.418832	0.274251	0.353549	0.260951	0.984417	0.376983	0.216226	0.022891
Rank	10	7	8	6	16	9	4	1
Group	A_2B_1	A_1B_2	A_1B_2	A_1B_2	A_2B_2	A_2B_1	A_1B_1	A_1B_1

ID	9	10	11	12	13	14	15	16
Random number	0.139578	0.690888	0.783236	0.553716	0.880478	0.224759	0.077282	0.716943
Rank	3	12	14	11	15	5	2	13
Group	A_1B_1	A_2B_1	A_2B_2	A_2B_1	A_2B_2	A_1B_2	A_1B_1	A_2B_2

For two factors with three levels each, the number of treatment groups is $3 \times 3 = 9$. Thus, a typical factorial design involves a full combination of levels of two or more factors, resembling a randomized block design. However, there are more than one replications in each combination level in a factorial design, making it possible to investigate potential interaction effects (i.e., whether a change in one factor affects the experimental effects of other factors). The interaction between two factors is called a primary interaction, and the interaction among three factors is called a secondary interaction. Although a higher order of interaction could be investigated, in practice, involving too many factors in a study can undermine the feasibility of the experimental design and the interpretation of the results.

Factorial designs are an efficient design method, which can not only analyze the differences among different levels within each factor (main effect), but can also detect interaction effects. However, factorial designs also have some disadvantages: i) extra time, compliance, and management are required for a factorial design; ii) a factorial design aiming to detect an interaction effect requires a much larger sample size to ensure sufficient power to detect an interaction effect. With an increased number of factors and levels, the sample size increases dramatically, and the interpretation of the results of higher-order interaction analysis is also complicated; and iii) the appropriateness biological and scientific grounds for combined interventions must be explored and determined.

The sample size determination method for testing interaction effects using a factorial design is relatively complex. If we focus only on the main effect, the principle is the same as in the completely randomized design and randomized block design.

20.5 Crossover Design

20.5.1 Concepts of Crossover Design

In a crossover design, subjects receive two or more interventions through randomizing to one of a set of pre-specified sequences which consists of a sequence of two or more treatments given consecutively. For instance, an $g \times j$ crossover design refers to g treatments administered at j different periods. Because subjects receive different treatments sequentially and the effects of one treatment might persist and impact responses to subsequent treatments (known as a carryover effect), a wash-out period is arranged between the periods in a crossover design to reduce the influence of the carryover effect. The length of the wash-out period can be determined based on the attenuation time of drugs in serum, determined by referring to the pharmacopoeia or pre-test results. The wash-out period is generally required to be equivalent to at least seven half-lives of the drug. For example, the half-life of insulin in the body is 2 hours. Considering the feasibility and patient compliance, the wash-out period can be set as 1 day. The simplest form (which is also the most common) of crossover design is a 2×2 design, as discussed in Example 10.4.

Because each research subject serves as their own control in crossover design, this design allows within-subject comparisons between treatments, and, therefore, inter-subject variability can be removed from the comparison between treatments. This can potentially lead to a more precise estimate of the treatment effect, meaning that the trial requires fewer participants. Moreover, a crossover design is more ethically attractive compared with a completely randomized because all patients have the opportunity to receive both treatments.

The disadvantage of crossover design is that not all diseases are suitable for being studied using this method. As a result, this approach is only suitable for investigating diseases with chronic conditions (such as asthma) rather than diseases with a self-healing tendency or short course, so that the circumstances at the beginning of each period are more likely to be the same and the course of the disease is less likely to bias the study findings. In addition, subjects receive more treatments, often corresponding to a longer research period compared with a completely randomized design, which could increase the likelihood of drop-out after finishing one period of treatment. Finally, if one or more subjects leave the study prematurely, a situation could arise in which very few treatment contrasts for both direct effects and carryover effects can be estimated, further complicating the interpretation and analysis.

20.5.2 Sample Size for 2×2 Crossover Design

Consider a 2×2 crossover design in which y_{ijg} represents the observed measure from the ith subject $(i = 1,2,\ldots,n)$ in the jth sequence $(j = 1,2)$ under the gth treatment $(g = 1,2)$. Let $\delta = \tau_1 - \tau_2$ (where τ_g is the gth treatment effect). Therefore, the null and alternative hypotheses are: $H_0 : \delta = 0,\ \ H_1 : \delta \neq 0$.

Let $d_{ij} = y_{ij1} - y_{ij2}$, then an unbiased estimate of δ is given by $\hat{\delta} = \frac{1}{2n}\sum_{j=1}^{2}\sum_{i=1}^{n} d_{ij}$, and follows a normal distribution with mean δ and variance $\sigma_d^2 = \sigma^2 / n$ (where σ^2 is the within-subject variance).

For a large enough n, the null hypothesis could be rejected at α level of significance if

$$\left| \frac{\hat{\delta}}{\sqrt{\sigma_d^2}} \right| > z_{1-\alpha/2}. \tag{20.3}$$

Under the alternative hypothesis that $\delta \neq 0$, the power $1-\beta$ of this test is given by:

$$\begin{aligned} 1-\beta &= \Phi\left(\frac{\delta}{\sqrt{\sigma_d^2}} - z_{1-\alpha/2}\right) + \Phi\left(-\frac{\delta}{\sqrt{\sigma_d^2}} - z_{1-\alpha/2}\right) \\ &= \Phi\left(\frac{\delta}{\sqrt{\sigma^2/n}} - z_{1-\alpha/2}\right) + \Phi\left(-\frac{\delta}{\sqrt{\sigma^2/n}} - z_{1-\alpha/2}\right). \\ &\approx \Phi\left(\frac{|\delta|}{\sqrt{\sigma^2/n}} - z_{1-\alpha/2}\right) \end{aligned}$$

As a result, the sample size needed to achieve power $1-\beta$ can be obtained by solving the n, therefore, the sample size for each sequence could be calculated using:

$$n = \frac{\left(z_{1-\alpha/2} + z_{1-\beta}\right)^2 \sigma^2}{\delta^2}. \tag{20.4}$$

Example 20.11 Let us consider the research described in Example 10.5. Suppose in the planning stage the investigator decided that a difference of at least 5 units on the dyspnea scale is of clinical significance. In addition, suppose that, according to the pilot study, the within-patient variance in mean PEFR scores was $\sigma^2 = 30$. How many patients would be required to detect a difference of a size of difference as 5 units with a power of 0.9 and two-sided significance level of $\alpha = 0.05$?

Solution

As $\alpha = 0.05$, $\beta = 0.1$, $\sigma^2 = 30$, $\delta = 5$,

using Formula 20.4, the sample size in each sequence could be calculated as:

$$n = \frac{\left(z_{1-\alpha/2} + z_{1-\beta}\right)^2 \sigma^2}{\delta^2} = \frac{(1.96 + 1.28)^2 \times 30}{5^2} = 12.60 \approx 13$$

Therefore, at least 13 patients are required for each sequence, and a total of 26 research subjects are needed.

20.6 Summary

In an experimental study, the researcher could manipulate one or more control variables of the research subject(s) and measure the effects of manipulation. An experimental design has three basic components: research subject, treatment factor, and experimental effect. To conduct an experimental study, several basic principles should be adhered to: control, randomization, and replication. The purpose of setting up control conditions is to serve as reference levels for the effects of treatment factors in the experimental group. Randomization ensures the balance and consistency between groups of subjects. Replication refers to multiple experiments under the same experimental conditions to improve the reliability and accuracy of experiments. Blindness aims to avoid the interference of subjective factors and psychological factors of researchers and subjects, to control the bias generated in the process of conducting the clinical trial and interpreting the results.

Common design methods for random allocation include: completely random design, randomized block design, factorial design, and crossover design. Choosing an appropriate design type is directly related to the accuracy and reliability of the research results. Choosing the most appropriate design type should take the research objective, ethics, resources, and other specific situations into consideration. Similar to observational studies, sample size determination is also a critical part of experimental design. Finally, specific calculation methods differ across different experimental designs.

20.7 Exercises

1. In an investigation of the effects of reduced glutathione tablets and adefovir dipivoxil and their potential interaction effects in the treatment of abnormal liver function, research subjects were randomly divided into three groups. Group *A* took adefovir dipivoxil, group *B* took reduced glutathione tablets, and group *C* took

both reduced glutathione tablets and adefovir dipivoxil at the same time. A transaminase test was performed to measure the effect of treatment, and the results were compared using t-tests.

(a) Is the research design appropriate in this study? If not, please propose your design to improve the research.

(b) How are the principles of control, randomization, and replication reflected in your design?

(c) Which statistical method should be employed in concordance with your design?

2. In a clinical study, the mouths of 60 patients with mild or moderate oral ulcers were pasted with a particular type of oral membrane. The membrane was gently pressed for several seconds, and was used after cleaning the oral cavity four times a day (after breakfast, lunch, dinner, and before going to bed). One piece was pasted onto each ulcer for 5 days. Taking the ulcer area as the main evaluation indicator, after 5 days of treatment, it was found that the ulcer area was significantly reduced, and this effect was statistically significant. Therefore, it was concluded that the oral membrane had a positive curative effect in the treatment of oral ulcers.

(a) Do you agree with the conclusion of this research? If not, please give your reasons and state how to improve the research?

(b) Could the research be randomized? What is the purpose of randomization in this case?

(c) Is there a control group in this research? Which kind of control discussed in this chapter could be adopted here? Please explain their advantages and downsides in the context of current research.

(d) Is the blindness principle appropriate in this research? Can a single-blind or double-blind approach be used? Can a third-party evaluation be used? Please give the reasons for your answer.

(e) How is the replication principle manifested in this research?

Appendix

Appendix Table 1 Table of 2500 random digits.

	1–10	11–20	21–30	31–40	41–50
1	22 17 68 65 81	68 95 23 92 35	87 02 22 57 51	61 09 43 95 06	58 24 82 03 47
2	19 36 27 59 46	13 79 93 37 55	39 77 32 77 09	85 52 05 30 62	47 83 51 62 74
3	16 77 23 02 77	09 61 87 25 21	28 06 24 25 93	16 71 13 59 78	23 05 47 47 25
4	78 43 76 71 61	20 44 90 32 64	97 67 63 99 61	46 38 03 93 22	69 81 21 99 21
5	03 28 28 26 08	73 37 32 04 05	69 30 16 09 05	88 69 58 28 99	35 07 44 75 47
6	93 22 53 64 39	07 10 63 76 35	87 03 04 79 88	08 13 13 85 51	55 34 57 72 69
7	78 76 58 54 74	92 38 70 96 92	52 06 79 79 45	82 63 18 27 44	69 66 92 19 09
8	23 68 35 26 00	99 53 93 61 28	52 70 05 48 34	56 65 05 61 86	90 92 10 70 80
9	15 39 25 70 99	93 86 52 77 65	15 33 59 05 28	22 87 26 07 47	86 96 98 29 06
10	58 71 96 30 24	18 46 23 34 27	85 13 99 24 44	49 18 09 79 49	74 16 32 23 02
11	57 35 27 33 72	24 53 63 94 09	41 10 76 47 91	44 04 95 49 66	39 60 04 59 81
12	48 50 86 54 48	22 06 34 72 52	82 21 15 65 20	33 29 94 71 11	15 91 29 12 03
13	61 96 48 95 03	07 16 39 33 66	98 56 10 56 79	77 21 30 27 12	90 49 22 23 62
14	36 93 89 41 26	29 70 83 63 51	99 74 20 52 36	87 09 41 15 09	98 60 16 03 03
15	18 87 00 42 31	57 90 12 02 07	23 47 37 17 31	54 08 01 88 63	39 41 88 92 10
16	88 56 53 27 59	33 35 72 67 47	77 34 55 45 70	08 18 27 38 90	16 95 86 70 75
17	09 72 95 84 29	49 41 31 06 70	42 38 06 45 18	64 84 73 31 65	52 53 37 97 15
18	12 96 88 17 31	65 19 69 02 83	60 75 86 90 68	24 64 19 35 51	56 61 87 39 12
19	85 94 57 24 16	92 09 84 38 76	22 00 27 69 85	29 81 94 78 70	21 94 47 90 12
20	38 64 43 59 98	98 77 87 68 07	91 51 67 62 44	40 98 05 93 78	23 32 65 41 18
21	53 44 09 42 72	00 41 86 79 79	68 47 22 00 20	35 55 31 51 51	00 83 63 22 55
22	40 76 66 26 84	57 99 99 90 37	36 63 32 08 58	37 40 13 68 97	87 64 81 07 83
23	02 17 79 18 05	12 59 52 57 02	22 07 90 47 03	28 14 11 30 79	20 69 22 40 98
24	95 17 82 06 53	31 51 10 96 46	92 06 88 07 77	56 11 50 81 69	40 23 72 51 39

(Continued)

Applied Medical Statistics, First Edition. Jingmei Jiang.

Companion website: www.wiley.com\go\jiang\appliedmedicalstatistics

Appendix Table 1 (Continued)

	1–10	11–20	21–30	31–40	41–50
25	35 76 22 42 92	96 11 83 44 80	34 68 35 48 77	33 42 40 90 60	73 96 53 97 86
26	26 29 31 56 41	85 47 04 66 08	34 72 57 59 13	82 43 80 46 15	38 26 61 70 04
27	77 80 20 75 82	72 82 32 99 90	63 95 73 76 63	89 73 44 99 05	48 67 26 43 18
28	46 40 66 44 52	91 36 74 43 53	30 82 13 54 00	78 45 63 98 35	55 03 36 67 68
29	37 56 08 18 09	77 53 84 46 47	31 91 18 95 58	24 16 74 11 53	44 10 13 85 57
30	61 65 61 68 66	37 27 47 39 19	84 83 70 07 48	53 21 40 06 71	95 06 79 88 54
31	93 43 69 64 07	34 18 04 52 35	56 27 09 24 86	61 85 53 83 45	19 90 70 99 00
32	21 96 60 12 99	11 20 99 45 18	48 13 93 55 34	18 37 79 49 90	65 97 38 20 46
33	95 20 47 97 97	27 37 83 28 71	00 06 41 41 74	45 89 09 39 84	51 67 11 52 49
34	97 86 21 78 73	10 65 81 92 59	58 76 17 14 97	04 76 62 16 17	17 95 70 45 80
35	69 92 06 34 13	59 71 74 17 32	27 55 10 24 19	23 71 82 13 74	63 52 52 01 41
36	04 31 17 21 56	33 73 99 19 87	26 72 39 27 67	53 77 57 68 93	60 61 97 22 61
37	61 06 98 03 91	87 14 77 43 96	43 00 65 98 50	45 60 33 01 07	98 99 46 50 47
38	85 93 85 86 88	72 87 08 62 40	16 06 10 89 20	23 21 34 74 97	76 38 03 29 63
39	21 74 32 47 45	73 96 07 94 52	09 65 90 77 47	25 76 16 19 33	53 05 70 53 30
40	15 69 53 82 80	79 96 23 53 10	65 39 07 16 29	45 33 02 43 70	02 87 40 41 45
41	02 89 08 04 49	20 21 14 68 86	87 63 93 95 17	11 29 01 95 80	35 14 97 35 33
42	87 18 15 89 79	85 43 01 72 73	08 61 74 51 69	89 74 39 82 15	94 51 33 41 67
43	98 83 71 94 22	59 97 50 99 52	08 52 85 08 40	87 80 61 65 31	91 51 80 32 44
44	10 08 58 21 66	72 68 49 29 31	89 85 84 46 06	59 73 19 85 23	65 09 29 75 63
45	47 90 56 10 08	88 02 84 27 83	42 29 72 23 19	66 56 45 65 79	20 71 53 20 25
46	22 85 61 68 90	49 64 92 85 44	16 40 12 89 88	50 14 49 81 06	01 82 77 45 12
47	67 80 43 79 33	12 83 11 41 16	25 58 19 68 70	77 02 54 00 52	53 43 37 15 26
48	27 62 50 96 72	79 44 61 40 15	14 53 40 65 39	27 31 58 50 28	11 39 03 34 25
49	33 78 80 87 15	38 30 06 38 21	14 47 47 07 26	54 96 87 53 32	40 36 40 96 76
50	13 13 92 66 99	47 24 49 57 74	32 25 43 62 17	10 97 11 69 84	99 63 22 32 98

Appendix Table 2 Table of random permutation.

	1	2	3	4	5	6	7	8	9	10	11	12	13	14	15	16	17	18	19	20
1	8	6	19	13	5	18	12	1	4	3	9	2	17	14	11	7	16	15	10	0
2	8	19	7	6	11	14	2	13	5	17	9	12	0	16	15	1	4	10	18	3
3	18	1	10	13	17	2	0	3	8	15	7	4	19	12	5	14	9	11	6	16
4	6	19	1	5	18	12	4	0	13	10	16	17	7	14	11	15	8	3	9	2
5	1	2	7	4	18	0	15	13	5	12	19	10	9	14	16	8	6	11	3	17
6	11	19	2	15	14	10	8	12	1	17	4	3	0	9	16	6	13	7	18	5
7	14	3	16	7	9	2	15	12	11	4	13	19	8	1	18	6	0	5	17	10
8	3	2	16	6	1	13	17	19	8	14	0	15	9	18	11	5	4	10	7	12
9	16	9	10	3	15	0	11	2	1	5	18	8	19	13	6	12	17	4	7	14

(Continued)

Appendix Table 2 (Continued)

10	4	11	18	6	0	8	12	16	17	3	2	9	5	7	19	10	15	13	14	1
11	5	15	18	13	7	3	10	14	16	1	8	2	17	6	9	4	0	12	19	11
12	0	18	10	15	11	12	3	13	14	1	17	2	6	9	16	4	7	8	19	5
13	10	9	14	18	12	17	15	3	5	2	11	19	8	0	1	4	7	13	6	16
14	11	9	13	0	14	12	18	7	2	10	4	17	19	6	5	8	3	15	1	16
15	17	1	0	16	9	12	2	4	5	18	14	15	7	19	6	8	11	3	10	13
16	17	1	5	2	8	12	15	13	19	14	7	16	6	3	9	10	4	11	0	18
17	5	16	15	7	18	10	12	9	11	6	13	17	14	1	0	4	3	2	19	8
18	16	19	0	8	6	10	13	17	4	3	15	18	11	1	12	9	5	7	2	14
19	13	9	17	12	15	4	3	1	16	2	10	18	8	6	7	19	14	11	0	5
20	11	12	8	16	3	19	14	17	9	7	4	1	10	0	18	15	6	5	13	2
21	19	12	13	8	4	15	16	7	0	11	1	5	14	18	3	6	10	9	2	17
22	2	18	8	14	6	11	1	9	15	0	17	10	4	7	13	3	12	5	16	19
23	9	16	17	18	5	7	12	2	4	10	0	13	8	3	14	15	6	11	1	19
24	15	0	14	6	1	2	9	8	18	4	10	17	3	12	16	11	19	13	7	5
25	14	0	9	18	6	16	10	4	5	1	19	2	12	3	11	13	7	8	17	15

Appendix Table 3 $\Phi(z)$ of the standard normal distribution.

z	0.00	0.01	0.02	0.03	0.04	0.05	0.06	0.07	0.08	0.09
-3.0	0.0013	0.0013	0.0013	0.0012	0.0012	0.0011	0.0011	0.0011	0.0010	0.0010
-2.9	0.0019	0.0018	0.0018	0.0017	0.0016	0.0016	0.0015	0.0015	0.0014	0.0014
-2.8	0.0026	0.0025	0.0024	0.0023	0.0023	0.0022	0.0021	0.0021	0.0020	0.0019
-2.7	0.0035	0.0034	0.0033	0.0032	0.0031	0.0030	0.0029	0.0028	0.0027	0.0026
-2.6	0.0047	0.0045	0.0044	0.0043	0.0041	0.0040	0.0039	0.0038	0.0037	0.0036
-2.5	0.0062	0.0060	0.0059	0.0057	0.0055	0.0054	0.0052	0.0051	0.0049	0.0048
-2.4	0.0082	0.0080	0.0078	0.0075	0.0073	0.0071	0.0069	0.0068	0.0066	0.0064
-2.3	0.0107	0.0104	0.0102	0.0099	0.0096	0.0094	0.0091	0.0089	0.0087	0.0084
-2.2	0.0139	0.0136	0.0132	0.0129	0.0125	0.0122	0.0119	0.0116	0.0113	0.0110
-2.1	0.0179	0.0174	0.0170	0.0166	0.0162	0.0158	0.0154	0.0150	0.0146	0.0143
-2.0	0.0228	0.0222	0.0217	0.0212	0.0207	0.0202	0.0197	0.0192	0.0188	0.0183
-1.9	0.0287	0.0281	0.0274	0.0268	0.0262	0.0256	0.0250	0.0244	0.0239	0.0233
-1.8	0.0359	0.0351	0.0344	0.0336	0.0329	0.0322	0.0314	0.0307	0.0301	0.0294
-1.7	0.0446	0.0436	0.0427	0.0418	0.0409	0.0401	0.0392	0.0384	0.0375	0.0367
-1.6	0.0548	0.0537	0.0526	0.0516	0.0505	0.0495	0.0485	0.0475	0.0465	0.0455
-1.5	0.0668	0.0655	0.0643	0.0630	0.0618	0.0606	0.0594	0.0582	0.0571	0.0559
-1.4	0.0808	0.0793	0.0778	0.0764	0.0749	0.0735	0.0721	0.0708	0.0694	0.0681
-1.3	0.0968	0.0951	0.0934	0.0918	0.0901	0.0885	0.0869	0.0853	0.0838	0.0823
-1.2	0.1151	0.1131	0.1112	0.1093	0.1075	0.1056	0.1038	0.1020	0.1003	0.0985
-1.1	0.1357	0.1335	0.1314	0.1292	0.1271	0.1251	0.1230	0.1210	0.1190	0.1170

(Continued)

Appendix Table 3 (Continued)

z	0.00	0.01	0.02	0.03	0.04	0.05	0.06	0.07	0.08	0.09
-1.0	0.1587	0.1562	0.1539	0.1515	0.1492	0.1469	0.1446	0.1423	0.1401	0.1379
-0.9	0.1841	0.1814	0.1788	0.1762	0.1736	0.1711	0.1685	0.1660	0.1635	0.1611
-0.8	0.2119	0.2090	0.2061	0.2033	0.2005	0.1977	0.1949	0.1922	0.1894	0.1867
-0.7	0.2420	0.2389	0.2358	0.2327	0.2296	0.2266	0.2236	0.2206	0.2177	0.2148
-0.6	0.2743	0.2709	0.2676	0.2643	0.2611	0.2578	0.2546	0.2514	0.2483	0.2451
-0.5	0.3085	0.3050	0.3015	0.2981	0.2946	0.2912	0.2877	0.2843	0.2810	0.2776
-0.4	0.3446	0.3409	0.3372	0.3336	0.3300	0.3264	0.3228	0.3192	0.3156	0.3121
-0.3	0.3821	0.3783	0.3745	0.3707	0.3669	0.3632	0.3594	0.3557	0.3520	0.3483
-0.2	0.4207	0.4168	0.4129	0.4090	0.4052	0.4013	0.3974	0.3936	0.3897	0.3859
-0.1	0.4602	0.4562	0.4522	0.4483	0.4443	0.4404	0.4364	0.4325	0.4286	0.4247
0.0	0.5000	0.4960	0.4920	0.4880	0.4840	0.4801	0.4761	0.4721	0.4681	0.4641

Note: $\Phi(-z) = 1 - \Phi(z)$

Appendix Table 4 Critical value of the t distribution.

Degrees of freedom v	α										
	One-sided	0.25	0.20	0.10	0.05	0.025	0.01	0.005	0.0025	0.001	0.0005
	Two-sided	0.50	0.40	0.20	0.10	0.05	0.02	0.01	0.005	0.002	0.001
1		1.000	1.376	3.078	6.314	12.706	31.821	63.657	127.321	318.309	636.619
2		0.816	1.061	1.886	2.920	4.303	6.965	9.925	14.089	22.327	31.599
3		0.765	0.978	1.638	2.353	3.182	4.541	5.841	7.453	10.215	12.924
4		0.741	0.941	1.533	2.132	2.776	3.747	4.604	5.598	7.173	8.610
5		0.727	0.920	1.476	2.015	2.571	3.365	4.032	4.773	5.893	6.869
6		0.718	0.906	1.440	1.943	2.447	3.143	3.707	4.317	5.208	5.959
7		0.711	0.896	1.415	1.895	2.365	2.998	3.499	4.029	4.785	5.408
8		0.706	0.889	1.397	1.860	2.306	2.896	3.355	3.833	4.501	5.041
9		0.703	0.883	1.383	1.833	2.262	2.821	3.250	3.690	4.297	4.781
10		0.700	0.879	1.372	1.812	2.228	2.764	3.169	3.581	4.144	4.587
11		0.697	0.876	1.363	1.796	2.201	2.718	3.106	3.497	4.025	4.437
12		0.695	0.873	1.356	1.782	2.179	2.681	3.055	3.428	3.930	4.318
13		0.694	0.870	1.350	1.771	2.160	2.650	3.012	3.372	3.852	4.221
14		0.692	0.868	1.345	1.761	2.145	2.624	2.977	3.326	3.787	4.140
15		0.691	0.866	1.341	1.753	2.131	2.602	2.947	3.286	3.733	4.073
16		0.690	0.865	1.337	1.746	2.120	2.583	2.921	3.252	3.686	4.015
17		0.689	0.863	1.333	1.740	2.110	2.567	2.898	3.222	3.646	3.965

(Continued)

Appendix Table 4 (Continued)

18	0.688	0.862	1.330	1.734	2.101	2.552	2.878	3.197	3.610	3.922
19	0.688	0.861	1.328	1.729	2.093	2.539	2.861	3.174	3.579	3.883
20	0.687	0.860	1.325	1.725	2.086	2.528	2.845	3.153	3.552	3.850
21	0.686	0.859	1.323	1.721	2.080	2.518	2.831	3.135	3.527	3.819
22	0.686	0.858	1.321	1.717	2.074	2.508	2.819	3.119	3.505	3.792
23	0.685	0.858	1.319	1.714	2.069	2.500	2.807	3.104	3.485	3.768
24	0.685	0.857	1.318	1.711	2.064	2.492	2.797	3.091	3.467	3.745
25	0.684	0.856	1.316	1.708	2.060	2.485	2.787	3.078	3.450	3.725
26	0.684	0.856	1.315	1.706	2.056	2.479	2.779	3.067	3.435	3.707
27	0.684	0.855	1.314	1.703	2.052	2.473	2.771	3.057	3.421	3.690
28	0.683	0.855	1.313	1.701	2.048	2.467	2.763	3.047	3.408	3.674
29	0.683	0.854	1.311	1.699	2.045	2.462	2.756	3.038	3.396	3.659
30	0.683	0.854	1.310	1.697	2.042	2.457	2.750	3.030	3.385	3.646
31	0.682	0.853	1.309	1.696	2.040	2.453	2.744	3.022	3.375	3.633
32	0.682	0.853	1.309	1.694	2.037	2.449	2.738	3.015	3.365	3.622
33	0.682	0.853	1.308	1.692	2.035	2.445	2.733	3.008	3.356	3.611
34	0.682	0.852	1.307	1.691	2.032	2.441	2.728	3.002	3.348	3.601
35	0.682	0.852	1.306	1.690	2.030	2.438	2.724	2.996	3.340	3.591
36	0.681	0.852	1.306	1.688	2.028	2.434	2.719	2.990	3.333	3.582
37	0.681	0.851	1.305	1.687	2.026	2.431	2.715	2.985	3.326	3.574
38	0.681	0.851	1.304	1.686	2.024	2.429	2.712	2.980	3.319	3.566
39	0.681	0.851	1.304	1.685	2.023	2.426	2.708	2.976	3.313	3.558
40	0.681	0.851	1.303	1.684	2.021	2.423	2.704	2.971	3.307	3.551
50	0.679	0.849	1.299	1.676	2.009	2.403	2.678	2.937	3.261	3.496
60	0.679	0.848	1.296	1.671	2.000	2.390	2.660	2.915	3.232	3.460
70	0.678	0.847	1.294	1.667	1.994	2.381	2.648	2.899	3.211	3.435
80	0.678	0.846	1.292	1.664	1.990	2.374	2.639	2.887	3.195	3.416
90	0.677	0.846	1.291	1.662	1.987	2.368	2.632	2.878	3.183	3.402
100	0.677	0.845	1.290	1.660	1.984	2.364	2.626	2.871	3.174	3.390
200	0.676	0.843	1.286	1.653	1.972	2.345	2.601	2.839	3.131	3.340
500	0.675	0.842	1.283	1.648	1.965	2.334	2.586	2.820	3.107	3.310
1000	0.675	0.842	1.282	1.646	1.962	2.330	2.581	2.813	3.098	3.300
∞	0.6745	0.8416	1.2816	1.6449	1.9600	2.3263	2.5758	2.8070	3.0902	3.2905

Appendix Table 5 Critical value of the χ^2 distribution.

Degrees of freedom ν	$1-\alpha$												
	0.005	0.010	0.025	0.050	0.100	0.250	0.500	0.750	0.900	0.950	0.975	0.990	0.995
1					0.02	0.10	0.45	1.32	2.71	3.84	5.02	6.63	7.88
2	0.01	0.02	0.05	0.10	0.21	0.58	1.39	2.77	4.61	5.99	7.38	9.21	10.60
3	0.07	0.11	0.22	0.35	0.58	1.21	2.37	4.11	6.25	7.81	9.35	11.34	12.84
4	0.21	0.30	0.48	0.71	1.06	1.92	3.36	5.39	7.78	9.49	11.14	13.28	14.86
5	0.41	0.55	0.83	1.15	1.61	2.67	4.35	6.63	9.24	11.07	12.83	15.09	16.75
6	0.68	0.87	1.24	1.64	2.20	3.45	5.35	7.84	10.64	12.59	14.45	16.81	18.55
7	0.99	1.24	1.69	2.17	2.83	4.25	6.35	9.04	12.02	14.07	16.01	18.48	20.28
8	1.34	1.65	2.18	2.73	3.49	5.07	7.34	10.22	13.36	15.51	17.53	20.09	21.95
9	1.73	2.09	2.70	3.33	4.17	5.90	8.34	11.39	14.68	16.92	19.02	21.67	23.59
10	2.16	2.56	3.25	3.94	4.87	6.74	9.34	12.55	15.99	18.31	20.48	23.21	25.19
11	2.60	3.05	3.82	4.57	5.58	7.58	10.34	13.70	17.28	19.68	21.92	24.72	26.76
12	3.07	3.57	4.40	5.23	6.30	8.44	11.34	14.85	18.55	21.03	23.34	26.22	28.30
13	3.57	4.11	5.01	5.89	7.04	9.30	12.34	15.98	19.81	22.36	24.74	27.69	29.82
14	4.07	4.66	5.63	6.57	7.79	10.17	13.34	17.12	21.06	23.68	26.12	29.14	31.32
15	4.60	5.23	6.26	7.26	8.55	11.04	14.34	18.25	22.31	25.00	27.49	30.58	32.80
16	5.14	5.81	6.91	7.96	9.31	11.91	15.34	19.37	23.54	26.30	28.85	32.00	34.27
17	5.70	6.41	7.56	8.67	10.09	12.79	16.34	20.49	24.77	27.59	30.19	33.41	35.72
18	6.26	7.01	8.23	9.39	10.86	13.68	17.34	21.60	25.99	28.87	31.53	34.81	37.16
19	6.84	7.63	8.91	10.12	11.65	14.56	18.34	22.72	27.20	30.14	32.85	36.19	38.58
20	7.43	8.26	9.59	10.85	12.44	15.45	19.34	23.83	28.41	31.41	34.17	37.57	40.00

21	8.03	8.90	10.28	11.59	13.24	16.34	20.34	24.93	29.62	32.67	35.48	38.93	41.40
22	8.64	9.54	10.98	12.34	14.04	17.24	21.34	26.04	30.81	33.92	36.78	40.29	42.80
23	9.26	10.20	11.69	13.09	14.85	18.14	22.34	27.14	32.01	35.17	38.08	41.64	44.18
24	9.89	10.86	12.40	13.85	15.66	19.04	23.34	28.24	33.20	36.42	39.36	42.98	45.56
25	10.52	11.52	13.12	14.61	16.47	19.94	24.34	29.34	34.38	37.65	40.65	44.31	46.93
26	11.16	12.20	13.84	15.38	17.29	20.84	25.34	30.43	35.56	38.89	41.92	45.64	48.29
27	11.81	12.88	14.57	16.15	18.11	21.75	26.34	31.53	36.74	40.11	43.19	46.96	49.64
28	12.46	13.56	15.31	16.93	18.94	22.66	27.34	32.62	37.92	41.34	44.46	48.28	50.99
29	13.12	14.26	16.05	17.71	19.77	23.57	28.34	33.71	39.09	42.56	45.72	49.59	52.34
30	13.79	14.95	16.79	18.49	20.60	24.48	29.34	34.80	40.26	43.77	46.98	50.89	53.67
40	20.71	22.16	24.43	26.51	29.05	33.66	39.34	45.62	51.81	55.76	59.34	63.69	66.77
50	27.99	29.71	32.36	34.76	37.69	42.94	49.33	56.33	63.17	67.50	71.42	76.15	79.49
60	35.53	37.48	40.48	43.19	46.46	52.29	59.33	66.98	74.40	79.08	83.30	88.38	91.95
70	43.28	45.44	48.76	51.74	55.33	61.70	69.33	77.58	85.53	90.53	95.02	100.43	104.21
80	51.17	53.54	57.15	60.39	64.28	71.14	79.33	88.13	96.58	101.88	106.63	112.33	116.32
90	59.20	61.75	65.65	69.13	73.29	80.62	89.33	98.65	107.57	113.15	118.14	124.12	128.30
100	67.33	70.06	74.22	77.93	82.36	90.13	99.33	109.14	118.50	124.34	129.56	135.81	140.17

Appendix Table 6 Critical value of the F distribution (ANOVA).

$\alpha = 0.10$

ν_2	ν_1																	
	1	**2**	**3**	**4**	**5**	**6**	**7**	**8**	**9**	**10**	**15**	**20**	**30**	**50**	**100**	**200**	**500**	∞
1	39.9	49.5	53.6	55.8	57.2	58.2	58.9	59.4	59.9	60.2	61.2	61.7	62.3	62.7	63.0	63.2	63.3	63.3
2	8.53	9.00	9.16	9.24	9.29	9.33	9.35	9.37	9.38	9.39	9.42	9.44	9.46	9.47	9.48	9.49	9.49	9.49
3	5.54	5.46	5.39	5.34	5.31	5.28	5.27	5.25	5.24	5.23	5.20	5.18	5.17	5.15	5.14	5.14	5.14	5.13
4	4.54	4.32	4.19	4.11	4.05	4.01	3.98	3.95	3.94	3.92	3.87	3.84	3.82	3.80	3.78	3.77	3.76	3.76
5	4.06	3.78	3.62	3.52	3.45	3.40	3.37	3.34	3.32	3.30	3.24	3.21	3.17	3.15	3.13	3.12	3.11	3.10
6	3.78	3.46	3.29	3.18	3.11	3.05	3.01	2.98	2.96	2.94	2.87	2.84	2.80	2.77	2.75	2.73	2.73	2.72
7	3.59	3.26	3.07	2.96	2.88	2.83	2.78	2.75	2.72	2.70	2.63	2.59	2.56	2.52	2.50	2.48	2.48	2.47
8	3.46	3.11	2.92	2.81	2.73	2.67	2.62	2.59	2.56	2.54	2.46	2.42	2.38	2.35	2.32	2.31	2.30	2.29
9	3.36	3.01	2.81	2.69	2.61	2.55	2.51	2.47	2.44	2.42	2.34	2.30	2.25	2.22	2.19	2.17	2.17	2.16
10	3.29	2.92	2.73	2.61	2.52	2.46	2.41	2.38	2.35	2.32	2.24	2.20	2.16	2.12	2.09	2.07	2.06	2.06
11	3.23	2.86	2.66	2.54	2.45	2.39	2.34	2.30	2.27	2.25	2.17	2.12	2.08	2.04	2.01	1.99	1.98	1.97
12	3.18	2.81	2.61	2.48	2.39	2.33	2.28	2.24	2.21	2.19	2.10	2.06	2.01	1.97	1.94	1.92	1.91	1.90
13	3.14	2.76	2.56	2.43	2.35	2.28	2.23	2.20	2.16	2.14	2.05	2.01	1.96	1.92	1.88	1.86	1.85	1.85
14	3.10	2.73	2.52	2.39	2.31	2.24	2.19	2.15	2.12	2.10	2.01	1.96	1.91	1.87	1.83	1.82	1.80	1.80
15	3.07	2.70	2.49	2.36	2.27	2.21	2.16	2.12	2.09	2.06	1.97	1.92	1.87	1.83	1.79	1.77	1.76	1.76
16	3.05	2.67	2.46	2.33	2.24	2.18	2.13	2.09	2.06	2.03	1.94	1.89	1.84	1.79	1.76	1.74	1.73	1.72
17	3.03	2.64	2.44	2.31	2.22	2.15	2.10	2.06	2.03	2.00	1.91	1.86	1.81	1.76	1.73	1.71	1.69	1.69
18	3.01	2.62	2.42	2.29	2.20	2.13	2.08	2.04	2.00	1.98	1.89	1.84	1.78	1.74	1.70	1.68	1.67	1.66
19	2.99	2.61	2.40	2.27	2.18	2.11	2.06	2.02	1.98	1.96	1.86	1.81	1.76	1.71	1.67	1.65	1.64	1.63
20	2.97	2.59	2.38	2.25	2.16	2.09	2.04	2.00	1.96	1.94	1.84	1.79	1.74	1.69	1.65	1.63	1.62	1.61

21	2.96	2.57	2.36	2.23	2.14	2.08	2.02	1.98	1.95	1.92	1.83	1.78	1.72	1.67	1.63	1.61	1.60	1.59
22	2.95	2.56	2.35	2.22	2.13	2.06	2.01	1.97	1.93	1.90	1.81	1.76	1.70	1.65	1.61	1.59	1.58	1.57
23	2.94	2.55	2.34	2.21	2.11	2.05	1.99	1.95	1.92	1.89	1.80	1.74	1.69	1.64	1.59	1.57	1.56	1.55
24	2.93	2.54	2.33	2.19	2.10	2.04	1.98	1.94	1.91	1.88	1.78	1.73	1.67	1.62	1.58	1.56	1.54	1.53
25	2.92	2.53	2.32	2.18	2.09	2.02	1.97	1.93	1.89	1.87	1.77	1.72	1.66	1.61	1.56	1.54	1.53	1.52
26	2.91	2.52	2.31	2.17	2.08	2.01	1.96	1.92	1.88	1.86	1.76	1.71	1.65	1.59	1.55	1.53	1.51	1.50
27	2.90	2.51	2.30	2.17	2.07	2.00	1.95	1.91	1.87	1.85	1.75	1.70	1.64	1.58	1.54	1.52	1.50	1.49
28	2.89	2.50	2.29	2.16	2.06	2.00	1.94	1.90	1.87	1.84	1.74	1.69	1.63	1.57	1.53	1.50	1.49	1.48
29	2.89	2.50	2.28	2.15	2.06	1.99	1.93	1.89	1.86	1.83	1.73	1.68	1.62	1.56	1.52	1.49	1.48	1.47
30	2.88	2.49	2.28	2.14	2.05	1.98	1.93	1.88	1.85	1.82	1.72	1.67	1.61	1.55	1.51	1.48	1.47	1.46
40	2.84	2.44	2.23	2.09	2.00	1.93	1.87	1.83	1.79	1.76	1.66	1.61	1.54	1.48	1.43	1.41	1.39	1.38
50	2.81	2.41	2.20	2.06	1.97	1.90	1.84	1.80	1.76	1.73	1.63	1.57	1.50	1.44	1.39	1.36	1.34	1.33
60	2.79	2.39	2.18	2.04	1.95	1.87	1.82	1.77	1.74	1.71	1.60	1.54	1.48	1.41	1.36	1.33	1.31	1.29
70	2.78	2.38	2.16	2.03	1.93	1.86	1.80	1.76	1.72	1.69	1.59	1.53	1.46	1.39	1.34	1.30	1.28	1.27
80	2.77	2.37	2.15	2.02	1.92	1.85	1.79	1.75	1.71	1.68	1.57	1.51	1.44	1.38	1.32	1.28	1.26	1.24
100	2.76	2.36	2.14	2.00	1.91	1.83	1.78	1.73	1.69	1.66	1.56	1.49	1.42	1.35	1.29	1.26	1.23	1.21
200	2.73	2.33	2.11	1.97	1.88	1.80	1.75	1.70	1.66	1.63	1.52	1.46	1.38	1.31	1.24	1.20	1.17	1.14
500	2.72	2.31	2.09	1.96	1.86	1.79	1.73	1.68	1.64	1.61	1.50	1.44	1.36	1.28	1.21	1.16	1.12	1.09
∞	2.71	2.30	2.08	1.94	1.85	1.77	1.72	1.67	1.63	1.60	1.49	1.42	1.34	1.25	1.18	1.13	1.08	1.00

(Continued)

Appendix Table 6 (Continued)

$\alpha = 0.05$

ν_2	ν_1 1	2	3	4	5	6	7	8	9	10	11	12	13	14	15
1	161.4	199.5	215.7	224.6	230.2	234.0	236.8	238.9	240.5	241.9	243.0	243.9	244.7	245.4	245.9
2	18.51	19.00	19.16	19.25	19.30	19.33	19.35	19.37	19.38	19.40	19.40	19.41	19.42	19.42	19.43
3	10.13	9.55	9.28	9.12	9.01	8.94	8.89	8.85	8.81	8.79	8.76	8.74	8.73	8.71	8.70
4	7.71	6.94	6.59	6.39	6.26	6.16	6.09	6.04	6.00	5.96	5.94	5.91	5.89	5.87	5.86
5	6.61	5.79	5.41	5.19	5.05	4.95	4.88	4.82	4.77	4.74	4.70	4.68	4.66	4.64	4.62
6	5.99	5.14	4.76	4.53	4.39	4.28	4.21	4.15	4.10	4.06	4.03	4.00	3.98	3.96	3.94
7	5.59	4.74	4.35	4.12	3.97	3.87	3.79	3.73	3.68	3.64	3.60	3.57	3.55	3.53	3.51
8	5.32	4.46	4.07	3.84	3.69	3.58	3.50	3.44	3.39	3.35	3.31	3.28	3.26	3.24	3.22
9	5.12	4.26	3.86	3.63	3.48	3.37	3.29	3.23	3.18	3.14	3.10	3.07	3.05	3.03	3.01
10	4.96	4.10	3.71	3.48	3.33	3.22	3.14	3.07	3.02	2.98	2.94	2.91	2.89	2.86	2.85
11	4.84	3.98	3.59	3.36	3.20	3.09	3.01	2.95	2.90	2.85	2.82	2.79	2.76	2.74	2.72
12	4.75	3.89	3.49	3.26	3.11	3.00	2.91	2.85	2.80	2.75	2.72	2.69	2.66	2.64	2.62
13	4.67	3.81	3.41	3.18	3.03	2.92	2.83	2.77	2.71	2.67	2.63	2.60	2.58	2.55	2.53
14	4.60	3.74	3.34	3.11	2.96	2.85	2.76	2.70	2.65	2.60	2.57	2.53	2.51	2.48	2.46
15	4.54	3.68	3.29	3.06	2.90	2.79	2.71	2.64	2.59	2.54	2.51	2.48	2.45	2.42	2.40
16	4.49	3.63	3.24	3.01	2.85	2.74	2.66	2.59	2.54	2.49	2.46	2.42	2.40	2.37	2.35
17	4.45	3.59	3.20	2.96	2.81	2.70	2.61	2.55	2.49	2.45	2.41	2.38	2.35	2.33	2.31
18	4.41	3.55	3.16	2.93	2.77	2.66	2.58	2.51	2.46	2.41	2.37	2.34	2.31	2.29	2.27
19	4.38	3.52	3.13	2.90	2.74	2.63	2.54	2.48	2.42	2.38	2.34	2.31	2.28	2.26	2.23
20	4.35	3.49	3.10	2.87	2.71	2.60	2.51	2.45	2.39	2.35	2.31	2.28	2.25	2.22	2.20

21	4.32	3.47	3.07	2.84	2.68	2.57	2.49	2.42	2.37	2.32	2.28	2.25	2.22	2.20	2.18
22	4.30	3.44	3.05	2.82	2.66	2.55	2.46	2.40	2.34	2.30	2.26	2.23	2.20	2.17	2.15
23	4.28	3.42	3.03	2.80	2.64	2.53	2.44	2.37	2.32	2.27	2.24	2.20	2.18	2.15	2.13
24	4.26	3.40	3.01	2.78	2.62	2.51	2.42	2.36	2.30	2.25	2.22	2.18	2.15	2.13	2.11
25	4.24	3.39	2.99	2.76	2.60	2.49	2.40	2.34	2.28	2.24	2.20	2.16	2.14	2.11	2.09
26	4.23	3.37	2.98	2.74	2.59	2.47	2.39	2.32	2.27	2.22	2.18	2.15	2.12	2.09	2.07
27	4.21	3.35	2.96	2.73	2.57	2.46	2.37	2.31	2.25	2.20	2.17	2.13	2.10	2.08	2.06
28	4.20	3.34	2.95	2.71	2.56	2.45	2.36	2.29	2.24	2.19	2.15	2.12	2.09	2.06	2.04
29	4.18	3.33	2.93	2.70	2.55	2.43	2.35	2.28	2.22	2.18	2.14	2.10	2.08	2.05	2.03
30	4.17	3.32	2.92	2.69	2.53	2.42	2.33	2.27	2.21	2.16	2.13	2.09	2.06	2.04	2.01
32	4.15	3.29	2.90	2.67	2.51	2.40	2.31	2.24	2.19	2.14	2.10	2.07	2.04	2.01	1.99
34	4.13	3.28	2.88	2.65	2.49	2.38	2.29	2.23	2.17	2.12	2.08	2.05	2.02	1.99	1.97
36	4.11	3.26	2.87	2.63	2.48	2.36	2.28	2.21	2.15	2.11	2.07	2.03	2.00	1.98	1.95
38	4.10	3.24	2.85	2.62	2.46	2.35	2.26	2.19	2.14	2.09	2.05	2.02	1.99	1.96	1.94
40	4.08	3.23	2.84	2.61	2.45	2.34	2.25	2.18	2.12	2.08	2.04	2.00	1.97	1.95	1.92
42	4.07	3.22	2.83	2.59	2.44	2.32	2.24	2.17	2.11	2.06	2.03	1.99	1.96	1.94	1.91
44	4.06	3.21	2.82	2.58	2.43	2.31	2.23	2.16	2.10	2.05	2.01	1.98	1.95	1.92	1.90
46	4.05	3.20	2.81	2.57	2.42	2.30	2.22	2.15	2.09	2.04	2.00	1.97	1.94	1.91	1.89
48	4.04	3.19	2.80	2.57	2.41	2.29	2.21	2.14	2.08	2.03	1.99	1.96	1.93	1.90	1.88
50	4.03	3.18	2.79	2.56	2.40	2.29	2.20	2.13	2.07	2.03	1.99	1.95	1.92	1.89	1.87
100	3.94	3.09	2.70	2.46	2.31	2.19	2.10	2.03	1.97	1.93	1.89	1.85	1.82	1.79	1.77
125	3.92	3.07	2.68	2.44	2.29	2.17	2.08	2.01	1.96	1.91	1.87	1.83	1.80	1.77	1.75
150	3.90	3.06	2.66	2.43	2.27	2.16	2.07	2.00	1.94	1.89	1.85	1.82	1.79	1.76	1.73

(Continued)

Appendix Table 6 (Continued)

ν_2	ν_1 1	2	3	4	5	6	7	8	9	10	11	12	13	14	15
200	3.89	3.04	2.65	2.42	2.26	2.14	2.06	1.98	1.93	1.88	1.84	1.80	1.77	1.74	1.72
300	3.87	3.03	2.63	2.40	2.24	2.13	2.04	1.97	1.91	1.86	1.82	1.78	1.75	1.72	1.70
500	3.86	3.01	2.62	2.39	2.23	2.12	2.03	1.96	1.90	1.85	1.81	1.77	1.74	1.71	1.69
1000	3.85	3.00	2.61	2.38	2.22	2.11	2.02	1.95	1.89	1.84	1.80	1.76	1.73	1.70	1.68
∞	3.84	3.00	2.60	2.37	2.21	2.10	2.01	1.94	1.88	1.83	1.79	1.75	1.72	1.69	1.67

$\alpha = 0.05$

ν_2	ν_1 16	18	20	25	30	35	40	45	50	100	200	300	400	500	∞
1	246.5	247.3	248.0	249.3	250.1	250.7	251.1	251.5	251.8	253.0	253.7	253.9	254.0	254.1	254.3
2	19.43	19.44	19.45	19.46	19.46	19.47	19.47	19.47	19.48	19.49	19.49	19.49	19.49	19.49	19.50
3	8.69	8.67	8.66	8.63	8.62	8.60	8.59	8.59	8.58	8.55	8.54	8.54	8.53	8.53	8.53
4	5.84	5.82	5.80	5.77	5.75	5.73	5.72	5.71	5.70	5.66	5.65	5.64	5.64	5.64	5.63
5	4.60	4.58	4.56	4.52	4.50	4.48	4.46	4.45	4.44	4.41	4.39	4.38	4.38	4.37	4.36
6	3.92	3.90	3.87	3.83	3.81	3.79	3.77	3.76	3.75	3.71	3.69	3.68	3.68	3.68	3.67
7	3.49	3.47	3.44	3.40	3.38	3.36	3.34	3.33	3.32	3.27	3.25	3.24	3.24	3.24	3.23
8	3.20	3.17	3.15	3.11	3.08	3.06	3.04	3.03	3.02	2.97	2.95	2.94	2.94	2.94	2.93
9	2.99	2.96	2.94	2.89	2.86	2.84	2.83	2.81	2.80	2.76	2.73	2.72	2.72	2.72	2.71
10	2.83	2.80	2.77	2.73	2.70	2.68	2.66	2.65	2.64	2.59	2.56	2.55	2.55	2.55	2.54
11	2.70	2.67	2.65	2.60	2.57	2.55	2.53	2.52	2.51	2.46	2.43	2.42	2.42	2.42	2.40

12	2.60	2.57	2.54	2.50	2.47	2.44	2.43	2.41	2.40	2.35	2.32	2.31	2.31	2.31	2.30
13	2.51	2.48	2.46	2.41	2.38	2.36	2.34	2.33	2.31	2.26	2.23	2.23	2.22	2.22	2.21
14	2.44	2.41	2.39	2.34	2.31	2.28	2.27	2.25	2.24	2.19	2.16	2.15	2.15	2.14	2.13
15	2.38	2.35	2.33	2.28	2.25	2.22	2.20	2.19	2.18	2.12	2.10	2.09	2.08	2.08	2.07
16	2.33	2.30	2.28	2.23	2.19	2.17	2.15	2.14	2.12	2.07	2.04	2.03	2.02	2.02	2.01
17	2.29	2.26	2.23	2.18	2.15	2.12	2.10	2.09	2.08	2.02	1.99	1.98	1.98	1.97	1.96
18	2.25	2.22	2.19	2.14	2.11	2.08	2.06	2.05	2.04	1.98	1.95	1.94	1.93	1.93	1.92
19	2.21	2.18	2.16	2.11	2.07	2.05	2.03	2.01	2.00	1.94	1.91	1.90	1.89	1.89	1.88
20	2.18	2.15	2.12	2.07	2.04	2.01	1.99	1.98	1.97	1.91	1.88	1.86	1.86	1.86	1.84
21	2.16	2.12	2.10	2.05	2.01	1.98	1.96	1.95	1.94	1.88	1.84	1.83	1.83	1.83	1.81
22	2.13	2.10	2.07	2.02	1.98	1.96	1.94	1.92	1.91	1.85	1.82	1.81	1.80	1.80	1.78
23	2.11	2.08	2.05	2.00	1.96	1.93	1.91	1.90	1.88	1.82	1.79	1.78	1.77	1.77	1.76
24	2.09	2.05	2.03	1.97	1.94	1.91	1.89	1.88	1.86	1.80	1.77	1.76	1.75	1.75	1.73
25	2.07	2.04	2.01	1.96	1.92	1.89	1.87	1.86	1.84	1.78	1.75	1.73	1.73	1.73	1.71
26	2.05	2.02	1.99	1.94	1.90	1.87	1.85	1.84	1.82	1.76	1.73	1.71	1.71	1.71	1.69
27	2.04	2.00	1.97	1.92	1.88	1.86	1.84	1.82	1.81	1.74	1.71	1.70	1.69	1.69	1.67
28	2.02	1.99	1.96	1.91	1.87	1.84	1.82	1.80	1.79	1.73	1.69	1.68	1.67	1.67	1.65
29	2.01	1.97	1.94	1.89	1.85	1.83	1.81	1.79	1.77	1.71	1.67	1.66	1.66	1.65	1.64
30	1.99	1.96	1.93	1.88	1.84	1.81	1.79	1.77	1.76	1.70	1.66	1.65	1.64	1.64	1.62
32	1.97	1.94	1.91	1.85	1.82	1.79	1.77	1.75	1.74	1.67	1.63	1.62	1.61	1.61	1.59
34	1.95	1.92	1.89	1.83	1.80	1.77	1.75	1.73	1.71	1.65	1.61	1.60	1.59	1.59	1.57
36	1.93	1.90	1.87	1.81	1.78	1.75	1.73	1.71	1.69	1.62	1.59	1.57	1.57	1.56	1.55
38	1.92	1.88	1.85	1.80	1.76	1.73	1.71	1.69	1.68	1.61	1.57	1.55	1.55	1.54	1.53

(Continued)

Appendix Table 6 (Continued)

40	1.90	1.87	1.84	1.78	1.74	1.72	1.69	1.67	1.66	1.59	1.55	1.54	1.53	1.53	1.51
42	1.89	1.86	1.83	1.77	1.73	1.70	1.68	1.66	1.65	1.57	1.53	1.52	1.51	1.51	1.49
44	1.88	1.84	1.81	1.76	1.72	1.69	1.67	1.65	1.63	1.56	1.52	1.51	1.50	1.49	1.48
46	1.87	1.83	1.80	1.75	1.71	1.68	1.65	1.64	1.62	1.55	1.51	1.49	1.49	1.48	1.46
48	1.86	1.82	1.79	1.74	1.70	1.67	1.64	1.62	1.61	1.54	1.49	1.48	1.47	1.47	1.45
50	1.85	1.81	1.78	1.73	1.69	1.66	1.63	1.61	1.60	1.52	1.48	1.47	1.46	1.46	1.44
100	1.82	1.78	1.75	1.69	1.65	1.62	1.59	1.57	1.56	1.48	1.44	1.42	1.41	1.41	1.39
125	1.77	1.73	1.70	1.64	1.60	1.57	1.54	1.52	1.51	1.43	1.38	1.36	1.35	1.35	1.32
150	1.75	1.71	1.68	1.62	1.57	1.54	1.52	1.49	1.48	1.39	1.34	1.32	1.31	1.31	1.28
200	1.73	1.69	1.66	1.59	1.55	1.52	1.49	1.47	1.45	1.36	1.31	1.29	1.28	1.27	1.25
300	1.71	1.67	1.64	1.58	1.54	1.50	1.48	1.45	1.44	1.34	1.29	1.27	1.26	1.25	1.22
500	1.69	1.66	1.62	1.56	1.52	1.48	1.46	1.43	1.41	1.32	1.26	1.24	1.23	1.22	1.19
1000	1.68	1.64	1.61	1.54	1.50	1.46	1.43	1.41	1.39	1.30	1.23	1.21	1.20	1.19	1.15
∞	1.66	1.62	1.59	1.53	1.48	1.45	1.42	1.40	1.38	1.28	1.21	1.18	1.17	1.16	1.11

$\alpha = 0.01$

ν_2	ν_1														
	1	**2**	**3**	**4**	**5**	**6**	**7**	**8**	**9**	**10**	**12**	**14**	**16**	**18**	**20**
1	4052	5000	5403	5625	5764	5859	5928	5981	6022	6056	6106	6143	6170	6192	6209
2	98.50	99.00	99.17	99.25	99.30	99.33	99.36	99.37	99.39	99.40	99.42	99.43	99.44	99.44	99.45
3	34.12	30.82	29.46	28.71	28.24	27.91	27.67	27.49	27.35	27.23	27.05	26.92	26.83	26.75	26.69

4	21.20	18.00	16.69	15.98	15.52	15.21	14.98	14.80	14.66	14.55	14.37	14.25	14.15	14.08	14.02
5	16.26	13.27	12.06	11.39	10.97	10.67	10.46	10.29	10.16	10.05	9.89	9.77	9.68	9.61	9.55
6	13.75	10.92	9.78	9.15	8.75	8.47	8.26	8.10	7.98	7.87	7.72	7.60	7.52	7.45	7.40
7	12.25	9.55	8.45	7.85	7.46	7.19	6.99	6.84	6.72	6.62	6.47	6.36	6.28	6.21	6.16
8	11.26	8.65	7.59	7.01	6.63	6.37	6.18	6.03	5.91	5.81	5.67	5.56	5.48	5.41	5.36
9	10.56	8.02	6.99	6.42	6.06	5.80	5.61	5.47	5.35	5.26	5.11	5.01	4.92	4.86	4.81
10	10.04	7.56	6.55	5.99	5.64	5.39	5.20	5.06	4.94	4.85	4.71	4.60	4.52	4.46	4.41
11	9.65	7.21	6.22	5.67	5.32	5.07	4.89	4.74	4.63	4.54	4.40	4.29	4.21	4.15	4.10
12	9.33	6.93	5.95	5.41	5.06	4.82	4.64	4.50	4.39	4.30	4.16	4.05	3.97	3.91	3.86
13	9.07	6.70	5.74	5.21	4.86	4.62	4.44	4.30	4.19	4.10	3.96	3.86	3.78	3.72	3.66
14	8.86	6.51	5.56	5.04	4.69	4.46	4.28	4.14	4.03	3.94	3.80	3.70	3.62	3.56	3.51
15	8.68	6.36	5.42	4.89	4.56	4.32	4.14	4.00	3.89	3.80	3.67	3.56	3.49	3.42	3.37
16	8.53	6.23	5.29	4.77	4.44	4.20	4.03	3.89	3.78	3.69	3.55	3.45	3.37	3.31	3.26
17	8.40	6.11	5.18	4.67	4.34	4.10	3.93	3.79	3.68	3.59	3.46	3.35	3.27	3.21	3.16
18	8.29	6.01	5.09	4.58	4.25	4.01	3.84	3.71	3.60	3.51	3.37	3.27	3.19	3.13	3.08
19	8.18	5.93	5.01	4.50	4.17	3.94	3.77	3.63	3.52	3.43	3.30	3.19	3.12	3.05	3.00
20	8.10	5.85	4.94	4.43	4.10	3.87	3.70	3.56	3.46	3.37	3.23	3.13	3.05	2.99	2.94
21	8.02	5.78	4.87	4.37	4.04	3.81	3.64	3.51	3.40	3.31	3.17	3.07	2.99	2.93	2.88
22	7.95	5.72	4.82	4.31	3.99	3.76	3.59	3.45	3.35	3.26	3.12	3.02	2.94	2.88	2.83
23	7.88	5.66	4.76	4.26	3.94	3.71	3.54	3.41	3.30	3.21	3.07	2.97	2.89	2.83	2.78
24	7.82	5.61	4.72	4.22	3.90	3.67	3.50	3.36	3.26	3.17	3.03	2.93	2.85	2.79	2.74
25	7.77	5.57	4.68	4.18	3.85	3.63	3.46	3.32	3.22	3.13	2.99	2.89	2.81	2.75	2.70
26	7.72	5.53	4.64	4.14	3.82	3.59	3.42	3.29	3.18	3.09	2.96	2.86	2.78	2.72	2.66
27	7.68	5.49	4.60	4.11	3.78	3.56	3.39	3.26	3.15	3.06	2.93	2.82	2.75	2.68	2.63

(Continued)

Appendix Table 6 (Continued)

ν_2	ν_1 1	2	3	4	5	6	7	8	9	10	12	14	16	18	20
28	7.64	5.45	4.57	4.07	3.75	3.53	3.36	3.23	3.12	3.03	2.90	2.79	2.72	2.65	2.60
29	7.60	5.42	4.54	4.04	3.73	3.50	3.33	3.20	3.09	3.00	2.87	2.77	2.69	2.63	2.57
30	7.56	5.39	4.51	4.02	3.70	3.47	3.30	3.17	3.07	2.98	2.84	2.74	2.66	2.60	2.55
32	7.50	5.34	4.46	3.97	3.65	3.43	3.26	3.13	3.02	2.93	2.80	2.70	2.62	2.55	2.50
34	7.44	5.29	4.42	3.93	3.61	3.39	3.22	3.09	2.98	2.89	2.76	2.66	2.58	2.51	2.46
36	7.40	5.25	4.38	3.89	3.57	3.35	3.18	3.05	2.95	2.86	2.72	2.62	2.54	2.48	2.43
38	7.35	5.21	4.34	3.86	3.54	3.32	3.15	3.02	2.92	2.83	2.69	2.59	2.51	2.45	2.40
40	7.31	5.18	4.31	3.83	3.51	3.29	3.12	2.99	2.89	2.80	2.66	2.56	2.48	2.42	2.37
42	7.28	5.15	4.29	3.80	3.49	3.27	3.10	2.97	2.86	2.78	2.64	2.54	2.46	2.40	2.34
44	7.25	5.12	4.26	3.78	3.47	3.24	3.08	2.95	2.84	2.75	2.62	2.52	2.44	2.37	2.32
46	7.22	5.10	4.24	3.76	3.44	3.22	3.06	2.93	2.82	2.73	2.60	2.50	2.42	2.35	2.30
48	7.19	5.08	4.22	3.74	3.43	3.20	3.04	2.91	2.80	2.71	2.58	2.48	2.40	2.33	2.28
50	7.17	5.06	4.20	3.72	3.41	3.19	3.02	2.89	2.78	2.70	2.56	2.46	2.38	2.32	2.27
60	7.08	4.98	4.13	3.65	3.34	3.12	2.95	2.82	2.72	2.63	2.50	2.39	2.31	2.25	2.20
80	6.96	4.88	4.04	3.56	3.26	3.04	2.87	2.74	2.64	2.55	2.42	2.31	2.23	2.17	2.12
100	6.90	4.82	3.98	3.51	3.21	2.99	2.82	2.69	2.59	2.50	2.37	2.27	2.19	2.12	2.07
125	6.84	4.78	3.94	3.47	3.17	2.95	2.79	2.66	2.55	2.47	2.33	2.23	2.15	2.08	2.03
150	6.81	4.75	3.91	3.45	3.14	2.92	2.76	2.63	2.53	2.44	2.31	2.20	2.12	2.06	2.00
200	6.76	4.71	3.88	3.41	3.11	2.89	2.73	2.60	2.50	2.41	2.27	2.17	2.09	2.03	1.97
300	6.72	4.68	3.85	3.38	3.08	2.86	2.70	2.57	2.47	2.38	2.24	2.14	2.06	1.99	1.94
500	6.69	4.65	3.82	3.36	3.05	2.84	2.68	2.55	2.44	2.36	2.22	2.12	2.04	1.97	1.92
1000	6.66	4.63	3.80	3.34	3.04	2.82	2.66	2.53	2.43	2.34	2.20	2.10	2.02	1.95	1.90
∞	6.63	4.61	3.78	3.32	3.02	2.80	2.64	2.51	2.41	2.32	2.18	2.08	2.00	1.93	1.88

$\alpha = 0.01$

ν_2	ν_1														
	22	24	26	28	30	35	40	45	50	60	80	100	200	500	∞
1	6223	6235	6245	6253	6261	6276	6287	6296	6303	6313	6326	6334	6350	6360	6366
2	99.45	99.46	99.46	99.46	99.47	99.47	99.47	99.48	99.48	99.48	99.49	99.49	99.49	99.50	99.50
3	26.64	26.60	26.56	26.53	26.50	26.45	26.41	26.38	26.35	26.32	26.27	26.24	26.18	26.15	26.13
4	13.97	13.93	13.89	13.86	13.84	13.79	13.75	13.71	13.69	13.65	13.61	13.58	13.52	13.49	13.46
5	9.51	9.47	9.43	9.40	9.38	9.33	9.29	9.26	9.24	9.20	9.16	9.13	9.08	9.04	9.02
6	7.35	7.31	7.28	7.25	7.23	7.18	7.14	7.11	7.09	7.06	7.01	6.99	6.93	6.90	6.88
7	6.11	6.07	6.04	6.02	5.99	5.94	5.91	5.88	5.86	5.82	5.78	5.75	5.70	5.67	5.65
8	5.32	5.28	5.25	5.22	5.20	5.15	5.12	5.09	5.07	5.03	4.99	4.96	4.91	4.88	4.86
9	4.77	4.73	4.70	4.67	4.65	4.60	4.57	4.54	4.52	4.48	4.44	4.41	4.36	4.33	4.31
10	4.36	4.33	4.30	4.27	4.25	4.20	4.17	4.14	4.12	4.08	4.04	4.01	3.96	3.93	3.91
11	4.06	4.02	3.99	3.96	3.94	3.89	3.86	3.83	3.81	3.78	3.73	3.71	3.66	3.62	3.60
12	3.82	3.78	3.75	3.72	3.70	3.65	3.62	3.59	3.57	3.54	3.49	3.47	3.41	3.38	3.36
13	3.62	3.59	3.56	3.53	3.51	3.46	3.43	3.40	3.38	3.34	3.30	3.27	3.22	3.19	3.17
14	3.46	3.43	3.40	3.37	3.35	3.30	3.27	3.24	3.22	3.18	3.14	3.11	3.06	3.03	3.01
15	3.33	3.29	3.26	3.24	3.21	3.17	3.13	3.10	3.08	3.05	3.00	2.98	2.92	2.89	2.87
16	3.22	3.18	3.15	3.12	3.10	3.05	3.02	2.99	2.97	2.93	2.89	2.86	2.81	2.78	2.75
17	3.12	3.08	3.05	3.03	3.00	2.96	2.92	2.89	2.87	2.83	2.79	2.76	2.71	2.68	2.65
18	3.03	3.00	2.97	2.94	2.92	2.87	2.84	2.81	2.78	2.75	2.70	2.68	2.62	2.59	2.57
19	2.96	2.92	2.89	2.87	2.84	2.80	2.76	2.73	2.71	2.67	2.63	2.60	2.55	2.51	2.49
20	2.90	2.86	2.83	2.80	2.78	2.73	2.69	2.67	2.64	2.61	2.56	2.54	2.48	2.44	2.42

(Continued)

Appendix Table 6 (Continued)

ν_2	ν_1														
	1	2	3	4	5	6	7	8	9	10	12	14	16	18	20
21	2.84	2.80	2.77	2.74	2.72	2.67	2.64	2.61	2.58	2.55	2.50	2.48	2.42	2.38	2.36
22	2.78	2.75	2.72	2.69	2.67	2.62	2.58	2.55	2.53	2.50	2.45	2.42	2.36	2.33	2.31
23	2.74	2.70	2.67	2.64	2.62	2.57	2.54	2.51	2.48	2.45	2.40	2.37	2.32	2.28	2.26
24	2.70	2.66	2.63	2.60	2.58	2.53	2.49	2.46	2.44	2.40	2.36	2.33	2.27	2.24	2.21
25	2.66	2.62	2.59	2.56	2.54	2.49	2.45	2.42	2.40	2.36	2.32	2.29	2.23	2.19	2.17
26	2.62	2.58	2.55	2.53	2.50	2.45	2.42	2.39	2.36	2.33	2.28	2.25	2.19	2.16	2.13
27	2.59	2.55	2.52	2.49	2.47	2.42	2.38	2.35	2.33	2.29	2.25	2.22	2.16	2.12	2.10
28	2.56	2.52	2.49	2.46	2.44	2.39	2.35	2.32	2.30	2.26	2.22	2.19	2.13	2.09	2.07
29	2.53	2.49	2.46	2.44	2.41	2.36	2.33	2.30	2.27	2.23	2.19	2.16	2.10	2.06	2.04
30	2.51	2.47	2.44	2.41	2.39	2.34	2.30	2.27	2.25	2.21	2.16	2.13	2.07	2.03	2.01
32	2.46	2.42	2.39	2.36	2.34	2.29	2.25	2.22	2.20	2.16	2.11	2.08	2.02	1.98	1.96
34	2.42	2.38	2.35	2.32	2.30	2.25	2.21	2.18	2.16	2.12	2.07	2.04	1.98	1.94	1.91
36	2.38	2.35	2.32	2.29	2.26	2.21	2.18	2.14	2.12	2.08	2.03	2.00	1.94	1.90	1.87
38	2.35	2.32	2.28	2.26	2.23	2.18	2.14	2.11	2.09	2.05	2.00	1.97	1.90	1.86	1.84
40	2.33	2.29	2.26	2.23	2.20	2.15	2.11	2.08	2.06	2.02	1.97	1.94	1.87	1.83	1.81
42	2.30	2.26	2.23	2.20	2.18	2.13	2.09	2.06	2.03	1.99	1.94	1.91	1.85	1.80	1.78
44	2.28	2.24	2.21	2.18	2.15	2.10	2.07	2.03	2.01	1.97	1.92	1.89	1.82	1.78	1.75
46	2.26	2.22	2.19	2.16	2.13	2.08	2.04	2.01	1.99	1.95	1.90	1.86	1.80	1.76	1.73
48	2.24	2.20	2.17	2.14	2.12	2.06	2.02	1.99	1.97	1.93	1.88	1.84	1.78	1.73	1.71
50	2.22	2.18	2.15	2.12	2.10	2.05	2.01	1.97	1.95	1.91	1.86	1.82	1.76	1.71	1.68

60	2.15	2.12	2.08	2.05	2.03	1.98	1.94	1.90	1.88	1.84	1.78	1.75	1.68	1.63	1.60
80	2.07	2.03	2.00	1.97	1.94	1.89	1.85	1.82	1.79	1.75	1.69	1.65	1.58	1.53	1.50
100	2.02	1.98	1.95	1.92	1.89	1.84	1.80	1.76	1.74	1.69	1.63	1.60	1.52	1.47	1.43
125	1.98	1.94	1.91	1.88	1.85	1.80	1.76	1.72	1.69	1.65	1.59	1.55	1.47	1.41	1.37
150	1.96	1.92	1.88	1.85	1.83	1.77	1.73	1.69	1.66	1.62	1.56	1.52	1.43	1.38	1.33
200	1.93	1.89	1.85	1.82	1.79	1.74	1.69	1.66	1.63	1.58	1.52	1.48	1.39	1.33	1.28
300	1.89	1.85	1.82	1.79	1.76	1.70	1.66	1.62	1.59	1.55	1.48	1.44	1.35	1.28	1.22
500	1.87	1.83	1.79	1.76	1.74	1.68	1.63	1.60	1.57	1.52	1.45	1.41	1.31	1.23	1.17
1000	1.85	1.81	1.77	1.74	1.72	1.66	1.61	1.58	1.54	1.50	1.43	1.38	1.28	1.19	1.12
∞	1.83	1.79	1.76	1.72	1.70	1.64	1.59	1.55	1.52	1.47	1.40	1.36	1.25	1.15	1.00

Appendix Table 7 Critical value of the F distribution (Test of homogeneity of variances, for two-sided test).

$\alpha = 0.10$

ν_2	ν_1														
	1	2	3	4	5	6	7	8	9	10	11	12	13	14	15
1	161.4	199.5	215.7	224.6	230.2	234.0	236.8	238.9	240.5	241.9	243.0	243.9	244.7	245.4	245.9
2	18.51	19.00	19.16	19.25	19.30	19.33	19.35	19.37	19.38	19.40	19.40	19.41	19.42	19.42	19.43
3	10.13	9.55	9.28	9.12	9.01	8.94	8.89	8.85	8.81	8.79	8.76	8.74	8.73	8.71	8.70
4	7.71	6.94	6.59	6.39	6.26	6.16	6.09	6.04	6.00	5.96	5.94	5.91	5.89	5.87	5.86
5	6.61	5.79	5.41	5.19	5.05	4.95	4.88	4.82	4.77	4.74	4.70	4.68	4.66	4.64	4.62
6	5.99	5.14	4.76	4.53	4.39	4.28	4.21	4.15	4.10	4.06	4.03	4.00	3.98	3.96	3.94
7	5.59	4.74	4.35	4.12	3.97	3.87	3.79	3.73	3.68	3.64	3.60	3.57	3.55	3.53	3.51
8	5.32	4.46	4.07	3.84	3.69	3.58	3.50	3.44	3.39	3.35	3.31	3.28	3.26	3.24	3.22
9	5.12	4.26	3.86	3.63	3.48	3.37	3.29	3.23	3.18	3.14	3.10	3.07	3.05	3.03	3.01
10	4.96	4.10	3.71	3.48	3.33	3.22	3.14	3.07	3.02	2.98	2.94	2.91	2.89	2.86	2.85
11	4.84	3.98	3.59	3.36	3.20	3.09	3.01	2.95	2.90	2.85	2.82	2.79	2.76	2.74	2.72
12	4.75	3.89	3.49	3.26	3.11	3.00	2.91	2.85	2.80	2.75	2.72	2.69	2.66	2.64	2.62
13	4.67	3.81	3.41	3.18	3.03	2.92	2.83	2.77	2.71	2.67	2.63	2.60	2.58	2.55	2.53
14	4.60	3.74	3.34	3.11	2.96	2.85	2.76	2.70	2.65	2.60	2.57	2.53	2.51	2.48	2.46
15	4.54	3.68	3.29	3.06	2.90	2.79	2.71	2.64	2.59	2.54	2.51	2.48	2.45	2.42	2.40
16	4.49	3.63	3.24	3.01	2.85	2.74	2.66	2.59	2.54	2.49	2.46	2.42	2.40	2.37	2.35
17	4.45	3.59	3.20	2.96	2.81	2.70	2.61	2.55	2.49	2.45	2.41	2.38	2.35	2.33	2.31
18	4.41	3.55	3.16	2.93	2.77	2.66	2.58	2.51	2.46	2.41	2.37	2.34	2.31	2.29	2.27
19	4.38	3.52	3.13	2.90	2.74	2.63	2.54	2.48	2.42	2.38	2.34	2.31	2.28	2.26	2.23

20	4.35	3.49	3.10	2.87	2.71	2.60	2.51	2.45	2.39	2.35	2.31	2.28	2.25	2.22	2.20
21	4.32	3.47	3.07	2.84	2.68	2.57	2.49	2.42	2.37	2.32	2.28	2.25	2.22	2.20	2.18
22	4.30	3.44	3.05	2.82	2.66	2.55	2.46	2.40	2.34	2.30	2.26	2.23	2.20	2.17	2.15
23	4.28	3.42	3.03	2.80	2.64	2.53	2.44	2.37	2.32	2.27	2.24	2.20	2.18	2.15	2.13
24	4.26	3.40	3.01	2.78	2.62	2.51	2.42	2.36	2.30	2.25	2.22	2.18	2.15	2.13	2.11
25	4.24	3.39	2.99	2.76	2.60	2.49	2.40	2.34	2.28	2.24	2.20	2.16	2.14	2.11	2.09
26	4.23	3.37	2.98	2.74	2.59	2.47	2.39	2.32	2.27	2.22	2.18	2.15	2.12	2.09	2.07
27	4.21	3.35	2.96	2.73	2.57	2.46	2.37	2.31	2.25	2.20	2.17	2.13	2.10	2.08	2.06
28	4.20	3.34	2.95	2.71	2.56	2.45	2.36	2.29	2.24	2.19	2.15	2.12	2.09	2.06	2.04
29	4.18	3.33	2.93	2.70	2.55	2.43	2.35	2.28	2.22	2.18	2.14	2.10	2.08	2.05	2.03
30	4.17	3.32	2.92	2.69	2.53	2.42	2.33	2.27	2.21	2.16	2.13	2.09	2.06	2.04	2.01
32	4.15	3.29	2.90	2.67	2.51	2.40	2.31	2.24	2.19	2.14	2.10	2.07	2.04	2.01	1.99
34	4.13	3.28	2.88	2.65	2.49	2.38	2.29	2.23	2.17	2.12	2.08	2.05	2.02	1.99	1.97
36	4.11	3.26	2.87	2.63	2.48	2.36	2.28	2.21	2.15	2.11	2.07	2.03	2.00	1.98	1.95
38	4.10	3.24	2.85	2.62	2.46	2.35	2.26	2.19	2.14	2.09	2.05	2.02	1.99	1.96	1.94
40	4.08	3.23	2.84	2.61	2.45	2.34	2.25	2.18	2.12	2.08	2.04	2.00	1.97	1.95	1.92
42	4.07	3.22	2.83	2.59	2.44	2.32	2.24	2.17	2.11	2.06	2.03	1.99	1.96	1.94	1.91
44	4.06	3.21	2.82	2.58	2.43	2.31	2.23	2.16	2.10	2.05	2.01	1.98	1.95	1.92	1.90
46	4.05	3.20	2.81	2.57	2.42	2.30	2.22	2.15	2.09	2.04	2.00	1.97	1.94	1.91	1.89
48	4.04	3.19	2.80	2.57	2.41	2.29	2.21	2.14	2.08	2.03	1.99	1.96	1.93	1.90	1.88
50	4.03	3.18	2.79	2.56	2.40	2.29	2.20	2.13	2.07	2.03	1.99	1.95	1.92	1.89	1.87
100	3.94	3.09	2.70	2.46	2.31	2.19	2.10	2.03	1.97	1.93	1.89	1.85	1.82	1.79	1.77
125	3.92	3.07	2.68	2.44	2.29	2.17	2.08	2.01	1.96	1.91	1.87	1.83	1.80	1.77	1.75
150	3.90	3.06	2.66	2.43	2.27	2.16	2.07	2.00	1.94	1.89	1.85	1.82	1.79	1.76	1.73

(Continued)

Appendix Table 7 (Continued)

ν_2	ν_1 1	2	3	4	5	6	7	8	9	10	11	12	13	14	15
200	3.89	3.04	2.65	2.42	2.26	2.14	2.06	1.98	1.93	1.88	1.84	1.80	1.77	1.74	1.72
300	3.87	3.03	2.63	2.40	2.24	2.13	2.04	1.97	1.91	1.86	1.82	1.78	1.75	1.72	1.70
500	3.86	3.01	2.62	2.39	2.23	2.12	2.03	1.96	1.90	1.85	1.81	1.77	1.74	1.71	1.69
1000	3.85	3.00	2.61	2.38	2.22	2.11	2.02	1.95	1.89	1.84	1.80	1.76	1.73	1.70	1.68
∞	3.84	3.00	2.60	2.37	2.21	2.10	2.01	1.94	1.88	1.83	1.79	1.75	1.72	1.69	1.67

$\alpha = 0.05$

ν_2	ν_1 16	18	20	25	30	35	40	45	50	100	200	300	400	500	∞
1	246.5	247.3	248.0	249.3	250.1	250.7	251.1	251.5	251.8	253.0	253.7	253.9	254.0	254.1	254.3
2	19.43	19.44	19.45	19.46	19.46	19.47	19.47	19.47	19.48	19.49	19.49	19.49	19.49	19.49	19.50
3	8.69	8.67	8.66	8.63	8.62	8.60	8.59	8.59	8.58	8.55	8.54	8.54	8.53	8.53	8.53
4	5.84	5.82	5.80	5.77	5.75	5.73	5.72	5.71	5.70	5.66	5.65	5.64	5.64	5.64	5.63
5	4.60	4.58	4.56	4.52	4.50	4.48	4.46	4.45	4.44	4.41	4.39	4.38	4.38	4.37	4.36
6	3.92	3.90	3.87	3.83	3.81	3.79	3.77	3.76	3.75	3.71	3.69	3.68	3.68	3.68	3.67
7	3.49	3.47	3.44	3.40	3.38	3.36	3.34	3.33	3.32	3.27	3.25	3.24	3.24	3.24	3.23
8	3.20	3.17	3.15	3.11	3.08	3.06	3.04	3.03	3.02	2.97	2.95	2.94	2.94	2.94	2.93
9	2.99	2.96	2.94	2.89	2.86	2.84	2.83	2.81	2.80	2.76	2.73	2.72	2.72	2.72	2.71
10	2.83	2.80	2.77	2.73	2.70	2.68	2.66	2.65	2.64	2.59	2.56	2.55	2.55	2.55	2.54
11	2.70	2.67	2.65	2.60	2.57	2.55	2.53	2.52	2.51	2.46	2.43	2.42	2.42	2.42	2.40

12	2.60	2.57	2.54	2.50	2.47	2.44	2.43	2.41	2.40	2.35	2.32	2.31	2.31	2.31	2.30
13	2.51	2.48	2.46	2.41	2.38	2.36	2.34	2.33	2.31	2.26	2.23	2.23	2.22	2.22	2.21
14	2.44	2.41	2.39	2.34	2.31	2.28	2.27	2.25	2.24	2.19	2.16	2.15	2.15	2.14	2.13
15	2.38	2.35	2.33	2.28	2.25	2.22	2.20	2.19	2.18	2.12	2.10	2.09	2.08	2.08	2.07
16	2.33	2.30	2.28	2.23	2.19	2.17	2.15	2.14	2.12	2.07	2.04	2.03	2.02	2.02	2.01
17	2.29	2.26	2.23	2.18	2.15	2.12	2.10	2.09	2.08	2.02	1.99	1.98	1.98	1.97	1.96
18	2.25	2.22	2.19	2.14	2.11	2.08	2.06	2.05	2.04	1.98	1.95	1.94	1.93	1.93	1.92
19	2.21	2.18	2.16	2.11	2.07	2.05	2.03	2.01	2.00	1.94	1.91	1.90	1.89	1.89	1.88
20	2.18	2.15	2.12	2.07	2.04	2.01	1.99	1.98	1.97	1.91	1.88	1.86	1.86	1.86	1.84
21	2.16	2.12	2.10	2.05	2.01	1.98	1.96	1.95	1.94	1.88	1.84	1.83	1.83	1.83	1.81
22	2.13	2.10	2.07	2.02	1.98	1.96	1.94	1.92	1.91	1.85	1.82	1.81	1.80	1.80	1.78
23	2.11	2.08	2.05	2.00	1.96	1.93	1.91	1.90	1.88	1.82	1.79	1.78	1.77	1.77	1.76
24	2.09	2.05	2.03	1.97	1.94	1.91	1.89	1.88	1.86	1.80	1.77	1.76	1.75	1.75	1.73
25	2.07	2.04	2.01	1.96	1.92	1.89	1.87	1.86	1.84	1.78	1.75	1.73	1.73	1.73	1.71
26	2.05	2.02	1.99	1.94	1.90	1.87	1.85	1.84	1.82	1.76	1.73	1.71	1.71	1.71	1.69
27	2.04	2.00	1.97	1.92	1.88	1.86	1.84	1.82	1.81	1.74	1.71	1.70	1.69	1.69	1.67
28	2.02	1.99	1.96	1.91	1.87	1.84	1.82	1.80	1.79	1.73	1.69	1.68	1.67	1.67	1.65
29	2.01	1.97	1.94	1.89	1.85	1.83	1.81	1.79	1.77	1.71	1.67	1.66	1.66	1.65	1.64
30	1.99	1.96	1.93	1.88	1.84	1.81	1.79	1.77	1.76	1.70	1.66	1.65	1.64	1.64	1.62
32	1.97	1.94	1.91	1.85	1.82	1.79	1.77	1.75	1.74	1.67	1.63	1.62	1.61	1.61	1.59
34	1.95	1.92	1.89	1.83	1.80	1.77	1.75	1.73	1.71	1.65	1.61	1.60	1.59	1.59	1.57
36	1.93	1.90	1.87	1.81	1.78	1.75	1.73	1.71	1.69	1.62	1.59	1.57	1.57	1.56	1.55
38	1.92	1.88	1.85	1.80	1.76	1.73	1.71	1.69	1.68	1.61	1.57	1.55	1.55	1.54	1.53
40	1.90	1.87	1.84	1.78	1.74	1.72	1.69	1.67	1.66	1.59	1.55	1.54	1.53	1.53	1.51

(Continued)

Appendix Table 7 (Continued)

ν_2	ν_1														
	16	**18**	**20**	**25**	**30**	**35**	**40**	**45**	**50**	**100**	**200**	**300**	**400**	**500**	∞
42	1.89	1.86	1.83	1.77	1.73	1.70	1.68	1.66	1.65	1.57	1.53	1.52	1.51	1.51	1.49
44	1.88	1.84	1.81	1.76	1.72	1.69	1.67	1.65	1.63	1.56	1.52	1.51	1.50	1.49	1.48
46	1.87	1.83	1.80	1.75	1.71	1.68	1.65	1.64	1.62	1.55	1.51	1.49	1.49	1.48	1.46
48	1.86	1.82	1.79	1.74	1.70	1.67	1.64	1.62	1.61	1.54	1.49	1.48	1.47	1.47	1.45
50	1.85	1.81	1.78	1.73	1.69	1.66	1.63	1.61	1.60	1.52	1.48	1.47	1.46	1.46	1.44
100	1.82	1.78	1.75	1.69	1.65	1.62	1.59	1.57	1.56	1.48	1.44	1.42	1.41	1.41	1.39
125	1.77	1.73	1.70	1.64	1.60	1.57	1.54	1.52	1.51	1.43	1.38	1.36	1.35	1.35	1.32
150	1.75	1.71	1.68	1.62	1.57	1.54	1.52	1.49	1.48	1.39	1.34	1.32	1.31	1.31	1.28
200	1.73	1.69	1.66	1.59	1.55	1.52	1.49	1.47	1.45	1.36	1.31	1.29	1.28	1.27	1.25
300	1.71	1.67	1.64	1.58	1.54	1.50	1.48	1.45	1.44	1.34	1.29	1.27	1.26	1.25	1.22
500	1.69	1.66	1.62	1.56	1.52	1.48	1.46	1.43	1.41	1.32	1.26	1.24	1.23	1.22	1.19
1000	1.68	1.64	1.61	1.54	1.50	1.46	1.43	1.41	1.39	1.30	1.23	1.21	1.20	1.19	1.15
∞	1.66	1.62	1.59	1.53	1.48	1.45	1.42	1.40	1.38	1.28	1.21	1.18	1.17	1.16	1.11

$\alpha = 0.05$

ν_2	ν_1														
	1	**2**	**3**	**4**	**5**	**6**	**7**	**8**	**9**	**10**	**11**	**12**	**13**	**14**	**15**
1	647.8	799.5	864.2	899.6	921.8	937.1	948.2	956.7	963.3	968.6	973.0	976.7	979.8	982.5	984.9
2	38.51	39.00	39.17	39.25	39.30	39.33	39.36	39.37	39.39	39.40	19.40	39.41	39.42	39.43	39.43
3	17.44	16.04	15.44	15.10	14.88	14.73	14.62	14.54	14.47	14.42	14.37	14.34	14.30	14.28	14.25
4	12.22	10.65	9.98	9.60	9.36	9.20	9.07	8.98	8.90	8.84	8.79	8.75	8.71	8.68	8.66
5	10.01	8.43	7.76	7.39	7.15	6.98	6.85	6.76	6.68	6.62	6.57	6.52	6.49	6.46	6.43

6	8.81	7.26	6.60	6.23	5.99	5.82	5.70	5.60	5.52	5.46	5.41	5.37	5.33	5.30	5.27
7	8.07	6.54	5.89	5.52	5.29	5.12	4.99	4.90	4.82	4.76	4.71	4.67	4.63	4.60	4.57
8	7.57	6.06	5.42	5.05	4.82	4.65	4.53	4.43	4.36	4.30	4.24	4.20	4.16	4.13	4.10
9	7.21	5.71	5.08	4.72	4.48	4.32	4.20	4.10	4.03	3.96	3.91	3.87	3.83	3.80	3.77
10	6.94	5.46	4.83	4.47	4.24	4.07	3.95	3.85	3.78	3.72	3.66	3.62	3.58	3.55	3.52
11	6.72	5.26	4.63	4.28	4.04	3.88	3.76	3.66	3.59	3.53	3.47	3.43	3.39	3.36	3.33
12	6.55	5.10	4.47	4.12	3.89	3.73	3.61	3.51	3.44	3.37	3.32	3.28	3.24	3.21	3.18
13	6.41	4.97	4.35	4.00	3.77	3.60	3.48	3.39	3.31	3.25	3.20	3.15	3.12	3.08	3.05
14	6.30	4.86	4.24	3.89	3.66	3.50	3.38	3.29	3.21	3.15	3.09	3.05	3.01	2.98	2.95
15	6.20	4.77	4.15	3.80	3.58	3.41	3.29	3.20	3.12	3.06	3.01	2.96	2.92	2.89	2.86
16	6.12	4.69	4.08	3.73	3.50	3.34	3.22	3.12	3.05	2.99	2.93	2.89	2.85	2.82	2.79
17	6.04	4.62	4.01	3.66	3.44	3.28	3.16	3.06	2.98	2.92	2.87	2.82	2.79	2.75	2.72
18	5.98	4.56	3.95	3.61	3.38	3.22	3.10	3.01	2.93	2.87	2.81	2.77	2.73	2.7	2.67
19	5.92	4.51	3.90	3.56	3.33	3.17	3.05	2.96	2.88	2.82	2.76	2.72	2.68	2.65	2.62
20	5.87	4.46	3.86	3.51	3.29	3.13	3.01	2.91	2.84	2.77	2.72	2.68	2.64	2.60	2.57
21	5.83	4.42	3.82	3.48	3.25	3.09	2.97	2.87	2.80	2.73	2.68	2.64	2.60	2.56	2.53
22	5.79	4.38	3.78	3.44	3.22	3.05	2.93	2.84	2.76	2.70	2.65	2.6	2.56	2.53	2.50
23	5.75	4.35	3.75	3.41	3.18	3.02	2.90	2.81	2.73	2.67	2.62	2.57	2.53	2.50	2.47
24	5.72	4.32	3.72	3.38	3.15	2.99	2.87	2.78	2.70	2.64	2.59	2.54	2.50	2.47	2.44
25	5.69	4.29	3.69	3.35	3.13	2.97	2.85	2.75	2.68	2.61	2.56	2.51	2.48	2.44	2.41
26	5.66	4.27	3.67	3.33	3.10	2.94	2.82	2.73	2.65	2.59	2.54	2.49	2.45	2.42	2.39
27	5.63	4.24	3.65	3.31	3.08	2.92	2.80	2.71	2.63	2.57	2.51	2.47	2.43	2.39	2.36
28	5.61	4.22	3.63	3.29	3.06	2.90	2.78	2.69	2.61	2.55	2.49	2.45	2.41	2.37	2.34
29	5.59	4.20	3.61	3.27	3.04	2.88	2.76	2.67	2.59	2.53	2.48	2.43	2.39	2.36	2.32

(Continued)

Appendix Table 7 (Continued)

ν_2	ν_1														
	1	**2**	**3**	**4**	**5**	**6**	**7**	**8**	**9**	**10**	**11**	**12**	**13**	**14**	**15**
30	5.57	4.18	3.59	3.25	3.03	2.87	2.75	2.65	2.57	2.51	2.46	2.41	2.37	2.34	2.31
32	5.53	4.15	3.56	3.22	3.00	2.84	2.71	2.62	2.54	2.48	2.43	2.38	2.34	2.31	2.28
34	5.50	4.12	3.53	3.19	2.97	2.81	2.69	2.59	2.52	2.45	2.40	2.35	2.31	2.28	2.25
36	5.47	4.09	3.50	3.17	2.94	2.78	2.66	2.57	2.49	2.43	2.43	2.33	2.29	2.25	2.22
38	5.45	4.07	3.48	3.15	2.92	2.76	2.64	2.55	2.47	2.41	2.35	2.31	2.27	2.23	2.20
40	5.42	4.05	3.46	3.13	2.90	2.74	2.62	2.53	2.45	2.39	2.33	2.29	2.25	2.21	2.18
42	5.40	4.03	3.45	3.11	2.89	2.73	2.61	2.51	2.43	2.37	2.32	2.27	2.23	2.20	2.16
44	5.39	4.02	3.43	3.09	2.87	2.71	2.59	2.50	2.42	2.36	2.30	2.26	2.22	2.18	2.15
46	5.37	4.00	3.42	3.08	2.86	2.70	2.58	2.48	2.41	2.34	2.29	2.24	2.20	2.17	2.13
48	5.35	3.99	3.40	3.07	2.84	2.69	2.56	2.47	2.39	2.33	2.27	2.23	2.19	2.15	2.12
50	5.34	3.97	3.39	3.05	2.83	2.67	2.55	2.46	2.38	2.32	2.26	2.22	2.18	2.14	2.11
60	5.29	3.93	3.34	3.01	2.79	2.63	2.51	2.41	2.33	2.27	2.22	2.17	2.13	2.09	2.06
80	5.22	3.86	3.28	2.95	2.73	2.57	2.45	2.35	2.28	2.21	2.16	2.11	2.07	2.03	2.00
100	5.18	3.83	3.25	2.92	2.70	2.54	2.42	2.32	2.24	2.18	2.12	2.08	2.04	2.00	1.97
125	5.15	3.80	3.22	2.89	2.67	2.51	2.39	2.30	2.22	2.15	2.10	2.05	2.01	1.97	1.94
150	5.13	3.78	3.20	2.87	2.65	2.49	2.37	2.28	2.20	2.13	2.02	2.03	1.99	1.95	1.92
200	5.10	3.76	3.18	2.85	2.63	2.47	2.35	2.26	2.18	2.11	2.06	2.01	1.97	1.93	1.90
300	5.07	3.73	3.16	2.83	2.61	2.45	2.33	2.23	2.16	2.09	2.04	1.99	1.95	1.91	1.88
500	5.05	3.72	3.14	2.81	2.59	2.43	2.31	2.22	2.14	2.07	2.02	1.97	1.93	1.89	1.86
1000	5.04	3.70	3.13	2.80	2.58	2.42	2.30	2.20	2.13	2.06	2.01	1.96	1.92	1.88	1.85
∞	5.03	3.69	3.12	2.79	2.57	2.41	2.29	2.19	2.11	2.05	1.99	1.94	1.90	1.87	1.83

$\alpha = 0.05$

ν_2	ν_1														
	16	18	20	25	30	35	40	45	50	100	200	300	400	500	∞
1	986.9	990.3	993.1	998.1	1001.4	1003.8	1005.6	1007.0	1008.1	1013.2	1015.7	1016.6	1017.0	1017	1018
2	39.44	39.44	39.45	39.46	39.46	39.47	39.47	39.48	39.48	39.49	39.49	39.49	39.50	39.50	39.50
3	14.23	14.2	14.17	14.12	14.08	14.06	14.04	14.02	14.01	13.96	13.93	13.92	13.92	13.91	13.90
4	8.63	8.59	8.56	8.50	8.46	8.43	8.41	8.39	8.38	8.32	8.29	8.28	8.27	8.27	8.26
5	6.40	6.36	6.33	6.27	6.23	6.20	6.18	6.16	6.14	6.08	6.05	6.04	6.03	6.03	6.02
6	5.24	5.20	5.17	5.11	5.07	5.04	5.01	4.99	4.98	4.92	4.88	4.87	4.87	4.86	4.85
7	4.54	4.50	4.47	4.40	4.36	4.33	4.31	4.29	4.28	4.21	4.18	4.17	4.16	4.16	4.14
8	4.08	4.03	4.00	3.94	3.89	3.86	3.84	3.82	3.81	3.74	3.70	3.69	3.69	3.68	3.67
9	3.74	3.70	3.67	3.60	3.56	3.53	3.51	3.49	3.47	3.40	3.37	3.36	3.35	3.35	3.33
10	3.50	3.45	3.42	3.35	3.31	3.28	3.26	3.24	3.22	3.15	3.12	3.10	3.10	3.09	3.08
11	3.30	3.26	3.23	3.16	3.12	3.09	3.06	3.04	3.03	2.96	2.92	2.91	2.90	2.90	2.88
12	3.15	3.11	3.07	3.01	2.96	2.93	2.91	2.89	2.87	2.80	2.76	2.75	2.74	2.74	2.73
13	3.03	2.98	2.95	2.88	2.84	2.80	2.78	2.76	2.74	2.67	2.63	2.62	2.61	2.61	2.60
14	2.92	2.88	2.84	2.78	2.73	2.70	2.67	2.65	2.64	2.56	2.53	2.51	2.51	2.50	2.49
15	2.84	2.79	2.76	2.69	2.64	2.61	2.59	2.56	2.55	2.47	2.44	2.42	2.42	2.41	2.40
16	2.76	2.72	2.68	2.61	2.57	2.53	2.51	2.49	2.47	2.40	2.36	2.34	2.34	2.33	2.32
17	2.70	2.65	2.62	2.55	2.50	2.47	2.44	2.42	2.41	2.33	2.29	2.27	2.27	2.26	2.25
18	2.64	2.60	2.56	2.49	2.44	2.41	2.38	2.36	2.35	2.27	2.23	2.21	2.21	2.20	2.19
19	2.59	2.55	2.51	2.44	2.39	2.36	2.33	2.31	2.30	2.22	2.18	2.16	2.15	2.15	2.13
20	2.55	2.50	2.46	2.40	2.35	2.31	2.29	2.27	2.25	2.17	2.13	2.11	2.11	2.10	2.09
21	2.51	2.46	2.42	2.36	2.31	2.27	2.25	2.23	2.21	2.13	2.09	2.07	2.06	2.06	2.04
22	2.47	2.43	2.39	2.32	2.27	2.24	2.21	2.19	2.17	2.09	2.05	2.03	2.03	2.02	2.00

(Continued)

Appendix Table 7 (Continued)

ν_2	ν_1														
	16	18	20	25	30	35	40	45	50	100	200	300	400	500	∞
23	2.44	2.39	2.36	2.29	2.24	2.20	2.18	2.15	2.14	2.06	2.01	2.00	1.99	1.99	1.97
24	2.41	2.36	2.33	2.26	2.21	2.17	2.15	2.12	2.11	2.02	1.98	1.97	1.96	1.95	1.94
25	2.38	2.34	2.30	2.23	2.18	2.15	2.12	2.10	2.08	2.00	1.95	1.94	1.93	1.92	1.91
26	2.36	2.31	2.28	2.21	2.16	2.12	2.09	2.07	2.05	1.97	1.92	1.91	1.90	1.90	1.88
27	2.34	2.29	2.25	2.18	2.13	2.10	2.07	2.05	2.03	1.94	1.90	1.88	1.88	1.87	1.85
28	2.32	2.27	2.23	2.16	2.11	2.08	2.05	2.03	2.01	1.92	1.88	1.86	1.85	1.85	1.83
29	2.30	2.25	2.21	2.14	2.09	2.06	2.03	2.01	1.99	1.90	1.86	1.84	1.83	1.83	1.81
30	2.28	2.23	2.20	2.12	2.07	2.04	2.01	1.99	1.97	1.88	1.84	1.82	1.81	1.81	1.79
32	2.25	2.20	2.16	2.09	2.04	2.00	1.98	1.95	1.93	1.85	1.80	1.78	1.77	1.77	1.75
34	2.22	2.17	2.13	2.06	2.01	1.97	1.95	1.92	1.90	1.82	1.77	1.75	1.74	1.74	1.72
36	2.20	2.15	2.11	2.04	1.99	1.95	1.92	1.90	1.88	1.79	1.74	1.72	1.71	1.71	1.69
38	2.17	2.13	2.09	2.01	1.96	1.93	1.90	1.87	1.85	1.76	1.71	1.70	1.69	1.68	1.66
40	2.15	2.11	2.07	1.99	1.94	1.90	1.88	1.85	1.83	1.74	1.69	1.67	1.66	1.66	1.64
42	2.14	2.09	2.05	1.98	1.92	1.89	1.86	1.83	1.81	1.72	1.67	1.65	1.64	1.64	1.62
44	2.12	2.07	2.03	1.96	1.91	1.87	1.84	1.82	1.80	1.70	1.65	1.63	1.62	1.62	1.60
46	2.11	2.06	2.02	1.94	1.89	1.85	1.82	1.80	1.78	1.69	1.63	1.62	1.61	1.60	1.58
48	2.09	2.05	2.01	1.93	1.88	1.84	1.81	1.79	1.77	1.67	1.62	1.60	1.59	1.58	1.56
50	2.08	2.03	1.99	1.92	1.87	1.83	1.80	1.77	1.75	1.66	1.60	1.58	1.57	1.57	1.55
60	2.03	1.98	1.94	1.87	1.82	1.78	1.74	1.72	1.70	1.60	1.54	1.52	1.51	1.51	1.48
80	1.97	1.92	1.88	1.81	1.75	1.71	1.68	1.65	1.63	1.53	1.47	1.45	1.43	1.43	1.40
100	1.94	1.89	1.85	1.77	1.71	1.67	1.64	1.61	1.59	1.48	1.42	1.40	1.39	1.38	1.35

125	1.91	1.86	1.82	1.74	1.68	1.64	1.61	1.58	1.56	1.45	1.38	1.36	1.34	1.34	1.30
150	1.89	1.84	1.80	1.72	1.67	1.62	1.59	1.56	1.54	1.42	1.35	1.33	1.32	1.31	1.27
200	1.87	1.82	1.78	1.70	1.64	1.60	1.56	1.53	1.51	1.39	1.32	1.29	1.28	1.27	1.23
300	1.85	1.80	1.75	1.67	1.62	1.57	1.54	1.51	1.48	1.36	1.28	1.25	1.24	1.23	1.18
500	1.83	1.78	1.74	1.65	1.60	1.55	1.52	1.49	1.46	1.34	1.25	1.22	1.20	1.19	1.14
1000	1.82	1.77	1.72	1.64	1.58	1.54	1.50	1.47	1.45	1.32	1.23	1.20	1.17	1.16	1.10
∞	1.80	1.75	1.71	1.63	1.57	1.52	1.48	1.45	1.43	1.30	1.21	1.17	1.14	1.13	1.04

$\alpha = 0.01$

ν_2	ν_1														
	1	**2**	**3**	**4**	**5**	**6**	**7**	**8**	**9**	**10**	**11**	**12**	**13**	**14**	**15**
1	16211	20000	21615	22500	23056	23437	23715	23925	24091	24224	24334	24426	24505	24572	24630
2	198.5	199.0	199.2	199.2	199.3	199.3	199.4	199.4	199.4	199.4	199.4	199.4	199.4	199.4	199.4
3	55.55	49.80	47.47	46.19	45.39	44.84	44.43	44.13	43.88	43.69	43.52	43.39	43.27	43.17	43.08
4	31.33	26.28	24.26	23.15	22.46	21.97	21.62	21.35	21.14	20.97	20.82	20.7	20.60	20.51	20.44
5	22.78	18.31	16.53	15.56	14.94	14.51	14.20	13.96	13.77	13.62	13.49	13.38	13.29	13.21	13.15
6	18.63	14.54	12.92	12.03	11.46	11.07	10.79	10.57	10.39	10.25	10.13	10.03	9.95	9.88	9.81
7	16.24	12.40	10.88	10.05	9.52	9.16	8.89	8.68	8.51	8.38	8.27	8.18	8.10	8.03	7.97
8	14.69	11.04	9.60	8.81	8.30	7.95	7.69	7.50	7.34	7.21	7.10	7.01	6.94	6.87	6.81
9	13.61	10.11	8.72	7.96	7.47	7.13	6.88	6.69	6.54	6.42	6.31	6.23	6.15	6.09	6.03
10	12.83	9.43	8.08	7.34	6.87	6.54	6.30	6.12	5.97	5.85	5.75	5.66	5.59	5.53	5.47
11	12.23	8.91	7.60	6.88	6.42	6.10	5.86	5.68	5.54	5.42	5.32	5.24	5.16	5.10	5.05
12	11.75	8.51	7.23	6.52	6.07	5.76	5.52	5.35	5.20	5.09	4.99	4.91	4.84	4.77	4.72

(Continued)

Appendix Table 7 (Continued)

ν_2	ν_1 1	2	3	4	5	6	7	8	9	10	11	12	13	14	15
13	11.37	8.19	6.93	6.23	5.79	5.48	5.25	5.08	4.94	4.82	4.72	4.64	4.57	4.51	4.46
14	11.06	7.92	6.68	6.00	5.56	5.26	5.03	4.86	4.72	4.60	4.51	4.43	4.36	4.30	4.25
15	10.80	7.70	6.48	5.80	5.37	5.07	4.85	4.67	4.54	4.42	4.33	4.25	4.18	4.12	4.07
16	10.58	7.51	6.30	5.64	5.21	4.91	4.69	4.52	4.38	4.27	4.18	4.10	4.03	3.97	3.92
17	10.38	7.35	6.16	5.50	5.07	4.78	4.56	4.39	4.25	4.14	4.05	3.97	3.90	3.84	3.79
18	10.22	7.21	6.03	5.37	4.96	4.66	4.44	4.28	4.14	4.03	3.94	3.86	3.79	3.73	3.68
19	10.07	7.09	5.92	5.27	4.85	4.56	4.34	4.18	4.04	3.93	3.84	3.76	3.70	3.64	3.59
20	9.94	6.99	5.82	5.17	4.76	4.47	4.26	4.09	3.96	3.85	3.76	3.68	3.61	3.55	3.50
21	9.83	6.89	5.73	5.09	4.68	4.39	4.18	4.01	3.88	3.77	3.68	3.60	3.54	3.48	3.43
22	9.73	6.81	5.65	5.02	4.61	4.32	4.11	3.94	3.81	3.70	3.61	3.54	3.47	3.41	3.36
23	9.63	6.73	5.58	4.95	4.54	4.26	4.05	3.88	3.75	3.64	3.55	3.47	3.41	3.35	3.30
24	9.55	6.66	5.52	4.89	4.49	4.20	3.99	3.83	3.69	3.59	3.50	3.42	3.35	3.30	3.25
25	9.48	6.60	5.46	4.84	4.43	4.15	3.94	3.78	3.64	3.54	3.45	3.37	3.30	3.25	3.20
26	9.41	6.54	5.41	4.79	4.38	4.10	3.89	3.73	3.60	3.49	3.40	3.33	3.26	3.20	3.15
27	9.34	6.49	5.36	4.74	4.34	4.06	3.85	3.69	3.56	3.45	3.36	3.28	3.22	3.16	3.11
28	9.28	6.44	5.32	4.70	4.30	4.02	3.81	3.65	3.52	3.41	3.32	3.25	3.18	3.12	3.07
29	9.23	6.40	5.28	4.66	4.26	3.98	3.77	3.61	3.48	3.38	3.29	3.21	3.15	3.09	3.04
30	9.18	6.35	5.24	4.62	4.23	3.95	3.74	3.58	3.45	3.34	3.25	3.18	3.11	3.06	3.01
32	9.09	6.28	5.17	4.56	4.17	3.89	3.68	3.52	3.39	3.29	3.20	3.12	3.06	3.00	2.95
34	9.01	6.22	5.11	4.50	4.11	3.84	3.63	3.47	3.34	3.24	3.15	3.07	3.01	2.95	2.90
36	8.94	6.16	5.06	4.46	4.06	3.79	3.58	3.42	3.30	3.19	3.10	3.03	2.96	2.9	2.85
38	8.88	6.11	5.02	4.41	4.02	3.75	3.54	3.39	3.26	3.15	3.06	2.99	2.92	2.87	2.82

40	8.83	6.07	4.98	4.37	3.99	3.71	3.51	3.35	3.22	3.12	3.03	2.95	2.89	2.83	2.78
42	8.78	6.03	4.94	4.34	3.95	3.68	3.48	3.32	3.19	3.09	3.00	2.92	2.86	2.80	2.75
44	8.74	5.99	4.91	4.31	3.92	3.65	3.45	3.29	3.16	3.06	2.97	2.89	2.83	2.77	2.72
46	8.70	5.96	4.88	4.28	3.90	3.62	3.42	3.26	3.14	3.03	2.94	2.87	2.80	2.75	2.70
48	8.66	5.93	4.85	4.25	3.87	3.60	3.40	3.24	3.11	3.01	2.92	2.85	2.78	2.72	2.67
50	8.63	5.90	4.83	4.23	3.85	3.58	3.38	3.22	3.09	2.99	2.90	2.82	2.76	2.70	2.65
60	8.49	5.79	4.73	4.14	3.76	3.49	3.29	3.13	3.01	2.90	2.82	2.74	2.68	2.62	2.57
80	8.33	5.67	4.61	4.03	3.65	3.39	3.19	3.03	2.91	2.80	2.72	2.64	2.58	2.52	2.47
100	8.24	5.59	4.54	3.96	3.59	3.33	3.13	2.97	2.85	2.74	2.66	2.58	2.52	2.46	2.41
125	8.17	5.53	4.49	3.91	3.54	3.28	3.08	2.93	2.80	2.70	2.61	2.54	2.47	2.42	2.37
150	8.12	5.49	4.45	3.88	3.51	3.25	3.05	2.89	2.77	2.67	2.58	2.51	2.44	2.38	2.33
200	8.06	5.44	4.41	3.84	3.47	3.21	3.01	2.86	2.73	2.63	2.54	2.47	2.40	2.35	2.30
300	8.00	5.39	4.36	3.80	3.43	3.17	2.97	2.82	2.69	2.59	2.51	2.43	2.37	2.31	2.26
500	7.95	5.35	4.33	3.76	3.40	3.14	2.94	2.79	2.66	2.56	2.48	2.4	2.34	2.28	2.23
1000	7.91	5.33	4.30	3.74	3.37	3.11	2.92	2.77	2.64	2.54	2.45	2.38	2.32	2.26	2.21
∞	7.88	5.30	4.28	3.72	3.35	3.09	2.90	2.75	2.62	2.52	2.43	2.36	2.29	2.24	2.19

$\alpha = 0.01$

ν_2	ν_1														
	16	**18**	**20**	**25**	**30**	**35**	**40**	**45**	**50**	**100**	**200**	**300**	**400**	**500**	**∞**
1	24681	24767	24836	24960	25044	25103	25148	25183	25211	25338	25401	25422	25433	25439	25463
2	199.4	199.4	199.4	199.5	199.5	199.5	199.5	199.5	199.5	199.5	199.5	199.5	199.5	199.5	199.5
3	43.01	42.88	42.78	42.59	42.47	42.38	42.31	42.26	42.21	42.02	41.93	41.89	41.88	41.87	41.83

(Continued)

Appendix Table 7 (Continued)

ν_2	ν_1 16	18	20	25	30	35	40	45	50	100	200	300	400	500	∞
4	20.37	20.26	20.17	20.00	19.89	19.81	19.75	19.70	19.67	19.50	19.41	19.38	19.37	19.36	19.33
5	13.09	12.98	12.90	12.76	12.66	12.58	12.53	12.49	12.45	12.30	12.22	12.20	12.18	12.17	12.15
6	9.76	9.66	9.59	9.45	9.36	9.29	9.24	9.20	9.17	9.03	8.95	8.93	8.92	8.91	8.88
7	7.91	7.83	7.75	7.62	7.53	7.47	7.42	7.38	7.35	7.22	7.15	7.12	7.11	7.10	7.08
8	6.76	6.68	6.61	6.48	6.40	6.33	6.29	6.25	6.22	6.09	6.02	6.00	5.99	5.98	5.95
9	5.98	5.90	5.83	5.71	5.62	5.56	5.52	5.48	5.45	5.32	5.26	5.23	5.22	5.21	5.19
10	5.42	5.34	5.27	5.15	5.07	5.01	4.97	4.93	4.90	4.77	4.71	4.68	4.67	4.67	4.64
11	5.00	4.92	4.86	4.74	4.65	4.60	4.55	4.52	4.49	4.36	4.29	4.27	4.26	4.25	4.23
12	4.67	4.59	4.53	4.41	4.33	4.27	4.23	4.19	4.17	4.04	3.97	3.95	3.94	3.93	3.91
13	4.41	4.33	4.27	4.15	4.07	4.01	3.97	3.94	3.91	3.78	3.71	3.69	3.68	3.67	3.65
14	4.20	4.12	4.06	3.94	3.86	3.80	3.76	3.73	3.70	3.57	3.50	3.48	3.47	3.46	3.44
15	4.02	3.95	3.88	3.77	3.69	3.63	3.58	3.55	3.52	3.39	3.33	3.31	3.29	3.29	3.26
16	3.87	3.80	3.73	3.62	3.54	3.48	3.44	3.40	3.37	3.25	3.18	3.16	3.15	3.14	3.11
17	3.75	3.67	3.61	3.49	3.41	3.35	3.31	3.28	3.25	3.12	3.05	3.03	3.02	3.01	2.99
18	3.64	3.56	3.50	3.38	3.30	3.25	3.20	3.17	3.14	3.01	2.94	2.92	2.91	2.90	2.87
19	3.54	3.46	3.40	3.29	3.21	3.15	3.11	3.07	3.04	2.91	2.85	2.82	2.81	2.80	2.78
20	3.46	3.38	3.32	3.20	3.12	3.07	3.02	2.99	2.96	2.83	2.76	2.74	2.73	2.72	2.69
21	3.38	3.31	3.24	3.13	3.05	2.99	2.95	2.91	2.88	2.75	2.68	2.66	2.65	2.64	2.62
22	3.31	3.24	3.18	3.06	2.98	2.92	2.88	2.84	2.82	2.69	2.62	2.59	2.58	2.57	2.55
23	3.25	3.18	3.12	3.00	2.92	2.86	2.82	2.78	2.76	2.62	2.56	2.53	2.52	2.51	2.49
24	3.20	3.12	3.06	2.95	2.87	2.81	2.77	2.73	2.70	2.57	2.50	2.48	2.46	2.46	2.43
25	3.15	3.08	3.01	2.90	2.82	2.76	2.72	2.68	2.65	2.52	2.45	2.43	2.41	2.41	2.38

26	3.11	3.03	2.97	2.85	2.77	2.72	2.67	2.64	2.61	2.47	2.40	2.38	2.37	2.36	2.33
27	3.07	2.99	2.93	2.81	2.73	2.67	2.63	2.59	2.57	2.43	2.36	2.34	2.32	2.32	2.29
28	3.03	2.95	2.89	2.77	2.69	2.64	2.59	2.56	2.53	2.39	2.32	2.30	2.28	2.28	2.25
29	2.99	2.92	2.86	2.74	2.66	2.60	2.56	2.52	2.49	2.36	2.29	2.26	2.25	2.24	2.21
30	2.96	2.89	2.82	2.71	2.63	2.57	2.52	2.49	2.46	2.32	2.25	2.23	2.21	2.21	2.18
32	2.90	2.83	2.77	2.65	2.57	2.51	2.47	2.43	2.40	2.26	2.19	2.17	2.15	2.15	2.12
34	2.85	2.78	2.72	2.60	2.52	2.46	2.42	2.38	2.35	2.21	2.14	2.11	2.10	2.09	2.06
36	2.81	2.73	2.67	2.56	2.48	2.42	2.37	2.33	2.30	2.17	2.09	2.07	2.05	2.04	2.01
38	2.77	2.70	2.63	2.52	2.44	2.38	2.33	2.29	2.27	2.12	2.05	2.02	2.01	2.00	1.97
40	2.74	2.66	2.60	2.48	2.40	2.34	2.30	2.26	2.23	2.09	2.01	1.99	1.97	1.96	1.93
42	2.71	2.63	2.57	2.45	2.37	2.31	2.26	2.23	2.20	2.06	1.98	1.95	1.94	1.93	1.90
44	2.68	2.60	2.54	2.42	2.34	2.28	2.24	2.20	2.17	2.03	1.95	1.92	1.91	1.90	1.87
46	2.65	2.58	2.51	2.40	2.32	2.26	2.21	2.17	2.14	2.00	1.92	1.89	1.88	1.87	1.84
48	2.63	2.55	2.49	2.37	2.29	2.23	2.19	2.15	2.12	1.97	1.90	1.87	1.85	1.85	1.81
50	2.61	2.53	2.47	2.35	2.27	2.21	2.16	2.13	2.10	1.95	1.87	1.84	1.83	1.82	1.79
60	2.53	2.45	2.39	2.27	2.19	2.13	2.08	2.04	2.01	1.86	1.78	1.75	1.73	1.73	1.69
80	2.43	2.35	2.29	2.17	2.08	2.02	1.97	1.94	1.90	1.75	1.66	1.63	1.61	1.60	1.57
100	2.37	2.29	2.23	2.11	2.02	1.96	1.91	1.87	1.84	1.68	1.59	1.56	1.54	1.53	1.49
125	2.32	2.24	2.18	2.06	1.98	1.91	1.86	1.82	1.79	1.63	1.53	1.50	1.48	1.47	1.42
150	2.29	2.21	2.15	2.03	1.94	1.88	1.83	1.79	1.76	1.59	1.49	1.46	1.44	1.42	1.38
200	2.25	2.18	2.11	1.99	1.91	1.84	1.79	1.75	1.71	1.54	1.44	1.40	1.38	1.37	1.32
300	2.21	2.14	2.07	1.95	1.87	1.80	1.75	1.71	1.67	1.50	1.39	1.35	1.32	1.31	1.25
500	2.19	2.11	2.04	1.92	1.84	1.77	1.72	1.67	1.64	1.46	1.35	1.30	1.28	1.26	1.19
1000	2.16	2.09	2.02	1.90	1.81	1.75	1.69	1.65	1.61	1.43	1.31	1.26	1.24	1.22	1.13
∞	2.14	2.06	2.00	1.88	1.79	1.72	1.67	1.63	1.59	1.40	1.28	1.22	1.19	1.18	1.05

Appendix Table 8 Confidence interval (CI) for rate (%).

First row 95% CI; Second row 99% CI

n	*X*													
	0	**1**	**2**	**3**	**4**	**5**	**6**	**7**	**8**	**9**	**10**	**11**	**12**	**13**
1	0–98													
	0–100													
2	0–84	1–99												
	0–93	0–100												
3	0–71	1–91	9–99											
	0–83	0–96	4–100											
4	0–60	1–81	7–93											
	0–73	0–89	3–97											
5	0–52	1–72	5–85	15–95										
	0–65	0–81	2–92	8–98										
6	0–46	0–64	4–78	12–88										
	0–59	0–75	2–86	7–93										
7	0–41	0–58	4–71	10–82	18–90									
	0–53	0–68	2–80	6–88	12–94									
8	0–37	0–53	3–65	9–76	16–64									
	0–48	0–63	1–74	5–83	10–90									
9	0–34	0–48	3–60	7–70	14–79	21–86								
	0–45	0–59	1–69	4–78	9–85	15–91								
10	0–31	0–45	3–56	7–65	12–74	19–81								
	0–41	0–54	1–65	4–74	8–81	13–87								

11	0–28	0–41	2–52	6–61	11–69	17–77	23–83				
	0–38	0–51	1–61	3–69	7–77	11–83	17–89				
12	0–26	0–38	2–48	5–57	10–65	15–72	21–79				
	0–36	0–48	1–57	3–66	6–73	10–79	18–85				
13	0–25	0–36	2–45	5–54	9–61	14–68	19–75	25–81			
	0–34	0–45	1–54	3–62	6–69	9–76	14–81	19–86			
14	0–23	0–34	2–43	5–51	8–58	16–65	8–71	23–77			
	0–32	0–42	1–51	3–59	5–66	9–72	13–78	17–83			
15	0–22	0–32	2–41	4–48	8–55	12–62	16–68	21–73	27–79		
	0–30	0–40	1–49	2–56	5–63	8–69	12–74	16–79	21–84		
16	0–21	0–30	2–38	4–46	7–52	11–59	15–65	20–70	25–75		
	0–28	0–38	1–46	2–53	5–60	8–66	11–71	15–76	19–81		
17	0–20	0–29	2–36	4–43	7–50	10–56	14–62	18–67	25–72	28–77	
	0–27	0–36	1–44	2–51	4–57	7–63	10–69	14–74	18–78	22–82	
18	0–19	0–27	1–35	4–41	6–48	10–54	13–59	17–64	22–69	26–74	
	0–26	0–35	1–42	2–49	4–55	7–61	10–66	13–71	17–75	21–79	
19	0–18	0–26	1–33	3–40	6–46	9–51	13–57	16–62	20–67	24–71	29–76
	0–24	0–33	1–40	2–47	4–53	6–58	9–63	12–68	16–73	19–77	23–81
20	0–17	0–25	1–32	3–38	6–44	9–49	12–54	15–59	19–64	23–69	27–73
	0–23	0–32	1–39	2–45	4–51	6–56	9–61	11–66	15–70	18–74	22–78
21	0–16	0–24	1–30	3–36	5–42	8–47	11–52	15–57	18–62	22–66	26–70	30–74
	0–22	0–30	1–37	2–43	3–49	6–54	8–59	11–63	14–68	17–71	21–76	24–80
22	0–15	0–23	1–29	3–35	5–40	8–45	11–50	14–55	17–59	21–64	24–68	28–72
	0–21	0–29	1–36	2–42	3–47	5–52	8–57	10–61	13–66	16–70	20–73	23–77

(Continued)

Appendix Table 8 (Continued)

n	*X*													
	0	1	2	3	4	5	6	7	8	9	10	11	12	13
23	0–15	0–22	1–28	3–34	5–39	8–44	10–48	13–53	16–57	20–62	23–66	27–69	31–73	
	0–21	0–28	1–35	2–40	3–45	5–50	7–55	10–59	13–63	15–67	19–71	22–75	25–78	
24	0–14	0–21	1–27	3–32	5–37	7–42	10–47	13–51	16–55	19–59	22–63	26–67	29–71	
	0–20	0–27	0–33	2–39	3–44	5–49	7–53	9–57	12–61	15–65	18–69	21–73	24–76	
25	0–14	0–20	1–26	3–31	5–36	7–41	9–45	12–49	15–54	18–58	21–61	24–65	28–69	31–72
	0–19	0–26	0–32	1–37	3–42	5–47	7–51	9–56	11–60	14–63	17–67	20–71	23–74	26–77
26	0–13	0–20	1–25	2–30	4–35	7–39	9–44	12–48	14–52	17–56	20–60	23–63	27–67	30–70
	0–18	0–25	0–31	1–36	3–41	4–46	6–50	9–54	11–58	13–62	16–65	19–69	22–72	25–75
27	0–13	0–19	1–24	2–29	4–34	6–38	9–42	11–46	14–50	17–54	19–58	22–61	26–65	27–68
	0–18	0–28	0–30	1–35	3–40	4–44	6–48	8–52	10–56	13–60	15–63	18–67	21–70	24–73
28	0–12	0–18	1–24	2–28	4–33	6–37	8–41	11–45	13–49	16–52	19–56	22–59	25–63	28–66
	0–17	0–24	0–29	1–34	3–39	4–43	6–47	8–51	10–55	12–58	15–62	17–65	20–68	23–71
29	0–12	0–18	1–23	2–27	4–32	6–36	8–40	10–44	13–47	15–51	18–54	21–58	24–61	26–64
	0–17	0–23	0–28	1–33	2–37	4–42	6–46	8–49	10–53	12–57	14–60	17–63	19–66	22–70
30	0–12	0–17	1–22	2–27	4–31	6–35	8–39	10–42	12–46	14–49	17–53	20–56	23–59	26–63
	0–16	0–22	0–27	1–32	2–36	4–40	5–44	7–48	9–52	1–55	14–58	16–62	19–65	21–68
31	0–11	0–17	1–22	2–26	4–30	6–34	8–38	10–41	12–45	14–48	17–51	19–55	22–58	25–61
	0–16	0–22	0–27	1–31	2–35	4–39	5–43	7–47	9–50	11–54	13–57	16–60	18–63	20–66
32	0–11	0–16	1–21	2–25	4–29	5–33	7–36	9–40	12–43	14–47	16–50	19–53	21–56	24–59
	0–15	0–21	0–26	1–30	2–34	4–38	5–42	7–46	9–49	11–52	13–56	15–59	17–62	20–65
33	0–11	0–15	1–20	2–24	3–28	5–32	7–36	9–39	11–42	13–46	16–49	18–52	20–55	23–58
	0–15	0–20	0–25	1–30	2–34	3–37	5–41	7–44	8–48	10–51	12–54	14–57	17–60	19–63

34	0–10	0–15	1–19	2–23	3–28	5–31	7–35	9–38	11–41	13–44	15–48	17–51	20–54	22–56
	0–14	0–20	0–25	1–29	2–33	3–36	5–40	6–43	8–47	10–50	12–53	14–56	16–59	18–62
35	0–10	0–15	1–19	2–23	3–27	5–30	7–34	8–37	10–40	13–43	15–46	17–49	19–52	22–55
	0–14	0–20	0–24	1–28	2–32	3–35	5–39	6–42	8–45	10–49	12–52	14–55	16–57	18–60
36	0–10	0–15	1–18	2–22	3–26	5–29	6–33	8–36	10–39	12–42	14–45	16–48	17–51	21–54
	0–14	0–19	0–23	1–27	2–31	3–35	5–38	6–41	8–44	9–47	11–50	13–53	15–56	17–59
37	0–10	0–14	1–18	2–22	3–25	5–28	6–32	8–35	10–38	12–41	14–44	16–47	18–50	20–53
	0–13	0–18	0–23	1–27	2–30	3–34	4–37	6–40	7–43	9–46	11–49	13–52	15–55	17–58
38	0–10	0–14	1–18	2–21	3–25	5–28	6–32	8–34	10–37	11–40	13–43	15–47	18–49	20–51
	0–13	0–18	0–22	1–26	2–30	3–33	4–36	6–39	7–42	9–45	11–48	12–51	14–54	16–56
39	0–9	0–14	1–17	2–21	3–24	4–27	6–31	8–33	9–36	11–39	13–42	15–45	17–48	19–50
	0–13	0–18	0–21	1–25	2–29	3–32	4–35	6–38	7–41	9–44	10–47	12–50	14–53	16–55
40	0–9	0–13	1–17	2–21	3–24	4–27	6–30	8–33	9–35	11–38	13–41	15–44	17–47	19–49
	0–12	0–17	0–21	1–25	2–28	3–32	4–35	5–38	7–40	9–43	10–46	12–49	13–52	15–54
41	0–9	0–13	1–17	2–20	3–23	4–26	6–29	7–32	9–35	11–37	12–40	14–43	16–46	18–48
	0–12	0–17	0–21	1–24	2–28	3–31	4–34	5–37	7–40	8–42	10–45	11–48	13–50	15–53
42	0–9	0–13	1–16	2–20	3–23	4–26	6–28	7–31	9–34	10–37	12–39	14–42	16–45	18–47
	0–12	0–17	0–20	1–24	2–27	3–30	4–33	5–36	7–39	8–42	9–44	11–47	13–49	15–52
43	0–9	0–12	1–16	2–19	3–23	4–25	5–28	7–31	8–33	10–36	12–39	14–41	15–44	17–46
	0–12	0–16	0–20	1–23	2–27	3–30	4–33	5–35	6–38	8–41	9–43	11–46	13–49	14–51
44	0–9	0–12	1–15	2–19	3–22	4–25	5–28	7–30	8–33	10–35	11–38	13–40	15–43	17–45
	0–11	0–16	0–19	1–23	2–26	3–29	4–32	5–35	6–37	8–40	9–42	11–45	12–47	14–50
45	0–8	0–12	1–15	2–18	3–21	4–24	5–27	7–30	8–32	9–34	11–37	13–39	14–42	16–44
	0–11	0–15	0–19	1–22	2–25	3–29	4–31	5–34	6–37	8–39	9–42	10–44	12–47	14–49

(Continued)

Appendix Table 8 (Continued)

n	X													
	0	1	2	3	4	5	6	7	8	9	10	11	12	13
46	0–8	0–12	1–15	2–18	3–21	4–24	5–26	7–29	8–31	9–34	11–36	13–39	14–41	16–43
	0–11	0–15	0–19	1–22	2–25	3–28	4–31	5–33	6–36	7–39	9–41	10–43	12–46	13–48
47	0–8	0–12	1–15	2–17	3–20	4–23	5–26	6–28	8–31	9–34	11–36	12–38	14–40	16–43
	0–11	0–15	0–18	1–21	2–24	2–27	3–30	5–33	6–35	7–38	9–40	10–42	11–45	13–47
48	0–8	0–11	1–14	2–17	3–20	4–22	5–25	6–28	8–30	9–33	11–35	12–37	14–39	15–42
	0–10	0–14	0–18	1–21	2–24	2–27	3–29	5–32	6–35	7–37	8–40	10–42	11–44	13–47
49	0–8	0–11	1–14	2–17	2–20	4–22	5–25	6–27	7–30	9–32	11–35	12–37	13–39	15–41
	0–10	0–14	0–17	1–20	2–24	2–26	3–29	4–32	6–34	7–36	8–39	9–41	11–44	12–46
50	0–7	0–11	1–14	2–17	2–19	3–22	5–24	6–26	7–29	9–31	10–34	11–36	13–38	15–41
	0–10	0–14	0–17	1–20	1–23	2–26	3–28	4–31	5–33	7–36	8–38	9–40	11–43	12–45

n	X											
	14	15	16	17	18	19	20	21	22	23	24	25
27	32–71											
	27–76											
28	31–69											
	26–74											
29	30–68	33–71										
	25–72	28–75										

30	28–66	31–69						
	24–71	27–74						
31	27–64	30–67	33–70					
	23–69	26–72	28–75					
32	26–62	29–65	32–68					
	22–67	25–70	27–73					
33	26–61	28–64	31–67	34–69				
	21–66	24–69	26–71	27–74				
34	25–59	27–62	30–65	32–68				
	21–64	23–67	25–70	28–82				
35	24–58	26–61	29–63	31–66	34–69			
	20–63	22–66	24–68	27–71	29–73			
36	23–57	26–59	28–62	30–65	33–67			
	19–62	22–64	23–67	26–69	28–72			
37	23–55	25–58	27–61	30–63	32–66	34–68		
	19–60	21–63	23–65	25–68	28–70	30–73		
38	22–54	24–57	26–59	29–62	31–64	33–67		
	18–59	20–61	22–64	25–66	27–69	29–71		
39	21–53	23–55	26–58	28–60	30–63	32–65	35–68	
	18–58	20–60	22–63	24–65	26–68	28–70	30–72	
40	21–52	23–54	25–57	27–59	29–62	32–64	34–66	
	17–57	19–59	21–61	23–64	25–66	27–68	30–71	
41	20–51	22–53	24–56	26–58	29–60	31–63	33–65	36–67
	17–55	19–58	21–60	23–63	25–65	27–67	29–69	31–71

(Continued)

Appendix Table 8 (Continued)

n	*X*											
	14	**15**	**16**	**17**	**18**	**19**	**20**	**21**	**22**	**23**	**24**	**25**
42	20–50	22–52	24–54	26–57	28–59	30–61	32–64	34–66				
	16–54	18–57	20–59	22–61	24–64	26–66	28–67	30–70				
43	19–49	21–51	23–53	25–56	27–58	29–60	31–62	33–65	36–67			
	16–53	18–56	19–58	21–60	23–62	25–65	27–66	29–69	31–71			
44	19–48	21–50	22–52	24–55	26–57	28–59	30–61	33–63	35–65			
	15–52	17–55	19–57	21–59	23–61	25–63	26–65	28–68	30–70			
45	18–47	20–49	22–51	24–54	26–56	28–58	30–60	32–62	34–64	36–66		
	15–51	17–54	19–56	20–58	22–60	24–62	26–64	28–66	30–68	32–70		
46	18–46	20–48	21–50	23–53	25–55	27–57	29–59	31–61	33–63	35–65		
	15–50	16–53	18–55	20–57	22–59	23–61	25–63	27–65	29–67	31–69		
47	18–45	19–47	21–49	23–52	25–54	26–56	28–58	30–60	32–62	34–64	36–66	
	14–19	16–52	18–54	19–56	21–58	23–60	25–62	26–64	28–66	30–68	32–70	
48	17–44	19–46	21–48	22–51	24–53	26–55	28–57	30–59	31–61	33–63	35–65	
	14–49	16–51	17–53	19–55	21–57	22–59	24–61	26–63	28–65	29–67	31–69	
49	17–43	18–45	20–47	22–50	24–52	25–54	27–56	29–58	31–60	33–62	34–64	36–66
	14–48	15–50	17–52	19–54	20–56	22–58	23–60	25–62	27–64	29–66	31–68	32–70
50	16–43	18–45	20–47	21–49	23–51	25–53	26–55	28–57	30–59	32–61	34–63	36–65
	14–47	15–49	17–51	18–53	20–55	21–57	23–59	25–61	26–63	28–65	30–67	32–68

Appendix Table 9 Critical values for the statistic q (Tukey's test).

Degrees of freedom v	Number of group k								
	2	3	4	5	6	7	8	9	10
$\alpha = 0.05$									
1	17.97	26.98	32.82	37.08	40.41	43.12	45.40	47.36	49.07
2	6.08	8.33	9.80	10.88	11.74	12.44	14.03	13.54	13.99
3	4.50	5.91	6.82	7.50	7.04	8.48	8.86	9.18	9.46
4	3.93	5.04	5.76	6.29	6.70	7.05	7.36	7.60	7.83
5	3.64	4.60	5.22	5.67	6.03	6.33	6.58	6.80	6.99
6	3.46	4.34	4.90	5.30	5.63	5.90	6.12	6.32	6.49
7	3.34	4.16	4.68	5.06	5.36	5.61	5.82	6.00	6.16
8	3.26	4.04	4.53	4.89	5.17	5.40	5.60	5.77	5.92
9	3.20	3.95	4.41	4.76	5.02	5.24	5.43	5.59	5.74
10	3.15	3.88	4.33	4.65	4.91	5.12	5.30	5.46	5.60
11	3.11	3.82	4.26	4.57	4.82	5.03	5.20	5.35	5.49
12	3.08	3.77	4.20	4.51	4.75	4.95	5.12	5.27	5.39
13	3.06	3.73	4.15	4.45	4.69	4.88	5.05	5.19	5.32
14	3.03	3.70	4.11	4.41	4.64	4.83	4.99	5.13	5.25
15	3.01	3.67	4.08	4.37	4.59	4.78	4.94	5.08	5.00
16	3.00	3.65	4.05	4.33	4.56	4.74	4.90	5.03	5.15
17	2.98	3.63	4.02	4.30	4.52	4.70	4.86	4.99	5.11
18	2.97	3.61	4.00	4.28	4.49	4.67	4.82	4.96	5.07
19	2.96	3.59	3.98	4.25	4.47	4.65	4.79	4.92	5.04
20	2.95	3.58	3.96	4.23	4.45	4.62	4.77	4.90	5.01
30	2.89	3.49	3.85	4.10	4.30	4.46	4.60	4.72	4.82
40	2.86	3.44	3.79	4.04	4.23	4.39	4.52	4.63	4.73
60	2.83	3.40	3.74	3.98	4.16	4.31	4.44	4.55	4.65
120	2.80	3.36	3.68	3.92	4.10	4.24	4.36	4.47	4.56
∞	2.77	3.31	3.63	3.86	4.03	4.17	4.29	4.39	4.47
$\alpha = 0.01$									
1	90.03	135.00	164.30	185.60	202.20	215.80	227.20	237.00	245.60
2	14.04	17.02	22.26	24.72	26.63	28.20	29.53	30.68	31.69
3	8.26	10.62	12.17	13.33	14.24	15.00	15.64	16.20	16.69
4	6.51	8.12	9.17	9.96	10.58	11.10	11.55	11.93	12.27
5	5.70	6.98	7.80	8.42	8.91	6.32	9.67	9.97	10.24
6	5.24	6.33	7.03	7.56	7.97	8.32	8.61	8.87	9.10
7	4.95	5.92	6.54	7.01	7.37	7.68	7.94	8.17	8.37
8	4.75	5.64	6.20	6.62	6.96	7.24	7.47	7.68	7.86
9	4.60	5.43	5.96	6.35	6.66	6.91	7.13	7.33	7.49
10	4.48	5.27	5.77	6.14	6.43	6.67	6.87	7.05	7.21
11	4.39	5.15	5.62	5.97	6.26	6.48	6.67	6.84	6.99

(Continued)

Appendix Table 9 (Continued)

Degrees of freedom v	Number of group k								
	2	3	4	5	6	7	8	9	10
12	4.32	5.05	5.50	5.84	6.10	6.32	6.51	6.67	6.81
13	4.26	4.96	5.40	5.73	5.98	6.19	6.37	6.53	6.67
14	4.21	4.89	5.32	5.63	5.88	6.08	6.26	6.41	6.54
15	4.17	4.84	5.25	5.56	5.80	5.99	6.16	6.31	6.44
16	4.13	4.79	5.19	5.49	5.72	5.92	6.08	6.22	6.35
17	4.10	4.74	5.14	5.43	5.66	5.85	6.01	6.15	6.27
18	4.07	4.70	5.09	5.38	5.60	5.79	5.94	6.08	6.20
19	4.05	4.67	5.06	5.33	5.55	5.73	5.89	6.02	6.14
20	4.02	4.64	5.02	5.29	5.51	5.69	5.84	5.97	6.09
30	3.89	4.45	4.80	5.05	5.24	5.40	5.54	5.65	5.76
40	3.82	4.37	4.70	4.93	5.11	5.26	5.39	5.50	5.60
60	3.76	4.28	4.59	4.82	4.99	5.13	5.25	5.36	5.45
120	3.70	4.20	4.50	4.71	4.87	5.01	5.12	5.21	5.30
∞	3.64	4.12	4.40	4.60	4.76	4.88	4.99	5.08	5.16

Degrees of freedom v	Number of groups k									
	11	12	13	14	15	16	17	18	19	20
$\alpha = 0.05$										
1	50.59	51.96	53.20	54.33	55.36	56.32	57.22	58.04	58.83	59.56
2	14.39	14.75	15.08	15.38	15.65	15.91	16.14	16.37	16.57	16.77
3	9.72	9.95	10.15	10.35	10.52	10.69	10.84	10.98	11.11	11.24
4	8.03	8.21	8.37	8.52	8.66	8.79	8.91	9.03	9.13	9.23
5	7.17	7.32	7.47	7.60	7.72	7.83	7.93	8.03	8.12	8.21
6	6.65	6.79	6.92	7.03	7.14	7.24	7.34	7.43	7.51	7.59
7	6.30	6.43	6.55	6.66	6.76	6.85	6.94	7.02	7.10	7.17
8	6.05	6.18	6.29	6.38	6.48	6.57	6.65	6.75	6.80	6.87
9	5.87	5.98	6.09	6.19	6.28	6.36	6.44	6.51	6.58	6.64
10	5.72	5.83	5.93	6.03	6.11	6.19	6.27	6.34	6.40	6.47
11	5.61	5.71	5.81	5.90	5.98	6.06	6.13	6.20	6.27	6.33
12	5.51	5.61	5.71	5.80	5.88	5.95	6.02	6.09	6.15	6.21
13	5.43	5.53	5.63	5.71	5.79	5.86	5.93	5.99	6.05	6.11
14	5.36	5.46	5.55	5.64	5.71	5.79	5.85	5.91	5.97	6.03
15	5.31	5.40	5.49	5.57	5.65	5.72	5.78	5.85	5.90	5.96
16	5.26	5.35	5.44	5.52	5.59	5.66	5.73	5.79	5.84	5.90
17	5.21	5.31	5.39	5.47	5.54	5.61	5.67	5.73	5.79	5.84
18	5.17	5.27	5.35	5.43	5.50	5.57	5.63	5.69	5.74	5.79

(Continued)

Appendix Table 9 (Continued)

Degrees of freedom *v*	Number of groups *k*									
	11	12	13	14	15	16	17	18	19	20
19	5.14	5.23	5.31	5.39	5.46	5.53	5.59	5.65	5.70	5.75
20	5.11	5.20	5.28	5.36	5.43	5.49	5.55	5.61	5.69	5.71
30	4.92	5.00	5.08	5.15	5.21	5.27	5.33	5.38	5.43	5.47
40	4.82	4.90	4.98	5.04	5.11	5.16	5.22	5.27	5.31	5.36
60	4.73	4.81	4.88	4.94	5.00	5.06	5.11	5.15	5.20	5.24
120	4.64	4.71	4.78	4.84	4.90	4.95	5.00	5.04	5.09	5.13
∞	4.55	4.62	4.68	4.74	4.80	4.85	4.89	4.93	4.97	5.01
$\alpha = 0.01$										
1	253.20	260.00	266.20	271.80	277.00	281.80	286.30	290.40	294.30	298.00
2	32.59	33.40	34.13	34.81	35.43	36.00	35.53	37.03	37.50	37.95
3	17.13	17.53	17.86	18.22	18.52	18.81	19.07	19.32	19.55	19.77
4	12.57	12.84	13.09	13.32	13.53	13.73	13.91	14.08	14.24	14.40
5	10.48	10.70	10.89	11.08	11.24	11.40	11.55	11.68	11.81	11.93
6	9.30	9.48	9.65	9.81	9.95	10.08	10.21	10.32	10.43	10.54
7	8.55	8.71	8.86	9.00	9.12	9.44	9.35	9.46	9.55	9.65
8	8.03	8.18	8.31	8.44	8.55	8.66	8.76	8.85	8.94	9.03
9	7.65	7.78	7.91	8.03	8.13	8.23	8.33	8.41	8.49	8.57
10	7.36	7.49	7.60	7.71	7.81	7.91	7.99	8.08	8.15	8.23
11	7.13	7.25	7.36	7.46	7.56	7.65	7.65	7.81	7.88	7.95
12	6.94	7.06	7.17	7.26	7.36	7.44	7.52	7.69	7.66	7.73
13	6.79	6.90	7.01	7.10	7.19	7.27	7.35	7.42	7.48	7.55
14	6.66	6.77	6.87	6.96	7.05	7.13	7.20	7.27	7.33	7.39
15	6.55	6.66	6.76	6.84	6.93	7.00	7.07	7.14	7.20	7.26
16	6.46	6.56	6.66	6.74	6.82	6.90	6.97	7.03	7.09	7.15
17	6.38	6.48	6.57	6.66	6.73	6.81	6.87	6.94	7.00	7.05
18	6.31	6.41	6.50	6.58	6.65	6.73	6.79	6.85	6.91	6.97
19	6.25	6.34	6.43	6.51	6.58	6.65	6.72	6.78	6.84	6.89
20	6.19	6.28	6.37	6.45	6.52	6.59	6.65	6.71	6.77	6.82
30	5.85	5.93	6.01	6.08	6.14	6.20	6.26	6.31	6.36	6.41
40	5.69	5.76	5.83	5.90	5.96	6.02	6.07	6.12	6.16	6.21
60	5.53	5.60	5.67	5.73	5.78	5.84	5.89	5.93	5.97	6.01
120	5.37	5.44	5.50	5.56	5.61	5.66	5.71	5.75	5.79	5.83
∞	5.23	5.29	5.35	5.40	5.45	5.49	5.54	5.57	5.61	5.65

Appendix Table 10 Critical values for the statistic q' (Dunnett's test).

One-sided

Degrees of freedom v	Number of treatment groups (including control group) a								
	2	3	4	5	6	7	8	9	10
$\alpha = 0.05$									
5	2.02	2.44	2.68	2.85	2.98	3.08	2.16	3.24	3.30
6	1.94	2.34	2.56	2.71	2.83	2.92	3.00	3.07	3.12
7	1.89	2.27	2.48	2.62	2.73	2.82	2.89	2.95	3.01
8	1.86	2.22	2.42	2.55	2.66	2.74	2.81	2.87	2.92
9	1.83	2.18	2.37	2.50	2.60	2.68	2.75	2.81	2.86
10	1.81	2.15	2.34	2.47	2.56	2.64	2.70	2.76	2.81
11	1.80	2.13	2.31	2.44	2.53	2.60	2.67	2.72	2.77
12	1.78	2.11	2.29	2.41	2.50	2.58	2.64	2.69	2.74
13	1.77	2.09	2.27	2.39	2.48	2.55	2.61	2.66	2.71
14	1.76	2.08	2.25	2.37	2.46	2.53	2.59	2.64	2.69
15	1.75	2.07	2.24	2.36	2.44	2.51	2.57	2.62	2.67
16	1.75	2.06	2.23	2.34	2.43	2.50	2.56	2.61	2.65
17	1.74	2.05	2.22	2.33	2.42	2.49	2.54	2.59	2.64
18	1.73	2.04	2.21	2.32	2.41	2.48	2.53	2.58	2.62
19	1.73	2.03	2.20	2.31	2.40	2.47	2.52	2.57	2.61
20	1.72	2.03	2.19	2.30	2.39	2.46	2.51	2.56	2.60
24	1.71	2.01	2.17	2.28	2.36	2.43	2.48	2.53	2.57
30	1.70	1.99	2.15	2.25	2.33	2.40	2.45	2.50	2.54
40	1.68	1.97	2.13	2.23	2.31	2.37	2.42	2.47	2.51
60	1.67	1.95	2.10	2.21	2.28	2.35	2.39	2.44	2.48
120	1.66	1.93	2.08	2.18	2.26	2.32	2.37	2.41	2.45
∞	1.64	1.92	2.06	2.16	2.23	2.29	2.34	2.38	2.42
$\alpha = 0.01$									
5	3.37	3.90	4.21	4.43	4.60	4.73	4.85	4.94	5.03
6	3.14	3.61	3.88	4.07	4.21	4.33	4.43	4.51	4.59
7	3.00	3.42	3.66	3.83	3.96	4.07	4.15	4.23	4.30
8	2.90	3.29	3.51	3.67	3.79	3.88	3.96	4.03	4.09
9	2.82	3.19	3.40	3.55	3.66	3.75	3.92	3.89	3.94
10	2.76	3.11	3.31	3.45	3.56	3.64	3.71	3.78	3.83
11	2.72	3.06	3.25	3.38	3.48	3.56	3.63	3.69	3.74
12	2.68	3.01	3.19	3.32	3.42	3.50	3.56	3.62	3.67
13	2.65	2.97	3.15	3.27	3.37	3.44	3.51	3.56	3.61
14	2.62	2.94	3.11	3.23	3.32	3.40	3.46	3.51	3.56
15	2.60	2.91	3.08	3.20	3.29	3.36	3.42	3.47	3.52
16	2.58	2.88	3.05	3.17	3.26	3.33	3.39	3.44	3.48

(Continued)

Appendix Table 10 (Continued)

Degrees of freedom v	Number of treatment groups (including control group) a								
	2	**3**	**4**	**5**	**6**	**7**	**8**	**9**	**10**
17	2.57	2.86	3.03	3.14	3.23	3.30	3.36	3.41	3.45
18	2.55	2.84	3.01	3.12	3.21	3.27	3.33	3.38	3.42
19	2.54	2.83	2.99	3.10	3.18	3.25	3.31	3.36	3.40
20	2.53	2.81	2.97	3.08	3.17	3.23	3.29	3.34	3.38
24	2.49	2.77	2.92	3.03	3.11	3.17	3.22	3.27	3.31
30	2.46	2.72	2.87	2.97	3.05	3.11	3.16	3.21	3.24
40	2.42	2.68	2.82	2.92	2.99	3.05	3.10	3.14	3.18
60	2.39	2.64	2.78	2.87	2.94	3.00	3.04	3.08	3.12
120	2.36	2.60	2.73	2.82	2.89	2.94	2.99	3.03	3.06
∞	2.33	2.56	2.68	2.77	2.84	2.89	2.93	2.97	3.00

Two-sided

Degrees of freedom v	Number of treatment groups (including control group) a								
	2	**3**	**4**	**5**	**6**	**7**	**8**	**9**	**10**
$\alpha = 0.05$									
5	2.57	3.03	3.29	3.48	3.62	3.73	3.82	3.90	3.97
6	2.45	2.86	3.10	3.26	3.39	3.49	3.57	3.64	3.71
7	2.36	2.75	2.97	3.12	3.24	3.33	3.41	3.47	3.53
8	2.31	2.67	2.88	3.02	3.13	3.22	3.29	3.35	3.41
9	2.26	2.61	2.81	2.95	3.05	3.14	3.20	3.26	3.32
10	2.23	2.57	2.76	2.89	2.99	3.07	3.14	3.19	3.24
11	2.20	2.53	2.72	2.84	2.94	3.02	3.08	3.14	3.19
12	2.18	2.50	2.68	2.81	2.90	2.98	3.04	3.09	3.14
13	2.16	2.48	2.65	2.78	2.87	2.94	3.00	3.06	3.10
14	2.14	2.46	2.63	2.75	2.84	2.91	2.97	3.02	3.07
15	2.13	2.44	2.61	2.73	2.82	2.89	2.95	3.00	3.04
16	2.12	2.42	2.59	2.71	2.80	2.87	2.92	2.97	3.02
17	2.11	2.41	2.58	2.69	2.78	2.85	2.90	2.95	3.00
18	2.10	2.40	2.56	2.68	2.76	2.83	2.89	2.94	2.98
19	2.09	2.39	2.55	2.66	2.75	2.81	2.87	2.92	2.96
20	2.09	2.38	2.54	2.65	2.73	2.80	2.86	2.90	2.95
24	2.06	2.35	2.51	2.61	2.70	2.76	2.81	2.86	2.90
30	2.04	2.32	2.47	2.58	2.66	2.72	2.77	2.82	2.86
40	2.02	2.29	2.44	2.54	2.62	2.68	2.73	2.77	2.81
60	2.00	2.27	2.41	2.51	2.58	2.64	2.69	2.73	2.77
120	1.98	2.24	2.38	2.47	2.55	2.60	2.65	2.69	2.73
∞	1.96	2.21	2.35	2.44	2.51	2.57	2.61	2.65	2.69

(Continued)

Appendix Table 10 (Continued)

Degrees of freedom v	Number of treatment groups (including control group) a								
	2	3	4	5	6	7	8	9	10
$\alpha = 0.01$									
5	4.03	4.63	4.98	5.22	5.41	5.56	5.69	5.80	5.89
6	3.71	4.21	4.51	4.71	4.87	5.00	5.10	5.20	5.28
7	3.50	3.95	4.21	4.39	4.53	4.64	4.74	4.82	4.89
8	3.36	3.77	4.00	4.17	4.29	4.40	4.48	4.56	4.62
9	3.25	3.63	3.85	4.01	4.12	4.22	4.30	4.37	4.43
10	3.17	3.53	3.74	3.88	3.99	4.08	4.16	4.22	4.28
11	3.11	3.45	3.65	3.79	3.89	3.98	4.05	4.11	4.16
12	3.05	3.39	3.58	3.71	3.81	3.89	3.96	4.02	4.07
13	3.01	3.33	3.52	3.65	3.74	3.82	3.89	3.94	3.99
14	2.98	3.29	3.47	3.59	3.69	3.76	3.83	3.88	3.93
15	2.95	3.25	3.43	3.55	3.64	3.71	3.78	3.83	3.88
16	2.92	3.22	3.39	3.51	3.60	3.67	3.73	3.78	3.83
17	2.90	3.19	3.36	3.47	3.56	3.63	3.69	3.74	3.79
18	2.88	3.17	3.33	3.44	3.53	3.60	3.66	3.71	3.75
19	2.86	3.15	3.31	3.42	3.50	3.57	3.63	3.68	3.72
20	2.85	3.13	3.29	3.40	3.48	3.55	3.60	3.65	3.69
24	2.80	3.07	3.22	3.32	3.40	3.47	3.52	3.57	3.61
30	2.75	3.01	3.15	3.25	3.33	3.39	3.44	3.49	3.52
40	2.70	2.95	3.09	3.19	3.26	3.32	3.37	3.41	3.44
60	2.66	2.90	3.03	3.12	3.19	3.25	3.29	3.33	3.37
120	2.62	2.85	2.97	3.06	3.12	3.18	3.22	3.26	3.29
∞	2.58	2.79	2.92	3.00	3.06	3.11	3.15	3.19	3.22

Source: Dunnett (1964)

Appendix Table 11 Critical values for Pearson correlation coefficient r.

Degrees of freedom v	α									
	One-sided	**0.25**	**0.10**	**0.05**	**0.025**	**0.01**	**0.005**	**0.0025**	**0.001**	**0.0005**
	Two-sided	**0.50**	**0.20**	**0.10**	**0.05**	**0.02**	**0.01**	**0.005**	**0.002**	**0.001**
1		0.707	0.951	0.988	0.997	1.000	1.000	1.000	1.000	1.000
2		0.500	0.800	0.900	0.950	0.980	0.990	0.995	0.998	0.999
3		0.404	0.687	0.805	0.878	0.934	0.959	0.974	0.986	0.991
4		0.347	0.608	0.729	0.811	0.882	0.917	0.942	0.963	0.974
5		0.309	0.551	0.669	0.755	0.833	0.875	0.906	0.935	0.951
6		0.282	0.507	0.621	0.707	0.789	0.834	0.870	0.905	0.925
7		0.260	0.472	0.582	0.666	0.750	0.798	0.836	0.875	0.898
8		0.242	0.443	0.549	0.632	0.715	0.765	0.805	0.847	0.872

(Continued)

Appendix Table 11 (Continued)

9	0.228	0.419	0.521	0.602	0.685	0.634	0.776	0.820	0.847
10	0.216	0.398	0.497	0.576	0.658	0.708	0.750	0.795	0.823
11	0.206	0.380	0.476	0.553	0.634	0.684	0.726	0.772	0.801
12	0.197	0.365	0.457	0.532	0.612	0.661	0.703	0.750	0.780
13	0.189	0.351	0.441	0.514	0.592	0.641	0.683	0.730	0.760
14	0.182	0.338	0.426	0.497	0.574	0.623	0.664	0.711	0.742
15	0.176	0.328	0.412	0.482	0.558	0.606	0.647	0.694	0.725
16	0.170	0.317	0.400	0.468	0.542	0.590	0.631	0.678	0.707
17	0.165	0.308	0.389	0.456	0.529	0.575	0.616	0.662	0.693
18	0.160	0.299	0.378	0.444	0.515	0.561	0.602	0.648	0.679
19	0.156	0.291	0.369	0.433	0.503	0.549	0.589	0.635	0.665
20	0.152	0.384	0.360	0.423	0.492	0.537	0.576	0.622	0.652
21	0.148	0.277	0.352	0.413	0.482	0.526	0.565	0.610	0.640
22	0.145	0.271	0.344	0.404	0.472	0.515	0.554	0.599	0.629
23	0.141	0.265	0.337	0.396	0.462	0.505	0.543	0.588	0.618
24	0.138	0.260	0.330	0.388	0.453	0.496	0.534	0.578	0.607
25	0.136	0.255	0.323	0.381	0.445	0.487	0.524	0.568	0.597
26	0.133	0.250	0.317	0.374	0.437	0.479	0.515	0.559	0.588
27	0.131	0.245	0.311	0.367	0.430	0.471	0.507	0.550	0.579
28	0.128	0.241	0.306	0.361	0.423	0.463	0.499	0.541	0.570
29	0.126	0.237	0.301	0.355	0.416	0.456	0.491	0.533	0.562
30	0.124	0.233	0.296	0.349	0.409	0.449	0.484	0.526	0.554
31	0.122	0.229	0.291	0.344	0.403	0.442	0.477	0.518	0.546
32	0.120	0.225	0.287	0.339	0.397	0.436	0.470	0.511	0.539
33	0.118	0.222	0.283	0.334	0.392	0.430	0.464	0.504	0.532
34	0.116	0.219	0.279	0.329	0.386	0.424	0.458	0.498	0.525
35	0.115	0.216	0.275	0.325	0.381	0.418	0.452	0.492	0.519
36	0.113	0.213	0.271	0.320	0.376	0.413	0.446	0.486	0.513
37	0.111	0.210	0.267	0.316	0.371	0.408	0.441	0.480	0.507
38	0.110	0.207	0.264	0.312	0.367	0.403	0.435	0.474	0.501
39	0.108	0.204	0.261	0.308	0.362	0.398	0.430	0.469	0.495
40	0.107	0.202	0.257	0.304	0.358	0.393	0.425	0.463	0.490
41	0.106	0.199	0.254	0.301	0.354	0.389	0.420	0.458	0.484
42	0.104	0.197	0.251	0.297	0.350	0.384	0.416	0.453	0.479
43	0.103	0.195	0.248	0.294	0.346	0.380	0.411	0.449	0.474
44	0.102	0.192	0.246	0.291	0.342	0.376	0.407	0.444	0.469
45	0.101	0.190	0.243	0.288	0.338	0.372	0.403	0.439	0.465
46	0.100	0.188	0.240	0.285	0.335	0.368	0.399	0.435	0.460
47	0.099	0.186	0.238	0.282	0.331	0.365	0.395	0.431	0.456
48	0.098	0.184	0.235	0.279	0.328	0.361	0.391	0.427	0.451
49	0.097	0.182	0.233	0.276	0.325	0.358	0.387	0.423	0.447
50	0.096	0.181	0.231	0.273	0.322	0.354	0.384	0.419	0.443

Appendix Table 12 Critical values for Spearman's rank correlation coefficient r_S.

Degrees of freedom v	a									
	One-sided	0.25	0.10	0.05	0.025	0.01	0.005	0.0025	0.001	0.0005
	Two-sided	0.50	0.20	0.10	0.05	0.02	0.01	0.005	0.002	0.001
4		0.600	1.000	1.000						
5		0.500	0.800	0.900	1.000	1.000				
6		0.371	0.657	0.829	0.886	0.943	1.000	1.000		
7		0.321	0.571	0.714	0.786	0.893	0.929	0.964	1.000	1.000
8		0.310	0.524	0.643	0.738	0.833	0.881	0.905	0.952	0.976
9		0.267	0.483	0.600	0.700	0.783	0.833	0.867	0.917	0.933
10		0.248	0.455	0.564	0.648	0.745	0.794	0.830	0.879	0.903
11		0.236	0.427	0.536	0.618	0.709	0.755	0.800	0.845	0.873
12		0.217	0.406	0.503	0.587	0.678	0.727	0.769	0.818	0.846
13		0.209	0.385	0.484	0.560	0.648	0.703	0.747	0.791	0.824
14		0.200	0.367	0.464	0.538	0.626	0.679	0.723	0.771	0.802
15		0.189	0.354	0.446	0.521	0.604	0.654	0.700	0.750	0.779
16		0.182	0.341	0.429	0.503	0.582	0.635	0.679	0.729	0.762
17		0.176	0.328	0.414	0.485	0.566	0.615	0.662	0.713	0.748
18		0.170	0.317	0.401	0.472	0.550	0.600	0.643	0.695	0.728
19		0.165	0.309	0.391	0.460	0.535	0.584	0.628	0.677	0.712
20		0.161	0.299	0.380	0.447	0.520	0.570	0.612	0.662	0.696
21		0.156	0.292	0.370	0.435	0.508	0.556	0.599	0.648	0.681
22		0.152	0.284	0.361	0.425	0.496	0.544	0.586	0.634	0.667
23		0.148	0.278	0.353	0.415	0.486	0.532	0.573	0.622	0.654
24		0.144	0.271	0.344	0.406	0.476	0.521	0.562	0.610	0.642
25		0.143	0.265	0.337	0.398	0.466	0.511	0.551	0.598	0.630
26		0.138	0.259	0.331	0.390	0.457	0.501	0.541	0.587	0.619
27		0.136	0.255	0.324	0.382	0.448	0.491	0.531	0.577	0.608
28		0.133	0.250	0.317	0.375	0.440	0.483	0.522	0.567	0.598
29		0.130	0.245	0.312	0.368	0.433	0.475	0.513	0.558	0.589
30		0.128	0.240	0.306	0.362	0.425	0.467	0.504	0.549	0.580
31		0.126	0.236	0.301	0.356	0.418	0.459	0.496	0.541	0.571
32		0.124	0.232	0.296	0.350	0.412	0.452	0.489	0.533	0.563
33		0.121	0.229	0.291	0.345	0.405	0.446	0.482	0.525	0.554
34		0.120	0.225	0.287	0.340	0.399	0.439	0.475	0.517	0.547
35		0.118	0.222	0.283	0.335	0.394	0.433	0.468	0.510	0.539
36		0.116	0.219	0.279	0.330	0.388	0.427	0.462	0.504	0.533
37		0.114	0.216	0.275	0.325	0.382	0.421	0.456	0.497	0.526
38		0.113	0.212	0.271	0.321	0.378	0.415	0.450	0.491	0.519

(Continued)

Appendix Table 12 (Continued)

39	0.111	0.210	0.267	0.317	0.373	0.410	0.444	0.485	0.513
40	0.110	0.207	0.264	0.313	0.368	0.405	0.439	0.479	0.507
41	0.108	0.204	0.261	0.309	0.364	0.400	0.433	0.473	0.501
42	0.107	0.202	0.257	0.305	0.359	0.395	0.428	0.468	0.495
43	0.105	0.199	0.254	0.301	0.355	0.391	0.423	0.463	0.490
44	0.104	0.197	0.251	0.298	0.351	0.386	0.419	0.458	0.484
45	0.103	0.194	0.248	0.294	0.347	0.382	0.414	0.453	0.479
46	0.102	0.192	0.246	0.291	0.343	0.378	0.410	0.448	0.474
47	0.101	0.190	0.243	0.288	0.340	0.374	0.405	0.443	0.469
48	0.100	0.188	0.240	0.285	0.336	0.370	0.401	0.439	0.465
49	0.098	0.186	0.238	0.282	0.333	0.366	0.397	0.434	0.460
50	0.097	0.184	0.235	0.279	0.329	0.363	0.393	0.430	0.456

Appendix Table 13 Critical values for the statistic T (Wilcoxon's signed rank test).

n	α				
	One-sided	**0.05**	**0.025**	**0.01**	**0.005**
	Two-sided	**0.10**	**0.05**	**0.02**	**0.01**
5		1			
6		2	1		
7		4	2	0	
8		6	4	2	0
9		8	6	3	2
10		11	8	5	3
11		14	11	7	5
12		17	14	10	7
13		21	17	13	10
14		26	21	16	13
15		30	25	20	16
16		36	30	24	19
17		41	35	28	23
18		47	40	33	28
19		54	46	38	32
20		60	52	43	37
21		68	59	49	43
22		75	66	56	49
23		83	73	62	55
24		92	81	69	61
25		101	90	77	68

(Continued)

Appendix Table 13 (Continued)

n	α				
	One-sided	**0.05**	**0.025**	**0.01**	**0.005**
	Two-sided	**0.10**	**0.05**	**0.02**	**0.01**
26		110	98	85	76
27		120	107	93	84
28		130	117	102	92
29		141	127	111	100
30		152	137	120	109
31		163	148	130	118
32		175	159	141	128
33		188	171	151	138
34		201	183	162	149
35		214	195	174	160
36		228	208	186	171
37		242	222	198	183
38		256	235	211	195
39		271	250	224	208
40		287	264	238	221
41		303	279	252	234
42		319	295	267	248
43		336	311	281	262
44		353	327	297	277
45		371	344	313	292
46		389	361	329	307
47		408	379	345	323
48		427	397	362	339
49		446	415	380	356
50		466	434	398	373

Appendix Table14 Critical values for the statistic T (Wilcoxon's rank sum test).

	One-sided	**Two-sided**
Row 1	$\alpha = 0.050$	$\alpha = 0.10$
Row2	$\alpha = 0.025$	$\alpha = 0.05$
Row3	$\alpha = 0.010$	$\alpha = 0.02$
Row4	$\alpha = 0.005$	$\alpha = 0.01$

(Continued)

Appendix Table 14 (Continued)

n_1	$n_1 - n_2$										
	0	1	2	3	4	5	6	7	8	9	10
2				3–13	3–15	3–17	4–18	4–20	4–22	4–24	5–25
							3–19	3–21	3–23	3–25	4–26
3	6–15	6–18	7–20	8–22	8–25	9–27	10–29	10–32	11–34	11–37	12–39
			6–21	7–23	7–26	8–28	8–31	9–33	9–36	10–38	10–41
					6–27	6–30	7–32	7–35	7–38	8–40	8–43
							6–33	6–36	6–39	7–41	7–44
4	11–25	12–28	13–31	14–34	15–37	16–40	17–43	18–46	19–49	20–52	21–55
	10–26	11–29	12–32	13–35	14–38	14–42	15–45	16–48	17–51	18–54	19–57
		10–30	11–33	11–37	12–40	13–43	13–47	14–50	15–53	15–57	16–60
			10–34	10–38	11–40	11–45	12–48	12–52	13–55	13–59	14–62
5	19–36	20–40	21–44	23–47	24–51	26–54	27–58	28–62	30–65	31–69	33–72
	17–38	18–42	20–45	21–49	22–53	23–57	24–61	26–64	27–68	28–72	29–76
	16–39	17–43	18–47	19–51	20–55	21–59	22–63	23–67	24–71	25–75	26–79
	15–40	16–44	16–49	17–53	18–57	19–61	20–65	21–69	22–73	22–78	23–82
6	28–50	29–55	31–59	33–63	35–67	37–71	38–76	40–80	42–84	44–88	46–92
	26–52	27–57	29–61	31–65	32–70	34–74	35–79	37–83	38–88	40–92	42–96
	24–54	25–59	27–63	28–68	29–73	30–78	32–82	33–87	34–92	36–96	37–101
	23–55	24–60	25–65	26–70	27–75	28–80	30–84	31–89	32–94	33–99	34–104
7	39–66	41–71	43–76	45–81	47–86	49–91	52–95	54–100	56–105	58–110	61–114
	36–69	38–74	40–79	42–84	44–89	46–94	48–99	50–104	52–109	54–114	56–119
	34–71	35–77	37–82	39–87	40–93	42–98	44–103	45–109	47–114	49–119	51–124

(Continued)

Appendix Table 14 (Continued)

n_1	n_2-n_1										
	0	1	2	3	4	5	6	7	8	9	10
	32–73	34–78	35–84	37–89	38–95	40–100	41–106	43–111	44–117	45–122	47–128
8	51–85	54–90	56–96	59–101	62–106	64–112	67–117	69–123	72–128	75–133	77–139
	49–87	51–93	53–99	55–105	58–110	60–116	62–122	65–127	67–133	70–138	72–144
	45–91	47–97	49–103	51–109	53–115	56–120	58–126	60–132	62–138	64–144	66–150
	43–93	45–99	47–105	49–111	51–117	53–123	54–130	56–136	58–142	60–148	62–154
9	66–105	69–111	72–117	75–123	78–129	81–135	84–141	87–147	90–153	93–159	96–165
	62–109	65–115	68–121	71–127	73–134	76–140	79–146	82–152	84–159	87–165	90–171
	59–112	61–119	63–126	66–132	68–139	71–145	73–152	76–158	78–165	81–171	83–178
	56–115	58–122	61–128	63–135	65–142	67–149	69–156	72–162	74–169	76–176	78–183
10	82–128	86–134	89–141	92–148	96–154	99–161	103–167	106–174	110–180	113–187	117–193
	78–132	81–139	84–146	88–152	91–159	94–166	97–173	100–180	103–187	107–193	110–200
	74–136	77–143	79–151	82–158	85–165	88–172	91–179	93–187	96–194	99–201	102–208
	71–139	73–147	76–154	79–161	81–169	84–176	86–184	89–191	92–198	94–206	97–213

Source: Yamauchi (1972)

Appendix Table 15 Critical values for the statistic H (Kruskal–Wallis test).

n	n_1	n_2	n_3	α		n	n_1	n_2	n_3	α	
				0.05	**0.01**					**0.05**	**0.01**
7	3	2	2	4.71			5	3	2	4.25	6.82
	3	3	1	5.14			5	4	1	4.99	6.95
8	3	3	2	5.36		11	4	4	3	5.60	7.14
	4	2	2	5.33			5	3	3	5.65	7.08
	4	3	1	5.21			5	4	2	5.27	7.12
	5	2	1	5.00			5	5	1	5.13	7.31
9	3	3	3	5.60	7.20	12	4	4	4	5.69	7.65
	4	3	2	5.44	6.44		5	4	3	5.63	7.44
	4	4	1	4.97	6.67		5	5	2	5.34	7.27
	5	2	2	5.16	6.53	13	5	4	4	5.62	7.76
	5	3	1	4.96			5	5	3	5.71	7.54
10	4	3	3	5.73	6.75	14	5	5	4	5.64	7.79
	4	4	2	5.45	7.04	15	5	5	5	5.78	7.98

Appendix Table 16 Critical values for the statistic M (Friedman's test).

Number of blocks b	$k=3$		$k=4$		$k=5$		$k=6$	
	$\alpha=0.10$	$\alpha=0.05$	$\alpha=0.10$	$\alpha=0.05$	$\alpha=0.10$	$\alpha=0.05$	$\alpha=0.10$	$\alpha=0.05$
2			6.000	6.000	7.200	7.600	8.286	9.143
3	6.000	6.000	6.600	7.400	7.467	8.533	8.714	9.857
4	6.000	6.500	6.300	7.800	7.600	8.800	9.000	10.286
5	5.200	6.400	6.360	7.800	7.680	8.960	9.000	10.486
6	5.333	7.000	6.400	7.600	7.733	9.067	9.048	10.571
7	5.429	7.143	6.429	7.800	7.771	9.143	9.122	10.674
8	5.250	6.250	6.300	7.650	7.800	9.300	9.143	10.714
9	5.556	6.222	6.467	7.800	7.733	9.244	9.127	10.778
10	5.000	6.200	6.360	7.800	7.760	9.280	9.143	10.800
11	4.909	6.545	6.382	7.909				
12	5.167	6.500	6.400	7.900				
13	4.769	6.000	6.415	7.985				
14	5.143	6.143	6.343	7.886				
15	4.933	6.400	6.440	8.040				

(Continued)

Appendix Table 16 (Continued)

Number of blocks b	$k = 3$		$k = 4$		$k = 5$		$k = 6$	
	$\alpha = 0.01$	$\alpha = 0.005$	$\alpha = 0.01$	$\alpha = 0.005$	$\alpha = 0.01$	$\alpha = 0.005$	$\alpha = 0.01$	$\alpha = 0.005$
2					8.000		9.714	10.000
3			9.000	9.000	10.133	10.667	11.762	12.524
4	8.000	8.000	9.600	10.200	11.200	12.000	12.714	13.571
5	8.400	10.000	9.960	10.920	11.680	12.480	13.229	14.257
6	9.000	10.333	10.200	11.400	11.867	13.067	13.619	14.762
7	8.857	10.286	10.371	11.400	12.114	13.257	13.857	15.000
8	9.000	9.750	10.500	11.850	12.300	13.500	14.000	15.286
9	8.667	10.667	10.867	12.067	12.444	13.689	14.143	15.476
10	9.600	10.400	10.800	12.000	12.480	13.840	14.229	15.600
11	9.455	10.364	11.073	12.273				
12	9.500	10.167	11.100	12.300				
13	9.385	10.308	11.123	12.323				
14	9.000	10.429	11.143	12.514				
15	8.933	10.000	11.240	12.520				

Source: Martin et al. (1993)

References

Agresti, A. (2018). *An Introduction to Categorical Data Analysis*, Hoboken, NJ: John Wiley & Sons.

Ahrens, W. and Pigeot, I. (2014). *Handbook of Epidemiology. 2nd ed*, New York: Springer.

Allison, P.D. (2012). *Logistic Regression Using SAS: Theory and Application*, Cary, NC: SAS Institute.

Armitage, P., Berry, G., and Matthews, J.N.S. (2001). *Statistical Methods in Medical Research. 4th ed*, Chichester, UK: Wiley-Blackwell.

Armitage, P. and Colton, T. (2005). *Encyclopedia of Biostatistics. 8 Volume Set. 2nd ed*, New York: Wiley.

Barton, B. and Peat, J. (2014). *Medical Statistics: A Guide to SPSS, Data Analysis and Critical Appraisal. 2nd ed*, New York: Wiley.

Bernard, R. (2015). *Fundamentals of Biostatistics. 8th ed*, Boston, MA: Cengage Learning.

Campbell, M.J. (2007). *Medical Statistics. 5th ed*, Hoboken, NJ: John Wiley & Sons.

Campbell, M.J., Machin, D., Walters, S.J. et al. (2007). *Medical Statistics: A Textbook for the Health Sciences. 4th ed*, New York: Wiley.

Chow, S.C. and Liu, J.P. (2013). *Design and Analysis of Clinical Trials: Concepts and Methodologies. 3rd ed*, New York: Wiley.

Chow, S.C., Shao, J., and Wang, H. (2003). *Sample Size Calculations in Clinical Research*, Abingdon, UK: Taylor & Francis.

D'Agostino, R., Sullivan, L.M., and Beiser, A. (2005). *Introductory Applied Biostatistics*, Boston, MA: Cengage Learning.

Daly, L.E. and Bourke, G.J. (2000). *Interpretation and Uses of Medical Statistics. 5th ed*, London: Blackwell Science.

Daniel, W.W. (1995). *Biostatistics. A Foundation for Analysis in the Health Sciences. 6th ed*, New York: Wiley & Sons.

Daniel, W.W. and Cross, C.L. (2013). *Biostatistics: A Foundation for Analysis in the Health Sciences. 10th ed*, New York: Wiley.

Davis, C.S. (2002). *Statistical Methods for the Analysis of Repeated Measurements (Springer Texts in Statistics)*, Berlin: Springer.

Dean, A., Voss, D., and Draguljić, D. (2017). *Design and Analysis of Experiments (Springer Texts in Statistics). 2nd ed*, Berlin: Springer.

DeGroot, M.H. and Schervish, M.J. (2011). *Probability and Statistics. 4th ed*, Boston, MA: Pearson Education.

Devore, J.L. (2015). *Probability and Statistics for Engineering and the Sciences. 9th ed*, Boston, MA: Cengage Learning.

Applied Medical Statistics, First Edition. Jingmei Jiang.

Companion website: www.wiley.com\go\jiang\appliedmedicalstatistics

Dobson, A.J. and Barnett, A.G. (2018). *An Introduction to Generalized Linear Models*, Boca Raton, FL: CRC Press.

Everitt, B.S. and Skrondal, A. (2010). *The Cambridge Dictionary of Statistics. 4th ed*, Cambridge UK: Cambridge University Press.

Fang, J.Q. (2007). *Statistical Methods of Biomedical Research*, Beijing: Advanced Education Press. (in Chinese)

Fang, J.Q. (2017). *Handbook of Medical Statistics. 1st ed*, Singapore: World Scientific.

Fei, Y. (2007). *Applied Mathematical Statistics – Basic Concepts and Methods*, Beijing: Science Press. (in Chinese)

Fisher, R.A. (1918). The correlation between relatives on the supposition of Mendelian inheritance. *Translations of the Royal Society, Edinburgh* 52: 399–433.

Fisher, R.A. (1921). On the "probable error" of a coefficient of correlation deduced from a small sample. *Metron* 1: 3–32.

Fisher, R.A. (1936). *The Design of Experiments*, Edinburgh: Oliver and Boyd.

Forthofer, R.N., Lee, E.S., and Hernandez, M. (2006). *Biostatistics: A Guide to Design, Analysis and Discovery. 2nd ed*, New York: Academic Press.

Friedman, L.M., Furberg, C.D., DeMets, D.L. et al. (2015). *Fundamentals of Clinical Trials*, Berlin: Springer.

Gao, H.X. (2001). *Practical Statistical Method and SAS System*, Beijing: Peking University Press. (in Chinese)

Ghadessi, M., Tang, R., Zhou, J. et al. (2020). A roadmap to using historical controls in clinical trials – By Drug Information Association Adaptive Design Scientific Working Group (DIA-ADSWG). *Orphanet Journal of Rare Diseases* 15(1): 69.

Girden, E.R. (1991). *ANOVA: Repeated Measures (Quantitative Applications in the Social Sciences)*, Thousand Oaks, CA: SAGE Publications.

Glover, T. and Mitchell, K. (2015). *An Introduction to Biostatistics. 3rd ed*, Long Grove, IL: Waveland Press, Inc.

Guo, Z.C. (1988). *Methods of Medical Mathematical Statistics. 3rd ed*, Beijing: People's Medical Publishing House. (in Chinese)

Harrell Jr, F.E. (2015). *Regression Modeling Strategies: With Applications to Linear Models, Logistic and Ordinal Regression, and Survival Analysis. 2nd ed*, Berlin: Springer International Publishing.

He, C.Q. (2007). *Modern Statistical Method and Application. 2nd ed*, Beijng: China Renmin University Press. (in Chinese)

He, J. and Lu, J. (2002). *SAS Statistical Analysis in Medical Statistics*, Shanghai: The Second Military Medical University Press. (in Chinese)

Hilbe, J.M. (2009). *Logistic Regression Models*, Boca Raton, FL: CRC Press.

Hoffman, J. and Julien, I.E. (2019). *Biostatistics for Medical and Biomedical Practitioners. 2nd ed*, New York: Academic Press.

Hogg, V.R., McKean, J., and Craig, A.T. (2018). *Introduction to Mathematical Statistics (What's New in Statistics). 8th ed*, Boston, MA: Pearson Education.

Hosmer Jr, D.W., Lemeshow, S., and Sturdivant, R.X. (2013). *Applied Logistic Regression*, Hoboken, NJ: John Wiley & Sons.

Hsu, J. (1996). *Multiple Comparisons: Theory and Methods*, Boca Raton, FL: CRC Press.

Huang, J.Q., Luo, X.X., Wang, S.W. et al. (2006). Effect of cinnamaldehyde on activity of tumor and immunological function of S180 sarcoma in mice. *Chinese Journal of Clinical Rehabilitation* 10(11): 107–110.

Hulley, S.B. (2007). *Designing Clinical Research*, New York: Lippincott Williams & Wilkins.

Jin, P.H. (1993). *Medical Statistical Methods*, Shanghai: Shanghai Medical College Publishing Company. (in Chinese)

Jin, P.H. and Chen, F. (2009). *Medical Statistical Methods. 3rd ed*, Shanghai: Science and Education Press. (in Chinese)

John, P.W. (1998). *Statistical Design and Analysis of Experiments*, Philadelphia, PA: Society for Industrial and Applied Mathematics.

John, P.K. and Meivin, L.M. (2003). *Survival Analysis Techniques for Censored and Truncated Data. 2nd ed*, New York: Springer-Verlag.

Kalbfleisch, D. and Prentice, R.L. (1980). *The Statistical Analysis of Failure Time Data*, New York: Wiley.

Kaps, M. and Lamberson, W.R. (2004). *Biostatistics for Animal Science*, New York: Oxford University Press.

Kleinbaum, D.G. and Klein, M. (2002). *Logistic Regression: A Self-learning Text. 3rd ed*, Berlin: Springer.

Kleinbaum, D.G. and Klein, M. (2005). *Survival Analysis: A Self-Learning Text. 2nd ed*, New York: Springer.

Kleinbaum, D.G. and Klein, M. (2011). *Survival Analysis: A Self-Learning Text. 3rd ed*, New York: Spring Science+ Business Media.

Kleinbaum, D.G. and Klein, M. (2012). *Survival Analysis: A Self-Learning Text. 3rd ed*, New York: Springer-Verlag.

Kuehl, R.O. (2000). *Design of Experiments: Statistical Principles of Research Design and Analysis*, Pacific Grove, CA: Duxbury Press.

Lawless, J.F. (2011). *Statistical Models and Methods for Lifetime Data*, Hoboken, NJ: John Wiley & Sons.

Le, C.T. (2003). *Introductory Biostatistics*, New York: Wiley.

Le, C.T. and Eberly, L.E. (2016). *Introductory Biostatistics. 2nd ed*, New York: Wiley.

Li, C.X. (2000). *Biostatistics. 2nd ed*, Beijing: Science Press. (in Chinese)

Li, X.S. (2008). *Medical Statistics. 2nd ed*, Beijing: Advanced Education Press. (in Chinese)

Liu, G.F. (2007). *Medical Statistics. 2nd ed*, Beijing: Peking Union Medical College Press. (in Chinese)

Liu, L.F., Cheng, S.X., and Li, Z.L. (2007). *Biostatistics*, Beijing: Beijing Normal University Press. (in Chinese)

Liu, Q. (2004). *Encyclopedia of Chinese Medical Statistics. Multivariate Statistics*, Beijing: People's Medical Publishing House. (in Chinese)

Liu, Q. and Jin, P.H. (2002). *Statistical Analysis of Classified Data and SAS Programming*, Shanghai: Fudan University Press. (in Chinese)

Lu, S.Z. and Chen, F. (2007). *Medical Statistics. 2nd ed*, Beijing: China Statistical Publishing House. (in Chinese)

Lui, K.J. (2016). *Crossover Designs: Testing, Estimation, and Sample Size (Statistics in Practice)*, New York: Wiley.

Luo, T.E. (2009). *Study Guidance of Medical Statistics. 2nd ed*, Beijing: Peking Union Medical College Press. (in Chinese)

Machin, D. and Campbell, M.J. (2005). *Design of Studies for Medical Research*, New York: Wiley.

Mann, H.B. (1949). *Analysis and Design of Experiments: Analysis of Variance and Analysis of Variance Designs*, New York: Dover Publications.

Mao, S.S., Wang, J.L., and Pu, X.L. (1998). *Advanced Mathematical Statistics*, Beijing: Advanced Education Press. (in Chinese)

Maxwell, S.E., Delaney, H.D., and Kelley, K. (2017). *Designing Experiments and Analyzing Data: A Model Comparison Perspective. 3rd ed*, London: Routledge.

McHugh, M.L. (2011). Multiple comparison analysis testing in ANOVA. *Biochemia medica* 21(3): 203–209.

Menard, S. (2001). *Applied Logistic Regression Analysis (Quantitative Applications in the Social Sciences)*, Thousand Oaks, CA: SAGE Publications.

Miquel, P. (2014). *A Dictionary of Epidemiology. 6th ed*, New York: Oxford University Press.

Monaghan, F. and Corcos, A. (1985). Chi-square and Mendel's experiments: Where's the bias? *Journal of Heredity* 76(4): 307.

Montgomery, D.C. (2017). *Design and Analysis of Experiments*, Hoboken, NJ: John Wiley & Sons.

Newman, S.C. (2001). *Biostatistical Methods in Epidemiology*, Hoboken, NJ: John Wiley & Sons.

Newman, T.B. and Kohn, M.A. (2020). *Evidence-based Diagnosis: An Introduction to Clinical Epidemiology*, Cambridge, UK: Cambridge University Press.

Neyman, J. (1992). *On the Two Different Aspects of the Representative Method: The Method of Stratified Sampling and the Method of Purposive Selection. Breakthroughs in Statistics*, Berlin: Springer.

Ogunnaike, B.A. (2009). *Random Phenomena: Fundamentals of Probability and Statistics for Engineers*, Boca Raton, FL: CRC Press.

Olkin, I. and Pratt, J.W. (1958). Unbiased estimation of certain correlation coefficients. *Annals of Mathematical Statistics* 29(1): 201–211.

Onyiah, L.C. (2008). *Design and Analysis of Experiments: Classical and Regression Approaches with SAS*, Boca Raton, FL: CRC Press.

Pagano, M. and Gauvreau, K. (2018). *Principles of Biostatistics. 2nd ed*, London: Chapman and Hall/CRC.

Pampel, F.C. (2000). *Logistic Regression: A Primer*, Thousand Oaks, CA: SAGE Publications.

Petrie, A. and Sabin, C. (2019). *Medical Statistics at a Glance. 4th ed*, Chichester, UK: Wiley-Blackwell.

Portney, L.G. (2020). *Foundations of Clinical Research: Applications to Evidence-based Practice*, Philadelphia, PA: F.A. Davis.

Queen, J.P., Quinn, G.P., and Keough, M.J. (2002). *Experimental Design and Data Analysis for Biologists*, Cambridge, UK: Cambridge University Press.

Rafter, J.A., Abell, M.L., and Braselton, J.P. (2002). Multiple comparison methods for means. *Siam Review* 44(2): 259–278.

Rao, C.R., Miller, J.P., and Rao, D.C. (2007). *Epidemiology and Medical Statistics (Handbook of Statistics, Volume 27)*, Amsterdam: North Holland.

Rasch, D., Verdooren, R., and Pilz, J. (2019). *Applied Statistics: Theory and Problem Solutions with R*, New York: Wiley.

Ratkowsky, D., Alldredge, R., and Evans, M.A. (1992). *Cross-Over Experiments: Design, Analysis and Application*, Boca Raton, FL: CRC Press.

Rosner, B. (1999). *Fundamentals of Biostatistics. 5th ed*, Pacific Grove, CA: Duxbury Press.

Rosner, B. (2011). *Foundamentals of Biostatistics. 7th ed*, Boston, MA: Cengage Learning.

Rosner, B. (2015). *Fundamentals of Biostatistics. 8th ed*, Boston, MA: Cengage Learning.
Ross, S. (2018). *A First Course in Probability. 10th ed*, Boston, MA: Pearson Education.
Rothman, K.J., Greenland, S., and Lash, T.L. (2008). *Modern Epidemiology*, New York: Lippincott Williams & Wilkins.
Samuels, M., Witmer, J., and Schaffner, A. (2015). *Statistics for the Life Sciences, Global Edition*, London: Pearson Education Limited.
Senn, S.S. (2002). *Cross-over Trials in Clinical Research. 2nd ed*, New York: Wiley.
Shi, L.Y. (2001). *A Dictionary of Epidemiology*, Beijing: Science Press. (in Chinese)
Shiraishi, T.A., Sugiura, H., and Matsuda, S.I. (2019). *Pairwise Multiple Comparisons: Theory and Computation*, Singapore: Springer Singapore.
Soper, H.E., Young, A.W., Cave, B.M. et al. (1917). On the distribution of the correlation coefficient in small samples. Appendix II to the papers of "Student" and R.A. Fisher. *Biometrika* 11(4): 328–413.
Stefan, D.C. (2016). *Cancer Research and Clinical Trials in Developing Countries*, Cham: Springer International Publishing.
Sun, Z.Q. (2006). *Medical Statistical*, Beijng: People's Medical Publishing House. (in Chinese)
Sun, Z.Q. and Xu, Y.Y. (2007). *Medical Statistical. 2nd ed*, Beijng: People's Medical Publishing House. (in Chinese)
Tamhane, A.C. (2009). *Statistical Analysis of Designed Experiments: Theory and Applications*, Hoboken, NJ: John Wiley & Sons.
Thompson, S.K. (2012). *Sampling*, New York: Wiley.
Twomey, P. (2012). *Oxford Handbook of Medical Statistics: Oxford Medical Handbooks*, New York: Oxford University Press.
Utts, J.M. and Heckard, R.F. (2011). *Mind on Statistics. 4th ed*, Boston, MA: Cengage Learning.
van Belle, G., Fisher, L.D., Heagerty, P.J. et al. (2004). *Biostatistics: A Methodology for the Health Sciences. 2nd ed*, New York: Wiley-Interscience.
Vittinghoff, E., Glidden, D.V., Shiboski, S.C. et al. (2011). *Regression Methods in Biostatistics: Linear, Logistic, Survival, and Repeated Measures Models*, New York: Springer Science & Business Media.
Wackerly, D.D., Mendenhall, W., and Scheaffer, R.L. (2007). *Mathematical Statistics With Applications. 7th ed*, Belmon: Thomson Brooks/Cole.
Westfall, P.H., Tobias, R.D., Wolfinger, R.D. et al. (2011). *Multiple Comparisons and Multiple Tests Using SAS. 2nd ed*, Cary, NC: SAS Institute.
White, S. (2019). *Basic & Clinical Biostatistics. 5th ed*, New York: McGraw-Hill Education/ Medical.
Woodward, M. (1999). *Epidemiology Study Design and Data Analysis*, Boca Raton, FL: Chapman & Hall/CRC.
Yan, H. (2010). *Medical Statistical. 2nd ed*, Beijng: People's Medical Publishing House. (in Chinese)
Yang, S.Q. (1985). *Encyclopedia of Chinese Medicine – Medical Statistics*, Shanghai: Shanghai Science and Technology Press. (in Chinese)
Yu, C.H. (2014). *SPSS and Statistical Analysis*, Beijing: Electronics Industry Publishing House. (in Chinese)
Yu, S.L. (2002). *Medical Statistical*, Beijng: People's Medical Publishing House. (in Chinese)

Zar, J.H. (2009). *Biostatistical Analysis. 5th ed*, London: Prentice Hall.
Zar, J.H. (2014). *Biostatistical Analysis: Pearson New International Edition*, London: Pearson Education Limited.
Zhang, W.T. and Kuang, C.W. (2011). *Basic Course of SPSS Statistical Analysis. 2nd ed*, Beijing: Advanced Education Press. (in Chinese)
Zhao, N.Q. and Yin, P. (2014). *Medical Data Analysis*, Shanghai: Fudan University Press. (in Chinese)

Methodology

Bartlett, M.S. (1937). Properties of sufficiency and statistical tests. *Proceedings of the Royal Statistical Society, Series A* 160: 268–282.
Bateson, W. (1914). Mendels principles of heredity 3. Impression. *Abstammungs Und Vererbungslehre* 11(1): 200.
Bayes, T. (1763). An essay towards solving a problem in the doctrine of chances. *Philosophical Transactions* 53: 370–418.
Breslow, N.E. (1974). Covariance analysis of censored survival data. *Biometrics* 30(1): 89–99.
Cochran, W.G. and Cox, G.M. (1950). *Experimental Designs*, New York: John Wiley & Sons.
Cox, D.R. (1972). Regression models and life-tables. *Journal of the Royal Statistical Society* 34(2): 187–220.
Dunnett, C.W. (1955). A multiple comparison procedure for comparing several treatments with a control. *Journal of the American Statistical Association* 50: 1096–1121.
Dunnett, C.W. (1964). New tables for multiple comparisons with a control. *Biometrics* 20(3): 482–491.
Efron, B. (1977). The efficiency of Cox's likelihood function for censored data. *Journal of American Statistical Association* 72: 557–565.
Fisher, R.A. (1924). On a distribution yielding the error functions of several well-known statistics. *Proceedings of the International Congress Mathematicians, Toronto* 2: 805–813.
Fisher, R.A. (1938). Presidential address. *Sankhyā: The Indian Journal of Statistics (1933–1960)* 4(1): 14–17.
Friedman, M. (1937). The use of ranks to avoid the assumption of normality implicit in the analysis of variance. *Journal of the American Statistical Association* 32(200): 675–701.
Helmert, F.R. (1876). Ueber die Wahrscheinlichkeit der Potenzsummen der Beobachtungsfehler und über einige damit im Zusam- menhange stehende Fragen. *Zeitschrift für Mathematik und Physik* 21: 192–218.
Hotelling, H. and Pabst, M.R. (1936). Rank correlation and tests of significance involving no assumption of normality. *Annals of Mathematical Statistics* 7(1): 29–43.
Kaplan, E.L. and Meier, P. (1958). Nonparametric estimation from incomplete observations. *Journal of the American Statistical Association* 53(282): 457–481.
Krupinski, E.A. (2017). Receiver Operating Characteristic (ROC) analysis. *Frontline Learning Research* 5(3): 31–42.
Kruskal, W.H. and Wallis, W.A. (1952). Use of ranks in one-criterion variance analysis. *Journal of the American Statistical Association* 47(260): 583–621.

Levene, H. (1960). Robust tests for equality of variances. In I. Olkin (Ed.), *Contributions to Probability and Statistics* (pp. 278–292), Stanford, CA: Stanford University Press.
Lu, Y., Fang, J.Q., Tian, L. et al. (2015). *Advanced Medical Statistics. 2nd ed*, Singapore: World Scientific.
Mantel, N. (1966). Evaluation of survival data and two new rank order statistics arising in its consideration. *Cancer Chemotherapy Reports* 50(3): 163–170.
National Academy of Sciences (1994). *Biographical Memoirs*, Washington, DC: The National Academies Press.
Pearson, K. (1900). On the criterion that a given system of deviations from the probable in the case of a correlated system of variables is such that it can be reasonably supposed to have arisen from random sampling. *Philosophical Magazine. Series 5* 50(302): 157–175.
Pires, A.M. and Branco, J.A. (2010). A statistical model to explain the Mendel–Fisher controversy. *Statistical Science* 25(4): 545–565.
Rao, C.R. (1997). *Statistics and Truth: Putting Chance to Work. 2nd ed*, Singapore: World Scientific.
Salkind, N.J. (2010). *Encyclopedia of Research Design*, Thousand Oaks, CA: SAGE Publications.
Satterthwaite, F.E. (1946). An approximate distribution of estimates of variance components. *Biometrics Bulletin* 2: 110–114.
Sonego, P., Kocsor, A., and Pongor, S. (2008). ROC analysis: Applications to the classification of biological sequences and 3D structures. *Briefings in Bioinformatics* 9(3): 198–209.
Spearman, C. (1904). "General intelligence," objectively determined and measured. *The American Journal of Psychology* 15(2): 201–292.
Stigler, S. (2005). Fisher in 1921. *Statistical Science* 20(1): 32–49.
Student (1908). The probable error of the mean. *Biometrika* 6(1): 1–25.

Application

Carson, J.L., Terrin, M.L., and Noveck, H. (2011). Liberal or restrictive transfusion in high-risk patients after hip surgery. *New England Journal of Medicine* 365: 2453–2462.
Chen, F.F., Wang, W.P., Teng, H.H. et al. (2012). Trends and determinants of birthweight among live births in Beijing 1996–2010. *Chinese Journal of Evidence-Based Pediatrics* 7(6): 418–423.
Guðjónsdóttir, H., Halldórsson, T.I., Gunnarsdóttir, I. et al. (2015). Urban-rural differences in diet, BMI and education of men and women in Iceland. *Laeknabladid* 101(1): 11–16.
Klein, J.P. and Moeschberger, M.L. (2003). *Survival Analysis: Techniques for Censored and Truncated Data. 2nd ed*, Berlin: Springer Science & Business Media.
Küchenhoff, H., Shalabh, S., and Heumann, C. (2008). Coin tossing and spinning – Useful classroom experiments for teaching statistics. In *Recent Advances in Linear Models and Related Areas* (pp. 417–426), Heidelberg: Physica-Verlag HD.
Martin, L., Leblanc, R., Toan, N.K. et al. (1993). Tables for the Friedman rank test. *Canadian Journal of Statistics* 21: 39–43.
Patel, G.P., Grahe, J.S., Sperry, M. et al. (2010). Efficacy and safety of dopamine versus norepinephrine in the management of septic shock. *Shock* 33(4): 375–380.

Xu, X., Sui, X., Zhong, W. et al. (2019). Clinical utility of quantitative dual-energy CT iodine maps and CT morphological features in distinguishing small-cell from non-small-cell lung cancer. *Clinical Radiology* 74(4): 268–277.

Yamauchi, J. (1972). *Statistical Numeric Table*, Tokyo: Japanese Standard Association. (in Japanese)

Yao, J.X., Lu, H.H., Wang, Z.H. et al. (2018). A sensitive method for the determination of the gender difference of neuroactive metabolites in tryptophan and dopamine pathways in mouse serum and brain by UHPLC-MS/MS. *Journal of Chromatography B* 1093–1094: 91–99.

Yu, X., Huang, Y., Guo, Q. et al. (2017). Clinical motivation and the surgical safety checklist. *British Journal of Surgery* 104(4): 472.

Yu, X., Jiang, J., Shang, H. et al. (2019). Effect of a risk-stratified intervention strategy on surgical complications: Experience from a multicentre prospective study in China. *BMJ Open* 9(6): e025401.

Zhu, L., Lang, J.H., Liu, C.Y. et al. (2009). Epidemiological study on the prevalence of urinary incontinence in adult women in my country. *Chinese Journal of Obstetrics and Gynecology* 44(10): 776–779. (in Chinese)

Index

Applied Medical Statistics, First Edition. Jingmei Jiang.

Companion website: www.wiley.com\go\jiang\appliedmedicalstatistics

d

e

n

o

p

r

t

u

v

w

y

z

Printed and bound by CPI Group (UK) Ltd, Croydon, CR0 4YY
16/04/2025
14658371-0003